Paramedic Care
Principles & Practice
TRAUMA EMERGENCIES

SECOND EDITION

BRYAN E. BLEDSOE, D.O., F.A.C.E.P., EMT-P

Emergency Physician
Midlothian, Texas
and
Adjunct Associate Professor of Emergency Medicine
The George Washington University Medical Center
Washington, DC

ROBERT S. PORTER, M.A., NREMT-P

Senior Advanced Life Support Educator
Madison County Emergency Medical Services
Canastota, New York
and
Flight Paramedic
AirOne, Onondaga County Sheriff's Department
Syracuse, New York

RICHARD A. CHERRY, M.S., NREMT-P

Clinical Assistant Professor of Emergency Medicine
Assistant Residency Director
Upstate Medical University
Syracuse, New York

PEARSON
Prentice Hall

Brady
Prentice Hall Health
Upper Saddle River, NJ 07458

Library of Congress Cataloging-in-Publication Data

Bledsoe, Bryan E., (date)
  Paramedic care: principles & practice / Bryan E. Bledsoe, Robert S. Porter, Richard A. Cherry. — 2nd ed.
    p.; cm.
  Includes bibliographical references and index.
  ISBN 0-13-117837-7 (v. 4 : alk. paper)
  1. Emergency medicine. 2. Emergency medical technicians. I. Porter, Robert S., 1950- . II. Cherry, Richard A. III. Title.
  [DNLM: 1. Emergencies. 2. Emergency Medical Technicians. 3. Emergency Treatment. WB 105 B646pa 2005]
RC86.7.B5964 2005
616.02'5—dc22   2004012985

Publisher: Julie Levin Alexander
Publisher's Assistant: Regina Bruno
Executive Editor: Marlene McHugh Pratt
Senior Managing Editor for Development: Lois Berlowitz
Editorial Assistant: Matthew Sirinides
Project Manager: Sandy Breuer
Managing Photography Editor: Michal Heron
Director of Marketing: Karen Allman
Executive Marketing Manager: Katrin Beacom
Senior Channel Marketing Manager: Rachele Strober
Marketing Coordinator: Michael Sirinides
Director of Production and Manufacturing: Bruce Johnson
Managing Editor for Production: Patrick Walsh
Production Liaison: Faye Gemmellaro
Production Editor: Lynn Steines, Carlisle Publishers Services
Manufacturing Manager: Ilene Sanford
Manufacturing Buyer: Pat Brown
Creative Director: Cheryl Asherman
Senior Design Coordinator: Christopher Weigand
Cover Design: Christopher Weigand
Cover Image: Eddie Sperling
Cover Image Manipulation: Studio Montage
Interior Photographers: Michael Gallitelli, Michal Heron, Richard Logan
Interior Illustrations: Rolin Graphics
Interior Design: Jill Little
Media Project Manager: John J. Jordan
Manager of Media Production: Amy Peltier
New Media Project Manager: Stephen J. Hartner
Composition: Carlisle Publishers Services
Printing and Binding: Courier/Kendallville
Cover Printer: Phoenix Color

Notices

It is the intent of the authors and publishers that this textbook be used as part of a formal paramedic education program taught by a qualified instructor and supervised by a licensed physician. The care procedures presented here represent accepted practices in the United States. They are not offered as a standard of care. Paramedic-level emergency care is to be performed only under the authority and guidance of a licensed physician. It is the reader's responsibility to know and follow local care protocols as provided by medical advisors directing the system to which he or she belongs. Also, it is the reader's responsibility to stay informed of emergency care procedure changes.

Notice on Drugs and Drug Dosages

Every effort has been made to ensure that the drug dosages presented in this textbook are in accordance with nationally accepted standards. When applicable, the dosages and routes are taken from the American Heart Association's *Advanced Cardiac Life Support Guidelines.* The American Medical Association's publication *Drug Evaluations,* the *Physicians' Desk Reference,* and the *Prentice Hall Health Professional's Drug Guide* are followed with regard to drug dosages not covered by the American Heart Association's guidelines. It is the responsibility of the reader to be familiar with the drugs used in his or her system, as well as the dosages specified by the medical director. The drugs presented in this book should only be administered by direct order, whether verbally or through accepted standing orders, of a licensed physician.

Notice on Gender Usage

The English language has historically given preference to the male gender. Among many words, the pronouns "he" and "his" are commonly used to describe both genders. Society evolves faster than language and the male pronouns still predominate in our speech. The authors have made great effort to treat the two genders equally, recognizing that a significant percentage of paramedics and patients are female. However, in some instances, male pronouns may be used to describe both male and female paramedics and patients solely for the purpose of brevity. This is not intended to offend any readers of the female gender.

Notice on Photographs

Please note that many of the photographs contained in this book are taken of actual emergency situations. As such, it is possible that they may not accurately depict current, appropriate, or advisable practices of emergency medical care. They have been included for the sole purpose of giving general insight into real-life emergency settings.

Notice on Case Studies

The names used and situations depicted in the case studies throughout this textbook are fictitious.

10 9 8 7 6 5 4 3 2 1
ISBN 0-13-117837-7

▼DEDICATION

This edition of *Paramedic Care: Principles & Practice* is dedicated to the memory and life of Jim Page. Few people have had such a positive impact on EMS and society in general. Jim was many things—attorney, publisher, EMT, firefighter, visionary, advocate, fire chief, and friend. Most of all, he was humble. He never knew how important he really was. Jim had the unique talent of remembering names and always made you feel that, regardless of what was going on around him, you had his undivided attention and ear. We mourn his passing and miss his warm handshake and booming voice. Each of the three authors of this textbook called Jim a close friend, and we are forever grateful for his years of advice, counsel, and friendship. An old Spanish proverb says, "Good men must die, but death cannot kill their names." We hope that every paramedic student who reads these textbooks will periodically turn to this page and quietly reflect on the impact this important yet humble man had on EMS and the fire service.

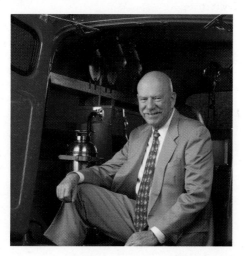

Tom Page/Jems Communications

James O. Page
1936–2004

No one's death comes to pass without making some impression, and those close to the deceased inherit part of the liberated soul, and thus become richer in their humaneness.

Robert Oxton Bolt

Content Overview

Volume I Introduction to Advanced Prehospital Care

Below is a brief content description of each chapter in Volume 1, *Introduction to Advanced Prehospital Care.*

continued

Content Overview

Volume I Introduction to Advanced Prehospital Care (continued)

Content Overview

Volume 2 Patient Assessment

Below is a brief content description of each chapter in Volume 2, *Patient Assessment.*

Content Overview

Volume 3 Medical Emergencies

Below is a brief content description of each chapter in Volume 3, *Medical Emergencies.*

Chapter 1   Pulmonology 2

★ Discusses respiratory system anatomy, physiology, and pathophysiology
★ Discusses respiratory system emergencies
★ Emphasizes recognition and treatment of reactive airway diseases such as asthma

Chapter 2   Cardiology 64

★ Discusses cardiovascular system anatomy, physiology, and pathophysiology
★ Presents material crucial to advanced prehospital cardiac care
★ Is presented in three parts: Part 1—essential cardiac anatomy, physiology, and electrophysiology; Part 2—cardiac and peripheral vascular system emergencies; Part 3—12-lead ECG monitoring and interpretation

Chapter 3   Neurology 246

★ Discusses nervous system anatomy, physiology, and pathophysiology
★ Discusses recognition and management of neurologic emergencies

Chapter 4   Endocrinology 300

★ Discusses endocrine system anatomy, physiology, and pathophysiology
★ Discusses recognition and management of endocrine emergencies, with emphasis on diabetic emergencies

Chapter 5   Allergies and Anaphylaxis 332

★ Reviews the immune system and the pathophysiology of allergic and anaphylactic reactions
★ Discusses recognition and treatment of allergic reactions, with emphasis on anaphylactic reactions

Chapter 6   Gastroenterology 348

★ Discusses gastrointestinal system anatomy, physiology, and pathophysiology
★ Discusses recognition and management of gastrointestinal emergencies

Chapter 7   Urology and Nephrology 380

★ Discusses genitourinary system anatomy, physiology, and pathophysiology
★ Discusses recognition and management of urinary system emergencies in males and females and male reproductive system emergencies

Chapter 8   Toxicology and Substance Abuse 414

★ Discusses basic toxicology and both common and uncommon causes of poisoning
★ Discusses overdose and substance abuse, including drug and alcohol abuse
★ Discusses recognition and management of poisoning, overdose, and substance abuse emergencies

Content Overview

Volume 3 Medical Emergencies

Content Overview

Volume 4 Trauma Emergencies

Below is a brief content description of each chapter in Volume 4, *Trauma Emergencies*.

Content Overview

Volume 4 Trauma Emergencies

Content Overview

Volume 5 Special Considerations/Operations

Below is a brief content description of each chapter in Volume 5, *Special Considerations/Operations*.

Content Overview

Volume 5 Special Considerations/Operations

▽Detailed Contents

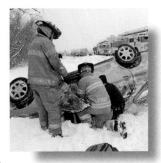
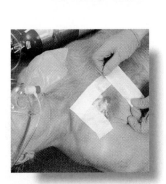

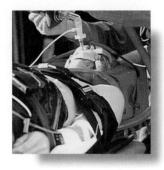

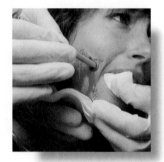

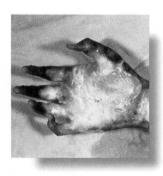

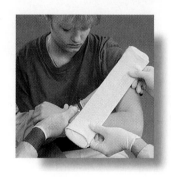

Chapter 7   Musculoskeletal Trauma 216

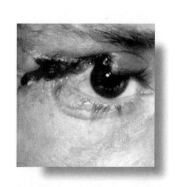

Chapter 8   Head, Facial, and Neck Trauma 270

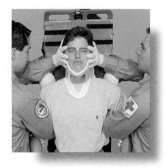

Chapter 9 Spinal Trauma 332

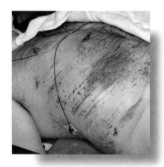

Chapter 10 Thoracic Trauma 378

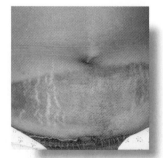

Chapter 11 Abdominal Trauma 426

Chapter 12   Shock Trauma Resuscitation   458

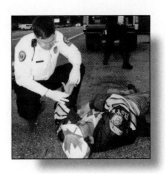

Photo Scans/Procedures

It's Your Profession

Dear Student:

Thank you for using Brady's ***Paramedic Care: Principles & Practice*** series. These five volumes, based on the widely used *Paramedic Emergency Care* text we developed more than 15 years ago, will provide the core foundation for your paramedic education. Coupled with quality classroom instruction and clinical rotations, you are assured of receiving the knowledge and skills required of a quality paramedic. We know you want to pass your certification exam, and you also want to be prepared for the challenges you'll encounter on the street. ***Paramedic Care: Principles & Practice*** is the textbook series that will help you accomplish both goals.

We are proud to tell you that Brady has made a top-down commitment to quality, a commitment that is evident in the book you now hold. William A. Foster once wrote, "Quality is never an accident; it is always the result of high intention, sincere effort, intelligent direction, and skilled execution; it represents the wise choice of many alternatives." Every person at Brady involved in the preparation of this text has made a sincere commitment to quality, beginning with our efforts as authors. We know you have made a significant investment in your program, and we have gone to great effort to ensure that our paramedic program is accurate, current, and complete. The second edition has been extensively reviewed and revised to reflect changes in EMS that have occurred since the first edition was published. The three of us, as well as contributors to this series, have made a tremendous effort to ensure that the material accurately reflects the current state of and best practices in EMS.

Brady makes a considerable investment in "development editing," and its development team is among the most dedicated and skilled in the publishing industry. Development editing ensures that content is reviewed appropriately for accuracy and currency, explanations are consistent, and the material remains at the appropriate level for the paramedic student. Brady's editors have worked hard toward these goals. Another of Brady's strongest assets is its production team. These publishing experts have many years of experience in the business and an undeniable commitment to producing books with distinctive designs and clear formatting. Working together, Brady's development and production teams help to ensure that our books are the best on the market. Brady's commitment to a standard of excellence continues with the customer service and feedback system provided by the sales team, the most experienced group in EMS publishing.

In summary, EMS is about quality. Welcome. Be safe. Have fun. We wish you all the best in your education and in the practice of EMS.

Sincerely,

Bryan Bledsoe   Robert Porter   Richard Cherry

Series Preface

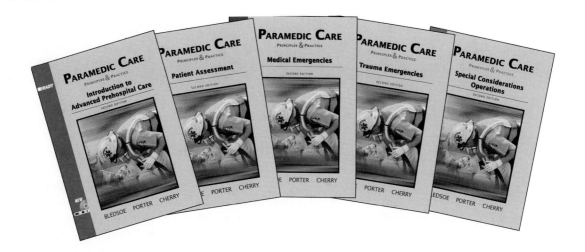

Congratulations on your decision to further your EMS career by undertaking the course of education required for certification as an Emergency Medical Technician–Paramedic! The world of paramedic emergency care is one that you will find both challenging and rewarding. Whether you will be working as a volunteer or a paid paramedic, you will find the field of advanced prehospital care very interesting.

This textbook, **the 2nd edition of *Paramedic Care: Principles & Practice,*** will serve as your guide and reference to advanced prehospital care. It is based on the 1998 U.S. Department of Transportation's *Emergency Medical Technician–Paramedic National Standard Curriculum* and is divided into five volumes:

Volume 1 *Introduction to Advanced Prehospital Care*
Volume 2 *Patient Assessment*
Volume 3 *Medical Emergencies*
Volume 4 *Trauma Emergencies*
Volume 5 *Special Considerations/Operations.*

Volume 1, *Introduction to Advanced Prehospital Care,* presents the foundations of paramedic practice as well as an introduction to pathophysiology, pharmacology, medication administration, and airway management and ventilation. **Volume 2, *Patient Assessment,*** adds the cognitive and psychomotor skills of patient assessment, communications, and documentation. This knowledge base expands as the series applies it to the medical patient in **Volume 3, *Medical Emergencies,*** and to the trauma patient in **Volume 4, *Trauma Emergencies.*** **Volume 5, *Special Considerations/ Operations***, enriches these general patient care concepts and principles with applications to special patients and circumstances we commonly see as paramedics. The product of this complete and integrated series is a set of principles of care you will be required to practice as a twenty-first-century paramedic.

Your paramedic education program should include ample classroom, practical laboratory, in-hospital clinical, and prehospital field experience. These educational experiences must be guided by instructors and preceptors with special training and experience in their areas of participation in your program.

DEVELOPING ADVANCED SKILLS

The psychomotor skills of fluid and medication administration, advanced airway care, ECG monitoring and defibrillation, and advanced medical and trauma patient care are best learned first in the classroom and the skills laboratory and then in the clinical and field settings. Commonly required advanced prehospital skills are discussed in the text as well as outlined in the accompanying procedure sheets. Review these before and while practicing each skill.

It is important to underscore that neither this nor any other text can teach skills. Care skills are learned only under the watchful eye of a paramedic instructor and perfected during your clinical and field internship.

CONTENT OF THE FIVE VOLUMES

It is intended that your program coordinator will assign reading from *Paramedic Care: Principles & Practice* in preparation for each classroom lecture and discussion section. The knowledge gained from reading this text will form the foundation of the information you will need in order to function effectively as a paramedic in your EMS system. Your instructors will build on this information to strengthen your knowledge and understanding of advanced prehospital care so that you may apply it in your practice.

The content of each volume of *Paramedic Care: Principles & Practice* is summarized below, with an emphasis on "what's new" in this 2nd edition.

VOLUME 1: INTRODUCTION TO ADVANCED PREHOSPITAL CARE

Volume 1 addresses the fundamentals of paramedic practice, including paramedic roles and responsibilities, pathophysiology, pharmacology, medication administration, and advanced airway management.

What's New in Volume 1?

★ In Chapter 2, "The Well-Being of the Paramedic," former discussions of critical incident stress management (a technique that is no longer recommended) have been replaced with new sections on specific **EMS stresses** and on **general mental health services** and **disaster mental health services** available to EMS personnel.

★ Chapter 6, "Medical/Legal Aspects of Advanced Prehospital Care," contains a new section on the **Health Insurance Portability and Accountability Act (HIPAA) privacy rules.**

★ Chapter 8, "General Principles of Pathophysiology," and Chapter 10, "Medication Administration," include new sections on **HBOCs (hemoglobin-based oxygen-carrying substances),** which are considered to have significant advantages over standard crystalloids and colloids for fluid resuscitation.

★ Chapter 9, "General Principles of Pharmacology," includes updated information on **insulin preparations,** an updated **immunization schedule,** and discussion of **new drugs for erectile dysfunction.**

★ Chapter 13, "Airway Management and Ventilation," includes a new section on **capnography,** particularly its uses in monitoring tube placement during endotracheal intubation. New sections are also included on the **Intubating LMA (laryngeal mask airway),** the **Cobra Perilaryngeal Airway,** and the **Ambu Laryngeal Mask.** For assistance in intubation, the **bougie** device is newly discussed and illustrated as are techniques for **nasotracheal auscultation.**

VOLUME 2: PATIENT ASSESSMENT

Volume 2 builds on the assessment skills taught in the basic EMT course, emphasizing advanced-level patient assessment and clinical decision-making at the scene.

What's New in Volume 2?

★ Chapter 2, "Physical Exam Techniques," includes much-expanded information and photos to illustrate the **ophthalmic (eye) exam** and the **otoscopic (ear) exam.**

★ Chapter 2, "Physical Exam Techniques," and Chapter 3, "Patient Assessment in the Field," feature new sections on **capnography** as an assessment tool.

★ Chapter 5, "Communications," includes new information on **wireless phones and 911 calls** (new technology for identifying locations and call-back numbers). There is a section on the promising new technology of **automatic collision notification (ACN)** and also a discussion of the importance of **speaking to medical direction on a recorded line** (which will help in the event of a lawsuit).

VOLUME 3: MEDICAL EMERGENCIES

Volume 3 addresses the paramedic level of care in medical emergencies. Particular emphasis is placed on respiratory and cardiovascular emergencies, which are the most common EMS medical calls.

What's New in Volume 3?

★ Chapter 1, "Pulmonology," features new information on **capnography** as a prehospital diagnostic tool and means of monitoring the patient's respiratory status, specifically in upper airway obstruction and asthma emergencies. New material on **severe acute respiratory syndrome (SARS)** is included.

★ Chapter 2, "Cardiology," introduces the use of the **15-lead and 18-lead ECGs in right ventricular and left ventricular posterior wall infarctions.**

★ Chapter 3, "Neurology," has added information on the **pediatric Glasgow Coma Scale.**

★ Chapter 7, "Urology and Nephrology," has a new section on **priapism.**

★ Chapter 11, "Infectious Disease"—like Chapter 1—includes new information on **SARS.**

★ Chapter 12, "Psychiatric and Behavior Disorders," features completely revised text and photos regarding **restraint of violent patients** to emphasize supine placement and monitoring the airway and breathing of the restrained patient.

VOLUME 4: TRAUMA EMERGENCIES

Volume 4 discusses advanced prehospital care of the trauma patient, from mechanism-of-injury analysis to care of specific types of trauma to general principles of shock/trauma resuscitation.

What's New in Volume 4?

★ Chapter 2, "Blunt Trauma," includes new information on **side air bags** and on **deactivation of undeployed air bags.** Notes are included regarding **terrorist use of explosives** that contain nails, screws, and other materials intended to cause maximum injury and destruction.

★ Chapter 4, "Hemorrhage and Shock," includes a new section on the use of **capnography** as a guide to ventilation rates and volumes as well as for ensuring proper tube placement. A new section has been added on the use of two techniques to improve ventilatory efficiency: **positive end-expiratory pressure (PEEP)** and **continuous positive airway pressure (CPAP).**

- ★ In Chapter 5, "Soft-Tissue Trauma," **fentanyl** is introduced as a drug for pain control.
- ★ Chapter 6, "Burns," includes new information on **keratitis,** an eye injury welders may suffer; on the unreliability of **pulse oximetry** to measure oxygen saturation in the burn patient and the patient who has inhaled carbon monoxide; and on **fentanyl** as a pain management drug. Illustrations and text on factors affecting **radiation exposure** have been revised to provide greater detail.
- ★ In Chapter 7, "Musculoskeletal Trauma," discussions and illustrations of the **vacuum splint** and the **pelvic sling** have been added. The Hare splint has been deleted from the section on traction splinting and the **Fernotrac splint** has been added. Under pain control medications, **fentanyl** has been added and nalbuphine has been de-emphasized.
- ★ Chapter 8, "Head, Facial, and Neck Trauma," has an added discussion of **capnography** as an assessment tool with the head injury patient and as a tool for confirmation of tube placement. A section on **recognition of brain herniation** is newly included. Both **adult and pediatric Glasgow Coma Scales** are now included. The importance of obtaining **blood glucose readings** in the head injury patient is newly emphasized. In the directed intubation section, the **bougie** device is introduced. Recommended **ventilation rates and volumes for the head injury patient** have been updated, as has information on **maintenance of blood pressure in the head injury patient.** Caveats regarding the use of **rapid sequence intubation** in the prehospital setting have been included. In the discussion of medications, mannitol has been deleted as a diuretic, **atracurium** has been added as a paralytic, and **etomidate** and **fentanyl** have been added as sedatives.
- ★ In Chapter 9, "Spinal Trauma," extensive discussions of **spinal clearance** and a spinal clearance protocol have been added. A term that is gaining acceptance, **spinal motion restriction,** is discussed. **Capnography** is now included, along with pulse oximetry, as an aid in ensuring adequate oxygenation. An explanation is included as to why routine use of **steroids in spine injury is no longer recommended.**
- ★ Chapter 12, "Shock Trauma Resuscitation," now includes **pediatric trauma scoring** in addition to adult trauma scoring.

VOLUME 5: SPECIAL CONSIDERATIONS/OPERATIONS

Volume 5 addresses such topics as neonatal, pediatric, and geriatric care; home health care and challenged patients; and incident command, ambulance service, rescue, hazardous material, crime scene operations, and responding to terrorist acts.

What's New in Volume 5?

- ★ Chapter 1, "Neonatology," includes expanded text regarding congenital anomalies and, in particular, more information on **congenital heart problems.**
- ★ Chapter 2, "Pediatrics," has a new section on **verification of tube placement in the pediatric patient.**
- ★ Chapter 4, "Abuse and Assault," features a new section on **date rape drugs.**
- ★ In Chapter 8, "Ambulance Operations," the **criteria for air medical dispatch** have been updated.
- ★ Chapter 9, "Medical Incident Management," makes reference to the new **U.S. Department of Homeland Security National Incident Management System (NIMS).** The former emphasis on critical incident stress debriefings has been deleted and replaced by new sections on **mental health support** and **disaster mental health services.**
- ★ **Chapter 14, "Responding to Terrorist Acts," is an entirely new chapter** that did not appear in the first (pre-September 11, 2001) edition of *Paramedic Care.* It includes information on **explosive, nuclear, chemical, and biological agents** as well as **scene safety, recognizing a terrorist attack,** and **responding to a terrorist attack.**

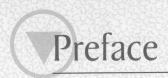

Preface

Until the late 1960s, the highest level of medical care available outside of the hospital was Red Cross First Aid. In 1966, the National Academy of Sciences commissioned a research study to examine the inadequacies of emergency medical care in this country. The findings of this study were published in a document called *Accidental Death and Disability: The Neglected Disease of Modern Society*. This document, commonly referred to as "The White Paper," was the impetus for development of EMS and emergency medicine as we know it today.

The initial emphasis of prehospital training was trauma care. Prehospital personnel received considerable training in bandaging, splinting, and rescue techniques. In the 1980s, prehospital trauma care was again improved through the development of Basic Trauma Life Support (BTLS) and Prehospital Trauma Life Support (PHTLS) training. These courses provided EMTs and paramedics with the additional information needed to care adequately for the trauma patient in the field.

The publication of **Paramedic Care: Principles & Practice**, *Volume 4, Trauma Emergencies* takes prehospital trauma care to the highest level yet. This volume details the anatomy, physiology, and pathophysiology of trauma. Although trauma is a surgical disease, and in many instances definitive care must be provided in the operating room, there is a significant amount of care that can be provided by prehospital personnel to help reduce both morbidity and mortality.

This volume addresses the various types of trauma based on the body systems involved. It is important to remember that many trauma patients have multiple injuries involving multiple body systems. Because of this, it is essential to consider the "whole patient" and not become distracted by a single injury.

OVERVIEW OF THE CHAPTERS

Chapter 1 "Trauma and Trauma Systems" introduces the paramedic student to trauma, the concept of trauma systems, and trauma triage protocols. It has been shown that trauma victims have the best chances of survival if they are cared for in a facility that routinely provides trauma care. In addition, certain patients will require very specialized trauma care, and it is often the responsibility of the paramedic to assure that the patient gets to the correct facility.

Chapter 2 "Blunt Trauma" presents the physics of blunt trauma and details the effects of blunt trauma on the various body tissues. Blunt trauma can often be very deceiving, as overt signs and symptoms of injury may not be evident at the time paramedics arrive. This chapter encourages the paramedic to evaluate the physics and mechanism of injury to help determine likely injuries.

Chapter 3 "Penetrating Trauma" provides a detailed discussion of the physics and pathophysiology of penetrating trauma. Formerly quite rare, penetrating trauma has become much more commonplace in our society. This chapter emphasizes the importance of considering the physics and mechanism of injury when assessing and treating a patient with penetrating trauma.

Chapter 4 "Hemorrhage and Shock" makes clear that regardless of the mechanism of injury, the final common denominator in most trauma patients is the fact that they are losing blood. Severe blood loss can result in the development of shock. The body's physiological responses to hemorrhage and shock are complex. This chapter details the physiological and pathophysiological response to hemorrhage and shock so that the paramedic can recognize the process early and intervene appropriately.

Chapter 5 "Soft-Tissue Trauma" explains that this is by far the most common form of trauma. Although most soft-tissue injuries are not life threatening, many can be. This chapter provides a detailed review of the anatomy and physiology of the integumentary system, a discussion of the pathophysiology of soft-tissue trauma, and a detailed discussion of soft-tissue treatment, including bandaging.

Chapter 6 "Burns" discusses the unique pathophysiology of burn injuries. The incidence of burn injuries is declining, but burn patients require specialized care. This chapter discusses the anatomy, physiology, and pathophysiology of burn injuries, including thermal, electrical, chemical, and radiation burns and inhalation injuries, with emphasis on management of the burn patient.

Chapter 7 "Musculoskeletal Trauma" notes that this type of trauma is second only to soft-tissue trauma in frequency. In this chapter, the student learns about various types of musculoskeletal trauma with special emphasis on treatment and pain control.

Chapter 8 "Head, Facial, and Neck Trauma" reviews the anatomy of the head, face, and neck and stresses that injuries to these areas can be severe and life threatening. The chapter places a special emphasis on recognizing injuries early and protecting the airway.

Chapter 9 "Spinal Trauma" concerns a type of trauma that, although relatively uncommon, can be devastating. The chapter reviews spinal anatomy and physiology, as well as prehospital precautions and treatment for possible spinal injuries.

Chapter 10 "Thoracic Trauma" details the impact of chest trauma on the body. Thoracic anatomy and physiology are unique and can require specialized treatment procedures. Special emphasis is placed on recognition and treatment of chest injuries, especially pneumothorax.

Chapter 11 "Abdominal Trauma" addresses the anatomy and physiology of the abdomen and discusses abdominal trauma pathology by organ and organ system. The chapter emphasizes the importance of maintaining a high index of suspicion when treating a trauma patient with possible internal injury.

Chapter 12 "Shock Trauma Resuscitation" ties together the underlying concepts regarding specific types of trauma addressed in the prior chapters. Most trauma patients will have more than one injured or affected body system. The paramedic must recognize all potential injuries, based on the physical exam and evaluation of the mechanism of injury. Then, the patient must be aggressively treated and transported to a hospital capable of providing the required care. This chapter reviews and underlines the effects of hemorrhage and shock and provides a detailed discussion of assessment and care of the trauma patient.

SUMMARY OF VOLUME 4

This volume, *Trauma Emergencies*, details the basic medical knowledge and skills expected of twenty-first century paramedics. This material should be mastered before undertaking actual care of a trauma patient.

Acknowledgments

CHAPTER CONTRIBUTORS

We wish to acknowledge the remarkable talents and efforts of the following people who contributed to this volume of *Paramedic Care: Principles & Practice.* Individually, they worked with extraordinary commitment on this new program. Together, they form a team of highly dedicated professionals who have upheld the highest standards of EMS instruction.

Chapter 1   Trauma and Trauma Systems
Robert Porter, MA, NREMT-P, Senior Advanced Life Support Educator, Madison County Emergency Medical Services Canastota, New York, and Flight Paramedic, AirOne, Onondaga County Sheriff's Department Syracuse, New York

Chapter 2   Blunt Trauma
Robert Porter, MA, NREMT-P, Senior Advanced Life Support Educator, Madison County Emergency Medical Services Canastota, New York, and Flight Paramedic, AirOne, Onondaga County Sheriff's Department Syracuse, New York

Chapter 3   Penetrating Trauma
Robert Porter, MA, NREMT-P, Senior Advanced Life Support Educator, Madison County Emergency Medical Services Canastota, New York, and Flight Paramedic, AirOne, Onondaga County Sheriff's Department Syracuse, New York

Chapter 4   Hemorrhage and Shock
Robert Porter, MA, NREMT-P, Senior Advanced Life Support Educator, Madison County Emergency Medical Services Canastota, New York, and Flight Paramedic, AirOne, Onondaga County Sheriff's Department Syracuse, New York

Chapter 5   Soft-Tissue Injuries
Robert A. De Lorenzo, MD, FACEP; Lieutenant Colonel, Medical Corps, U.S. Army; Associate Clinical Professor of Military and Emergency Medicine; Uniformed Services University of the Health Sciences, Bethesda, Maryland

Chapter 6   Burns
Robert A. De Lorenzo, MD, FACEP; Lieutenant Colonel, Medical Corps, U.S. Army; Associate Clinical Professor of Military and Emergency Medicine; Uniformed Services University of the Health Sciences, Bethesda, Maryland

Chapter 7   Musculoskeletal Trauma
Eric Heckerson, RN, MA, NREMT-P, EMS Coordinator, Mesa Fire Department, Mesa, Arizona

Chapter 8 Head, Facial, and Neck Trauma

Lawrence C. Brilliant, MD, FACEP, Clinical Assistant Professor, Department of Primary Care Education and Community Services, Hahnemann University; Emergency Physician, Doylestown Hospital, Doylestown, Pennsylvania

Chapter 9 Spinal Trauma

Robert Reinberg, EMT-P, PA-C, Emergency Medicine, Wayne, Pennsylvania

Chapter 10 Thoracic Trauma

Craig A. Soltis, MD, FACEP, Assistant Professor of Clinical Emergency Medicine, Northeastern Ohio Universities College of Medicine; Chairman, Department of Emergency Medicine, Forum Health, Youngstown, Ohio

Chapter 11 Abdominal Trauma

William Marx, DO; Associate Professor of Surgery and Critical Care; Director, Surgical Critical Care SUNY Upstate Medical University, Syracuse, New York

Chapter 12 Shock Trauma Resuscitation

Robert Porter, MA, NREMT-P, Senior Advanced Life Support Educator, Madison County Emergency Medical Services Canastota, New York, and Flight Paramedic, AirOne, Onondaga County Sheriff's Department Syracuse, New York

REVIEW BOARDS

Our special thanks to Joseph J. Mistovich, Chairperson and Associate Professor, Department of Health Professions, Youngstown State University, Youngstown, Ohio, for his review of the 1st edition of *Trauma Emergencies*. We appreciate the comments and suggestions he offered, a result of his knowledge of the paramedic curriculum, experience, and high standards. Our special thanks also to Robert A. De Lorenzo, MD, FACEP; Lieutenant Colonel, Medical Corps, U.S. Army; Associate Clinical Professor of Military and Emergency Medicine; Uniformed Services University of the Health Sciences. Dr. De Lorenzo's reviews of first edition material were carefully prepared, and we appreciate the thoughtful advice and keen insight he shared with us. We are additionally grateful to Christopher W. Lentz, MD, FACS, Associate Professor of Surgery and Pediatrics and Medical Director, Strong Regional Burn Center, University of Rochester Department of Surgery, Rochester, New York. Dr. Lentz reviewed the chapter on burn emergencies and offered valuable suggestions for revision.

INSTRUCTOR REVIEWERS

The reviewers of *Paramedic Care: Principles & Practice* have provided many excellent suggestions and ideas for improving the text. The quality of the reviews has been outstanding, and the reviews have been a major aid in the preparation and revision of the manuscript. The assistance provided by these EMS experts is deeply appreciated.

Brenda M. Beasley, RN, BS, EMT-P
Department Chair, Allied Health
Calhoun College
Decatur, AL

E. James Cole, MA, NREMT-P,
WEMTI, EMS 1
Lead EMS Instructor
Cleveland Clinic Health System
Cleveland, Ohio

Robert A. De Lorenzo, MD, FACEP
Brooke Army Medical Center
Ft. Sam Houston, TX

Bill Doss, Paramedic/Firefighter
Miami Twp Fire and EMS
Cleremont County, OH

John Dudte, MPA
Director, Emergency Health Services
The George Washington University
Washington, DC

Jeff Fritz, BS, NREMT-P
Temple College
Temple, TX

John Gosford
EMS Training Coordinator
Tallahassee, FL

Anthony S. Harbour, MEd, NREMT-P
Virginia PHTLS State Coordinator, NAEMT
EMS Instructor, Center for Emergency
   Health Services
Richmond, VA

Jane E. Hill, AAS, LP
Director, Shackelford County EMS
Coordinator, TechPro EMS Academy
Consultant, Hill Gandy Associates
Albany, TX

Carl Homa, BSN, RN, EMT-P
Lafayette Ambulance Squad
King of Prussia, PA

David M. LaCombe, NREMT-P
National EMS Academy
Lafayette, LA

Christopher W. Lentz, MD, FACS
Associate Professor of Surgery and Pediatrics
Medical Director, Strong Regional Burn
   Center
University of Rochester—Department
   of Surgery
Rochester, NY 14642

Jason R. Light
Boston University
Boston, MA

Lawrence Linder, BA, NREMT-P
EMS Faculty
St. Petersburg College
Pinellas Park, FL

Keith A. Monosky, MPM, EMT-P
Assistant Professor
Department of Emergency Medicine
The George Washington University
Washington, DC

Robert B. Morris
Clackamas Community College
Mt. Angel, OR

Allen O. Patterson
Holmes Community College
Ridgeland, MS

Randy Perkins, CEP
Paramedic Program Director
Scottsdale Community College
Scottsdale, AZ

Katharine P. Rickey, NREMT-P
NHCTC
Laconia, NH
Barnstead Fire-Rescue
Barnstead, NH

Janet L. Schulte, BS, AS, NR-CDEMT-P
IHM Health Studies Center
St. Louis, MO

Andrew R. Turcotte, NREMT-P, EMS I/C
Old Orchard Beach Fire Department
Old Orchard Beach, ME

We also wish to express appreciation to the following EMS professionals who reviewed the 1st edition of *Paramedic Care: Principles & Practice.* Their suggestions and perspectives helped to make this program a successful teaching tool.

Philip Adams, EMT-P, RN, BSN
Paramedic Course Coordinator
Paducah Community College
Paducah, KY

Rudy Garrett
Paramedic Training Coordinator
Somerset-Pulaski County EMS
Somerset, KY

Ted S. Goldman, EMT-P
City of Philadelphia Fire Department
Director of EMS Programs
Star Technical Institute
Philadelphia, PA

Linda Groarke, MPH/MS, NREMT-P
Paramedic Program Director
Assistant Professor
Natural and Applied Sciences
LaGuardia Community College/CUNY
New York, NY

Theresa Jordan, RN, TNS, EMT
Arkansas Emergency Transport
Jacksonville, AR

Scott Karr, MEd, NREMT-P
Bevill State Paramedic Program
Sumiton, AZ

David LaCombe, NREMT-P
Center for Research in Medical Education
University of Miami School of Medicine
Miami, FL

Shelby Louden, BS, EMT-P
Safety and Compliance Coordinator
Butler County Joint Vocational Schools
Hamilton, Ohio

Becky A. Morris, BS, NREMT-P, IC
EMS Department Head
Trenholm State College
Montgomery, AL

John Eric Powell, MS, NREMT-P
Flight Paramedic
UT-Lifestar Aeromedical Service
University of Tennessee Medical Center
Level 1 Trauma Facility
Knoxville, TN

Larry Richmond
Mountain Plains Health Consortium
Fort Meade, SD

Tom Rothrock, RN, BSN, CEN, PHRN
Flight Nurse, University Medevac
Paramedic Coordinator, Lehigh Valley
    Hospital
Allentown, PA

Andrew W. Stern, NREMT-P, MPA, MA
Senior Paramedic/Flightmedic
Town of Colonie Emergency Medical
    Services
Colonie, NY

Michael Tretola, BS, EMT-P
Administrative Coordinator
EMS Institute/Department of Emergency
    Medicine
Catholic Medical Center for Brooklyn
    and Queens, NY

Peter H. Viele, MS, NREMT-P
Operations Manager
Action Ambulance Service, Inc.
Stoneham, MA

PHOTO ACKNOWLEDGMENTS

All photographs not credited adjacent to the photograph or in the photo credit section below were photographed on assignment for Brady/Prentice Hall Pearson Education.

Organizations

We wish to thank the following people and organizations for their valuable assistance in creating the photo program for the paramedic volumes.

Marshall Eiss, REMT
Special Events Coordinator
Indian Rocks Volunteer Firemen's Association
Indian Rocks Beach, FL

Steve Fravel, NREMT-P
Pinellas County EMS & Fire Administration
Largo, FL

C.T. "Chuck" Kearns, MBA, EMT-P
Director, Pinellas County EMS / Sunstar
Largo, FL

Chief John R. Leahy, Jr.
Pinellas Suncoast Fire & Rescue
Indian Rocks Beach, FL

Darryl Quigley
TLC Ambulance Service
Dallas, TX

Rural/Metro Medical Services,
 Syracuse, NY
North Area Volunteer Ambulance
 Corps (NAVAC)
North Syracuse, NY

Chief David Schrodt
Midlothian Fire Department
Midlothian, TX

Rev. Robert A. Wagenseil, Jr.
Chaplain—Pinellas Suncoast Fire &
 Rescue
Rector—Calvary Episcopal Church
Indian Rocks Beach, FL

Robert A. Walley, REMT
District Chief
Pinellas Suncoast Fire & Rescue
Indian Rocks Beach, FL

Special thanks to Jeff Goethe of Phillips Medical Systems for provision of electronic monitors.

Technical Advisors

Thanks to the following people for providing valuable technical support during the photo shoots:

Richard A. Cherry, MS, NREMT-P
Clinical Assistant Professor of Emergency
 Medicine
Assistant Residency Director
Upstate Medical University
Syracuse, NY

Michael Cox, Instructor
Division of State Fire Marshal
Florida Bureau of Fire Standards and Training
Florida State Fire College
Ocala, FL

Richard T. Walker, EMT-P
District Chief
Pinellas Suncoast Fire & Rescue
Indian Rocks Beach, FL

Digital postproduction:
 Richard Carter, Tampa, FL

About the Authors

BRYAN E. BLEDSOE, D.O., F.A.C.E.P., EMT-P

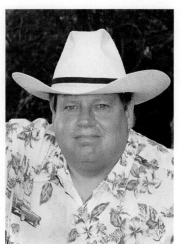

Dr. Bryan Bledsoe is an emergency physician with a special interest in prehospital care. He received his B.S. degree from the University of Texas at Arlington and his medical degree from the University of North Texas Health Sciences Center/Texas College of Osteopathic Medicine. He completed his internship at Texas Tech University and residency training at Scott and White Memorial Hospital/Texas A&M College of Medicine. Dr. Bledsoe is board certified in emergency medicine. Dr. Bledsoe is an Adjunct Associate Professor of Emergency Medicine at The George Washington University Medical Center in Washington, DC.

Prior to attending medical school, Dr. Bledsoe worked as an EMT, a paramedic, and a paramedic instructor. He completed EMT training in 1974 and paramedic training in 1976 and worked for 6 years as a field paramedic in Fort Worth, Texas. In 1979, he joined the faculty of the University of North Texas Health Sciences Center and served as coordinator of EMT and paramedic education programs at the university. Dr. Bledsoe is active in emergency medicine and EMS research. He is a popular speaker at state, national, and international seminars and writes regularly for numerous EMS journals.

Dr. Bledsoe has authored several EMS books published by Brady including *Paramedic Care: Principles & Practice, Essentials of Paramedic Care, Intermediate Emergency Care: Principles & Practice, Anatomy & Physiology for Emergency Care, Prehospital Emergency Pharmacology,* and *Pocket Reference for EMTs and Paramedics.* He is married to Emma Bledsoe. They have two children, Bryan and Andrea, and a grandson, Andrew, and live on a ranch south of Dallas, Texas. He enjoys saltwater fishing and warm latitudes.

ROBERT S. PORTER, M.A., NREMT-P

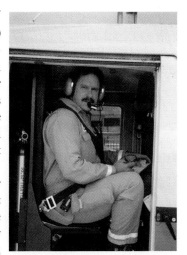

Robert Porter has been teaching in emergency medical services for 30 years and currently serves as the Senior Advanced Life Support Educator for Madison County, New York, and as a Flight Paramedic with the Onondaga, New York, County Sheriff's Department helicopter service, AirOne. Mr. Porter is a Wisconsin native and received his bachelor's degree in education from the University of Wisconsin. He completed his paramedic training at Northeast Wisconsin Technical Institute in 1978 and earned a master's degree in health education at Central Michigan University in 1990.

Mr. Porter has been an EMT and EMS educator and administrator since 1973 and obtained his national registration as an EMT-Paramedic in 1978. He has taught both basic and advanced EMS courses in the states of Wisconsin, Michigan, Louisiana, Pennsylvania, and New York. Mr. Porter served for more than 10 years as a paramedic program accreditation-site evaluator for the American Medical Association and is a past chair of the National Society of EMT Instructor/Coordinators. He has authored Brady's

Paramedic Care: Principles & Practice, Essentials of Paramedic Care, Intermediate Emergency Care: Principles & Practice, Tactical Emergency Care, and *Weapons of Mass Destruction: Emergency Care,* as well as the workbooks accompanying this text, *Paramedic Emergency Care,* and *Intermediate Emergency Care.* When not writing or teaching, Mr. Porter enjoys offshore sailboat racing and historic home restoration.

RICHARD A. CHERRY, M.S., NREMT-P

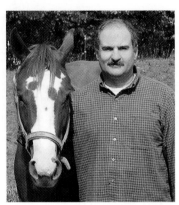

Richard Cherry is Clinical Assistant Professor of Emergency Medicine and Assistant Residency Director at Upstate Medical University in Syracuse, New York. His experience includes years of classroom teaching and emergency fieldwork. A native of Buffalo, Mr. Cherry earned his bachelor's degree at nearby St. Bonaventure University in 1972. He taught high school for the next 10 years while he earned his master's degree in education from Oswego State University in 1977. He holds a permanent teaching license in New York State.

Mr. Cherry entered the emergency medical services field in 1974 with the DeWitt Volunteer Fire Department, where he served his community as a firefighter and EMS provider for more than 15 years. He took his first EMT course in 1977 and became an ALS provider 2 years later. He earned his paramedic certificate in 1985 as a member of the area's first paramedic class.

Mr. Cherry has authored several books for Brady. Most notable are *Paramedic Care: Principles & Practice, Essentials of Paramedic Care, Intermediate Emergency Care: Principles & Practice,* and *EMT Teaching: A Common Sense Approach.* He has made presentations at many state, national, and international EMS conferences on a variety of teaching topics. He regularly teaches in the paramedic program he helped establish and is Regional Faculty for ACLS and PALS. As Assistant Residency Director he is responsible for implementing the 3-year emergency medicine core curriculum through weekly conferences. He and his wife Sue run a horse-riding camp for children with cancer and other life-threatening diseases on their property in West Monroe, New York. He also plays guitar in a Christian band.

Welcome to Paramedic Care

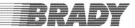

Brady
Prentice Hall Health
Upper Saddle River, NJ 07458

Dear Instructor:

Brady, your partner in education, is pleased to present the 2nd edition of our best-selling *Paramedic Care: Principles & Practice.* This revision is one of the most important we've published to date. Since we published the 1st edition, changes in education, publishing, technology, and the EMS profession have been occurring at a greater rate than ever. Indeed, the world is a different place today. Responding to these changes in a meaningful way required us to look at this series from several perspectives—its history, its quality, its experience, and its commitment. Getting to the next edition meant taking a close look at the past and discovering the things that make us a unique choice.

PCPP has a rich and long history. Since the advent of the EMS profession, several things have happened in the Advanced Life Support arena: a curriculum emerged; care is more widely available; care is more consistent; and it's now beginning to benefit from research. Our authors have been associated with this product all along the way, taking care to ensure that the latest and safest practices are taught. This edition is an extension of that care.

When the 1st edition of *PCPP* was published, two unique things happened: 1) the series went to the #1 position in the market; and 2) there were very few errors. This is an exceptional success story in the publishing world. What made this happen? In a word, quality. The authoring, developmental, and production acumen on this series is second to none. They take no shortcuts, and they never compromise the needs of their customers. This new edition has the same individuals at work together to create an even better solution.

Quality also comes from experience. Our authors have been known for their clear, comprehensive, and accurate style of presentation for more than 25 years. They are active, accessible teachers, writers, and practitioners who enjoy respect among their peers. At Brady, our combined editorial experience is 70 years, with more than 20 years focused on EMS exclusively. Our production and design experience totals more than 70 years. Finally, our EMS-exclusive sales and marketing experience is over 100 years! This means that we're specialists; we have in-depth product knowledge; and we can truly understand what we can offer our customers based on their individual needs.

Last is our commitment. The people—inside and outside Brady—affiliated with this series can't think of anything they'd rather be doing. This dedication comes through, every step of the way, in our writing, reviewing, photography, marketing, and selling. We truly believe we have an obligation to provide the best possible product, so that you can teach students to provide the best possible care. In the world of educational publishing, there are few equals to this combination. We believe it translates into what you'll see as you take a look inside this series. We also believe it represents the work of professionals and hope that our work enables your students to become the same—professionals.

We know you have many choices when it comes to choosing a textbook and appreciate the support you've given us over the years. This support has enabled us to continue to bring you up-to-date, accurate, consistent, comprehensive, and relevant products for EMS education. We're committed to helping students learn to become the best professionals possible. After all, it's they who may help us in an emergency some day. This new edition is an extension of our promise to you and to them.

Sincerely,

Julie Levin Alexander
VP/Publisher

Katrin Beacom
Senior Marketing Manager

Marlene McHugh Pratt
Executive Editor

Thomas Kennally
National Sales Manager

Lois Berlowitz
Senior Managing Editor

Emphasizing Principles

Objectives

Part 1: Cardiovascular Anatomy and Physiology, ECG Monitoring, and Dysrhythmia Analysis (begins on p. 73)

After reading Part 1 of this chapter, you should be able to:

1. Describe the incidence, morbidity, and mortality of cardiovascular disease. (pp. 71, 241)
2. Discuss prevention strategies that may reduce the morbidity and mortality of cardiovascular disease. (pp. 71–72)
3. Identify the risk factors most predisposing to coronary artery disease. (pp. 71–72)

◀ **Chapter Objectives with Page References.** List the objectives that form the basis of each chapter, in addition to the page on which each objective is covered.

One of your most important skills as a paramedic will be obtaining and interpreting ECG rhythm strips.

▲ **Key Points.** Help students identify and learn fundamental points.

cardiovascular disease (CVD) *disease affecting the heart, peripheral blood vessels, or both.*

▲ **Key Terms.** Located in margins near the paragraphs in which they first appear, these help students master new terminology.

✓ Review

Factors Affecting Stroke Volume

- Preload
- Cardiac contractility
- Afterload

▲ **Content Review.** Summarizes important content, giving students a format for quick review.

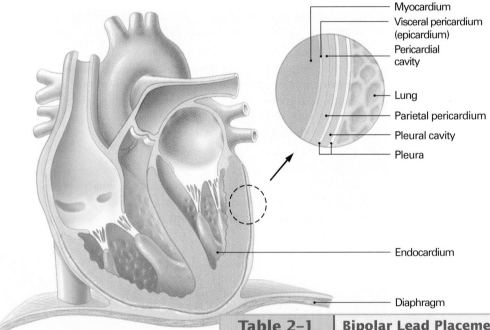

■ Figure 2-2   Layers of the heart.

Labels: Myocardium; Visceral pericardium (epicardium); Pericardial cavity; Lung; Parietal pericardium; Pleural cavity; Pleura; Endocardium; Diaphragm

◀▼ **Tables and Illustrations.** Provide visual support to enhance understanding.

Table 2–1	Bipolar Lead Placement Sites	
Lead	Positive Electrode	Negative Electrode
I	Left arm	Right arm
II	Left leg	Right arm
III	Left leg	Left arm

Emphasizing Principles ▼

Summary

▶ **Summary.** Provides students with a concise review of important chapter information.

Cardiovascular disease is the number-one cause of death in the United States and Canada. Many deaths from heart attack occur within the first 24 hours—frequently within the first hour. With the advent of fibrinolytic therapy, time is of the essence when managing the patient with suspected ischemic heart disease. EMS plays an ever-increasing role in the early recognition of patients suffering coronary ischemia. In certain areas, EMS provides definitive care by initiating fibrinolytic therapy in the field. This is especially important in cases where transport times can be long. With cardiovascular disease, EMS can truly mean the difference between life and death.

Review Questions

1. The _____ is a protective sac surrounding the heart and consists of two layers, visceral and parietal.
   a. myocardium
   b. pericardium
   c. mesocardium
   d. endocardium

2. The outermost lining of the walls of arteries and veins is the _____ _____, a fibrous tissue covering that gives the vessel strength to withstand the pressures generated by the heart's contractions.
   a. tunica media
   b. tunica intima
   c. tunica adventitia
   d. visceral media

◀ **NEW Review Questions.** Ask students to recall information and to apply the principles they've just learned.

Further Reading

▶ **Further Reading.** Recommendations for books and journal articles.

Beasley, B. M. *Understanding 12-Lead EKGs: A Practical Approach.* 2nd ed. Upper Saddle River, N.J.: Pearson/Prentice Hall, 2001.

Beasley, B. M. *Understanding EKGs: A Practical Approach.* 2nd ed. Upper Saddle River, N.J.: Pearson/Prentice Hall, 2003.

Bledsoe, B. E., and D. E. Clayden. *Prehospital Emergency Pharmacology.* 6th ed. Upper Saddle River, N.J.: Pearson/Prentice Hall, 2005.

On the Web

Visit Brady's Paramedic Website at **www.bradybooks.com/paramedic**.

◀ **On the Web.** www.bradybooks.com/paramedic refers students to a Companion Website, where additional activities and information can be found on the chapter's topics. Also, links to other topic-specific website are listed.

Emphasizing Practice

Case Study

The crew of Paramedic Unit 112 is called to a local nursing home to evaluate Mr. Evan Henry, an 80-year-old male with chest pain. It is Sunday afternoon, and Mr. Henry's family has been visiting from out of town. Not used to all the attention and excitement, Mr. Henry has developed substernal chest pain that radiates to his left arm. He has a history of this type of pain, but it usually resolves after one or two sublingual nitroglycerin tablets. This time, however, the nitroglycerin tablets have failed to alleviate his pain. Because of this, the nursing home staff has activated the EMS system.

◀ **Case Study.** Draws students into the reading and creates a link between the text content and real-life situations and experiences.

You Make the Call

▶ **You Make the Call.** Promotes critical thinking by requiring students to apply principles to actual practice.

You and your partner on Medic 3 are dispatched to a well-kept residence about three blocks from the station. The dispatch information relates the nature of the call as a medical emergency. On your arrival at the residence, the patient's wife meets you and shows you to a back room. The patient is a male who appears to be in his late 60s. He is complaining of severe back pain that began approximately 30 minutes ago. He thinks it may be due to some light yard work he did earlier in the day. The patient appears in severe distress, however, and is sweaty and diaphoretic.

Procedure 2–5 **12-Lead Prehospital ECG Monitoring**

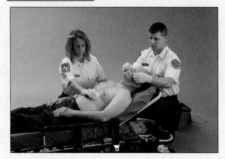

2-5a   Prep the skin.

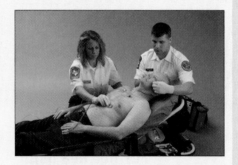

2-5b   Place the four limb leads according to the manufacturer's recommendations.

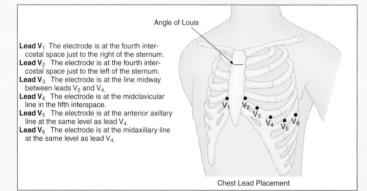

Angle of Louis

Lead V₁ The electrode is at the fourth intercostal space just to the right of the sternum.
Lead V₂ The electrode is at the fourth intercostal space just to the left of the sternum.
Lead V₃ The electrode is at the line midway between leads V₂ and V₄.
Lead V₄ The electrode is at the midclavicular line in the fifth interspace.
Lead V₅ The electrode is at the anterior axillary line at the same level as lead V₄.
Lead V₆ The electrode is at the midaxillary line at the same level as lead V₄.

V₁ V₂ V₃ V₄ V₅ V₆

Chest Lead Placement

2-5c   Proper placement of the precordial leads.

◀ **Procedure Scans.** Provide step-by-step visual support on how to perform skills.

Emphasizing Practice ▽

► **Patient Care Algorithms.** Provide graphic "pathways" that integrate assessment and care procedures.

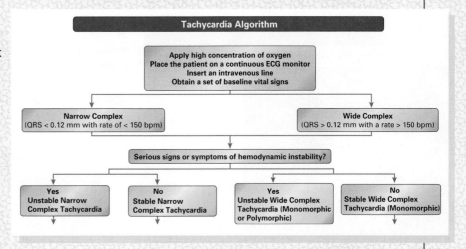

Tachycardia Algorithm

Apply high concentration of oxygen
Place the patient on a continuous ECG monitor
Insert an intravenous line
Obtain a set of baseline vital signs

| Narrow Complex (QRS < 0.12 mm with rate of < 150 bpm) | Wide Complex (QRS > 0.12 mm with a rate > 150 bpm) |

Serious signs or symptoms of hemodynamic instability?

Yes Unstable Narrow Complex Tachycardia

No Stable Narrow Complex Tachycardia

Yes Unstable Wide Complex Tachycardia (Monomorphic or Polymorphic)

No Stable Wide Complex Tachycardia (Monomorphic)

Patho Pearls

The Best Treatment for Stroke Despite the great strides in medicine, there is still very little that can be provided to help minimize the effects of a stroke. Stroke therapy usually involves medically stabilizing the patient after the stroke and then getting him into a physical rehabilitation program where he can regain as much motor function as possible.

◄ **NEW Patho Pearls.** Offer a snapshot of pathological considerations students will encounter in the field.

► **NEW Legal Notes.** Present instances in which legal or ethical considerations should be evaluated.

Legal Notes

Reporting Contagious Diseases All states have provisions for reporting contagious diseases without fear of violating the patient's privacy or confidentiality issues. Even the Health Insurance Portability and Accountability Act (HIPAA) has provisions in place for reporting contagious disease without violating provisions of the act. There are over 60 diseases in the United States that are reportable at a national level. In addition, there are state-reportable diseases which vary from state to state. Some illnesses, including anthrax, brucellosis, diphtheria, pertussis, plague, and others, must be immediately reported. Others, including AIDS, gonorrhea, leprosy, and syphilis, must be reported within 1 week. Some require reporting of individual cases and others require reporting of numbers only.

Cultural Considerations

Culture and Cardiovascular Disease Cardiovascular disease remains the number-one cause of death in the United States and Canada. The incidence of cardiovascular disease increased steadily during the twentieth century although it has stabilized somewhat over the last decade or so.

◄ **NEW Cultural Considerations.** Provide an awareness of beliefs that might affect patient care.

Student CD

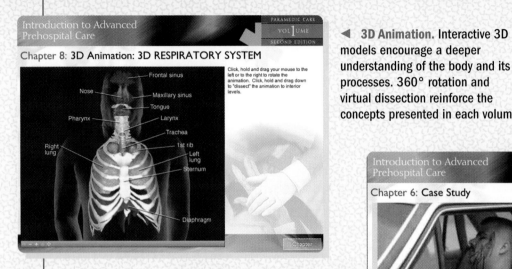

3D Animation. Interactive 3D models encourage a deeper understanding of the body and its processes. 360° rotation and virtual dissection reinforce the concepts presented in each volume.

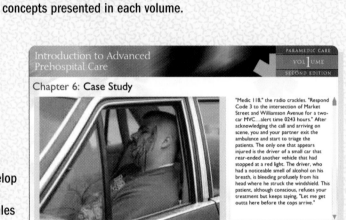

Case Study. Designed to develop critical thinking skills, each case study offers questions and rationales that help to hone the student's assessment skills.

Drug Guide. A valuable reference tool, this hotlinked PDF allows quick access to important information regarding the drugs most commonly used by today's paramedic.

EMS Scenes. Video clips of real-life situations put you in the action. See what you might encounter at an actual emergency scene.

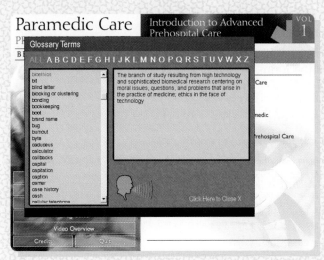

◄ **Glossary.** This interactive, indexed glossary contains the definitions and audio pronunciations of the key terms presented in each volume.

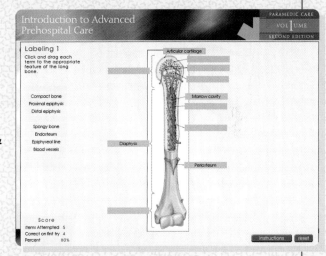

► **Interactives.** From Bone Structure to Body Cavities, drag & drop interactive exercises make learning both engaging and fun.

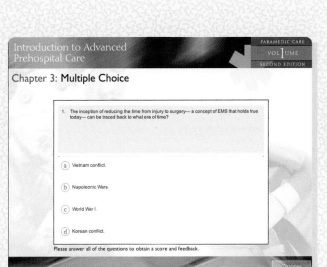

◄ **Multiple Choice.** Each chapter offers self-testing in a multiple-choice format. Upon completion, a score and feedback are provided for post-assessment.

► **Virtual Tours.** Including the airway, cardiovascular system, muscle-skeletal system, nervous system and heart, these narrated tours guide you through the intricate workings of the body systems in an easy-to-understand presentation.

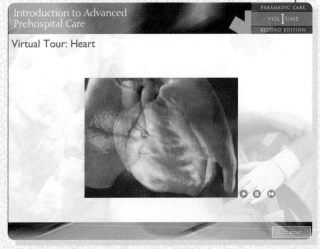

▼ Student Workbook

A student workbook with review and practice activities accompanies each volume of the Paramedic Care series. The workbooks include multiple-choice questions, other exercises, case studies, and special projects, along with an answer key with text page references. National Registry Practical Evaluation forms and Flash Cards are also provided in each volume.

Review of Chapter Objectives

▶ **Review of Chapter Objectives.** Reviews important content elements addressed by chapter objectives.

After reading this part of the chapter, you should be able to:

1. Describe the incidence, morbidity, and mortality of cardiovascular disease.　　　pp. 71, 241

Cardiovascular disease (CVD) is serious and extremely common, with more than 60 million Americans affected. Morbidity is considerable: An American has a nonfatal heart attack (myocardial infarction, MI) roughly every 29 seconds. Coronary heart disease (CHD), one type of CVD, is the single largest killer of Americans and Canadians. Roughly 466,000 Americans die annually from CHD, half of them before reaching a hospital. Many deaths from CHD are sudden and involve lethal cardiac dysrhythmias. Many deaths from MI occur within the first 24 hours, frequently within the first hour.

Case Study Review

Reread the case study in Chapter 2 of Paramedic Care: Medical Emergencies *before reading the discussion below.*

　　This case study demonstrates how paramedics react to a typical medical emergency involving chest pain. In addition to observing how the team conducts the patient's initial assessment, note how they respond as the situation quickly changes into a more complex and urgent one.

◀ **Case Study Review.** Reviews and points out essential information and applied principles.

Content Self-Evaluation

▶▼ **Content Self-Evaluation.** Multiple-choice, matching, and short-answer questions to test reading comprehension.

MULTIPLE CHOICE

_____ 1. From innermost to outermost, the three tissue layers of the heart are:
A. the endocardium, the pericardium, and the myocardium.
B. the endocardium, the myocardium, and the syncytium.
C. the endocardium, the myocardium, and the pericardium.
D. the myocardium, the epicardium, and the pericardium.
E. the epicardium, the myocardium, and the endocardium.

MATCHING

Write the letter of the ECG leads in the space provided next to the type of leads they are.

A. I, II, III

B. V_1, V_2, V_3, V_4, V_5, V_6

C. aVR, aVL, aVF

_____ 9. unipolar (augmented)

_____ 10. bipolar

_____ 11. precordial

Fill-in-the-Blanks

56. The _____ valves lie between the atria and ventricles, whereas the _____ valves lie between the ventricles and the arteries into which they open.

57. The four properties of cells in the cardiac conductive system are _____ , _____ , _____ , and _____ .

Special Project

Assessing Respiratory Emergencies

Read the assessment written for each of three patients evaluated in a prehospital setting and identify the probable cause for each emergency. Check the Assessment section of the textbook for each disorder to refamiliarize yourself with characteristic findings on history and physical examination.

Scenario 1: You are called to an elementary school where a student has become "suddenly ill" during a class birthday party. You find a distressed seven-year-old child who is breathing rapidly and shallowly and whose skin tone is becoming dusky. The use of accessory muscles to breathe is evident. The school nurse offers you a box containing an inhaler that she says the child uses on an "as needed" basis and states she isn't sure what ingredients were in the cupcakes brought for the party. She adds that the boy has several severe food allergies.

Probable cause: _____

Scenario 2: You are called to a home where an elderly man is "short of breath." On arrival, you find a thin, elderly man with a broad chest whose breathing is labored despite use of a home supplemental oxygen setup. His daughter tells you that he has had a cold recently, and he suddenly became "shorter of breath" this morning. On exam, the man has a fever of

◄ **Special Projects.** Experiences designed to help students remember information and principles.

EMT-Paramedic Form

National Registry of Emergency Medical Technicians
Advanced Level Practical Examination

PATIENT ASSESSMENT - TRAUMA

Candidate: _____ Examiner: _____

Date: _____ Signature: _____

Scenario # _____

Time Start: NOTE: Areas denoted by "**" may be integrated within sequence of Initial Assessment	Possible Points	Points Awarded
Takes or verbalizes body substance isolation precautions	1	
SCENE SIZE-UP		
Determines the scene/situation is safe	1	
Determines the mechanism of injury/nature of illness	1	
Determines the number of patients	1	
Requests additional help if necessary	1	
Considers stabilization of spine	1	

► **National Registry Practical Evaluation Forms.** Gives a clearer picture of what is expected during the practical exam.

CARD 1 PATIENT HISTORY

Dispatch Information: Responding to a residence for a patient complaining of chest pain.

Scene Size-Up: Small but clean home with the patient seated on the couch, in obvious pain, and clutching his chest; no hazards noted.

Medical History
A—anesthetic at the dentist's office ("caine" family)
M—nitroglycerin and calcium supplements
P—sees his doctor yearly but doesn't have any medical problems
L—breakfast an hour ago, 2 eggs, toast, and coffee
E—watching television, nothing unusual

◄ **Patient Scenario Flash Cards.** Present scenarios with signs and symptoms and information to make field diagnoses.

Teaching and Learning Package

FOR THE INSTRUCTOR

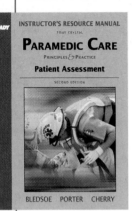

Instructor's Resource Manual. The Instructor's Resource Manual for each volume contains everything needed to teach the 1998 U.S. DOT National Standard Curriculum for Paramedics. It fully covers the DOT curriculum with:

- Time estimates for various topics
- Listing of additional resources
- Lecture outlines
- Student activities handouts
- Answers to student review questions
- Case study discussion questions
- Transition guides from current edition and competing text

This manual is also available on disk in Word and PDF format so instructors can customize resources to their individual needs.

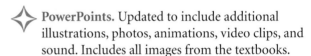

★ **TestGen.** Thoroughly updated and reviewed. Contains more than 2,000 exam-style questions, including DOT objectives and book page references.

PowerPoints. Updated to include additional illustrations, photos, animations, video clips, and sound. Includes all images from the textbooks.

FOR THE STUDENT

NEW Student CD. In-text CD contains quizzes, a virtual airway tour, animations, case study exercises, video skills clips, on-scene video footage, and audio glossary.

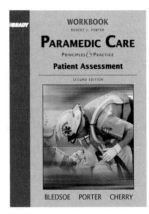

Workbook. Contains review of chapter objectives with summary information; case study review; content self-evaluation that includes multiple-choice, matching, and short-answer questions; special projects; content review; practical evaluation forms; and patient scenario flash cards.

ONLINE RESOURCES

Companion Website. Contains quizzes, labeling exercises, state EMS directories, *New York Times* link, weblinks, and trauma gallery.

OneKey. A distance learning program to support the series, offered on one of three platforms: Course Compass, Blackboard, or WebCT. Includes the IRM, PowerPoints, Test Manager, and Companion Website for instruction. Features include:

- Course outline
- Online gradebook, which automatically keeps track of students' performance on quizzes, class participation, and attendance
- Ability to upload questions authored offline and to randomize question order for each student
- Ability to add your own URLs and course links, set up discussion boards, modify navigation features
- A virtual classroom for real-time sessions and communication with students
- Weblinks
- Ability to include your teaching assistants into course creation/management

Other Titles of Interest

SKILLS

Brady Skills Series: Advanced Life Support
(0-13-119307-4—video; 0-13-119326-0—CD)
26 skills presented in step-by-step format with
introduction, equipment, overview, and close-up, including
assessment.

Advanced Life Support Skills (0-13-093874-2)
26 skills presented in full color, with step-by-step photos and
rationales.

ALS Skills Review (0-13-193637-9)
Close-ups for 26 skills, for student review.

REVIEW & REFERENCE

Beasley, Mistovich, *EMT Achieve: Paramedic Test
Preparation* (0-13-119269-8)
Online test preparation, with full-length exams and quizzes,
with rationales and supporting text, artwork, and video.

Cherry, Mistovich, *EMT-Paramedic Self-
Assessment Exam Review*, 3rd edition
(0-13-112869-8)
Best-selling review, containing test questions with DOT and
text page references and rationales.

Miller, *Paramedic National Standards Self-Test*,
4th edition (0-13-110500-0)
Based on the 1998 DOT curriculum, uses self-test format to
target areas students need to study further. Includes multiple-
choice and scenario-based questions.

Bledsoe, Clayden, *Pocket Reference for ALS Providers*,
3rd edition (0-13-170728-0)
Drugs, dosages, algorithms, tables and charts, pediatric emergencies, advanced skills, and home medications provided in
an easy-to-use field guide.

Cherry, Bledsoe, *Drug Guide for Paramedics*
(0-13-028798-9)
Handy field resource for accurate, easily accessed information
about patient medication.

Cherry, *Patient Assessment Handbook* (0-13-061578-1)
Concise, illustrated, step-by-step procedures for assessment
techniques.

ANATOMY & PHYSIOLOGY

Martini, Bartholemew, Bledsoe, *Anatomy &
Physiology for Emergency Care* (0-13-042298-3)
EMS-specific applications at the end of every chapter provide
an emergency care focus to A&P discussions.

CARDIAC/EKG

Walraven, *Basic Arrhythmias*, 6th edition
(0-13-117591-2)
Classic best-seller covers all the basics of EKG and includes a
new student CD. Also contains appendices on clinical
implications, cardiac anatomy & physiology, 12-lead EKG,
basic 12-lead interpretation, and pacemakers.

Beasley, *Understanding EKGs: A Practical Approach*,
2nd edition (0-13-045215-7)
A direct approach to EKG interpretation that presents all the
essential concepts for mastering the basics of this challenging
field, while assuming no prior knowledge of EKGs.

Page, *12-Lead ECG for Acute and Critical Care
Providers* (0-13-022460-X)
This full-color text presents ECG interpretation in a practical,
easy-to-understand, and user-friendly manner.

Beasley, *Understanding 12-Lead EKGs: A Practical
Approach*, 2nd edition (0-13-170789-2)
This comprehensive, reader-friendly text teaches beginning
students basic 12-lead EKG interpretation.

Mistovich, et al., *Prehospital Advanced Cardiac Life
Support*, 2nd edition (0-13-110143-9)
Straightforward and easy to follow, this text offers clear
explanations, a colorful design, and covers all of the core
concepts covered in an advanced cardiac life support course.

MEDICAL

Dalton, et al., *Advanced Medical Life Support*,
2nd edition (0-13-098632-1)
This groundbreaking text offers a practical approach to
adult medical emergencies. Each chapter discusses realistic
methods that a seasoned EMS practitioner would use.

▼ Teaching and Learning Package

MEDICAL TERMINOLOGY

Rice, *Medical Terminology with Human Anatomy,* **5th edition (0-13-048706-6)**
Providing comprehensive coverage of all aspects of medical terminology, along with overviews of anatomy and physiology, this popular text is arranged by body systems and specialty areas.

PEDIATRICS

Markenson, et al., *Pediatric Prehospital Care* **(0-13-022618-1)**
Written for all levels of EMS providers, this text presents a physiological approach to rapid and accurate pediatric assessment, identification of potential problems, establishing treatment priorities with effective on-going assessment, and rapid and safe transport.

PHARMACOLOGY

Bledsoe, Clayden, *Prehospital Emergency Pharmacology,* **6th edition (0-13-150711-7)**
This text and handy reference is a complete guide to the most common medications used in prehospital care.

TRAUMA

Campbell, *Basic Trauma Life Support for Paramedics and Advanced Providers,* **5th edition (0-13-112351-3)**
Best-selling BTLS text provides a complete course that covers all the skills necessary for rapid assessment, resuscitation, stabilization, and transportation of the trauma patient.

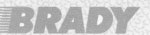

Paramedic Care
Principles & Practice
TRAUMA EMERGENCIES

SECOND EDITION

Trauma and Trauma Systems

Objectives

After reading this chapter, you should be able to:

1. Describe the prevalence and significance of trauma. (pp. 4–6)
2. List the components of a comprehensive trauma system. (pp. 6–8)
3. Identify the characteristics of community, area, and regional trauma centers. (pp. 6–8)
4. Identify the trauma triage criteria and apply them to narrative descriptions of trauma patients. (pp. 8–11)
5. Describe how trauma emergencies differ from medical emergencies in the scene size-up, assessment, prehospital emergency care, and transport. (pp. 8–11)
6. Explain the "Golden Hour" concept, and describe how it applies to prehospital emergency medical service. (p. 10)
7. Explain the value of air medical service in trauma patient care and transport. (p. 10)

Key Terms

Case Study

On a sunny and warm mid-summer day, the annunciator sounds and requests that the fly car with paramedic Earl Antak and the Hamilton Area Volunteer Ambulance respond to a bicycle/auto collision 3 miles south of Amble Corners. It is a 10-minute trip for Earl, and about the same for the volunteer ambulance. While the vehicles are en route, the dispatcher radios that the sheriff's department is on scene and that they have reported an unresponsive bicyclist.

Arriving at the location of the collision, Earl notes that members of the sheriff's department have secured the scene and are directing traffic. As he begins the scene size-up, he notices that several other cars are parked along the shoulder of the highway. Earl also sees a bicycle with a mangled front wheel resting against the open door of one of the cars. An officer from the sheriff's department is attending to a young adult who is lying on the roadside about 45 feet in front of the car. As Earl studies the scene more closely, he observes that the car's open door has been bent forward and that glass from the car is strewn along the highway.

The officer tells Earl that the person he is attending to is named John. He reports that John was unresponsive when the officer arrived but is now responsive, but somewhat confused. Earl's general impression is that the patient is a well-developed male in his early 20s. He is wearing a bicycle helmet, shorts, and a t-shirt. He has several abrasions to his right shoulder, arm, and forearm as well as to his right thigh. His helmet is badly scraped and deformed. Earl asks the officer to continue holding manual head immobilization while the paramedic applies a cervical collar.

Earl's initial assessment reveals that John is responsive and oriented to person but not to place or time. John reports that he was riding along at about 22 miles per hour when "this lady opened her door right in front of me." He flew through the window of that door and onto the pavement. He asks, "How's my bike?" His pulse rate is about 100 and his respirations are about 22 and full. Both lung fields are clear and his skin is warm and very wet. Earl applies oxygen via nonrebreather mask at 15 liters per minute.

The rapid trauma assessment reveals a small deformity just medial to the right upper anterior shoulder and some crepitus and pain with any movement of the right shoulder. There is a large abrasion to the right thigh. The upper and lower extremities have reduced sensation to pain and touch, good pulses and temperature, bilaterally equal but limited strength, and no pain with motion, except in the right upper extremity (suspected clavicle fracture). There are no signs of soft-tissue injuries to the head and John denies any pain other than to his right shoulder and thigh, a "twinge" in his neck, and a sensation of "pins and needles" in his extremities. When vital signs are taken, John's pulse is still 100, his respirations are still 22 and full, and his blood pressure is 132/84.

As the volunteer ambulance arrives, Earl uses his cell phone to contact medical direction for trauma center assignment. He is directed to Mercy Hospital, the closest Level 2 trauma center, and speaks to the trauma triage nurse. Earl tells the nurse that John meets the system's trauma triage criteria—initial unresponsiveness and a serious mechanism of injury—and relates his assessment findings and the patient's vital signs. Since the ground transport time is projected to be 35 minutes, he requests a helicopter intercept.

After about 8 minutes at the patient's side, Earl and the EMTs from the volunteer ambulance have applied a cervical collar, immobilized John onto a spine board, and loaded him into the ambulance. As transport begins, Earl establishes a 16-gauge IV access site, begins to administer normal saline at a to-keep-open rate, and continues to provide ongoing assessment. He notices that John can no longer remember what happened to him or who the paramedic is. He begins to mumble incoherently.

Earl and the ambulance intercept with a Central State Medevac helicopter at the pre-designated landing zone, a parking lot at the county community college. The flight paramedic greets Earl, takes his report, and quickly begins her assessment. She readies John for flight and Earl helps load him into the helicopter. Within minutes of the ambulance's arrival, the helicopter takes off en route to Mercy Hospital.

Later that day, Earl gets a follow-up phone call from the flight paramedic, thanking him for providing good care for John and a good patient report. She says that John had a fracture of the right clavicle; an epidural bleed, which was managed by surgery; and a confirmed C2 and C3 fracture. Because of John's age and physical condition, he is expected to recover quickly.

INTRODUCTION TO TRAUMA AND TRAUMA CARE

trauma   *a physical injury or wound caused by external force or violence.*

Trauma is the leading killer of persons under age 44 in the United States.

Trauma is a physical injury or wound caused by external force or violence. It is the number four killer in the United States today behind cardiovascular disease, stroke, and cancer. It is, however, the leading killer of persons under age 44. As such, trauma steals the greatest number of productive years from its victims. It also may be the most expensive medical problem because of the productivity losses it causes in its victims and the high cost of initial care, rehabilitation, and often lifelong maintenance of those victims.

Trauma accounts for about 150,000 deaths per year, with auto crashes responsible for about 44,000 and gunshot wounds another 28,000. Other trauma deaths are attributed to falls, blasts, stabbings, crush injuries, and sports injuries. In addition to the great death toll from trauma, many more of its victims are injured and carry lifelong physical reminders of their experiences with it.

Your role in trauma care, as a member of the Emergency Medical Services team, is to understand the structure and objectives of the trauma care system, to promote injury prevention, and to provide the seriously injured trauma patient with proper assessment, aggressive care, and rapid transport to the most appropriate facility. The remainder of this chapter will help you with these responsibilities as it further defines trauma, explains the components of trauma care systems, identifies the capabilities of different levels of trauma centers, and more fully defines your role as a care provider in the trauma system.

TRAUMA

The types of trauma can range from slight abrasions or scratches to the fatal, multiple-system injuries that might result from a high-speed automobile-versus-pedestrian collision. Trauma is broken down into two major categories, blunt and penetrating. **Penetrating trauma** occurs when an arrow, bullet, knife, or other object enters the body and exchanges energy with human tissue, thereby causing injury. **Blunt trauma** is injury that occurs as the energy and forces of collision with an object—not the object itself—enter the body and damage tissue. These two categories of trauma are discussed in greater detail in the next two chapters of this book.

Although trauma poses a serious threat to life, its presentation often masks the patient's true condition. Extremity injuries, for example, infrequently cause death. Yet they are often obvious and grotesque (Figure 1-1). However, life-threatening problems such as internal bleeding and shock may occur with only subtle signs and symptoms. When assessing a trauma patient, you must look beyond obvious injuries for evidence that suggests a life-threatening condition. When such a condition is found, you must assure rapid access to the trauma system for your patient.

Serious and life-threatening injury occurs in fewer than 10 percent of trauma patients. In most patients with life-threatening injury the injury is internal and is likely to involve the head or body cavity hemorrhage. Prehospital care can neither properly nor definitively stabilize these patients and their injuries in the field. The best care you as a paramedic can offer is to stabilize the cervical spine, secure the airway, assure adequate respirations, control any significant external hemorrhage, and rapidly transport the patient to definitive trauma care. That care is only available at a specialized treatment facility with rapid access to surgery—a trauma center.

Some 90 percent of trauma patients do not have serious, life-threatening injuries. You can best care for these patients by providing thorough on-scene assessment and stabilization followed by conservative transport to the nearest general hospital or other appropriate health care facility.

penetrating trauma *injury caused by an object breaking the skin and entering the body.*

blunt trauma *injury caused by the collision of an object with the body in which the object does not enter the body.*

 Life-threatening problems, such as internal bleeding and shock, may occur with only subtle signs and symptoms.

Image description: a small key icon appears here. When assessing a trauma patient, look beyond obvious injuries for evidence that suggests a life-threatening condition.

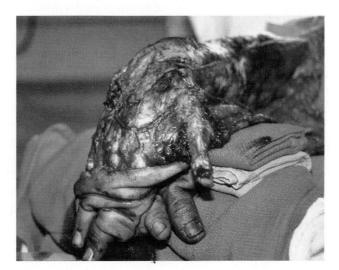

■ Figure 1-1   In prehospital care, it is essential that gruesome, non-life-threatening injuries do not distract you from more subtle, life-threatening problems. (© *Edward T. Dickinson, MD*)

It is essential that you determine the difference between trauma patients with serious, life-threatening conditions and those less seriously injured during your assessment. You will be aided in making this determination by using guidelines known as trauma triage criteria. These criteria involve consideration of the mechanisms by which patients are injured and of the physical or clinical findings indicating internal injury. Using these criteria, which will be discussed in detail later in this chapter, will help you properly direct patients as they enter the trauma care system.

THE TRAUMA CARE SYSTEM

In the mid-to-late 1960s, several medically oriented groups investigated the death toll on U.S. highways. Their studies revealed that victims of vehicle collisions suffered not only from the injuries received in the crashes but also from the lack of an organized approach to bringing these victims into the health care system. The studies also demonstrated that most hospitals were inadequately equipped and staffed to care for the victims of these crashes. These investigations led to passage of the Highway Safety Act of 1966 and to the development of today's Emergency Medical Services (EMS) system.

More than two decades later, the American College of Surgeons, recognizing that the system of caring for severely injured trauma victims was still inadequate, successfully worked to achieve passage of the Trauma Care Systems Planning and Development Act of 1990. This act helped establish guidelines, funding, and state-level leadership and support for the development of trauma systems.

The trauma system is predicated on the principle that serious trauma is a *surgical disease*. This means that the proper care for serious internal trauma is often immediate surgical intervention to repair internal hemorrhage sites. While patients with life-threatening injuries account for less than 10 percent of all trauma patients, immediate surgical care of these patients can drastically reduce trauma mortality and morbidity.

Care for seriously injured trauma patients is expensive and complicated. A well-designed EMS system will allocate trauma resources in a way that provides these patients with the most efficient and effective care. Such a system utilizes hospitals with special resources and commitment to trauma patient care. These hospitals are designated as trauma centers.

Serious trauma is a surgical disease; its proper care is immediate surgical intervention to repair internal hemorrhage sites.

TRAUMA CENTER DESIGNATION

The current model for a trauma system includes three levels of **trauma center,** with an increased ability and commitment to provide trauma care at each level (Table 1–1).

The Level I, or regional, trauma center is a hospital, usually a university teaching center, that is prepared and committed to handle all types of specialty trauma (Figure 1-2 ■). These centers provide neurosurgery, microsurgery (limb replantation), pediatric care, burn care, and care for multisystem trauma. They also provide leadership and resource support to other levels of the regional trauma system through system coordination and continuing medical and public education programs. When population density does not permit a commitment to the requirements of a Level I trauma center, a Level II trauma center may act as the regional trauma center.

The Level II, or area, trauma center has an increased commitment to trauma care, but not as great as a Level I facility. It has surgical care capability available at all times for incoming trauma patients. Level II centers can handle all but the most seriously injured specialty and multisystem trauma patients. Staff at these facilities can stabilize those patients in preparation for transport to a Level I trauma center.

The Level III, or community, trauma center is a general hospital with a commitment to special staff training and resource allocation for trauma patients. These centers

trauma center *a hospital that has the capability of caring for acutely injured patients; trauma centers must meet strict criteria to use this designation.*

The modern trauma system includes three levels of trauma center, each with an increased ability and commitment to providing trauma care.

Table 1-1	Criteria for Trauma Center Designation

Level I—Regional Trauma Center

Commits resources to address all types of specialty trauma 24 hours a day, 7 days a week.

Level II—Area Trauma Center

Commits the resources to address the most common trauma emergencies with surgical capability available 24 hours a day, 7 days a week; will stabilize and transport specialty cases to the regional trauma center.

Level III—Community Trauma Center

Commits to special emergency department training and has some surgical capability, but will usually stabilize and transfer seriously injured trauma patients to a higher level trauma center as needed.

Level IV—Trauma Facility

In remote areas, a small community hospital or medical care facility may be designated a trauma receiving facility, meaning that it will stabilize and prepare seriously injured trauma patients for transport to a higher level facility.

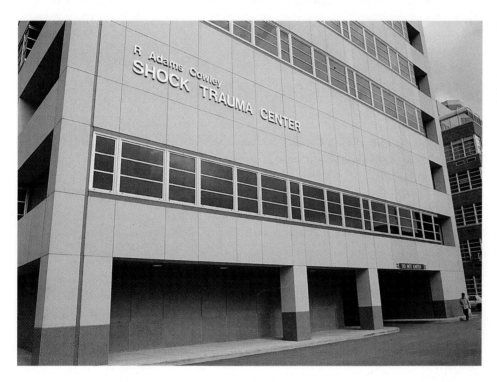

Figure 1-2 The R. Adams Cowley Shock Trauma Center in Baltimore, Maryland, is an example of a Level I trauma facility.

are located in smaller cities situated in generally rural areas. They are well prepared to care for most trauma victims and to stabilize and triage more seriously injured ones for transport to higher level trauma centers.

In some remote areas, there is provision for an additional level of trauma patient destination, a Level IV trauma facility, where seriously injured trauma patients may be taken for stabilization and care before transport, often by helicopter, to a more distant, higher level trauma center. In these areas, the incidence of trauma does not support the resource allocation necessary to meet the requirements of a trauma center, so, by default, some other type of health care facility is identified as a trauma transport destination.

The design of a trauma system should be flexible in order to meet the needs of the region it serves. In urban and suburban areas, there are just a few trauma centers to assure that each receives adequate patient volume to maintain staff proficiency and to assure that resources are being effectively used. In rural regions, a Level III center may act as the regional trauma center because the incidence of serious trauma does not support any greater commitment. In some areas, a Level IV facility may be all that is available and thus becomes the default destination for seriously injured trauma patients. Consult your EMS system plan to determine the intended patient flow patterns in your region.

SPECIALTY CENTERS

Beyond classification as trauma centers, certain medical facilities may be designated as specialty centers. Such facilities may include neurocenters, burn centers, pediatric trauma centers, and centers specializing in hand and limb replantation by microsurgery. One other specialty service is hyperbaric oxygenation, which is important in the treatment of carbon monoxide poisoning and problems related to scuba diving.

Specialty centers have made a commitment of trained personnel, equipment, and other resources to provide services not usually available at a general or trauma hospital. These centers are also more likely to provide a higher level of intensive care and state-of-the-art injury management than other facilities are able to. Be aware of the specialty services available in your system as well as the protocols defining when patients should be directed to them.

YOUR ROLE AS AN EMT-PARAMEDIC

As an EMT-Paramedic, your tasks in the trauma system are likely to include triage of trauma patients against standards established by your medical direction authority (trauma triage criteria) and assurance of the rapid assessment, care, and transport of patients to the closest appropriate medical facility (Figure 1-3 ■). For those patients who meet trauma triage criteria, the appropriate facility is the nearest trauma center.

Legal Notes

The Cost of Trauma Care Trauma systems and hospital designations are an important part of prehospital care. Trauma triage protocols help direct trauma patients to a facility that can adequately care for their injuries. However, now that it is the twenty-first century, several confounding factors are complicating these systems. For example, in most cases, trauma care is a cost for which most hospitals are not adequately reimbursed. In fact, they might actually lose money. In a time of shrinking health care dollars, many hospitals have found that they can no longer afford to provide costly trauma care.

Likewise, skyrocketing malpractice insurance premiums have driven many physicians from trauma practice—especially neurosurgeons. Trauma patients are often difficult to care for, and patient outcome is often determined more by the injury than by the care provided. However, many physicians and surgeons are finding that malpractice allegations come more frequently from trauma patients than from other classes of patients and, because of this, have elected not to provide trauma care. This, of course, has begun to create a signicant problem for EMS.

With trauma centers closing and physicians closing their practice to trauma, ambulances must often travel greater distances to get their patients to a proper facility. Although these issues are community issues, EMS personnel must stay informed and stay involved in order to make sure their patients receive the best possible care at the closest possible facility.

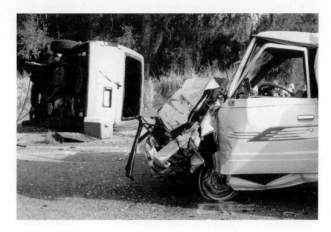

Trauma triage criteria are guidelines established to help you determine which patients require the services of a trauma center and which do not. The presence of certain mechanisms of injury and clinical findings have been proven, by research, to accurately reflect the potential for serious injury and the need for the intensive services available only at a trauma center. Compare your patient's mechanism of injury and any physical assessment findings to these preestablished criteria.

trauma triage criteria *guidelines to aid prehospital personnel in determining which trauma patients require urgent transportation to a trauma center.*

MECHANISM OF INJURY ANALYSIS

To help determine the **mechanism of injury,** mentally recreate the accident from evidence available at the scene. You should identify the forces involved in the incident, the direction from which they came, and the areas of the patient's body most likely to have been affected by these forces. In an automobile collision, for example, the mechanism of injury includes the energy exchange process between the auto and what it struck, between the patient and the auto's interior, and among the various tissues and organs as they collide, one with another, within the patient. Close inspection of the mangled auto reveals evidence about the collision and the forces at work within it. (See Chapter 2, Blunt Trauma, and Chapter 3, Penetrating Trauma.)

mechanism of injury *the processes and forces that cause trauma.*

Consideration of the mechanism of injury begins during the scene size-up. The mechanism of injury should be reconsidered as the first step of the focused history and physical exam for trauma patients.

You will begin your consideration of the mechanism of injury during the scene size-up. Later, you should reconsider the mechanism of injury as the first step of the focused history and physical exam for the trauma patient.

INDEX OF SUSPICION

The information you gather during your consideration and reconsideration of the mechanism of injury suggests an **index of suspicion** for possible injuries. This index is an anticipation of possible injuries based on analysis of the event. For example, a pedestrian struck by a car can be expected to have lower extremity fractures. Further, if the auto were moving at 20 miles per hour, fracture severity would be less than if it were moving at 55 miles per hour. Also, the probability of internal injury at lower speeds is less than it would be at higher speeds. By evaluating the strength of the impact and its nature, you can anticipate the structures and organs damaged and the degree to which they have been damaged.

index of suspicion *the anticipation of injury to a body region, organ, or structure based on analysis of the mechanism of injury.*

In addition to developing an index of suspicion for specific injuries, you will also examine the trauma patient for physical signs of injury, both during the initial assessment and during the rapid trauma assessment or the focused history and physical exam. The physical signs suggesting serious trauma include the signs and symptoms of shock and those of internal head injury. Because shock and head injury are the great

If you have any reason to suspect that the patient has sustained serious internal injury, move to enter him or her rapidly into the trauma system.

Golden Hour *the 60-minute period after a severe injury; it is the maximum acceptable time between the injury and initiation of surgery for the seriously injured trauma patient.*

Initial patient assessment, emergency stabilization, patient packaging, and initiation of transport should ideally take less than 10 minutes.

killers in trauma, be watchful for the earliest evidence of their existence. It is important to note that the body compensates well for the internal loss of blood and hides serious signs of injury until late in the shock process. If you have any reason to suspect that a patient has sustained serious internal injury, move to enter that patient rapidly into the trauma system. Otherwise, provide frequent ongoing assessment to assure that progressive signs of shock and internal head injury are discovered as early as possible.

THE GOLDEN HOUR

Time is a very important consideration in the survival of seriously injured trauma patients. Research has demonstrated that patient survival rates increase dramatically as time from the trauma incident to the beginning of surgery decreases. The current goal for incident-to-surgery time is 1 hour, often referred to as the **Golden Hour.**

Factors such as response time to the incident and the time needed to extricate a patient all consume a portion of the Golden Hour. Many of these factors will be beyond your control; for that reason, it is vital to keep time spent on factors over which you do have control to the minimum. Ideally, you should provide the initial and rapid trauma assessments, emergency stabilization, patient packaging, and initiation of transport in under 10 minutes. When distances or traffic conditions present prolonged ground transport times, reduce transport times by using an air medical service if possible.

Air medical service, usually provided by helicopter, has added a weapon in the race against time for the seriously injured trauma patient (Figure 1-4 ■). The helicopter often travels much faster than ground transport and in a straight line from the crash scene to the trauma center.

Be aware, however, that air medical transport is not appropriate in all cases. A trauma patient must be in relatively stable condition for it to be utilized. Additionally, the limited space within the aircraft and its associated engine noise make in-flight care difficult. Further, a combative patient may endanger the safety of the flight crew and the aircraft. Adverse weather conditions can also limit the use of air medical transport. In many cases, ground transport is as fast or faster. Finally, air medical transport services are very expensive and can be used most effectively only as part of a comprehensive EMS trauma system. Follow local protocols about when and how to request air medical transport.

THE DECISION TO TRANSPORT

The decision either to transport a patient immediately or to attempt more extensive on-scene care is among the most difficult you must make. The trauma triage criteria are designed to help you with this decision. As a rule, transport patients who experience certain mechanisms of injury and display key clinical findings quickly, with intravenous access and other time-consuming procedures attempted en route. Indicators for immediate transport are given in Table 1–2.

■ Figure 1-4 An air medical services helicopter can sometimes reduce transport time from the accident scene to the trauma center. (© *Craig Jackson/In the Dark Photography*)

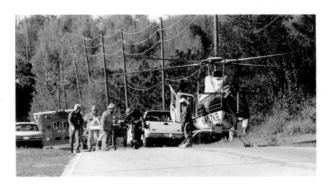

Table 1-2	Trauma Triage Criteria Indicating Need for Immediate Transport

Mechanism of Injury

- Falls greater than 20 feet (3 times the patient's height)
- Pedestrian/bicyclist versus auto collisions
  —Struck by a vehicle traveling over 5 mph
  —Thrown or run over by vehicle
- Motorcycle impact at greater than 20 mph
- Ejection from a vehicle
- Severe vehicle impact
  —Speed at impact greater than 40 mph
  —Intrusion of more than 12 inches into occupant compartment
  —Vehicle deformity greater than 20 inches
- Rollover with signs of serious impact
- Death of another occupant in the vehicle
- Extrication time greater than 20 minutes

Significant mechanism of injury considerations with infants and children include the following:

- A fall of greater than 10 feet (3 times the patient's height)
- A bicycle/vehicle collision
- A vehicle collision at medium speed
- Any vehicle collision where the infant or child was unrestrained

Physical Findings

- Revised Trauma Score less than 11 (see Chapter 12)
- Glasgow Coma Scale less than 14 (see Chapter 8)
- Systolic blood pressure less than 90
- Respiratory rate less than 10 or greater than 29
- Pulse less than 50 or greater than 120
- Penetrating trauma (except distal extremities)
- Two or more proximal long-bone fractures
- Flail chest
- Pelvic fractures
- Limb paralysis
- Burns to more than 15 percent of body surface area
- Burns to face or airway

In applying trauma triage criteria, it is best to err on the side of precaution. If a patient does not fit the stated criteria, be suspicious. Remember, you often arrive at the patient's side only minutes after the accident. The patient may not yet have lost enough blood internally to exhibit signs of shock or progressive head injury. If in doubt, transport to a trauma center without delay.

These criteria are designed for the "over-triage" of trauma patients. They assure that patients with very subtle signs and symptoms, yet with significant and serious injuries, are not missed during assessment. Use of these criteria means that you will transport some patients to trauma centers unnecessarily. However, transporting a patient

In applying trauma triage criteria, it is best to err on the side of precaution.

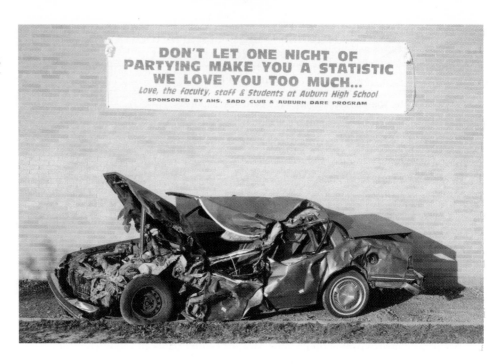

■ Figure 1-5 Public education programs can increase people's awareness of the role of the EMS system and of the importance of safe behaviors.

who may not need the resources of a trauma center is far better than not transporting a patient who truly needs the care available only there.

INJURY PREVENTION

One of the best and most cost-effective ways of reducing mortality and morbidity is to prevent trauma in the first place.

One of the best, most cost-effective ways of reducing mortality and morbidity is to prevent trauma in the first place. Several programs in this vein have been very effective. Programs promoting seat belt use and awareness of the dangers of drinking and driving have encouraged teenagers and adults to drive more safely and responsibly. Other programs, like "let's not meet by accident," increase society's awareness of trauma systems as well as an appreciation for safety-oriented behaviors (Figure 1-5 ■). Safety programs for users of boats and firearms also raise safety awareness and assist in injury prevention. The EMS system has a responsibility to support such programs and to promote their development where they do not exist. As an EMS provider, you should participate in these types of programs and encourage your peers to take part in them as well.

Technical developments such as better highway design, air bag restraint systems, and vehicles constructed to absorb the energy of crashes have also played major parts in greatly reducing the yearly highway death toll. Paramedics have a responsibility to support the development and use of these new designs and technologies as a way of further reducing trauma deaths and injuries.

DATA AND THE TRAUMA REGISTRY

trauma registry *a data retrieval system for trauma patient information, used to evaluate and improve the trauma system.*

As with all emergency medical services, research is the only way to recognize those trauma care practices and procedures that benefit patients and those that do not. In the trauma system, there is a data recovery system called the **trauma registry.** It is a uniform and standard set of data collected by regional trauma centers. These data are analyzed to determine how well the system is performing and to identify factors that may contribute to or lessen chances of patient survival.

It is important that you do all that you can to support this research effort by assuring that your prehospital care reports accurately and completely describe the findings of your assessments, the care you provide to patients, the results of ongoing assessments, and the times associated with calls. You should also consider taking part in and supporting prehospital research projects if the opportunity presents itself. By doing so, you can help establish the value of new field techniques and equipment.

QUALITY IMPROVEMENT

Trauma system Quality Improvement (QI), or Quality Management (QM), is another way of examining system performance with the aim of providing better patient care. In the QI process, committees look at selected care modalities (called indicators) to determine if designated standards of care are being met. For trauma system QI, the committees would study the application of trauma triage criteria, performance of field skills, and amounts of time spent in various aspects of response, care, and transport of patients. QI committees may also look at select calls to determine if their documentation accurately reflects the results of assessment and the care given. If the system standards are not being met, the committees may suggest such steps as continuing education programs for system personnel or modification of current care protocols. QI is a significant method of assessing system quality and providing for its improvement. As a prehospital member of the trauma system, you should become actively involved in and encourage the participation of your peers in these or similar programs.

Summary

Trauma remains one of the greatest tragedies of our modern society. It accounts for large numbers of deaths and disabling injuries and often affects individuals who are in their most productive years of life. A well-designed and well-implemented trauma system offers a way of lessening the impact of these traumas. Such a trauma system consists of several levels of trauma centers, with each level possessing an increasing commitment to immediate and intensive trauma care.

As a paramedic, you are a part of the trauma system. You are charged with evaluating trauma patients by comparing their mechanisms of injury and the physical signs of their injuries to preestablished trauma triage criteria in order to determine which patients should enter the trauma system and which could be best cared for at a general hospital. In the presence of severe, life-threatening trauma, you must assure rapid assessment, on-scene care, and appropriate transport to provide your patients with the best chances for survival.

You Make the Call

Just as you are about to move a seriously injured 12-year-old patient who has been in a bicycle/auto collision, her mother, Janet, emerges from the crowd. She is quite distraught and becomes even more so when you tell her that you'll be transporting her daughter to the Great Meadows Trauma Center on the far side of town. Janet informs you that she is a "lab tech" at Livingston Community Hospital just a few minutes from your location and wants her child transported there.

1. What authority does Janet have regarding the decision to transport her daughter?
2. What will you be telling her regarding your choice for a hospital destination?

See Suggested Responses at the back of this book.

Review Questions

1. The leading killer of persons under age 44 in the United States is:
   a. cancer.
   b. stroke.
   c. trauma.
   d. cardiovascular disease.

2. The best care you, as a paramedic, can offer the trauma patient is to stabilize the cervical spine, secure the airway, and:
   a. assure adequate respirations.
   b. control any significant external hemorrhage.
   c. rapidly transport the patient to definitive trauma care.
   d. all of the above.

3. Certain trauma centers commit to special emergency department training and have a degree of surgical capability but usually stabilize and transfer seriously injured patients. These centers are designated:
   a. Level II.
   b. Level I.
   c. Level IV.
   d. Level III.

4. One specialty service important in the treatment of carbon monoxide poisoning and problems related to scuba diving is the:
   a. neurocenters.
   b. hyperbaric oxygenation centers.
   c. burn centers.
   d. pediatric trauma centers.

5. When determining the mechanism of injury, you will identify the:
   a. forces involved in the accident.
   b. person who caused the accident.
   c. number of patients.
   d. need for additional resources.

6. You will begin your consideration of the mechanism of injury:
   a. during the scene size-up.
   b. during the detailed physical exam.
   c. during the focused physical exam.
   d. during the ongoing assessment.

7. The goal of EMS when dealing with the serious trauma patient is to get the patient quickly to definitive care. The objective time frame, describing the period of time from the incident to the patient's arrival at surgery, is the:
   a. transport time.
   b. Golden Hour.
   c. chronological limit.
   d. maximum time of run.

8. In the ideal scenario, you should provide the initial and rapid trauma assessments, emergency stabilization, patient packaging, and initiation of transport in under _____ minutes.
   a. 15
   b. 20
   c. 10
   d. 12

9. Limitations of the use of air medical transport include all of the following except:
   a. limited space within the aircraft.
   b. associated engine noise.
   c. indirect route of travel.
   d. combative and unruly patients.

10. In the Quality Improvement process, committees look at selected care modalities to determine if designated standards of care are being met. These modalities are also called:
    a. tips.
    b. pointers.
    c. indicators.
    d. suggestions.

See Answers to Review Questions at the back of this book.

Further Reading

American College of Surgeons, Committee on Trauma. *Advanced Trauma Life Support Course: Student Manual.* Chicago: American College of Surgeons, 1997.

American College of Surgeons, Committee on Trauma. *Resources for Optimal Care of the Injured Patient.* Chicago: American College of Surgeons, 1998.

Baxt, William G. *Trauma, The First Hour.* Upper Saddle River, N.J.: Pearson/Prentice Hall, 1985.

On the Web

Visit Brady's Paramedic Website at **www.bradybooks.com/paramedic**.

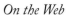

Blunt Trauma

Objectives

After reading this chapter, you should be able to:

1. Identify, and explain by example, the laws of inertia and conservation of energy. (pp. 19–20)
2. Define kinetic energy and force as they relate to trauma. (pp. 20–21)
3. Compare and contrast the types of vehicle impacts and their expected injuries. (pp. 22–24, 28–39)
4. Discuss the benefits of auto restraint and motorcycle helmet use. (pp. 25–28, 37)
5. Describe the mechanisms of injury associated with falls, crush injuries, and sports injuries. (pp. 47–50)
6. Identify the common blast injuries and any special considerations regarding their assessment and proper care. (pp. 40–47)
7. Identify and explain any special assessment and care considerations for patients with blunt trauma. (pp. 21–50)
8. Given several preprogrammed and moulaged blunt trauma patients, provide the appropriate scene size-up, initial assessment, rapid trauma assessment or focused physical exam and history, detailed exam, and ongoing assessment and provide appropriate patient care and transportation. (pp. 21–50)

Key Terms

Case Study

A call comes in to City Ambulance Unit 2 staffed by paramedic Kris and BLS provider Bob. The dispatcher reports multiple injuries in a two-car collision on the freeway at interchange 20. Because of backed-up traffic, the dispatcher tells the unit to take the road that intersects the freeway at that point and use the freeway exit ramp to access the scene.

Police arrive at the scene and provide Unit 2 with an update while it is en route. A green auto traveling at freeway speed has plowed into a red car stalled at the interchange. The wreck involves three injured parties—one in the red car and two in the green.

When Unit 2 reaches the scene, the police have secured it and are directing traffic around the vehicles involved. Kris and Bob approach the vehicles and begin the scene size-up, noting that about 100 yards now separate the two vehicles. The green car has severe front-end damage. Two "spider-web" cracks run across the windshield, the steering column is deformed, and the older model car has no air bags. The police officer in charge reports that both people in the car had failed to wear seat belts. The red car has severe rear-end damage, but the windshield is intact. The driver in this vehicle wore a seat belt and the head-rest is in the up position. Before acting, Kris calls for another unit to back up Unit 2. Kris and Bob now proceed to the green car, where they expect to find the worst injuries.

Kris and Bob perform initial assessments on the two occupants of that vehicle. The driver has suffered chest trauma caused by impact with the steering wheel. Although she is experiencing difficult and painful breathing, her airway is clear. She is oriented to time and place and denies any period of unconsciousness. Her pulses are strong, regular, and at a moderate rate. The physical exam reveals a forehead contusion, a reddened anterior chest with crepitus, and clear breath sounds bilaterally.

The passenger is unresponsive and cannot be aroused. She has shallow, rapid breaths and a rapid, barely palpable pulse. Her forehead is badly contused with moderate bleeding. Her thighs appear noticeably shortened. The rapid trauma assessment reveals instability of the pelvis and both femurs.

A police officer who has been trained as a First Responder indicates that the driver of the red car is conscious and alert. Although "shaken up," he has a blood pressure of 126/84 and a pulse of 86. He is breathing normally at a rate of 20. As the paramedic in charge, Kris asks the officer to stay with the driver until the second ambulance arrives.

Meanwhile, Bob has told the driver of the green car not to move. He immobilizes the passenger's head manually while Kris applies oxygen, then a cervical collar. Next, Kris prepares a long spine board with straps and a pelvic sling. They place the passenger on the board, strap her securely, firmly apply the sling, and affix her head with the cervical immobilization device. They then load her into the ambulance.

When the second ambulance arrives, Kris briefs that crew and assigns the remaining patients, the two drivers. Kris and Bob then rush the passenger, who is the most critical victim, to a nearby trauma center. En route, vital signs, taken quickly, reveal a blood pressure of 82 by palpation and a weak radial pulse of 130. The legs look ashen, feel cool to the touch, and show no palpable pulses. Capillary refill time is 3 seconds in the upper extremities, longer in the lower ones. The pulse oximeter reading is 92 percent.

Kris gives a brief report to medical direction and receives orders in response. Kris starts a large-bore IV and quickly administers a 250-mL bolus of normal saline. Kris then readies intubation equipment and hyperventilates the patient using the bag-valve mask. The ambulance stops briefly while Kris attempts orotracheal intubation, with the patient's head held fixed in the neutral position. When the effort proves unsuccessful, Kris withdraws the tube, hyperventilates the patient again, and tries to insert an LMA. The technique works and Kris infuses two more 250-mL boluses of fluid. Lung sounds are clear, chest excursion improves, capnography displays a proper waveform, and oximetry readings begin to rise.

The patient arrives at the trauma center with just under 1,500 mL of fluid infused, an end-tidal CO_2 reading of 35 mmHg, and an oxygen saturation of 96 percent. The operating room has been prepared for her. Doctors clear the C-spine, repair vascular injuries associated with the pelvic fracture, and infuse 6 units of typed and cross-matched whole blood. The patient recovers after a few weeks of hospitalization and will walk again with only slight reminders of the injuries and care she received.

Based on the speed of impact and the vehicle damage, the second ambulance crew decides to transport the other two patients to the trauma center. The driver of the green car has two fractured ribs, a C-spine cleared by X-ray and CT scan, and no neurologic deficit. She stays overnight for observation and is released the next afternoon with some medication for rib fracture pain. The other driver has a clear C-spine and returns home shortly after the emergency department evaluation.

INTRODUCTION TO KINETICS

Blunt trauma is the most common cause of trauma death and disability.

Blunt trauma can be deceptive because the true nature of the injury is often hidden and evidence of the serious injury is very subtle or even absent.

Blunt trauma is the most common cause of trauma death and disability. It results from an energy exchange between an object and the human body, without intrusion of the object through the skin (Figure 2-1 ■). The energy exchange causes a chain reaction within various body tissues that crushes and stretches their structures, resulting in injury beneath the surface. Blunt trauma is especially confounding because the true nature of the injury is often hidden, and evidence of the serious injury is very subtle or even absent.

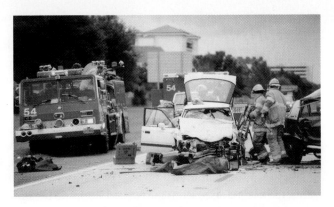

■ Figure 2-1   Blunt trauma is the most common cause of injury and trauma-related death. It is a physical exchange of energy from an object or surface transmitted through the skin into the body's interior. *(© Craig Jackson/In the Dark Photography)*

To properly care for victims of blunt and penetrating trauma, you should understand the injury process and its results. Study of this process, called kinetics of trauma, gives insight into the events that produce injury, known as the mechanism of injury. This insight then helps you develop an index of suspicion, an anticipation of the nature and severity of likely injuries. Armed with an index of suspicion, you can better focus your trauma patient assessment, triage, and care because you know what happened and the injuries the event is likely to have produced.

Let us look at the kinetics of blunt trauma, vehicular collisions, blast injuries, and other types of blunt trauma to develop an understanding of these prevalent mechanisms of injury and their pathophysiological results.

KINETICS OF BLUNT TRAUMA

Kinetics is a branch of physics dealing with forces of objects in motion and the energy exchanges that occur as objects collide. These collisions, or impacts, are the events that induce injury in patients. An understanding of kinetics helps you appreciate and anticipate the results of auto and other impacts. The two basic principles of kinetics are the law of inertia and the law of energy conservation. Further, kinetic energy and force formulas quantify the energy exchange process between the moving object and the human body. These laws and formulas best describe what happens during impact and help in our understanding of blunt trauma.

kinetics   *the branch of physics that deals with motion, taking into consideration mass, velocity, and force.*

INERTIA

The law of **inertia,** as described by Sir Isaac Newton and also known as Newton's first law, helps explain what happens during blunt trauma. The first part of his first law states: "A body in **motion** will remain in motion unless acted upon by an outside force." As an example, think of identical autos moving at 55 miles per hour. One car brakes for a red light; the other rams into a bridge abutment. An "outside force" stops the motion of both vehicles, but with very different results. In the first case, the car's brakes absorb the energy of motion. In the second, the front bumper and grill, the frame, and eventually the occupants of the car absorb the energy as the car stops.

The second part of the law states: "A body at rest will remain at rest unless acted upon by an outside force." Examples of this include an auto accelerating from a stop sign or a stopped vehicle propelled forward by a rear-end collision. In the first case, the auto engine provides the force to initiate movement. In the second, the energy of the moving vehicle provides the force as the stopped car absorbs the energy and jolts ahead.

inertia   *tendency of an object to remain at rest or in motion unless acted upon by an external force.*

motion   *the process of changing place; movement.*

CONSERVATION OF ENERGY

energy *the capacity to do work in the strict physical sense.*

The law of conservation of energy states: "**Energy** can neither be created nor destroyed. It can only be changed from one form to another." In an auto crash, as in other trauma, identifying probable energy changes helps you assess the impacts of various collisions. Kinetic energy, possessed by a moving car and its passengers, transforms into other energy forms whenever a car stops.

If an auto slows down gradually for a stop sign, the brakes develop friction to slow the turning wheels, producing heat. During an auto crash, however, the energy of motion is converted at a much faster rate into different forms. This conversion of energy is manifested in the sound of impact, the deformation of the auto's structural components, the heat released from the twisted steel, and the injuries to passengers as they collide with the vehicle interior. As all the kinetic energy converts to other energy forms, the auto and its passengers come to a stop.

KINETIC ENERGY

kinetic energy *the energy an object has while it is in motion. It is related to the object's mass and velocity.*

Kinetic energy is the energy of an object in motion. It is a function of the object's **mass** and its **velocity** (Figure 2-2 ▪). (While mass and weight, and velocity and speed, are not identical, we will consider them as such for these discussions.) The kinetic energy of an object while in motion is measured by the following formula:

mass *a measure of the matter that an object contains; the property of a physical body that gives the body inertia.*

$$\text{Kinetic Energy} = \frac{\text{Mass (Weight)} \times \text{Velocity (Speed)}^2}{2}$$

velocity *the rate of motion in a particular direction in relation to time.*

This formula illustrates that if you double an object's weight, you double its kinetic energy. It is twice as damaging to be hit by a 2-pound baseball as to be hit by a 1-pound ball. It is three times as damaging to be hit by a 3-pound ball, and so on.

As speed (velocity) increases, there is a larger (squared) increase in kinetic energy. Being hit with a 1-pound baseball traveling at 20 miles per hour is four times as injurious as being hit with the same ball moving at 10 miles per hour. If speed increases to 30 miles per hour, trauma is nine times worse. This concept plays a key role in understanding the devastating effects of a gunshot wound in which a small bullet, traveling very fast, can do great damage (as discussed in Chapter 3, Penetrating Trauma).

▪ Figure 2-2 Increasing mass directly increases kinetic energy, while increasing velocity exponentially increases kinetic energy.

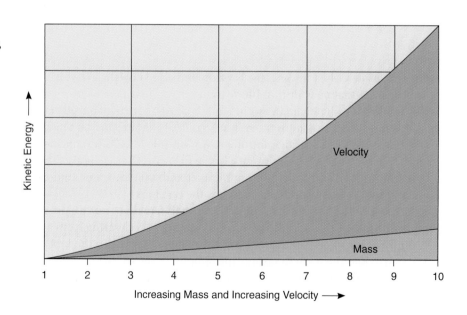

Kinetic energy is the measure of how much energy an object in motion has, not necessarily how much injury occurs. Two autos traveling at 55 miles per hour have about the same kinetic energy. The same two autos would have the same kinetic energy once they have stopped, even if one came to rest by hitting a bridge and the other through slow braking. The difference between these two events is the rate of slowing. The crash force is proportional to this rate.

FORCE

Newton's second law of motion explains the forces at work during a collision. It is summarized by the formula below:

$$\text{Force} = \text{Mass (Weight)} \times \text{Acceleration (or Deceleration)}$$

The formula emphasizes the importance of the rate at which an object changes speed, either increasing (**acceleration**) or decreasing (**deceleration**). Gradual changes in speed are usually uneventful. Normal deceleration, such as slowing for a stop sign, covers about 120 feet (from 55 miles per hour to 0 miles per hour at a braking rate of 22 feet/10 miles per hour). It therefore rarely results in injury. However, colliding with a bridge abutment and slowing from 55 miles per hour to 0 miles per hour in a matter of inches (and a fraction of a second) produces tremendous force and devastating injuries.

When significant kinetic energy is applied to human anatomy, we call it trauma. Trauma is defined as a wound or injury that is violently produced by some external force. The injury may be either blunt (closed) or penetrating (open) (Figure 2-3 ■).

acceleration *the rate at which speed or velocity increases.*

deceleration *the rate at which speed or velocity decreases.*

Trauma can be categorized as either blunt or penetrating.

BLUNT TRAUMA

Blunt trauma occurs when a body area is struck by, or strikes, an object. The transmission of energy, rather than the object, damages the tissues and organs beneath the skin as they collide with one another. An example of this is hitting your thumb with a hammer. The thumb is compressed between the hammer (which pushes the tissue) and the board (which resists the motion). Tissue injury results as flesh and bone are trapped between these two forces (acceleration and deceleration). Skin and muscle cells stretch and crush, blood vessels tear, and bone may fracture.

Blunt trauma can also induce injury deep within the body cavity. Forces of compression cause hollow organs like the bladder or bowel to rupture, spilling their contents and hemorrhaging. In the thorax, alveoli or small airways may burst, permitting air to enter the pleural space. Solid organs, such as the spleen, liver, pancreas, and kidneys, may contuse or lacerate, leading to swelling, blood loss, or both.

Other blunt trauma may result from the effects of rapid speed change on organ attachment. An example is the liver, which is suspended in the abdomen by the *ligamentum teres*. During severe deceleration, the liver may be sliced by the ligament in a way similar to cheese when cut by a wire cheese cutter. Similarly, the aorta may be injured as the chest slows and the heart, which is suspended from the great vessels, twists upon impact. Layers of the vessel are torn apart, and blood enters the injury with the force of the systolic blood pressure. The aorta balloons like a defective tire, leading to a tearing chest pain, circulatory compromise, and immediate or delayed **exsanguination** (severe blood loss).

Wounds that break the skin are classified as penetrating trauma. Penetrating trauma occurs when the energy source (such as a knife or bullet) progresses into the body. Energy may also be transmitted to surrounding body tissue, thus extending the trauma beyond the pathway of the object. This frequently happens with high-velocity gunshot wounds.

exsanguination *the draining of blood to the point at which life cannot be sustained.*

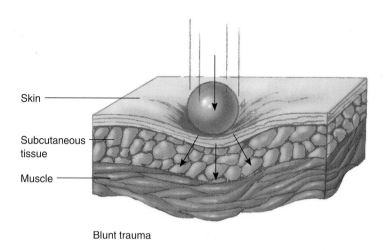

Figure 2-3a Blunt trauma results when an object or force impacts the body and kinetic energy is transferred to the involved body tissues.

Skin

Subcutaneous tissue

Muscle

Blunt trauma

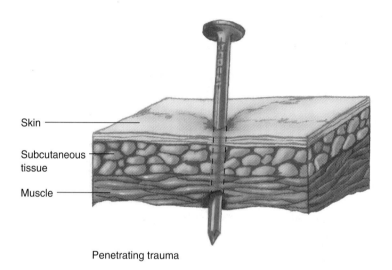

Figure 2-3b Penetrating injury is produced when an object enters the body resulting in direct injury

Skin

Subcutaneous tissue

Muscle

Penetrating trauma

As a paramedic, you will encounter both blunt and penetrating trauma. The balance of this chapter deals with examples of blunt trauma. Examples of penetrating trauma are discussed in Chapter 3. Blunt trauma most commonly results from motor vehicle collisions involving automobiles, motorcycles, pedestrians, or recreational vehicles (all-terrain vehicles, watercraft, snowmobiles). It can also result from explosions, falls, crush injuries, and sports injuries.

AUTOMOBILE COLLISIONS

Vehicular collisions—sometimes called motor vehicle collisions or motor vehicle crashes (MVCs)—account for a large proportion of paramedic responses. Each year over 100,000 serious collisions occur on U.S. highways. Some 44,000 people lose their lives in these collisions, while many more are seriously injured or permanently disabled. As a paramedic, you must be prepared to offer rapid assessment and appropriate care to victims of these collisions. To this end, you must recognize the various types of vehicular impacts, identify possible mechanisms of injury, and form a reasonable index of suspicion for specific injuries. Analysis of the types of impacts and the events associated with them help you form this index of suspicion.

Trauma and the Laws of Physics The laws of physics play a significant role in the pathophysiology of both blunt and penetrating injuries. In blunt trauma, the energy tends to be more widely distributed than with penetrating injuries. Also, as discussed in this chapter, solid organs are at greater risk of injury following blunt trauma than hollow organs because they tend to absorb more of the energy of impact.

Any patient who has sustained a blunt-force injury to the abdomen should increase your index of suspicion of solid organ injury. Injuries to the liver, spleen, pancreas, or even the kidneys can result in massive blood loss. Once at the trauma center, surgeons may elect to manage some blunt-force injuries conservatively, whereas others will require immediate surgical repair. However, it is important to remember that some hollow organs will begin to react in a way similar to solid organs when they are full or distended. For example, the urinary bladder may be full at the time of injury. Blunt-force trauma may result in its rupture with subsequent spillage of urine into the abdomen. Likewise, immediately after a meal, the stomach may be full and rupture or tear, spilling its contents into the abdomen.

Thus, questions about recent meals, alcohol and fluid intake, and similar factors must be taken into consideration when caring for a victim of blunt trauma.

Events of Impact

There are basically five types of vehicle impacts—frontal, lateral, rotational, rear-end, and rollover. Each type progresses through a series of four events (Figure 2-4 ■). These events are:

1. *Vehicle Collision.* Vehicle collision begins when the auto strikes an object (or an object strikes the auto). Kinetic energy causes vehicle damage as it is transferred to the object hit by the auto. The force developed in the collision depends on the velocity of travel and the stopping distance. If the auto slides into a snow bank, damage is limited. If the auto strikes a concrete retaining wall, the damage is much greater. The degree of auto deformity is a good indicator of the strength and direction of forces experienced by its occupants. The auto collision slows or stops the vehicle.

2. *Body Collision.* Body collision occurs when a vehicle occupant strikes the vehicle's interior. The vehicle and its interior have slowed dramatically during the collision, but an unrestrained occupant remains at or close to the initial speed. As the occupant contacts the interior, energy is transferred to the vehicle or is transformed into the initial tissue deformity, compression, stretching, and trauma. If the vehicle collision causes intrusion into the passenger compartment, this displacement may further injure occupants or otherwise worsen the injury process.

3. *Organ Collisions.* Organ collision results as the occupant contacts the vehicle's interior and slows or stops. Tissues behind the contacting surface collide, one into another, as the occupant's body comes to a halt. This causes compression and stretching as tissues and organs violently press into each other. In the process, organs may also twist or decelerate, and tear at their attachments or at blood vessels. The result is blunt trauma.

4. *Secondary Collisions.* Secondary collisions occur when a vehicle occupant is impacted by objects traveling within the auto. During the collision, objects—such as those in the back seat, on the back window ledge, or in the back of a van—or other unrestrained passengers may continue to

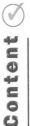

✓ Review

Events of Vehicle Collision

Vehicle collision
Body collision
Organ collision
Secondary collisions
Additional impacts

Secondary collisions may increase the severity of a patient's initial injuries or create new ones.

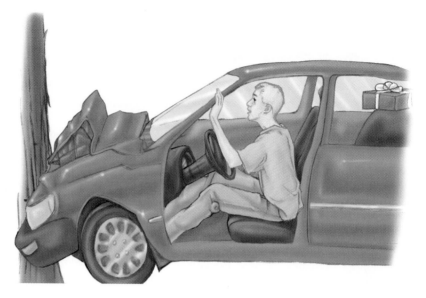

a. Vehicle collision

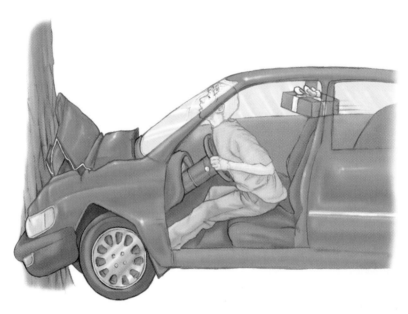

b. Body collision

travel at the auto's initial speed. They then impact an occupant who has come to rest within the auto. It is important to consider the possibility of any secondary collisions and their effects on occupants when developing an index of suspicion for injuries.

Additional impacts occur when a vehicle receives a second impact—for example, when it hits a vehicle, is deflected, then hits a parked car. This second impact may induce additional patient injuries or increase the seriousness of those already received. Consider someone who sustains a femur fracture. It takes a great deal of energy to break the bone initially. Once the bone is broken, however, the energy now needed to move those bone ends around and cause further, possibly more severe, injury to nerves and blood vessels is small. It is important to consider what effect any additional impacts may have on the initial injuries and overall patient condition.

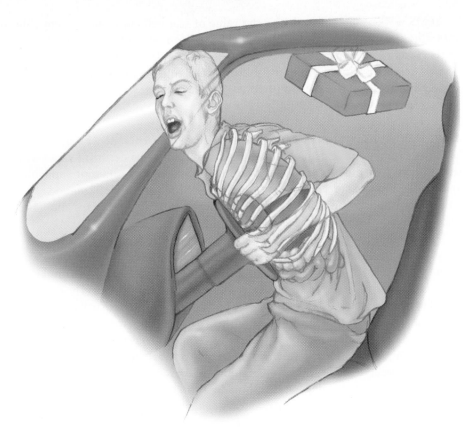

c. Organ collision

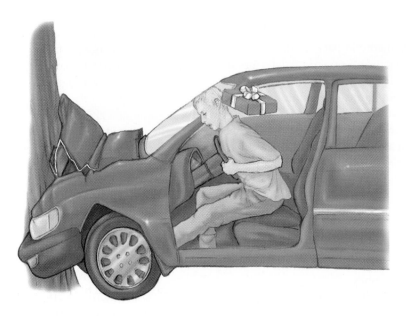

d. Secondary collision

Restraints

Restraints such as seat belts, shoulder straps, air bags, and child safety seats have a profound effect on the injuries associated with auto collisions. They have played a substantial role in reducing collision-related deaths from about 55,000 a year in the early 1970s to about 44,000 in recent years. It is important that you determine if restraints were used—and used properly—as you anticipate the possible results of an auto collision.

Restraints have had a profound effect in reducing collision-related deaths.

EMS workers should recognize the value of seat belts in reducing auto collision mortality and morbidity. Hence, all ambulance personnel must employ seat belts when in the patient care area of the vehicle and especially while driving. Securing the lap belt firmly provides positive positioning so drivers and other crew members are not as adversely affected by the gravitational-equivalent forces (G forces) sometimes associated with emergency driving.

Seat Belts   Use of seat belts and shoulder straps prevents the wearer's continuing and independent movement during a vehicle collision. The occupant slows with the auto rather than moving rapidly forward and impacting the interior suddenly. The occupant's ultimate deceleration rate is thus reduced, lessening the likelihood of serious injury from collisions within the vehicle. Seat belts and shoulder straps also lessen the chances that the wearer will be ejected from the vehicle.

Although seat belts and shoulder straps significantly reduce injury severity, they may cause some, usually much less serious, injuries. A lap belt worn alone does not restrain the torso, neck, or head from continuing forward. These body regions may impact the dash or steering wheel, resulting in chest, neck, and head injuries. The sudden folding of the body at the waist during extreme impacts when only a lap belt is worn may result in intra-abdominal or lower spine injuries. If the lap belt is worn alone and too high, abdominal compression and spinal (T12 to L2) fractures may result. If worn too low, it may cause hip dislocations. If the shoulder strap is worn alone, it may cause severe neck contusions, lacerations, possible spinal injury, and even decapitation in more violent collisions. In very strong impacts, the shoulder strap may induce chest contusions and, in some cases, rib fractures. Further, the seat belt and/or shoulder strap do not protect against intrusions into the passenger compartment. In severe collisions, the dashboard may displace into the front seat, trapping or crushing the lower extremities of occupants.

Air Bags   Air bags, also called supplemental restraint systems (SRS), work much differently than seat belts and are extremely effective for frontal collisions. They inflate explosively on auto impact, producing a cushion to absorb the energy exchange. Their ignition is dependent on several detectors sensing a very strong frontal deceleration, as can only occur with serious vehicle impact. Only after these detectors all agree does the explosive agent ignite. The ignition instantaneously fills the bag, slightly before or just as the occupant collides with it. The explosive gases escape quickly as the occupant compresses the bag, cushioning the impact much as the inflated bags used by pole-vaulters and movie stuntmen do. Like seat belts, air bags are credited with dramatically reducing vehicular death and trauma (Figure 2-5 ■).

Air bags are positioned in the steering wheel, and their presence is indicated by an "SRS" (supplemental restraint system) insignia on the windshield and/or on the steering wheel itself. They may also be located in the dash for the front seat passenger. Many cars are now equipped with side air bags and air curtains, which deploy with lateral collisions and rollovers. Steering wheel and dash-mounted air bags offer significant protection only in frontal impact collisions. This protection is only for the first impact and not subsequent ones.

Air bags may induce injury during their ignition and rapid inflation. As the bag inflates, especially from the steering wheel, it may impact the driver's fingers, hands, and forearms, possibly causing dislocations and fractures. In persons of small stature seated very close to the steering wheel, air bag inflation may also cause nasal fractures, minor facial lacerations, and contusions. The residue from air bag inflation may cause some irritation of the eyes; this can be relieved with gentle irrigation. Whenever an air bag has deployed, check beneath it for steering wheel deformity, which is indicative of possible injury to the driver.

Passenger air bags have inflated in minor impacts and pushed infant and child safety seats into seats with tremendous force. In some cases, infants and children have

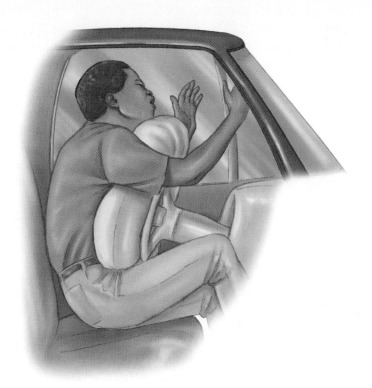

been severely injured or killed by inflation of the bags. For this reason, it is recommended that parents secure child carriers in the back seat when a passenger air bag system is in place.

Auto manufacturers are starting to install air bags in the seat sides, adjacent to the doors in some cars, for protection in lateral impact collisions. Some manufacturers also install air bags in the headliners above doors to provide protection for the head in such collisions. Because little experience is available for these types of restraints, their benefits and potential drawbacks are not well known. However, lateral impacts do account for a very high mortality rate that may be mediated with lateral-impact and head-protection air bags. Undeployed air bags and curtains may present a hazard at the auto crash scene and may cause serious injury to rescuers or to the patient if they unexpectedly inflate. Fire, rescue, and extrication personnel should be trained in air bag deactivation and should deactivate any undeployed devices at the crash scene.

Child Safety Seats The anatomy of children makes their protection in vehicle collisions difficult. Because a child's size changes so quickly with increasing age, normal restraint systems are designed for adults only. Small children should be placed in appropriate child safety seats to assure their relative safety during an auto impact. With infants and very small children, the child safety seat is positioned facing to the rear and held firmly to the seat with the seat belt. This positioning best distributes frontal impact forces and prevents unrestrained infant movement. As the child grows in size, the child carrier is turned facing forward and used as a small seat. The seat belt then crosses the child at the waistline.

Properly used child safety seats provide the best protection for infants and small children riding in vehicles.

Children held in an adult's lap or arms are not well protected during a collision. The holder may grasp them too tightly during impact or, more likely, will not (or cannot) hold on tightly enough. If the child is not held, he becomes an unrestrained moving object and will impact the vehicle interior suffering serious, possibly fatal, injury.

When evaluating the results of an auto impact, always be sure to examine for and ask questions about the use of restraints. Determine if seat belts and shoulder straps

■ Figure 2-6 Incidence of
motor vehicle impacts.

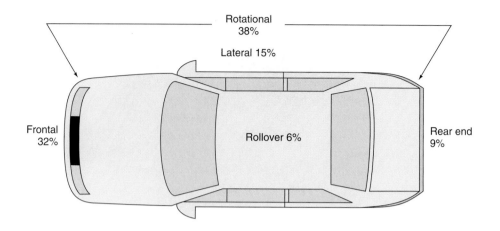

■ Review

**Types of Vehicle
Impact**

Rotational
Frontal
Lateral
Rear-end
Rollover

Frontal impact is one of the
most common types of
vehicle collision.

■ Review

**Mechanisms
Associated with
Frontal Impacts**

Up-and-over pathway
Down-and-under pathway
Ejection

The up-and-over pathway
accounts for over half of the
deaths in vehicular collisions.

were used and used properly, if air bags deployed during the collision, and if child carriers were properly positioned and secured. If these restraints were properly employed,
the severity of injuries to the vehicle occupants will very likely be reduced.

Types of Impact

As you have read, there are five general types of auto impacts. They are listed below with
frequency percentages in parentheses (illustrated in Figure 2-6 ■).

- ★ Rotational (38 percent)
- ★ Frontal (32 percent)
- ★ Lateral (15 percent)
- ★ Rear-end (9 percent)
- ★ Rollover (6 percent)

The listed percentages reflect an urban setting. In a more rural area, anticipate a greater
percentage of frontal impacts with corresponding reductions in other categories. Note
that rotational impact includes four subcategories: left front, right front, left rear, and
right rear.

Frontal Impact Frontal impact is one of the most common types of impact (Figure
2-7 ■) and produces three pathways of patient travel. They are:

1. *Up-and-Over Pathway.* In the up-and-over pathway, the unrestrained
   occupant tenses the legs in preparation for impact (Figure 2-8 ■). With
   vehicle slowing, the unrestrained body's upper half pivots forward and
   upward. The steering wheel impinges the femurs, causing possible
   bilateral fractures. In addition, it compresses and decelerates the
   abdominal contents, causing hollow-organ rupture and liver laceration.
   Traumatic compression may also force abdominal contents against the
   diaphragm, causing it to rupture and allowing organs to enter the thoracic
   cavity. As the body continues forward, the lower chest impacts the steering
   wheel and may account for the same thoracic injuries seen with the down-
   and-under pathway.

   The same forward motion propels the head into the windshield,
   leading to soft-tissue injury, skull or facial fractures, and internal head
   injury. Neck injury may result from hyperextension, hyperflexion, or the
   compressional forces of windshield impact. As the body is thrown upward
   and forward, the head contacts the windshield. The rest of the body tries
   to push the head through the windshield. The result is a compressional

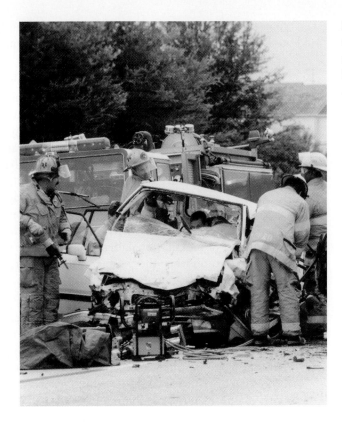

■ Figure 2-7 Frontal impact often results in a significant exchange of energy and serious injuries. (© *Craig Jackson/In the Dark Photography*)

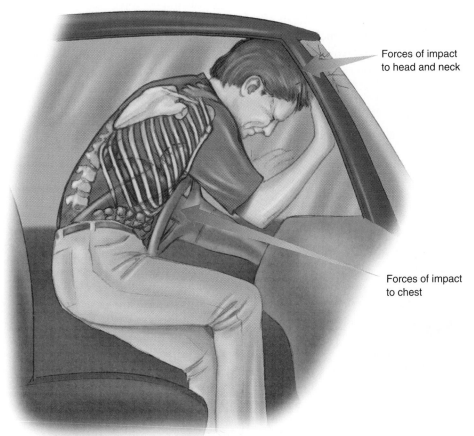

Forces of impact to head and neck

Forces of impact to chest

■ Figure 2-8 The up-and-over pathway is associated with frontal impact collisions.

force on the cervical spine called **axial loading.** This loading may result in collapse of support elements of the vertebral column. Over half of vehicular deaths are attributed to the up-and-over pathway.

2. *Down-and-Under Pathway.* In the down-and-under pathway, the unrestrained occupant slides downward as the vehicle comes to a stop. The knees contact the fire wall, under the dash, and absorb the initial impact. Knee, femur, and hip dislocations or fractures are common. Once the lower body slows, the upper body rotates forward, pivoting at the hip, and crashing against the steering wheel or dash. Chest injuries like flail chest, myocardial contusion, and aortic tears result. If the neck contacts the steering wheel, tracheal and vascular injury may occur. An injury process frequently associated with steering wheel impact is the "paper bag" syndrome (Figure 2-9 ■). The driver takes a deep breath in anticipation of the collision. Lung tissue (alveoli, bronchioles, and larger airways) ruptures when the chest impacts the steering wheel, much like an inflated paper bag caught between clapping hands. Pneumothorax and pulmonary contusion may result.

3. *Ejection.* The up-and-over pathway may lead to ejection of an unrestrained occupant. Such a victim experiences two impacts: (1) contact with the vehicle interior and windshield and (2) impact with the ground, tree, or other object. This mechanism of injury is responsible for about 27 percent of vehicular fatalities. While ejection may occur with other types of impact, it is most commonly associated with frontal impact.

Recognize that a frontal impact collision interposes more vehicle between the point of impact and the vehicle occupants. Modern vehicle design techniques use this area of the vehicle (called the **crumple zone**) to absorb the impact forces and limit occupant injury (Figure 2-10 ■). Patients in vehicle collisions such as those involving vans and lateral impacts do not benefit from these energy-absorbing crumple zones. In these circumstances, the apparent vehicle damage may be less than in a frontal impact collision, even though the forces delivered to the occupants are greater.

Lateral Impact   The kinetics of lateral impact are the same as for frontal impact with two exceptions. First, occupants present a different profile (turned 90 degrees) to collision forces. Second, the amount of structural steel between the impact site and the

crumple zone *the region of a vehicle designed to absorb the energy of impact.*

⚷

Occupants of a vehicle with a limited crumple zone may experience greater forces in a collision even though damage to the vehicle itself may not appear as severe as damage to a vehicle with a greater crumple zone involved in a similar collision.

■ Figure 2-9   The "paper bag" syndrome results from compression of the chest against the steering column.

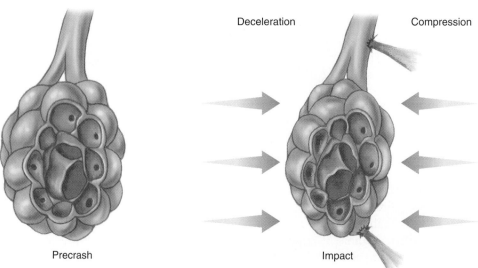

Deceleration   Compression

Precrash   Impact

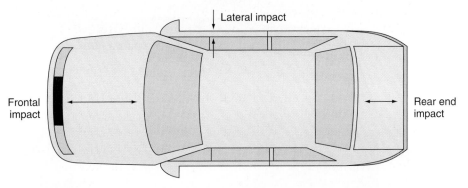

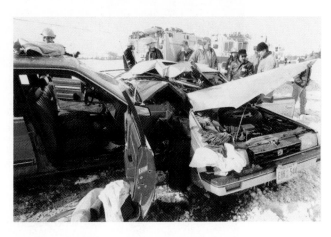

■ Figure 2-11 A lateral impact collision presents the least amount of crumple zone between the vehicle's exterior and its passenger compartment. (© *Craig Jackson/In the Dark Photography*)

vehicle interior is greatly reduced (Figure 2-11 ■). Lateral impacts account for 15 percent of all auto collisions, yet they are responsible for 22 percent of vehicular fatalities. When a lateral impact occurs, the index of suspicion for serious and life-threatening internal injuries must be higher than vehicle damage alone suggests.

With lateral impacts, there is an increase in upper extremity injuries (Figure 2-12 ■). The ribs fracture laterally on the side of impact instead of anteriorly. The clavicle, humerus, pelvis, and femur may fracture on the impact side. Cervical spine injury occurs as the body moves laterally while the head remains stationary. Vertebrae may fracture with the rapid lateral motion as may the skull as it smashes into the window. Lateral compression, affecting the body cavity, may give rise to diaphragm rupture, pulmonary contusion, splenic injury (to the driver), and much more. Aortic aneurysm may occur with this injury mechanism. The heart, which is not firmly attached in the central thorax, moves violently toward the impact as the body accelerates. This twists the aorta, tearing its inner layer, the intima. Blood seeps between the connective tissue layers and the vessel begins to delaminate. The aorta may rupture immediately or over the next few hours.

Evaluation of lateral impact collisions should take into consideration any unrestrained passenger opposite the impact site. If the driver's side is struck and such a passenger is not belted, the passenger becomes an object that will strike and injure the driver shortly after initial impact.

Rotational Impact In rotational impact, the auto is struck at an **oblique** angle and rotates as the collision forces are expended (Figure 2-13 ■). The ensuing rotation causes injuries similar to those from frontal and lateral impacts. Acceleration (or deceleration) is greatest farther from the center of the auto and closest to impact. Autos involved are deflected from their paths rather than being stopped abruptly. While rotational impact injuries can be serious, they are often less than vehicle damage might suggest. With the

⌐●─────────

Maintain a higher index of suspicion of serious injury when assessing lateral impact collisions because the degree of injury may be greater than the damage alone would indicate.

oblique *having a slanted position or direction.*

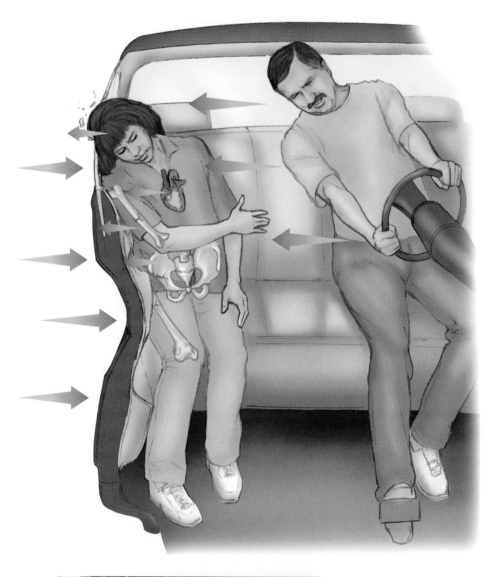

■ Figure 2-12 In a lateral impact collision, an occupant may experience lateral impact to the head, lateral bending of the neck, twisting of the heart and the aorta, and fractures of the humerus, clavicle, pelvis, and femur.

■ Figure 2-13 In rotational impacts, the energy exchange is more gradual and there may be less injury than vehicle damage suggests. There may, however, be multiple impacts. (© *Mark C. Ide*)

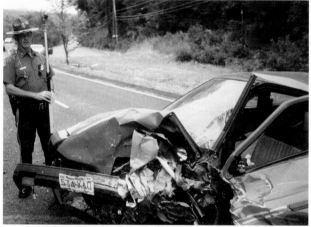

deflection of the impact, the occupant's stopping distance is much greater, deceleration is more gradual, and injuries are generally less serious.

Rear-End Impact In rear-end impact, the collision force pushes the auto forward (Figure 2-14 ■). Within the vehicle, the seat propels the occupant forward. If the

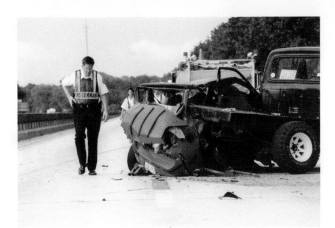

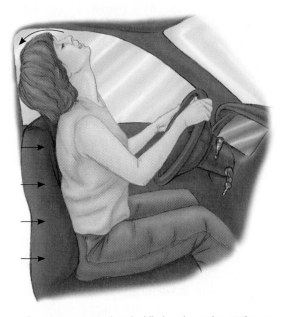

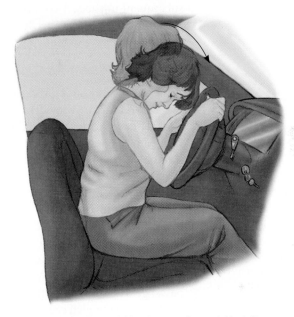

a. Occupant moves ahead while head remains stationary. Head rotates backward. Neck extends.

b. Head snaps forward. Head rotates forward. Neck flexes.

■ Figure 2-15 A rear-end collision affects the occupant of a vehicle.

headrest is not up, the head is unsupported and remains stationary. The neck extends severely, stretching the neck muscles and ligaments while the head rotates backward. Once acceleration ceases, the head snaps forward and the neck flexes. This rapid and extreme hyperextension followed by hyperflexion may result in severe connective tissue and cervical vertebra injuries (Figure 2-15 ■). There is also risk of injury when the auto finally ends its acceleration and an unrestrained occupant is thrown forward. However, rear-impact collisions usually result in limited injuries, especially if the headrest is positioned properly.

Rollover Auto rollover is normally caused by a change in elevation and/or a vehicle with a high center of gravity (Figure 2-16 ■). As the vehicle rolls, it impacts the ground at various points. The occupant experiences an impact with each impact of the vehicle. These impacts can be especially violent due to the absence of crumple zones and internal padding at the multiple points of impact (vehicle sides and roof). The type of injuries expected with a rollover relate to the specific vehicle impacts involved. Remember, any injury occurring with the first collision is likely to be compounded with

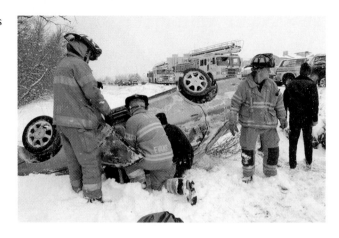

subsequent impacts. A common result of rollover is ejection or partial ejection with a limb or head trapped between the rolling vehicle and the ground. Restraints are especially effective in reducing ejection and injury during rollover.

Vehicle Collision Analysis

Vehicle collisions often produce hazards not only to the vehicle occupants but also to bystanders and care providers. Be alert for these hazards during the scene size-up. Such hazards may include hot engine and transmission parts, hot fluids such as radiator coolant or engine oil, caustic substances such as battery acid and automatic transmission or steering fluids, and the sharp, jagged edges of torn metal or broken glass. Also remain aware of the potential for danger from traffic moving near the crash site or from electrical power lines that may have been downed by the collision.

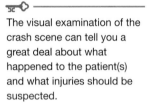

The visual examination of the crash scene can tell you a great deal about what happened to the patient(s) and what injuries should be suspected.

During the scene size-up, evaluate the vehicle to determine the direction of impact and the amount of vehicle damage. From the angle of impact, visualize the direction of forces expressed on the collision patients and the strength of those forces. Realize that the front and rear structures of the modern cars are designed to crumple during impact to absorb kinetic forces. While moderate-speed impacts may destroy the vehicle, the passengers may escape with little injury. Occupants in lateral and rollover impacts do not benefit from such crumple zones and frequently suffer injuries more directly related to the kinetic forces.

As you evaluate the collision, consider the relative sizes of the impacting vehicles or objects. A large, heavy vehicle impacting a smaller, lighter one will experience lesser acceleration or deceleration forces than the smaller vehicle. In this case, there is likely to be more severe vehicle damage to the smaller vehicle and more serious injuries to its occupants as well. Similar considerations apply with objects impacted by vehicles. For example, a large, well-rooted tree that does not move will cause much more damage during an impact than will a telephone pole that shears off.

When evaluation of the outside of the vehicle is complete, look at the passenger compartment (Figure 2-17 ■). Determine if there is any intrusion, which indicates the presence of forces greater than those that could be absorbed by the crumple zones. Quickly look for signs of occupant/interior impacts. A spider-webbed windshield suggests a severe impact between the occupant's head and the glass. A deformed steering wheel suggests injury to the driver's chest or upper abdomen. A dented dash suggests injury to the knees or injuries transmitted to the femur or hip. Deformities of the gas, brake, or clutch pedals suggest foot injury. Deployed and deflated air bags may indicate chest, forearm, or hand injury.

In very severe impacts, collision forces may push the dashboard and firewall into the passenger compartment, entrapping and crushing the lower extremities of occupants against the seat. In such cases, parts of the vehicle, such as foot pedals, turn indi-

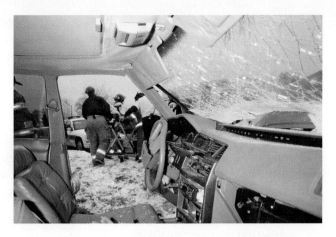

■ Figure 2-17 Study the interior of a crashed vehicle carefully to identify the strength and direction of forces expressed to the patient. (© *Jeff Forster*)

cator arms, shift levers, and instrument panel knobs or switches, may be physically imbedded in collision patients. This complicates extrication because the seat and the dash must be separated carefully to free the trapped occupant. In these cases, the area should be carefully examined before and while any extrication equipment is used. Ongoing examinations should be provided frequently during extrication in order to ensure that the process does not result in further, unnecessary harm to the patient.

Assess whether restraints have been used or air bags deployed. Use of these devices may limit the severity of injuries in frontal impacts. Conversely, their non-use may suggest more severe injuries. Check the positions of headrests in rear-impact collisions. Their proper positioning may limit neck hyperextension and injury.

Intoxication Whenever you evaluate motor vehicle trauma, consider the possibility of alcohol intoxication. Statistics from states requiring mandatory alcohol-level testing after fatal auto collisions reveal that more than 50 percent of the drivers were legally intoxicated. Alcohol use also contributes to many off-road-vehicle collisions, boating collisions, and accidental drownings.

Whenever you suspect alcohol intoxication, your assessment must be more diligent. Remember, alcohol interferes with the patient's level of consciousness and masks signs and symptoms of injury. Intoxication may be hard to differentiate from the signs of head injury. It also anesthetizes the patient somewhat to trauma pain. These factors make the mechanism of injury analysis and the resultant index of suspicion even more important. Otherwise, significant injuries may be overlooked or assumed to be symptoms of alcohol intoxication.

Alcohol intoxication is associated with most serious crashes.

Vehicular Mortality Examination of the effects of motor vehicle trauma on the human anatomy reveals certain areas to be especially prone to life-threatening injury. A study of the incidence of mortality and the associated location of trauma provides the findings in Table 2–1.

Table 2–1	Motor Vehicle Fatalities
Incidence by Body Area	
Head	47.7%
Internal (chest/abdominal/pelvic)	37.3%
Spinal and chest fracture	8.3%
Fractures to the extremities	2.0%
All other	4.7%

Head and body cavity trauma account for 85 percent of deaths in vehicular collisions.

Trauma to the head and body cavity accounts for 85 percent of vehicular mortality. For this reason, the rapid trauma assessment should be directed at the head, neck, thorax, abdomen, and pelvis. Once you secure the airway, breathing, and circulation, proceed to the rapid trauma assessment, looking at areas where your index of suspicion suggests injury. Examine the head, chest, and abdomen first to identify any evidence of life-threatening injuries.

Collision Evaluation   As a paramedic, you must be thoroughly practiced in the assessment of trauma patients, especially because of the high incidence of serious injury associated with auto collisions. Whenever you respond to a collision, analyze the five types of collisions associated with vehicle impact. In each case, ask yourself these questions:

★ How did the objects collide?

★ From what direction did they come?

★ At what speed were they traveling?

★ Were the objects similarly sized or grossly different? (For example, did a car and a semi-truck collide?)

★ Were any secondary collisions or additional transfers of energy involved?

In analyzing the mechanisms of injury, also consider the cause of the collision.

★ Did wet pavement or poor visibility contribute to the collision?

★ Was alcohol involved?

★ Is there an absence of skid marks? If so, what happened to the driver to prevent him from braking?

Examine the auto interior, which is the mass struck by the moving occupant.

★ Does the windshield show evidence of impact by the victim's head?
  –Is it bloody or broken in the characteristic spider web or star shape?
  –Has it been penetrated by the patient's head or body?

★ Is the steering wheel deformed or collapsed?

★ Is the dash indented where the knees or head hit it?

★ Has the impact damage extended into the passenger compartment (intrusion)?

Answers to such questions complement your mechanism of injury analysis and help you to develop accurate indices of suspicion.

MOTORCYCLE COLLISIONS

Serious trauma is likely with even low-speed motorcycle crashes because of the lack of protective vehicle structure.

In addition to auto collisions, as a paramedic you will respond to many motorcycle collisions. Because of the lack of protective vehicle structure, motorcycle collisions often result in serious trauma, even at lower speeds. The rider, rather than the structural steel, absorbs much of the crash energy (Figure 2-18 ■). Injuries can be severe, with an especially high incidence of head trauma. The motorcycle collision impacts differ somewhat from those of an auto collision. The four types of motorcycle impacts include the following: frontal, angular, sliding, and ejection.

Frontal   In a frontal, or head-on, impact the front of the bike dips downward, propelling the rider upward and forward. The handlebars catch the rider's lower abdomen

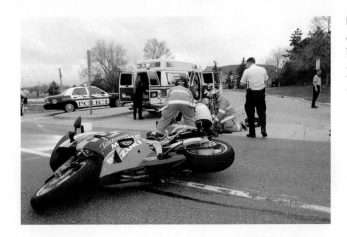

or pelvis, causing abdominal and/or pelvic injury. Occasionally, the rider travels through a higher trajectory. In such cases, the handlebars can trap the femurs, often resulting in bilateral fractures.

Angular An angular impact occurs when the bike strikes an object at an oblique angle. The rider's lower extremity is trapped between the object struck and the bike. This may fracture or crush the foot, ankle, knee, and femur. Open wounds often result.

Sliding Sliding impact occurs when an experienced rider, facing an imminent collision, "lays the bike down." The rider slides the bike sideways into the object, so that the bike hits the object first, absorbing much of the energy. Laying the bike down also reduces the chances of ejection. The result is an increase in lacerations, abrasions, and minor fractures, with a decrease in more serious injuries.

Ejection Ejection is common and usually results in serious injury. It may occur with any of the mechanisms previously described and result in the following impacts:

★ Initial bike/object collision

★ Rider/object impact

★ Rider/ground impact

Likely injuries include skull fracture and/or head injury, spinal fractures and paralysis, internal thoracic or abdominal injury, and extremity fractures.

In assessing a motorcycle crash, remember that protective equipment affects injury patterns. A helmet can reduce the incidence and severity of head injury by about 50 percent. Use of a helmet, however, neither increases nor decreases the incidence of spinal trauma. Leather clothing and boots protect the rider against open soft-tissue injury, but they can also hide underlying contusions and fractures.

Helmets reduce the incidence and severity of head injuries in motorcycle crashes, but they have no effect on the incidence of spinal trauma.

PEDESTRIAN COLLISIONS

Some vehicular collisions involve pedestrians, who are often severely injured because of the mass and speed of the object hitting them and because of their lack of protection. Adults and children suffer different types of injuries because of differing anatomical size and differing responses to the impending collision. Recognition of these differences helps you anticipate injuries and provide the necessary treatment.

Adult pedestrians generally turn away from oncoming vehicles and present a lateral surface to impact. Anatomically, impact is low. The bumper strikes the lower leg first, fracturing the tibia and fibula. Energy transmitted to the opposing knee can lead

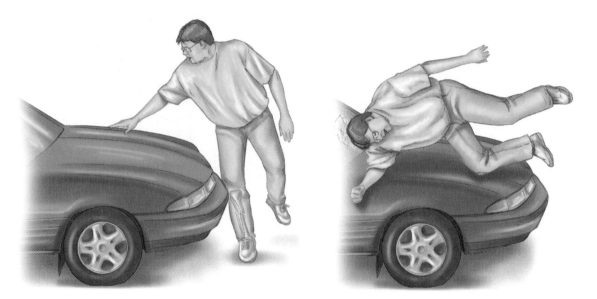

■ Figure 2-19   An adult frequently turns away from a collision with an automobile and thus impacts the vehicle first with a leg. Because of a higher center of gravity, such patients are often thrown onto the hood and into the windshield.

to ligament injury. As the lower extremities are propelled forward with the car, the upper and lateral body crashes into the hood causing femur, lateral chest, or upper extremity fractures. The victim then slides into the windshield, leading to head, neck, and shoulder trauma. The adult may be further injured when thrown to the ground. This secondary collision may cause additional injury or compound those already received (Figure 2-19 ■).

In contrast to adults, children usually turn toward an oncoming vehicle. Because of their smaller anatomy, injuries are located higher on children's bodies. The bumper impacts the femurs or pelvis, causing fracture. Children are frequently thrown in front of the vehicle because of their smaller size and lower center of gravity. They may then be run over or pushed to the side by the vehicle. If a child is thrown upward, injuries are similar to those of an adult (Figure 2-20 ■).

When evaluating the injuries associated with auto-vs.-pedestrian collisions, look carefully at the scene. Try to determine the speed of the vehicle at the time of impact and the distance the pedestrian was thrown. This information may be useful to the emergency department personnel in their determination of suspected injuries.

In pedestrian-vs.-automobile collisions, adults tend to turn away from the oncoming vehicle before impact, while children turn toward it.

■ Figure 2-20   In collisions with autos, children often turn toward the impact and, because of their lower body heights, are frequently thrown in front of the vehicle.

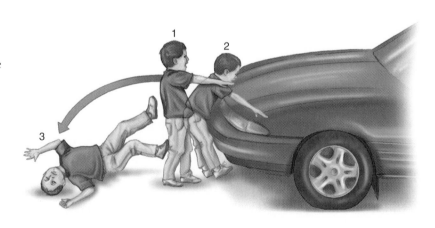

RECREATIONAL VEHICLE COLLISIONS

Over the past years, recreational vehicle usage has increased, and with it, the incidence of related trauma. Recreational vehicle collisions often cause injuries similar to those associated with auto collisions. Drivers and passengers of recreational vehicles, however, do not have the structural protections and restraint systems found in autos. Complicating injuries is the fact that recreational vehicles travel off road, which means there is often difficulty in reaching and retrieving victims once collisions are detected. The major types of vehicles most often involved in recreational vehicle collisions are snowmobiles, personal watercraft, and all-terrain vehicles (ATVs).

Snowmobile collisions can be very violent because the speeds at which snowmobiles travel can approach those of cars. In addition, snowmobiles offer very limited crumple zones for impact absorption. These collisions commonly result in ejections, crush injuries secondary to rollover, and glancing blows against obstructions in the snow. Riders also experience severe head and neck injuries from collisions with other vehicles, including autos, other snowmobiles, or with stationary objects such as trees. Snowmobile trauma may include severe neck injury when the rider runs into an unseen wire fence. The anterior neck is deeply lacerated, causing airway compromise, severe bleeding, and, in some cases, complete decapitation. Injuries to snowmobilers may be compounded by the effects of cold exposure and hypothermia.

Watercraft crashes commonly result from impact with other boats or obstructions, submerged or otherwise (Figure 2-21 ■). These vehicles are not designed to absorb the energy of impacts nor are the occupants provided with restraint systems. As a result, watercraft crashes can cause serious injuries, even though the speeds of typical watercraft are substantially lower than those of autos. Trauma in these crashes is further complicated by the potential for drowning if the occupants are thrown into the water or the boat sinks. In northern areas, water temperatures can also rapidly induce hypothermia. Alcohol is frequently associated with watercraft crashes.

The use of personal watercraft, commonly called jet skis, for water recreation has increased greatly in recent years, as has the incidence of watercraft accidents. Jet skis are especially dangerous in the hands of inexperienced riders. The high speeds attained by these watercraft contribute to the incidence and severity of injury associated with crashes. Although the craft's propulsion unit is protected and unlikely to cause trauma, collision with other watercraft, as well as objects and people in the water, lead to blunt trauma, again complicated by the potential for drowning.

The ATV (Figure 2-22 ■) accounts for many serious recreational injuries. Its driver may be young and not required to prove his driving skills or to maintain a license. The vehicle by its very nature travels off road at relatively high speeds and over rough and rugged terrain. The ATV's center of gravity is relatively high, contributing to the likelihood of rollover during quick turns. As with snowmobiles, a significant incidence of

⚷—

Recreational vehicles usually lack the structure and the restraint systems that offer significant protection to automobile drivers and passengers.

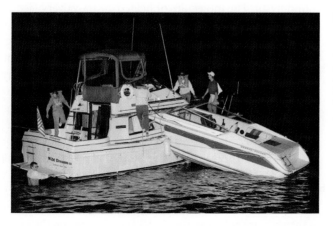

■ Figure 2-21 Watercraft crashes are common, may involve either objects on the surface or submerged, and present the risks of drowning or hypothermia. (© *Craig Jackson/ In the Dark Photography*)

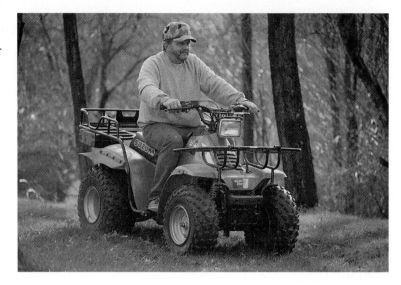

■ Figure 2-22 All-terrain vehicles (ATVs) can cause a multitude of injuries due to their speed and instability and lack of rider protection.

frontal collision is common with both types of ATVs. The injuries expected might include upper and lower extremity fracture and head and spine injury.

BLAST INJURIES

oxidizer *an agent that enhances combustion of a fuel.*

Explosions can be caused by dust, as in a grain elevator; by fumes, such as gasoline or natural gas; or by explosive compounds (combustible and **oxidizer** mixes), such as dynamite, gun powder, and TNT. The explosion may be the result of an accident or intentional act of terrorism or warfare. The blast magnitude may range from that of a small firecracker in the hands of a teenager to a nuclear detonation.

Explosion

An explosion occurs when an agent or environment combusts. During a conventional (non-nuclear) explosion, the fuel and oxidizing agent combine instantaneously. Chemical bonds are broken down and reestablished, releasing tremendous energy in the form of rapidly moving molecules, known to us as heat. This heat creates a great pressure differential between the exploding agent and the surrounding air. This heat and the pressure differential produce several mechanisms of injury including a pressure wave, blast wind, projectiles, heat, and displacement of persons near the blast (Figure 2-23 ■).

pressure wave *area of overpressure that radiates outward from an explosion.*

overpressure *a rapid increase, then decrease, in atmospheric pressure created by an explosion.*

Pressure Wave

As the combustible agent ignites and burns explosively, it immediately heats the surrounding air. The molecules of heated air move very fast, increasing the pressure of the exploding cloud. The rapid increase in pressure compresses adjacent air. Adjacent air, in turn, pushes against air farther out from the point of ignition, and a **pressure wave** begins to move away from the blast epicenter. This is not a gross air movement but rather a narrow compression wave moving rapidly outward, similar to a wave through water (where the wave and not the water moves). This narrow wave, called **overpressure,** results in a drastic but brief increase, then decrease, in air pressure as it passes. The blast overpressure wave moves outward slightly faster than the speed of sound through the air or water, and its strength decreases quickly.

When the explosion involves a dust, aerosol, or gas cloud, the result is an area, not a single point, of detonation. The exploding cloud's pressure is extremely lethal, and the area it involves can be extensive. A bomb's casing or confined spaces, such as a building interior, contain the pressure of an explosion until the structure ruptures. The ensuing rapid release of the pressure enhances the peak overpressure and the potential for injury and death.

 Review

Mechanisms Associated with Blasts

Pressure wave
Blast wind
Projectiles
Personnel displacement
Confined spaces and structural collapses
Burns

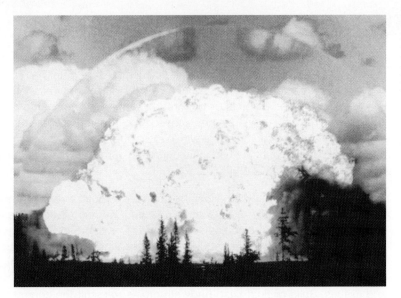

■ Figure 2-23 An explosion releases tremendous amounts of heat energy, generating a pressure wave, blast wind, and projection of debris.

Underwater detonation also greatly enhances the potential for injury and death associated with the pressure wave. Water is a noncompressible medium that transmits the overpressure efficiently. Any submerged portion of the victim is subject to the rapid compression and then decompression. The lethal range for an explosive charge increases threefold with an underwater detonation.

Upon striking the body, the overpressure wave instantly compresses, then decompresses, the body's air-filled spaces, causing trauma. This rapid compression/decompression may produce injury to the middle ear, sinuses, bowel, or lungs. Because overpressure intensity diminishes rapidly as the wave travels outward, most life-threatening compression injuries are usually limited to people in proximity to the detonation, with the exceptions of gas-cloud ignitions and underwater detonations.

A victim's orientation to the blast wave is also an important factor in the production of injuries. The greater the surface a victim presents to the blast wave, the greater the impact and damage. People standing and facing directly toward or away from the blast experience the greatest pressure effect. People lying on the ground, with their heads away from or toward the blast, experience the least pressure effects. In water, the same is true, although the more deeply submerged a victim is, the greater the damaging effects of the overpressure.

> Underwater detonation increases the lethal range of an explosion threefold.

Blast Wind

Following the pressure wave and traveling just behind it is the **blast wind.** This is the actual outward movement of heated and expanding combustion gases from the explosion epicenter. The blast wind has less strength but greater duration than the pressure wave. It causes much less direct injury, although in powerful blasts it may propel debris or displace victims, which will, in turn, produce injuries.

blast wind *the air movement caused as the heated and pressurized products of an explosion move outward.*

Projectiles

If the exploding material is contained by a casing, as with military **ordnance** or a pipe bomb, or by a structure, as with a garage filled with gas fumes, the container holds the explosive force until the container breaks apart. The parts of the container then become high-speed projectiles, behaving much like bullets and bound by the same laws of physics. Although they are not as fast as bullets and they lack good aerodynamic properties, they can cause serious injury beyond the injury zone of the blast's pressure wave itself. Some military ordnance contains special arrow-shaped missiles called **flechettes.** Their design gives the flechettes a greater following surface and aligns the missiles in flight, reducing their wind resistance and increasing their range and penetrating ability.

ordnance *military weapons and munitions.*

flechettes *arrow-shaped projectiles found in some military ordnance.*

Anatomy of an Explosion Natural gas from a ruptured pipe gathers in a basement until the explosive gas-air mixture reaches the hot-water heater's pilot light. The gas-air cloud immediately ignites, and the resulting flame instantaneously heats the air in several rooms of the house by hundreds of degrees. The heated air contains molecules, which are now moving at great speed. The collision of these molecules with others greatly increases the pressure within the cloud. Contained by walls and windows, the pressure builds until the windows burst and some of the walls collapse.

The Pressure Wave

As the windows collapse and allow the pressure to push outward, the rapidly moving molecules contact those of adjacent air, setting them in motion. These molecules in turn contact adjacent molecules and a wave of pressure moves outward at a speed just slightly faster than that of sound. The presenting surface of a person standing in the path of this wave is impacted and compressed, then decompressed. This wave of compression/decompression progresses through the person's body, affecting organs and tissues. Solid or fluid-filled body structures transmit the energy without damage while air-filled structures are compressed and then decompressed violently. The lungs, auditory canals, sinuses, and bowel sustain the most significant injury. Other victims within the structure and caught by the blast experience the same compression/decompression wave and associated injuries.

Burns

People caught within the confines of the blast are affected by the explosion's great heat. Because the heat energy is released very rapidly and because people's bodies are predominantly water, primary burn injuries are generally superficial. The blast heat often produces secondary combustion of materials such as clothing and blast debris. These ignited materials can produce burns ranging from superficial to full thickness in victims.

Projectiles

Breaking glass and parts of the collapsing walls are propelled outward with the release of the blast energy. These materials travel at great speed and contain great kinetic energy. As a result, these projectiles may penetrate and impale themselves in victims in their path. Unless such projectiles are heavy, they do not generally penetrate deeply.

Personnel Displacement

As the explosive gases move outward from the building, they create a blast of wind that moves more slowly than the pressure wave. The blast wind and the pressure wave push victims outward from the blast center, turning them into projectiles. The victims then impact other surfaces, objects, or debris and sustain further injuries.

Structural Collapse

As the explosion tears apart the walls of the structure, the debris and the building above collapse on victims within. Trapped by debris, the victims sustain severe crush injuries. The entrapment and crushing damage tissues and blood vessels and may restrict or stop circulation to a limb. The reduced blood flow results in the build up of toxic by-products of metabolism. When victims are released from entrapment and circulation is restored, hemorrhage from numerous damaged blood vessels and the entry of toxins into the central circulation results.

The conventional explosive used by a terrorist may also contain nails, screws, or other materials to enhance the weapon's effective range and potential for causing injury.

If the person is very close to a strong blast, the casing and debris may move forcefully enough to tear off limbs or cause serious open wounds. The blast debris—glass fragments, building materials, or casing elements—may also impale itself in the skin and soft tissue. While the wounds caused by blast debris are normally small, large and heavy fragments may penetrate deeply into personnel and cause serious tissue damage and hemorrhage.

Personnel Displacement

The pressure wave and blast wind may be strong enough to physically propel personnel away from the center of the blast. Those personnel then become projectiles and impact the ground, objects, debris, or other personnel, resulting in blunt or, in some cases, penetrating trauma. While the effects of this mechanism of injury are limited when compared to those produced by the pressure wave, blast wind, or projectiles, significant injuries can occur.

Confined Space Explosions and Structural Collapses

The effects of explosive devices are usually limited in range because the pressure wave and debris radiate outward in all directions from a central point. This rapidly reduces the overpressure and the concentration and, to a lesser degree, the velocity of projectiles. When an explosion occurs in a confined space, however, the pressure wave maintains its energy longer. There is also danger of structural collapse, and debris from the confining structure can increase the blast's projectile content. The blast overpressure also bounces off walls and, where pressure waves meet, the pressure greatly increases. The result can be extremely deadly overpressures. The most lethal blasts are those causing structural collapses followed by those involving confined spaces.

Structural collapse may cause severe crush-type injuries. The collapse may also make victims difficult to locate and, once found, difficult to extricate because of the weight of the material entrapping them. Damage to structures may present further hazards to rescuers and victims, including the possibility of additional collapse, electrocution, fire, or secondary explosion due to gas or fuel leaks.

The most lethal explosions are those causing structural collapses followed by those in confined spaces.

Burns

An explosion can create tremendous heat. This heat may cause flash burns to those very close to the detonation. These injuries are generally superficial or partial thickness burns and may occur in conjunction with other trauma. However, people may also be burned as the heat of the blast ignites combustibles such as clothing, debris, other munitions, or fuel. These secondary burns may be full thickness and extensive.

Some military and terrorist devices are designed to induce damage and injury through combustion. Napalm, for example, is a highly **incendiary,** jellylike substance that clings to people or structures when spread by a blast. It can produce severe or fatal full-thickness burns. Other ordnance uses materials, such as phosphorus, that spontaneously combust when exposed to air.

incendiary *an agent that combusts easily or creates combustion.*

Blast Injury Phases

The injuries produced by explosions are usually classified into three types depending on the phases of the blast that caused them: primary, secondary, and tertiary (Figure 2-24 ■).

Primary Blast Injuries Primary blast injuries are caused by the heat of the explosion and the overpressure wave. The pressure injuries are the most serious and life-threatening injuries associated with the explosion. Burn injuries are generally limited unless caused by secondary combustion.

Review

Content Blast Injury Phases

Primary—caused by heat of explosion and overpressure wave
Secondary—caused by blast projectiles
Tertiary—caused by personnel displacement and structural collapse

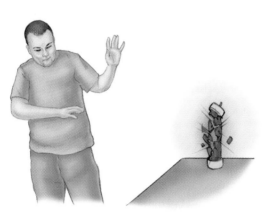

(a) Explosion
Instantaneous combustion of the explosive agent creates superheated gases. The resulting pressure blows the bomb casing apart.

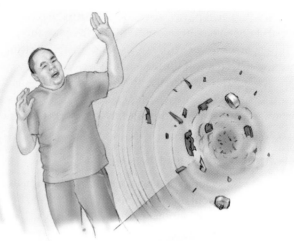

(b) Pressure Wave/Primary Injury
Air molecules slam into one another, creating a pressure wave moving outward from the blast center, causing pressure injuries.

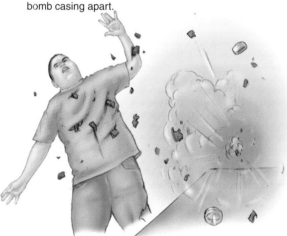

(c) Blast Wave/Secondary Injury
Instantaneous combustion of the explosive agent creates superheated gases. The resulting pressure blows the bomb casing apart. Pieces of the bomb become projectiles that cause injuries by impacting the victim.

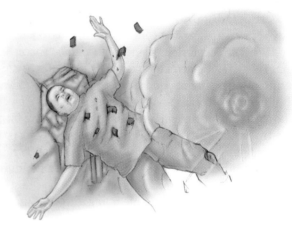

(d) Victim Displacement/Tertiary Injury
The blast wind may propel the victim to the ground or against objects, causing further injuries.

■ Figure 2-24   Blasts can cause injury with the initial blast, when the victim is struck by debris, or when the victim is thrown by the blast or injured by structural collapse.

Secondary Blast Injuries   Secondary blast injuries include trauma caused by projectiles. These injuries may be as or more severe than the primary blast injuries. Projectiles from an explosive blast do have the ability to extend the range of injury beyond that caused by the blast wave and wind. High concentrations of projectiles may also create multiple body penetrations and impalements over large areas of a person's body. The resulting injuries may produce severe bleeding.

Tertiary Blast Injuries   Tertiary blast injuries include those injuries resulting from personnel displacement and structural collapse. Blast victims may be thrown against walls, the ground, or other obstructions and suffer blunt and/or penetrating trauma. When the blast results in a structural collapse, crush injuries may also result. These injuries can be extensive and result in soft, skeletal, nervous, and vascular tissue and organ destruction.

Blast Injury Assessment

Blast injuries produce extreme trauma in those who are close to the blast epicenter. Blasts in densely populated areas may also involve large numbers of victims. Your role as an EMT-Paramedic is to survey and size up the scene and do what you can to secure it for further EMS operations. This normally involves implementing and assuring overall scene management. Once scene management is established and operational, you will likely begin caring for patients by applying the normal assessment priorities (the ABCs of the initial assessment) and then focusing on the seriously injured but salvageable blast victims. If the number of patients exceeds the immediate capabilities of your EMS system, employ disaster triage.

Employ disaster triage and activate the jurisdiction's disaster plan if the number of blast patients exceeds EMS system capacities.

Determine, if possible, whether the blast was the result of terrorist action. If you suspect that it was, be alert to the possibility that other explosive devices may be set or the area may be booby-trapped to endanger rescuers. Assure that police and bomb squad personnel sweep the area before you and your team enter it.

Carefully evaluate the scene for secondary hazards. Look for such things as gas leaks, disrupted electrical wiring, sharp debris, and the possibility of further structural collapse. During the scene size-up, determine the location of the epicenter of the blast. Note the presence of greater destruction and injury as you progress toward the epicenter. As you get closer, your index of suspicion for serious injury increases. When an explosion occurs in a confined space, remember that the bouncing of the pressure wave may concentrate its energy and cause regions of increased mortality at a greater distance from the epicenter.

The most common and serious trauma associated with explosions is lung injury. Pulmonary injury may not manifest itself immediately, so anticipate it in anyone with any other significant signs or symptoms of blast trauma. Evaluate breathing and breath sounds frequently, carefully watching and listening for any dyspnea and crackles or other signs of respiratory congestion. At the first sign of breathing problems, consider high-flow, high-concentration oxygen and rapid transport.

Pulmonary injuries are the most common and serious trauma associated with explosions.

Some blast victims may experience hearing loss due to the pressure wave. After experiencing the emotional impact of the blast itself, this injury can be extremely anxiety producing for patients. Do your best to calm and reassure these patients. Remember that they will find it difficult to understand what others are saying and will not be able to follow spoken commands.

Blast Injury Care

The effects of a serious explosion can produce injuries to the lungs, abdomen, and ears that involve special care considerations. Otherwise, care for blunt trauma, punctures/penetrations, and burns as you would for these injuries if they were produced by other mechanisms.

Lungs Pulmonary blast trauma is the most frequent and life-threatening pressure injury associated with an explosion. The blast-induced pressure wave rapidly and forcefully compresses and distorts the chest cavity, individual air passages, and the alveoli. During compression/decompression, the air pressures in these areas do not have time to equalize, as they do with normal respiration. The extreme pressure damages or ruptures the thin and delicate alveolar walls, resulting in fluid accumulation, hemorrhage, and possibly even the entry of air directly into the bloodstream from the alveoli. Fluid accumulation (pulmonary edema) makes the lungs less elastic and air movement more difficult. The patient finds it more laborious and energy consuming to breathe. Alveolar wall rupture releases blood into the alveoli and may allow air to enter the capillaries. The patient may spit or cough up blood or a frothy mixture of blood and air. If the air enters the bloodstream, it may then travel through the pulmonary circulation to the heart and then to other critical organs causing small obstructions to circulation called **emboli.** These emboli may cause strokelike signs, myocardial infarction, or even death.

emboli *undissolved solid, liquid, or gaseous matter in the bloodstream that may cause blockage of blood vessels.*

A patient history of exposure to a detonation should leave you suspicious of the possibility of lung injury. Since lung injury occurs more frequently with blasts than other pressure injuries and is usually more serious, assess carefully for signs and symptoms of lung injury in patients with any signs of abdominal and ear injuries. Lung injury

dyspnea *labored or difficult breathing.*

hemoptysis *expectoration of blood from the respiratory tract.*

pneumothorax *collection of air or gas in the pleural cavity between the chest wall and lung.*

Provide careful positive-pressure ventilations to any blast injury patient with serious dyspnea.

patients may have progressively worsening crackles, difficulty breathing (**dyspnea**), and, in extreme cases, may cough up blood or blood-tinged sputum (**hemoptysis**). Patients occasionally experience a reduced level of consciousness or small, strokelike episodes. If there is any reason to suspect lung injury from a blast, transport the victim immediately to the closest trauma center or other appropriate facility.

If it becomes necessary to ventilate a blast injury patient, do so with caution. The mechanism of injury may have damaged the alveolar-capillary walls and opened small blood vessels to the alveolar space. Positive-pressure ventilations may push small air bubbles into the vascular system and create emboli. These emboli may quickly travel to the heart and brain, where they can cause further injury or death. The pressure of the ventilations may also induce **pneumothorax** by pushing air past blast-induced lung defects and into the pleural space. If possible, place a patient in the left lateral recumbent position with the head somewhat down. This positioning will discourage emboli from traveling up the carotid arteries and toward the brain.

Despite the risks associated with ventilating blast injury patients, always provide positive-pressure ventilations to any casualty with serious dyspnea. Use only the pressure needed to obtain moderate chest rise and respiratory volumes. High-flow, high-concentration oxygen, as supplied with a reservoir, is also helpful because the bloodstream absorbs small oxygen bubbles more easily than the nitrogen of room air.

Abdomen The blast wave's sudden compression/decompression may also damage the air-filled bowel. Violent movements of the bowel wall cause hemorrhage and possible wall rupture. Rupture releases bowel contents into the abdominal cavity leading, over time, to severe infection and irritation (peritonitis).

Blast injuries to the abdomen require no special attention in the early stages of care. The impact of associated injuries—the bowel hemorrhage and spillage of bowel contents—on the patient's overall condition takes time to develop and is not usually apparent at the emergency scene. The only exceptions are when the blast is extremely powerful or the patient was very close to the detonation. In these cases, be alert for signs and symptoms of developing shock and provide rapid transport and fluid resuscitation as needed.

Ears The ears suffer greatly from blast wave forces associated with ordnance explosion, artillery fire, and even repeated small-arms fire at close range. The structure of the ears explains this. The middle ear is an air-filled cavity containing the organs of hearing (cochlea and stapes) and of positional sense (semicircular canals). The pina (the external portion of the ear) focuses and directs pressure waves (normally, sound waves) through the external auditory canal to the eardrum. The eardrum (tympanic membrane) permits the passage of sound waves but excludes the movement of air into the middle ear. The eustachian tube provides a mechanism for equalizing small and gradual changes in atmospheric pressure between the middle ear and the outside atmosphere. During blast overpressure, however, the eustachian tube cannot equalize the rapid pressure changes. The pressure on the tympanic membrane becomes so great that the membrane stretches or ruptures, resulting in acute hearing loss. The pressure change may be so great as to fracture the delicate bones of hearing, also resulting in acute hearing loss. Hearing losses associated with blasts may be temporary or permanent.

Often ear injuries, even with as much as a third of the eardrum torn, will improve over time without much attention. Direct your care to supporting the victim and assuring that the ear canal remains uncontaminated.

Penetrating Wounds Care for penetrating wounds as you would for any serious open wound. Remove as much of the contaminating material as is practical, and cover the site with a sterile dressing. If you encounter a large embedded or impaled object, stabilize the object by securing gauze pads around it or cover it with a non-Styrofoam paper cup to prevent movement during transport. Large areas of damaged tissue are prone to infection, so keep the wound as clean as possible. Care of penetrating trauma will be discussed at greater length in Chapter 3.

Burns Blasts can also cause extensive burn injuries either from the explosions themselves or from the ignition of other munitions or fuels or of debris or clothing. Care for burn injuries is discussed in detail in Chapter 6.

OTHER TYPES OF BLUNT TRAUMA

Blunt trauma can be caused by still other mechanisms. These include falls, sports injuries, and crush injuries.

Falls

In terms of physics, falls are a release of stored gravitational energy. The greater the distance a person falls, the greater the impact velocity, the greater the exchange of energy, and the greater the resultant trauma. As with auto impacts, stopping distance may be more important than the height of the fall. A person may dive pleasurably from a 12-foot platform into deep water, but a fall from a second story window to a concrete sidewalk results in serious injury. Newton's second law illustrates that the more rapid the deceleration (the shorter the stopping distance), the greater the force and resultant injury. The nature of the impact surface contour may also affect the nature of the injury. An irregular surface, like building rubble or a stairway, may focus the force of impact, increasing the seriousness of the injury.

Trauma resulting from a fall is dependent on the area of contact and the pathway of energy transmission. If the person lands feet first, energy is transmitted up the skeletal structure through the calcaneus, tibia, femur, pelvis, and lumbar spine (Figure 2-25 ■). Fractures along this skeletal pathway are common. The lumbar spine is especially prone to compression injury because it is the only skeletal component supporting the entire upper body. As the victim continues the collision, he may fall forward or backward. In

The potential for injury from a fall depends on the height and stopping distance.

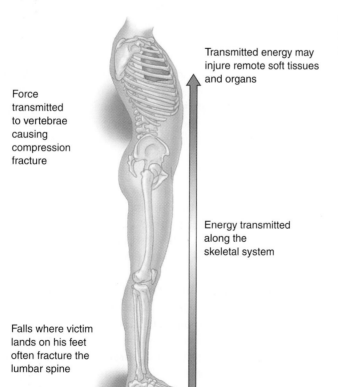

Force transmitted to vertebrae causing compression fracture

Transmitted energy may injure remote soft tissues and organs

Energy transmitted along the skeletal system

Falls where victim lands on his feet often fracture the lumbar spine

■ Figure 2-25　In falls, energy is transmitted along the skeletal system.

forward falls, an outstretched arm may attempt to break the impact, resulting in shoulder, clavicle, and wrist fractures. Pelvic, thoracic, and head injury may result from a backward fall. In some cases, the fall will progress with the patient continuing a straight impact. The tongue may be bitten deeply as the weight of the cranium pushes the maxilla against the mandible as it impacts the sternum.

The initial impact may involve other body surfaces with kinetic energy transmitted from the contact point toward the body's center of mass. In diving injuries, the patient's head meets with the lake or pool bottom, while the rest of the body compresses the cervical spine between the head and shoulders. Axial loading crushes the vertebrae, disrupts the spinal cord, and paralyzes the patient. This may result from even a very shallow dive, as from poolside or from within the water.

If the victim falls on outstretched arms, the impact energy is transmitted along the skeletal system from the hand and wrist, to the forearm, elbow, arm, and shoulder. In these cases, the clavicle often fractures because it is the smallest weight-bearing bone along the pathway of impact transmission. With collapse of the upper extremities, the head and neck may experience energy exchange and injury as may the shoulders upon collision with the impact surface.

In severe falls, with a person dropping more than three times his own height (20 feet for the adult, 10 feet for the small child), focus your attention on potential internal injuries. Rapid deceleration causes many organs to be compressed, displaced, and twisted. The heart, for example, is held in the center of the thorax by the aorta, the vena cavae, and the *ligamentum arteriosum*. When the victim contacts the ground, the heart is pulled downward with such force that it may tear from its aortic attachments, thus leading to immediate exsanguination.

In evaluating a fall, determine the point of impact, the fall height or velocity or force of impact, the impact surface, and the transmission pathway of forces along the skeleton. Then anticipate fracture sites and possible internal injuries. During your physical assessment, pay particular attention to the areas where you expect trauma for further signs of injury.

Falls are a common injury mechanism for older or geriatric patients. With increasing age comes decreases in coordination, deficits in eyesight and depth perception, and weakening bones. Often, the forces required to break bones are much less in geriatric patients than in younger ones. A brittle bone, like the femur, may actually break during ordinary activities, such as walking down a step, and result in a fall. Assess the circumstances surrounding the fall and the trauma involved, remembering that some fractures in the elderly can occur without the application of serious kinetic forces. Provide careful immobilization and gentle transport for these patients and assure that they are comforted and reassured.

Sports Injuries

Sports medicine is a rapidly growing and extensive field, one that certainly cannot be covered completely in this chapter or text. Understanding some basic principles of sports medicine, however, may help you to better understand and care for the injured athlete.

Sports injuries are most commonly produced by extreme exertion, fatigue, or by direct trauma forces. Injuries can be secondary to acceleration, deceleration, compression, rotation, hyperextension, or hyperflexion. These forces leave behind soft-tissue damage to muscle, connective tissue injury to tendons and ligaments, skeletal trauma to long bones or the spinal column, as well as internal damage to either hollow or solid organs.

When a debilitating sports-related injury occurs, transport the athlete to an emergency department for a complete examination before further participation in the sport is allowed. Injuries that present with minimal pain may be significantly worsened by the stress of further competition. Such stress may cause complete ligament rupture or other soft-tissue injury and increase the potential for permanent disability.

In some contact sports, athletes may experience severe impacts (Figure 2-26 ■). If collision leads to any period of unconsciousness, neurologic deficit, or lowered level of

If a collision leads to any loss of consciousness, neurologic deficit, or altered level of consciousness, the athlete should be evaluated by emergency department personnel.

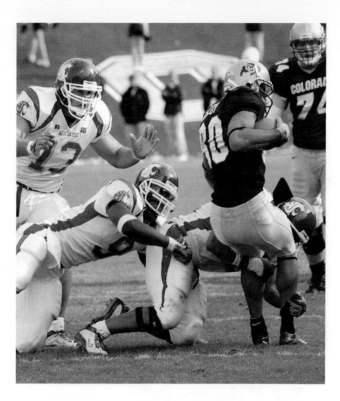

■ Figure 2-26 Contact sports may result in the exchange of great kinetic forces and produce serious injuries. (© *Jeff Forster*)

orientation, assure that the individual is evaluated by emergency department personnel. There is often a strong desire by coaches and players alike for the athlete's return to the game. Until head and cervical spine injury can be ruled out, however, discourage such action.

Protective gear reduces the chance for and significance of injuries. Gear, however, can sometimes be a contributing factor in sports injuries. In major contact sports, for example, shoes are designed to give maximum traction, using cleats to lock the foot firmly in position. In football, a player might be struck, forcing the body to turn on an immobile foot. Ligaments in the knee may tear, resulting in severe and disabling leg injury. In other cases, protective gear may hinder your complete assessment and patient stabilization.

A newer helmet design for high-school contact sports uses an air-filled bladder to immobilize the head within the device. This fixation may be adequate to immobilize the head within the helmet in cases of suspected spinal injuries. While it is difficult to immobilize a spherical helmet to the flat surface of a spine board, it may be preferable to attempting helmet removal. If your protocols require, attempt to immobilize the head and helmet to the long spine board, leaving the shoulder pads in place to help maintain the head and neck in a neutral position.

Crush Injuries

Crush injuries are common types of trauma. They may result from mechanisms such as structural collapse as in an explosion, an industrial or agricultural accident where a limb is caught in machinery, or an instance when a limb is caught under a vehicle. These mechanisms direct great force to soft tissues and bones, compressing surfaces together while stretching semifluid soft tissues laterally. The result may be severe tissue disruption and serious associated hemorrhage.

The injury may be further compounded if the crushing pressure remains in place for an extended period of time. The pressure can disrupt blood flow to and through the limb, causing anaerobic metabolism and some tissue death. This causes a buildup of toxins in the bloodstream. If blood flow returns to the limb, the blood may carry these toxins back to the central circulation. This acidic and toxic blood may then induce cardiac dysrhythmias or seriously damage the kidneys. Another consequence of the release of the crushing pressure is severe and difficult-to-control hemorrhage. The blood vessels within the limb are severely damaged, and bleeding results from many difficult-to-identify locations. With severe and prolonged crush injury entrapment, prehospital care may include the administration of sodium bicarbonate and other medications to combat the effects of acidosis, limit damage, and improve kidney function.

Summary

Blunt trauma accounts for most injury deaths and disabilities. While vehicle collisions are the most frequent cause of blunt trauma, blast injuries, sports injuries, crush injuries, and falls also account for significant mortality and morbidity. Blunt trauma is difficult to assess accurately so you, as the care provider, must look carefully at the mechanism of injury and subtle physical signs to help anticipate serious internal injury. Careful analysis of the mechanism of injury, followed by development of indices of suspicion for injury, can help guide you to recognize those patients needing rapid entry into the trauma system and those best served by on-scene care and transport to the nearest appropriate care facility.

You Make the Call

Arriving at the intersection that is the scene of a vehicle collision, you notice an auto that received a significant lateral impact to the driver's side. The door is pushed into the vehicle about 12 inches and the side window is broken out.
1. What scene hazards would you expect on this call?
2. What injuries would you suspect?
3. What care would you expect to provide?

See Suggested Responses at the back of this book.

Review Questions

1. The first tissue of the body to experience the effects of trauma is:
   a. bone.
   b. skin.
   c. pulmonary.
   d. cardiac.

2. The most common causes(s) of blunt trauma is/are:
   a. burns.
   b. motor vehicle crashes.
   c. sports injuries.
   d. falls.

3. A physical exchange of energy from an object or surface transmitted through the skin into the body's interior describes:
   a. blunt trauma.
   b. penetrating trauma.
   c. gunshot wound.
   d. abdominal trauma.

4. As you double the speed of an object, its ability to cause trauma is:
   a. reduced by one half.
   b. doubled.
   c. tripled.
   d. quadrupled.

5. In determining the potential for trauma caused by an object, you need to examine:
   a. the object's speed.
   b. the object's weight.
   c. the stopping distance.
   d. all of the above.

6. Examples of solid organs include all of the following except:
   a. spleen.
   b. stomach.
   c. pancreas.
   d. kidneys.

7. Blunt trauma can create internal injuries due to the movement of organs inside the body cavities. Which organs(s) can be lacerated by the ligamentum teres?
   a. the heart
   b. the liver
   c. the lungs
   d. the bladder

8. The draining of blood to the point at which life cannot be sustained is called:
   a. cavitation.
   b. third space loss.
   c. exsanguination.
   d. passive inertia.

9. Air bags work much differently than seat belts and are extremely effective for _____ crashes.
   a. frontal
   b. rear-end
   c. rollover
   d. rotational

10. The child's _____ makes protection in vehicle crashes difficult.
    a. age
    b. anatomy
    c. height
    d. weight

11. Frontal impacts produce three pathways of patient travel. Injuries in the down-and-under pathway most commonly include:
    a. skull fractures.
    b. hip fractures.
    c. diaphragm ruptures.
    d. hollow-organ ruptures.

12. The _____ pathway accounts for over half of the deaths in vehicular crashes.
    a. ejection
    b. rotational
    c. up-and-over
    d. down-and-under

13. When a _____ impact occurs, the index of suspicion for serious and life-threatening internal injuries must be higher than vehicle damage alone suggests.
    a. frontal
    b. rear-end
    c. lateral
    d. rollover

14. The anatomical region most commonly injured in the rear-end impact is the:
    a. head.
    b. neck.
    c. chest.
    d. extremities.

15. Blasts create overpressure waves that move outward from the source of the explosion. As an overpressure wave passes by the human body, a brief but drastic increase in air pressure occurs. Because of this, the paramedic needs to concentrate on:
    a. muscle injuries.
    b. solid organ injuries.
    c. hollow organ injuries.
    d. bone injuries.

16. In trauma associated with a blast, assessment should include a high index of suspicion for:
    a. lung injury.
    b. internal bleeding.
    c. fractures.
    d. head injury.

17. When a patient has respiratory compromise due to a blast injury, aggressive ventilation can create:
    a. hyperventilation.
    b. hyperperfusion.
    c. emboli.
    d. altered mental status.

18. In crush injuries, the release of toxins into the central circulation can cause:
    a. increased liver function.
    b. cardiac dysrhythmias.
    c. increased kidney output.
    d. severe alkalosis.

See Answers to Review Questions at the back of this book.

Further Reading

American College of Surgeons, Committee on Trauma. *Advanced Trauma Life Support Course: Student Manual.* Chicago: American College of Surgeons, 1997.

American College of Surgeons, Committee on Trauma. *Resources for Optimal Care of the Injured Patient.* Chicago: American College of Surgeons, 1998.

Baxt, William G. *Trauma, The First Hour.* Upper Saddle River, N.J.: Pearson/Prentice Hall, 1985.

Butman, Alexander M., and James L. Paturas. *Pre-Hospital Trauma Life Support.* Akron, Ohio: Emergency Training, 1999.

Campbell, John E., and the Alabama ACEP. *Basic Trauma Life Support for Paramedics and Other Advanced Providers.* 5th ed. Upper Saddle River, N.J.: Pearson/Prentice Hall, 2004.

De Lorenzo, Robert A., and Robert S. Porter. *Tactical Emergency Care: Military and Operational Out-of-Hospital Medicine.* Upper Saddle River, N.J.: Pearson/Prentice Hall, 1999.

Maull, Kimball Kirby, and Jackie and Dennis Rowe. *Trauma Update for the EMT.* Upper Saddle River, N.J.: Pearson/Prentice Hall, 1992.

On the Web

Visit Brady's Paramedic Website at **www.bradybooks.com/paramedic**.

Penetrating Trauma

Objectives

After reading this chapter, you should be able to:

1. Explain the energy exchange process between a penetrating object or projectile and the object it strikes. (pp. 56–61)

2. Determine the effects that profile, yaw, tumble, expansion, and fragmentation have on projectile energy transfer. (pp. 59–60)

3. Describe elements of the ballistic injury process including direct injury, cavitation, temporary cavity, permanent cavity, and zone of injury. (pp. 57–59, 64–66)

4. Identify the relative effects a penetrating object or projectile has when striking various body regions and tissues. (pp. 66–71)

5. Anticipate the injury types and the extent of damage associated with high-velocity/high-energy projectiles, such as rifle bullets; with medium-energy/medium-velocity projectiles such as handgun and shotgun bullets, slugs, or pellets; and with low-energy/low-velocity penetrating objects, such as knives and arrows. (pp. 61–63)

6. Identify important elements of the scene size-up associated with shootings or stabbings. (pp. 71–72)

7. Identify and explain any special assessment and care considerations for patients with penetrating trauma. (pp. 72–74)

8. Given several preprogrammed and moulaged penetrating trauma patients, provide the appropriate scene size-up, initial assessment, rapid trauma or focused physical exam and history, detailed exam, and ongoing assessment and provide appropriate patient care and transportation. (pp. 56–74)

Key Terms

Case Study

An early morning traffic stop results in a gun battle between a police officer and the armed driver of a car. EMS 7 is dispatched to care for the driver, who has been shot once in the chest. The dispatch report informs the unit that officers have the victim in custody and that all weapons have been secured.

Upon arrival at the shooting scene, paramedic Sandy O'Donnell notices several officers clustered around a male approximately 30 years old who is seated on the ground leaning back against a car. There are several shell casings on the ground near the man, and he appears to be bleeding from a small wound in his left anterior chest. The man's hands are cuffed behind his back. The man's skin color is somewhat ashen and pale, his facial expression reveals anxiety, and he appears to be breathing in an exaggerated fashion.

The arresting officer states that the man drew a weapon, a small-caliber handgun, pointed it, and fired at the officer. In response, the officer drew his weapon and fired three times, hitting the victim once in the chest. The victim dropped his weapon and slumped to his current position. The arresting officer took the victim's gun, and the weapon is now in that officer's custody.

Sandy asks if the victim was searched for other weapons and the officer replies, "No." An officer performs a quick search, discovering and taking into custody a small knife. He then clears Sandy to care for the victim.

The victim seems alert and oriented to person, place, and time and does not interrupt speech to breathe. He complains of mild chest pain that increases with deep breathing. He denies any significant medical history.

Initial assessment reveals a strong pulse with a rate of about 90, respirations about 20, and full and normal chest excursion. During the rapid trauma exam, Sandy notes a medium-to-large-caliber bullet hole in the left anterior chest at about the fourth intercostal space along the mid-clavicular line. No air appears to be moving through the wound with respirations, and hemorrhage is very minor. Assessment of the victim's back reveals a larger wound with a more "blown-out" appearance. Again, no air seems to be moving through the wound with respirations, although hemorrhage is more significant than from the anterior wound.

Sandy quickly applies oxygen via nonrebreather mask at 15 liters per minute and listens for breath sounds. The chest sounds are reasonably clear, though there are slight crackles in the left chest near the wounds. Sandy quickly seals both anterior and posterior wounds with occlusive dressings secured on three sides while her partner takes a quick blood pressure. She reports a finding of 122/86 and a regular and strong pulse at a rate of 92. Other findings are normal, including a pulse oximeter reading of 98 percent.

Sandy alerts the nearby trauma center to the patient's injury mechanism and the assessment findings. They request rapid transport with one IV of normal saline run at a to-keep-open rate. Sandy initiates the IV en route with a 14-gauge catheter, blood tubing, and a 1,000-mL bag of normal saline.

During transport to the trauma center, the ongoing assessment reveals no significant changes in the patient's condition. Upon arrival at the trauma center, Sandy provides an update on the patient's condition and vital signs to the trauma triage nurse while the patient is moved to the trauma suite for evaluation by the trauma surgical team.

INTRODUCTION TO PENETRATING TRAUMA

Modern society is experiencing a great increase in the number and severity of penetrating traumas, especially gunshot wounds. About 28,000 deaths occur each year as a result of shootings, and the number is growing. Many additional mechanisms, including knives, arrows, nails, and pieces of glass or wire, can also cause penetrating trauma. As is the case with auto crashes, physical laws govern the energy exchange process associated with penetrating trauma. Therefore, the types of weapons and projectiles involved and the characteristics of the tissue they impact all affect the severity of injury with penetrating trauma. Understanding the principles of energy exchange and projectile travel will help you to anticipate the potential for injuries, to recognize the injuries that have occurred, and, ultimately, to adequately assess and care for victims of penetrating trauma.

PHYSICS OF PENETRATING TRAUMA

The basic principles of physics that you read about in association with blunt trauma in the last chapter also apply to instances of penetrating trauma. When a projectile strikes a target, it exchanges its energy of motion, more properly called kinetic energy, with the

Legal Notes

Crime, Terrorism, and You Unfortunately, with the exception of war, the increased incidence of penetrating trauma in the world has been primarily due to an increase in crime, terrorism, and the availability of weapons. Any scene where there is a reported case of penetrating trauma should heighten your awareness of scene hazards and safety. Never approach a scene until law enforcement personnel tell you it is safe to do so. Likewise, if you are providing care to a victim of penetrating trauma and you feel the scene is becoming unsafe, you should retreat immediately to a safe distance—even if that requires you to leave the patient.

Our world is much different than it was 100 years ago, or even 50 years ago for that matter. Crime and terrorism pose real threats to both the public and EMS personnel. *Always* put personal safety and scene safety above all other priorities. Live to see another day.

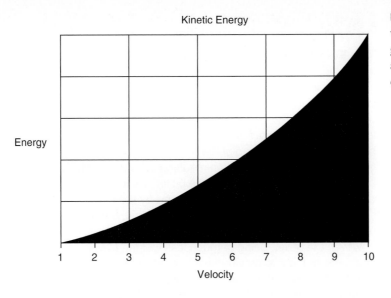

Kinetic Energy

Energy

1   2   3   4   5   6   7   8   9   10

Velocity

■ Figure 3-1 The extreme velocity of firearm projectiles gives them great kinetic energy and the potential to do great damage.

object struck. As you recall, an object's kinetic energy is equal to its mass times the square of its velocity:

$$\text{Kinetic Energy} = \frac{\text{Mass (Weight)} \times \text{Velocity (Speed)}^2}{2}$$

Thus, the greater the mass of an object, the greater the energy. If you double the mass of an object, it will have twice the kinetic energy if the speed of the object remains the same. However, the speed (or velocity) of an object has a squared relationship to its kinetic energy. If you double the speed of an object, its kinetic energy increases by fourfold. If the speed triples, the energy increases by ninefold, and so on (Figure 3-1 ■).

This relationship between mass and velocity explains why very small and relatively light bullets traveling very fast have the potential to do great harm. It also makes clear why different weights of bullets traveling at different velocities cause different amounts of damage. For example, handguns, shotguns, and low-powered rifles are considered to be medium-energy/medium-velocity weapons. They deliver their bullets, slugs, and pellets much faster than low-energy/low-velocity objects like knives and arrows but still are slower than bullets delivered by high-energy/high-velocity weapons like assault rifles. Thus, a handgun bullet is generally smaller and much slower (250 to 400 meters per second) than a rifle bullet. A hunting rifle, however, commonly expels a slightly heavier bullet at speeds of 600 to 1,000 meters per second. Hence, the high-energy rifle bullet's kinetic energy is three to nine times greater than the medium-energy handgun bullet's and can be expected to do significantly more damage. Incidents in Northern Ireland suggested that rifle bullets are between two and four times as lethal as handgun bullets.

The law of conservation of energy (energy can be neither created nor destroyed) explains why the projectile kinetic energy is transformed into damage as it slows. If a projectile like a bullet remains within the object struck, then all its energy is transferred to the object. If the projectile passes completely through the object, then the energy transferred to the object is equal to the kinetic energy just prior to entry minus the energy remaining in the projectile as it exits.

BALLISTICS

The study of the characteristics of projectiles in motion and their effects upon objects they impact is called **ballistics.** The basic physics previously described create the

Incidents in Northern Ireland suggested that wounds from rifle bullets are two to four times as lethal as wounds from handgun bullets.

ballistics *the study of projectile motion and its interactions with the gun, the air, and the object it contacts.*

The Bullet's Travel When the gun's firing pin strikes the shell casing primer, the resulting flash ignites the powder charge. The rapidly burning powder pressurizes the space behind the bullet and pushes the bullet forward. The gun barrel, which is slightly smaller than the bullet, resists its movement while the explosive pressure behind the bullet grows. As the bullet travels down the barrel, its velocity rapidly increases. The bullet also begins to spin, following the small lands and grooves, called rifling, in the gun's barrel. As it leaves the end of the gun barrel, the bullet is spinning rapidly and is pushed on by the barrel exhaust, often resulting in a slight wobble. For the first several inches beyond the mouth of the barrel, the bullet is followed by the very hot exhaust gases that drove the bullet down the gun barrel and by the residue of the spent explosive charge.

While the bullet moves down the gun barrel, the rifle is propelled in the opposite direction. The energy of motion, called kinetic energy, is equal between the two objects; however, the bullet, being of much less weight, travels at a much, much higher speed. The force of the rifle moving away from the target is called recoil and is absorbed by the shooter. The impact produced by a bullet striking an object (or person) cannot be greater than the energy absorbed by the shooter as he stops the recoiling gun. Remember, the bullet is accelerated along the distance of the gun barrel and causes the gun and then the shooter to be propelled backward. This distance is greater and the rate of bullet acceleration is more gradual than when the bullet impacts the victim.

The bullet's spin, induced by the rifling, causes it to track very straight and generally prevents serious wobble, or yaw, during flight. The bullet's speed slows gradually as it meets resistance from the air it must push out of its way. The bullet is also accelerated toward earth by gravity, dropping faster and faster with time. This effect gives a bullet's trajectory a curved shape. The trajectory of a very fast bullet is flatter or much less curved than that of a slower projectile.

As the bullet impacts its target, it exchanges its energy of motion by deforming the target and creating a shock wave within it. This kinetic energy transfer causes the damage associated with projectile injury.

---

trajectory *the path a projectile follows.*

starting point for this study. One aspect of ballistics is **trajectory,** or the curved path that a bullet follows once fired from a gun. As it travels through the air, the bullet is constantly pulled downward by gravity. The faster the bullet, the flatter its curve of travel and the straighter its trajectory.

A second, more significant, aspect of projectile travel is energy dissipation. Factors that affect energy dissipation include drag, cavitation, profile, stability, expansion, and shape. As a bullet travels through the air, it experiences wind resistance, or **drag.** The faster it travels, the more drag it experiences and the greater the slowing effect. Since this represents a reduction in bullet speed, it also means, if all else is equal, that the damage caused by a bullet fired at close range will be more severe than from one fired at a distance.

drag *the forces acting on a projectile in motion to slow its progress.*

Objects traveling relatively slowly and without much kinetic energy, like knives or arrows, will affect only the tissue they contact. High- or medium-velocity projectiles, like rifle or handgun bullets, however, set a portion of the semifluid body tissue in motion, creating a shock wave and a temporary cavity in the tissue. This stage of the destruction process is known as **cavitation** and is related to the bullet's velocity and how quickly it gives up its energy. The energy exchange rate is related to the size of the projectile's contacting surface, called its profile, and to its shape.

cavitation *the outward motion of tissue due to a projectile's passage, resulting in a temporary cavity and vacuum.*

Profile

The **profile** is the portion of the bullet you would see if you looked at it as it traveled toward you. The larger this surface profile, the greater the energy exchange rate, the more quickly the bullet slows, and the more extensive the damage to surrounding tissue. For bullets that remain stable during their travel and do not deform, the profile is the bullet's diameter, or **caliber.** To increase the energy exchange rate, bullets are designed to become unstable as they pass from one medium to another or to deform through expansion or fragmentation.

Stability

The location of a bullet's center of mass affects its stability both during its flight and when it impacts a solid or semisolid object. The longer the bullet, the farther the center of mass is from its leading edge. If the bullet is deflected from straight flight—for example, by the barrel exhaust or by a gust of wind—the lift created by the projectile's tip passing through air at an angle will cause the bullet to tumble. If it continues to tumble, the bullet will slow and the accuracy of the shot will be diminished. To prevent tumbling, bullets are sent spinning through the air by the gun barrel's rifling. This rotation gives a bullet gyroscopic stability like a spinning top. If the spinning bullet is slightly deflected, it will wobble, or **yaw,** then slowly return to straight flight.

When a bullet impacts a dense substance, several things happen. If there is already a yaw, the yaw greatly increases as the bullet begins its penetration. This occurs as the bullet's mass tries to overrun the leading edge. Secondly, the gyroscopic spin designed for stability in air becomes insufficient. A bullet would need to spin at a rate 30 times greater in body tissue than in air to maintain the same stability. The result may be tumbling and a great increase in the bullet's presenting profile. Since a rifle bullet is generally longer than a handgun bullet and has its center of mass farther back from the leading edge, it is more likely to tumble once it hits body tissue (Figure 3-2 ■). With increased tumbling and a larger presenting profile, a rifle bullet's kinetic energy exchange rate increases, as does its potential for causing damage. In human tissue, a rifle bullet generally rotates 180 degrees and then continues its travel base first.

Expansion and Fragmentation

Projectiles also may increase their profile and their energy exchange rate by deforming when they strike a medium denser than air. As the bullet's nose contacts the target, it is

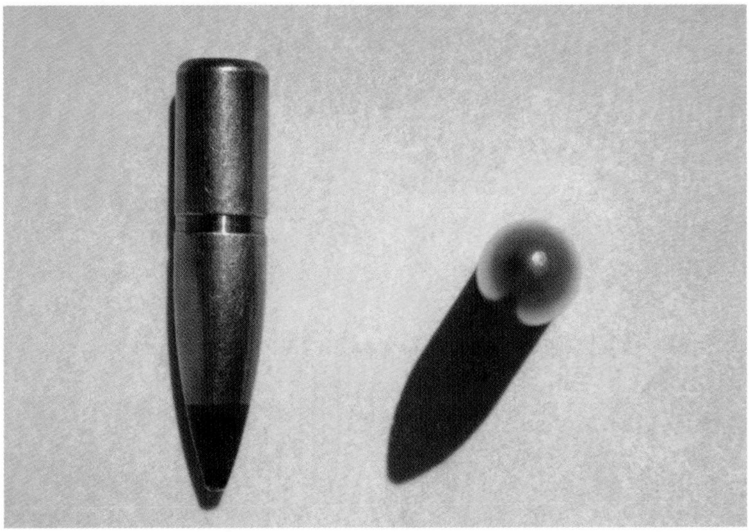

profile *the size and shape of a projectile as it contacts a target; it is the energy exchange surface of the contact.*

caliber *the diameter of a bullet expressed in hundredths of an inch (.22 caliber = 0.22 inches); the inside diameter of the barrel of a handgun, shotgun, or rifle.*

yaw *swing or wobble around the axis of a projectile's travel.*

■ Figure 3-2   The presenting surface, or profile, of a bullet changes as it tumbles when it contacts human tissue. *(Collection of Robert Porter)*

compressed by the weight of the rest of the bullet behind it. The nose of the bullet mushrooms outward as the rear of the bullet pushes into it, increasing the projectile's diameter (Figure 3-3 ■). In some cases, the initial impact forces are so great that the bullet separates into several pieces or fragments. This fragmentation increases the energy exchange rate of impact because the total surface area of the fragments is much greater than that of the original bullet profile (Figure 3-4 ■). While handgun bullets are made of relatively soft lead, their velocity, and hence their kinetic energy, is generally not sufficient to cause significant deformity. However, some bullets (dum-dums or wad-cutters) are specifically designed to mushroom and/or fragment upon impact and thereby increase the damage they cause. Rifle bullets have much greater velocities than handgun bullets and much more kinetic energy. They are more prone to deform when contacting human tissue, especially bullets used for big-game hunting. Most military ammunition is fully jacketed with impact-resistant metal and seldom deforms solely with soft tissue collision.

Secondary Impacts

The energy exchange between a projectile and body tissue can also be affected by any object the projectile strikes during its travel. Branches, window glass, or articles of clothing may all deflect a bullet and induce yaw and tumble. They may also cause bullet deformity, and thereby increase the energy exchange rate once the bullet impacts the victim.

■ Figure 3-3   Some bullets are designed to mushroom on impact, thus increasing their profile, energy exchange rate, and damage potential. *(Collection of Robert Porter)*

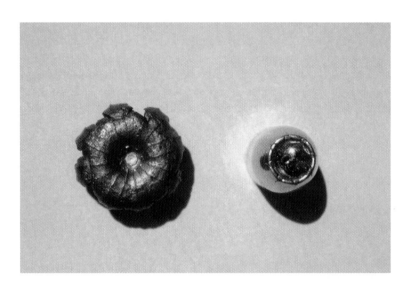

■ Figure 3-4   Some firearm projectiles may break apart, or fragment, on contact, greatly increasing their profile and damage potential. *(Collection of Robert Porter)*

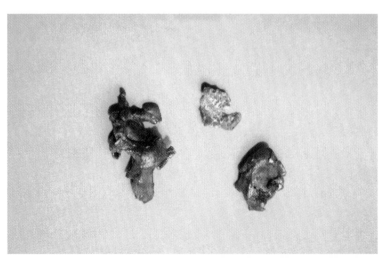

A special type of secondary impact occurs when the bullet collides with body armor. Kevlar™ and other synthetic fabrics can effectively resist the kinetic energy generated by medium-energy projectiles. This energy is absorbed by the armor and distributed to the victim in much the same way that the recoil of a gun is distributed to the shooter. The impact of the bullet may produce blunt trauma in the person hit (for example, myocardial contusion), but such injuries are generally less damaging than penetration by the bullet would have been. High-energy projectiles may pass through body armor, but in doing so they dissipate some of their energy as blunt trauma, thereby reducing the penetrating kinetic energy as the bullet strikes body tissue. Bullet deformity may increase the rate of energy exchange, but the reduction in kinetic energy reduces the overall injury potential. Ceramic inserts for body armor will stop penetration of most rifle bullets but not without causing significant, but less lethal, blunt trauma.

Shape

In addition to profile, other aspects of the shape of the bullet affect the energy exchange rate and the resulting damage. Handgun ammunition is rather blunt, is more resistant to travel through human tissue, and releases kinetic energy more quickly. Rifle bullets are more pointed and cut through the tissue more efficiently. However, if the rifle bullet tumbles, it will present a different shape and may exchange energy more rapidly both because of the shape and the increase in profile. If a bullet fragments, the irregular shape of the fragments means that the projectile will give up its energy more rapidly and through more erratic pathways than either an intact handgun or rifle bullet.

SPECIFIC WEAPON CHARACTERISTICS

Weapons that commonly cause wounds encountered by paramedics include handguns, domestic rifles, assault rifles, shotguns, and knives and arrows. Each type of weapon has certain characteristics associated with the injuries it produces (Figure 3-5 ■).

Handgun

The handgun is often a small-caliber, short-barreled, medium-velocity weapon with limited accuracy that is most effective at close range. Because a handgun does not fire a high-velocity, high-energy projectile as a rifle does, its potential for causing damage is limited. The blunter shape of the bullet and, less frequently, its softer composition and associated mushrooming and fragmentation may release the bullet's energy more rapidly. The damage is still, however, less than that of the higher energy rifle bullet. The

While body armor protects against penetration, impact may result in less lethal but still serious blunt injury.

 Review

Factors Affecting Energy Exchange Between a Projectile and Body Tissue

Velocity
Profile
Stability
Expansion and fragmentation
Secondary impacts
Shape

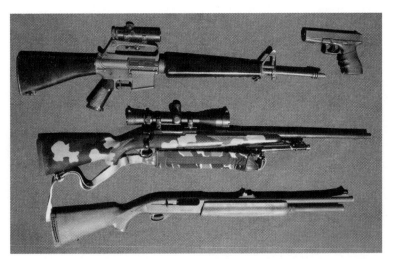

■ Figure 3-5 Firearms include (top to bottom) handguns, assault rifles, domestic rifles, and shotguns. (*Collection of Robert Porter*)

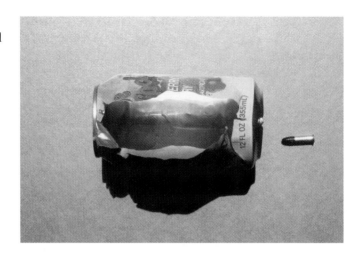

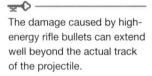

Figure 3-6 The energy of the handgun projectile is limited by low projectile weight and its relatively slow velocity. *(Collection of Robert Porter)*

severity of injury is usually related to the organs directly damaged by the bullet's passage (Figure 3-6 ■).

Some handguns fire automatically (machine pistols). They continue to discharge bullets until the trigger is released or the magazine empties. While the energy for each projectile remains the same, the damage potential associated with automatic weapons is increased because of the likelihood of multiple impacts or multiple victims.

Rifle

The domestic hunting rifle fires a heavier projectile than the handgun, through a much longer barrel, and with much greater muzzle velocity. It is either a manually loaded, single-shot weapon with some mechanical loading action to advance the next shell, or a semiautomatic weapon, in which the next shell is fed into the chamber by recoil or exhaust gases. However, no more than one bullet is expelled by each squeeze of the domestic hunting rifle's trigger. The high-energy rifle bullet travels much farther, with greater accuracy, and retains much more of its kinetic energy than does the handgun projectile. Due to the rifle bullet's high speed and energy, it transfers great damaging energy to the target (Figure 3-7 ■). This results in extensive wounds with injuries that extend beyond the projectile's immediate track. Domestic hunting ammunition is especially lethal. It is often designed to expand dramatically on impact, greatly increasing the energy delivery rate and the size of both the temporary cavity and the wound pathway.

The damage caused by high-energy rifle bullets can extend well beyond the actual track of the projectile.

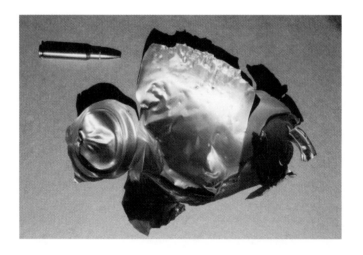

Figure 3-7 The energy carried by a rifle bullet is very damaging because of its heavier weight and very high velocity. *(Collection of Robert Porter)*

Assault Rifle

The assault rifle differs from the domestic hunting rifle in that it generally has a larger magazine capacity and will fire in both the semiautomatic and automatic mode. Examples of these weapons include the M16 and the AK47. The resulting injuries are similar to injuries produced by domestic hunting rifles, although multiple wounds and casualties can be expected. Military ammunition is fully jacketed and not designed for expansion; while still very deadly, the energy delivery is not as severe as with domestic hunting ammunition. Assault weapons in terrorist hands, however, may be loaded with domestic hunting-type ammunition. This greatly increases their injury potential.

Shotgun

The shotgun expels a single projectile (a slug) or numerous spheres (pellets or shot) at medium velocity. The shell is loaded with a slug or a particular size of lead shot, varying from 00 (about 1/3 inch in diameter) to #9 shot (about the size of a pin head). The size of the projectile compartment is approximately the same with various types of loads. This means that the larger the shot, the smaller the number of projectiles. Each projectile shares a portion of the total muzzle energy and adds to the resistance as it moves through air. The shotgun is limited in range and accuracy; however, injuries sustained at close range can be very severe or lethal (Figure 3-8 ■).

Knives and Arrows

In contrast to high- or medium-velocity projectiles such as rifle or handgun bullets, knives, arrows, and other slow-moving, penetrating objects cause low-velocity, low-energy wounds. Because low-velocity objects do not produce either a pressure shock wave or cavitation, damage is usually limited to physical injury caused by direct contact between the blade or object and the victim's tissue. The severity of a low-velocity penetrating wound, however, can often be difficult to assess because the depth and angle of the object's insertion cannot be determined from the visible wound. In addition, an attacker may move the penetrating object about inside the victim, then leave it in place or withdraw it. The penetration can result in serious internal hemorrhage or injury to individual or multiple body organs.

The hunting tips designed for arrows can be especially damaging. These feature three razor-tipped, pointed barbs that are intended to smoothly cut tissue. These tips produce severe internal hemorrhage. Also, any movement of an arrow while it is impaled in the victim increases both the tissue damage and hemorrhage rate.

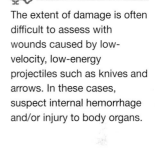

The extent of damage is often difficult to assess with wounds caused by low-velocity, low-energy projectiles such as knives and arrows. In these cases, suspect internal hemorrhage and/or injury to body organs.

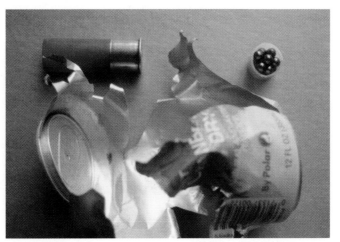

■ Figure 3-8   A shotgun propels small projectiles with limited velocity. However, because of the large number of projectiles, the weapon can be extremely damaging at close range. *(Collection of Robert Porter)*

When a Projectile Enters the Body The spinning bullet smashes into a semifluid target (such as human tissue) with great speed and kinetic energy. The tip of the bullet impacts tissue, pushing the tissue forward and to the side along the pathway of its travel. This tissue collides with adjacent tissue, ultimately creating a shock wave of pressure moving forward and lateral to the projectile. This shock wave continues to move perpendicular to the bullet's path as it passes. The rapid compression of tissue laterally and the stretching of the tissue as it moves outward from the bullet path crushes and tears the tissue structure. The motion creates a pocket, or cavity, behind the bullet. The pressure within this cavity is reduced, creating suction. This suction draws air and debris into the cavity from the entrance wound and from the exit wound, if one is present. The body tissue's elasticity then draws the sides of the cavity back together, causing the entrance wound, exit wound, and wound pathway to close completely or remain only partially open.

The bullet's exchange of energy with the body leaves various tissues disrupted and injured. Tissue in the direct pathway of the bullet suffers most. It is severely contused and likely to have been torn from its attachments. In addition to the directly injured tissue, other debris, blood, and air are found along the bullet's pathway. The cavitational wave stretches and tears adjacent tissue, damaging cell walls and small blood vessels. The adjacent tissue is injured, but will likely regain its normal function slowly. Larger blood vessels torn by the bullet and the cavitational wave release their precious fluid in large quantities into the damage pathway. Over time, this pathway, because of the disruption in circulation and the introduction of infectious material with the drawing-in of debris, may experience severe infection, which will prolong the healing process.

Review

Factors Associated with the Damage Pathway of a Projectile Wound

- Direct injury
- Pressure shock wave
- Cavitation
  - Temporary cavity
  - Permanent cavity
  - Zone of injury

DAMAGE PATHWAY

The damage pathway that a high-velocity projectile inflicts results from three specific factors. They are the direct injury, the pressure shock wave, and cavitation, or the creation of a temporary cavity. These three factors can also create a permanent cavity and a zone of injury (Figure 3-9 ■).

Direct Injury

Direct injury is the damage done as the projectile strikes tissue, contuses and tears that tissue, and pushes the tissue out of its way. The direct injury pathway is limited to the profile of the bullet as it moves through the body or the profiles of resulting fragments

■ Figure 3-9   As a bullet passes through a gel designed to simulate human tissue, it demonstrates the wounding process. *(Collection of Robert Porter)*

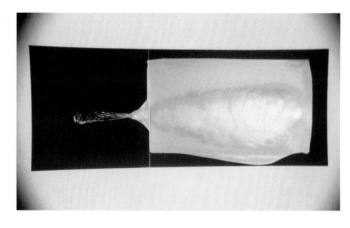

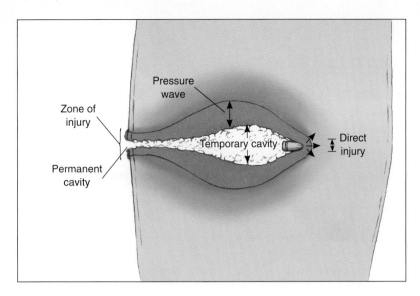

Figure 3-10 As a projectile passes through tissue it creates a pressure wave and temporary cavity, with results that include direct injury, a permanent cavity, and a zone of injury.

as the bullet breaks apart. Except for magnum rounds (generating particularly high velocities), handgun bullet damage is usually limited to direct injury.

Pressure Shock Wave

When a high-velocity high-energy projectile strikes human flesh, it creates a pressure shock wave (Figure 3-10 ■). Since most human tissue is semifluid and elastic, the impact of the projectile transmits energy outward very quickly. The tissue cells in front of the bullet are pushed forward and to the side at great speed. They push adjacent cells forward and outward, creating a moving wave of pressure and tissue. The faster and blunter the bullet, the greater the effect. With high-velocity rifle bullets, pressures are extreme, approaching 100 times normal atmospheric pressure.

The pressure wave travels very well through fluid, such as blood, and may injure blood vessels distant from the projectile pathway. Air-filled cavities, such as the small air sacs (alveoli) of the lung, compress very easily and absorb the pressure, quickly limiting the shock wave and the resulting temporary cavity. Solid and dense organs, like the liver and spleen, suffer greatly as the pressure wave moves through them, causing internal hemorrhage and, in extreme cases, fracture.

Temporary Cavity

The temporary cavity is a space created behind the high-energy bullet as tissue moves rapidly away from the bullet's path. The size of the cavity depends upon the amount of energy transferred during the bullet's passage. With rifle bullets, the temporary cavity may be as much as 12 times larger than the projectile's profile. After the bullet's passage, tissue elasticity causes the temporary cavity to close.

Cavitation also produces a subatmospheric pressure within the cavity as it expands. This means that air is drawn in from the entrance wound and the exit wound, if one exists. Debris and contamination enter the cavity with the in-flowing air, adding to the risk of infection.

Permanent Cavity

The movement that creates the temporary cavity crushes, stretches, and tears the affected tissues. These processes seriously damage the area in and adjacent to the bullet's path and may also damage the tissue's elasticity. The tissue thus may not return to its normal orientation, resulting in a permanent cavity that in some cases may be larger

The severity of injury in cases of bullet wounds usually depends on the organs damaged by the bullet's passage.

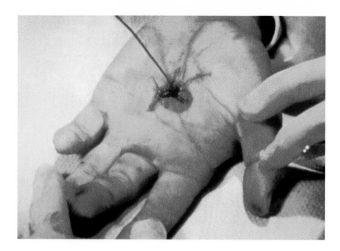

■ Figure 3-11 Damage caused by a low-velocity wounding process, such as that caused by a wire thrown by a lawn mower, is limited to the object's path of travel.

than the bullet's diameter. This cavity is not a void but is filled with disrupted tissues, some air, fluid, and debris.

Zone of Injury

Associated with most projectile wounds is a zone of injury that extends beyond the permanent cavity. This zone contains contused tissue that does not function normally and may be slow to heal because of cell and tissue damage, disrupted blood flow, and infection.

LOW-VELOCITY WOUNDS

Weapons such as knives, ice picks, arrows, or flying objects such as blast debris or wires thrown by a lawn mower can cause low-velocity penetrating trauma. The relatively slow speed of these objects limits the kinetic energy exchange rate as they enter the victim's body. Consider, for example, the stabbing of a victim by a 150-pound attacker who strikes with a knife moving at about 3 meters per second. Although the mass behind the penetration of the knife blade is significantly greater than a rifle bullet's, the velocity of the knife is vastly lower. This means that injury in such cases is usually restricted to the tissue actually contacted by the penetrating object (Figure 3-11 ■).

While the injury is limited to the penetrating object's pathway, that object may be twisted, moved about, or inserted at an oblique angle. As a result, the entrance wound may not reflect the depth of the object's penetration, the extent of its motion within the body, or the actual organs and tissues it contacts and injures.

Characteristics of the attacker and victim are important to keep in mind when assessing cases of low-velocity penetrating trauma. Knife-wielding males, for example, most often strike with a forward, outward, or crosswise stroke. Females usually strike with an overhand and downward stroke. Victims of these attacks initially attempt to protect themselves by using their arms. This means they often receive deep upper-extremity lacerations (commonly called defense wounds). If an attack continues, injuries are often directed to the chest, abdomen, face, neck, or back.

SPECIFIC TISSUE/ORGAN INJURIES

The extent of damage that a penetrating projectile causes within the body varies with the particular type of tissue it encounters. The density of an organ affects how efficiently the projectile's energy is transmitted to surrounding tissues. The tissue's connective strength and elasticity, called **resiliency,** also influence how much tissue damage occurs with the kinetic energy transfer. Structures and tissues within the body that behave differently during projectile passage include connective tissue, solid organs, hollow organs, lungs, and bone.

resiliency *the connective strength and elasticity of an object or fabric.*

CONNECTIVE TISSUE

Muscles, the skin, and other connective tissues are dense, elastic, and hold together very well. When exposed to the pressure and stretching of the cavitational wave, these types of tissue characteristically absorb energy while limiting tissue damage. The wound track closes due to the resiliency of the tissue, and serious injury is frequently limited to the projectile's pathway.

ORGANS

Another factor that has profound effects on the victim's potential for survival is the particular organ involved in a penetrating injury. Some organs, like the heart and brain, are immediately necessary for life functions, and serious injury may cause immediate death. When large blood vessels are involved, the hemorrhage can be rapid and severe. A penetrating injury to the urinary bladder, however, may not receive surgical intervention for several hours without threatening the patient's life. When evaluating a wound's seriousness, anticipate the organs injured and the effect their injury is likely to have on the patient's condition and survivability.

Solid Organs

Solid organs such as the liver, spleen, kidneys, pancreas, and brain have the density but not the resiliency of muscle and other connective tissues. When struck by the forces of bullet impact, these tissues compress and stretch, resulting in greater damage more closely associated with the size of the temporary cavity than with the bullet's profile. The tissue returns to its original location, not because of its own elasticity but because of the resiliency of surrounding tissues or the organ capsule. Hemorrhage associated with solid organ projectile damage is often severe.

Be alert to the possibility of severe hemorrhage if you suspect that a projectile has damaged a solid organ.

Hollow Organs

Hollow organs such as the bowel, stomach, urinary bladder, and heart are muscular containers holding fluid. The fluid within is noncompressible and rapidly transmits the impact energy outward. If the container is filled and distended with fluid at the time of impact, the energy released can tear the organ apart explosively (Figure 3-12 ■). Slower and smaller projectiles may produce small holes in an organ and permit slow leakage of its contents. If this occurs with the heart, it may produce **pericardial tamponade** (blood filling the pericardial sac, thus limiting heart function) or moderate and slowly life-threatening hemorrhage. If the container is not distended, it is more tolerant of cavitational forces. If a hollow organ, such as the bowel or stomach, holds air, the air compresses with the passage of the pressure wave and somewhat limits the extent of injury. (Large blood vessels respond to projectile passage much like hollow, fluid-distended organs.)

pericardial tamponade *filling of the pericardial sac with fluid, which in turn limits the filling and function of the heart.*

LUNGS

The lungs consist of millions of small, elastic, air-filled sacs. As the bullet and its associated pressure wave pass, the air is compressed, thereby slowing and limiting the

Injury to lung tissue in cases of penetrating trauma is generally less extensive than can be expected with any other body tissue.

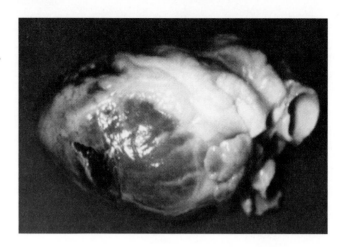

■ Figure 3-12 If a high-velocity bullet impacts the heart during maximum cardiac filling, cardiac rupture and rapid exsanguination may occur. *(Hamilton County, NY Coroner's Office, Dorothy E. Dean, MD)*

transmission of the cavitational wave. Injury to lung tissue in cases of penetrating trauma is generally less extensive than can be expected with any other body tissue.

A bullet may, however, open the chest wall or disrupt larger airways, thus permitting air to escape into the thorax (pneumothorax) or creating a valve-like defect that results in accumulating pressure within the chest (tension pneumothorax). Bullet wounds only infrequently induce an open pneumothorax (sucking chest wound) because the entrance wound diameter is usually limited to the bullet caliber. Close-range shotgun blasts and explosive exit wounds of high-powered rifles, however, may be large and cause significant disruption of the chest wall integrity. In these cases, a pneumothorax is a more likely outcome.

Suspect the possibility of pneumothorax when there has been a significant disruption of chest wall integrity.

BONE

In contrast to lung tissue, bone is some of the body's densest, most rigid, and nonelastic tissue of all. When struck by a projectile or its associated pressure wave, bone resists displacement until it fractures, often into numerous pieces. These bone fragments then may distribute the impact energy to surrounding tissue. The projectile's contact with bone may also significantly alter the projectile's path through the body.

GENERAL BODY REGIONS

Several body regions deserve special attention regarding projectile wounds. They include the extremities, abdomen, thorax, neck, and head (Figure 3-13 ■). A projectile's passage also has a special effect on the first and last tissue contacted, the sites of the entrance and the exit wounds.

Extremities

The extremities consist of skin covering muscles and surrounding large long bones. An extremity injury may be debilitating but does not immediately threaten life unless there is severe hemorrhage associated with it. The severity of injury is limited by the resiliency of the skin and muscle, although if the bone is involved, the degree of soft-tissue damage may be increased. In recent military experience, extremity injuries account for between 60 and 80 percent of injuries yet result in less than 10 percent of fatalities. The remaining 20 to 40 percent of penetrating injuries are divided among wounds of the abdomen, thorax, and head and account for more than 90 percent of mortality.

⊘ **Review**

Body Regions Deserving Special Attention with Penetrating Trauma

Extremities
Abdomen
Thorax
Neck
Head

Some 90 percent of penetrating trauma mortality involves the head, thorax, and abdomen.

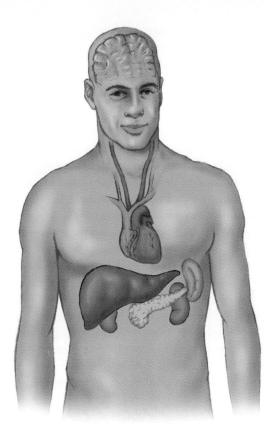

■ Figure 3-13 Critical structures in which the seriousness of a bullet's impact is increased include the brain, great vessels, heart, liver, kidneys, and pancreas.

Abdomen

The abdomen (including the pelvic cavity) is the largest body cavity and contains most of the human organs. The area is not well protected by skeletal structures other than the upper pelvic ring, the lower rib cage border, and the lumbar vertebral column. The passage of a projectile through the abdominal cavity can produce a significant cavitational wave. The major occupant of the cavity, the bowel, is very tolerant of compression and stretching, but the liver, spleen, kidneys, and pancreas are highly susceptible to injury and hemorrhage. Since these organs occupy the upper abdominal quadrants, you should consider any penetrating projectile injury to this area to be serious and to have the potential to cause severe internal hemorrhage. Serious consequences should also be anticipated with injuries to the abdominal aorta and inferior vena cava, which are located along the spinal column in the posterior and central abdomen.

Consider any penetrating projectile injury to the abdomen to be serious and to have the potential to cause severe internal hemorrhage.

If a projectile perforates the small or large bowel, those organs may spill their contents into the abdominal cavity. This spillage results in serious peritoneal irritation due to chemical action or infection, although the signs and symptoms take some time to develop. If the injury process disrupts the blood vessels, the free blood will result in only limited abdominal irritation.

Thorax

Within the chest is a cavity formed by the ribs, spine, sternum, clavicles, and the diaphragm's strong muscle. This thoracic cavity houses the lungs, heart, and major blood vessels as well as the esophagus and part of the trachea. The impact of a bullet with the ribs may induce an explosive energy exchange that injures the surrounding tissue with numerous bony fragments. Lung tissue can absorb much of the cavitational energy while sustaining limited injury itself. However, the heart and great vessels, as fluid-filled containers, may suffer greatly from the energy of the bullet's passage. The damage to these structures and the associated massive hemorrhage may cause almost instant death. Because of the pressure-driven dynamics of respiration, any large chest wound may compromise breathing. Air may pass through a wound instead of the normal airway (pneumothorax) or may build up under pressure within the chest wall (tension pneumothorax).

Neck

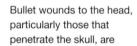

Monitor the airway closely in any patient with a penetrating wound to the neck.

The neck is an anatomical area traversed by several critical structures. These include the larynx, the trachea, the esophagus, several major blood vessels (the carotid and vertebral arteries and the jugular veins), and the spinal cord. Penetrating trauma in this area is very likely to damage vital structures and lead to airway compromise, severe bleeding, and/or neurological dysfunction. Associated swelling and hematoma formation may compromise circulation and the airway. Additionally, any large penetrating wound may permit air to be drawn into an open external jugular vein and immediately threaten life due to the resulting pulmonary emboli.

Head

Bullet wounds to the head, particularly those that penetrate the skull, are especially lethal.

The skull is a hollow, strong, and rigid container, housing the brain's delicate semisolid tissue. It is highly susceptible to projectile injury. If a bullet penetrates the skull, its cavitational energy is trapped within the cavity and subjects the brain to extreme pressures. If the released kinetic energy is great enough, the skull may rupture outward. In some cases, a bullet may enter the skull and not have enough energy to exit; in such a case, the bullet may continue to travel along the interior of the skull, disrupting more and more brain matter. Bullet wounds to the head, particularly those that penetrate the skull, are especially lethal.

The destructive forces released by a projectile wound to the head may also disrupt the airway and/or the victim's ability to control his own airway. The head and face are also areas with an extensive supply of blood vessels. Penetrating trauma may damage these vessels and result in serious and difficult-to-control hemorrhage.

Suspect the possibility of airway compromise in patients with projectile wounds to the head and face.

A frequent occurrence associated with suicide attempts is severe damage to the facial region. As the individual places a shotgun or rifle under the chin and pulls the trigger, the head tilts up and back. This directs the blast entirely to the facial region, but the projectile(s) may not enter the cranium or strike any immediately life-threatening structures. There is, however, serious bleeding. The bleeding and the associated damage can make the airway very hard to control. In these cases, use of an endotracheal tube to secure the airway can be difficult because many airway structures and landmarks are often obliterated by the blast.

Entrance Wound

Entrance wounds are usually the size of the bullet's profile. At this point, cavitational wave energy has not had time to develop and contribute to the wounding process (Figure 3-14 ■). The situation is different, however, with bullets that deform or tumble during flight. With these projectiles, the initial impact can be especially violent, producing a much larger and more disrupted entry wound than the caliber of the bullet alone would suggest.

Bullet entry wounds sustained at close range, a few feet or less, display special characteristics. Such wounds may be marked by elements of the barrel exhaust and bullet passage. Tattooing from the propellant residue may form a darkened circle or an oval (if the gun is held at an angle) around the entry wound and contaminate the wound itself. At the wound site, you may notice a small (usually 1- to 2-mm) ridge of discoloration around the entrance caused by the spinning bullet. If the gun barrel is held very close or against the skin as the weapon is fired, it may push the barrel exhaust into the

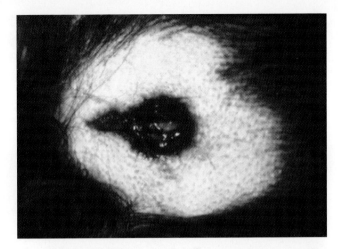

Figure 3-14 The entrance wound is often the same size as the projectile's profile and may demonstrate some bruising on the inner border of the wound. *(Hamilton County, NY Coroner's Office, Dorothy E. Dean, MD)*

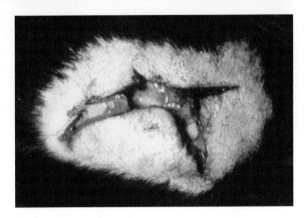

Figure 3-15 A bullet's exit wound often has a "blown outward" appearance, with stellate tears. *(Hamilton County, NY Coroner's Office, Dorothy E. Dean, MD)*

wound producing subcutaneous emphysema (air within the skin's tissue) and crepitus to the touch. If the barrel is held a few inches from the skin, you may notice some burns caused by the hot gases of the barrel exhaust.

Exit Wound

The exit wound is caused by the physical damage from both the passage of the bullet itself and from the cavitational wave. Since the pressure wave is moving forward and outward, the wound may have a "blown outward" appearance. The exit wound may appear as stellate, referring to the tears radiating outward in a star-like fashion (Figure 3-15). Because the cavitational wave has had time to develop, the exit wound may more accurately reflect the potential for damage caused by the bullet's passage than the entrance wound. If the bullet expends all its kinetic energy before it can exit the body, there is no exit wound and the bullet remains within the body. If the bullet does exit, the kinetic energy expended within the body is equal to the kinetic energy before impact minus the energy that remains in the bullet as it leaves the body.

An exit wound may more accurately reflect the potential damage caused by a bullet's passage through the body than an entrance wound.

SPECIAL CONCERNS WITH PENETRATING TRAUMA

SCENE SIZE-UP

The scene size-up for a shooting or stabbing raises special concerns not associated with most other emergency care situations. The very nature of these injuries should suggest the possibility of danger from further violence and potential injury to you and your

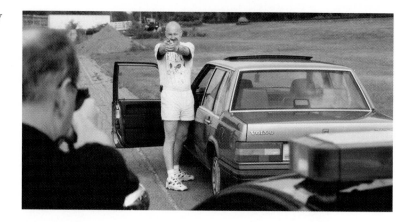

Figure 3-16 Assure that any potentially violent scene is safe and secured by police before entering. *(Collection of Robert Porter)*

In cases involving shootings or stabbings, always be sure that police have secured the scene before you enter it.

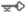

Consider the possibility that the patient may be carrying a weapon and have the police search him if necessary.

Make every effort to preserve evidence at a crime scene, but remember that care of the patient takes priority.

crew. Do not approach a shooting or stabbing scene unless and until law-enforcement personnel arrive and secure it and direct you to enter and provide care. If law-enforcement personnel are not yet on the scene when you arrive, stage your vehicle at least a block away and out of sight of the scene. Once police or other law-enforcement personnel arrive, bring your vehicle closer to the scene but keep the police and their vehicles between you and the shooting or stabbing site. Wait there for the police to indicate that it is safe to approach the patient (Figure 3-16 ■).

Once you reach the patient, survey carefully to determine that there are no weapons within the patient's reach. Consider the possibility that the victim may be carrying a knife or other weapon. If you have any doubts, request that the police search the victim for weapons before you begin to provide care.

As you carefully survey the scene of a shooting, try to reconstruct the event. Attempt to determine the victim's original position and his or her angle to and distance from the shooter. This helps you determine the angle at which the bullet entered the patient (which may not otherwise be revealed by the entrance wound) and whether the wound was received at point blank range or from a distance. Also try to determine the caliber of weapon and its type—handgun, rifle, or shotgun.

If the call involves a knifing injury, attempt to determine the gender and approximate weight of the attacker and the length of the blade. (You probably will not be able to determine the wound depth.) This information will help the emergency department determine the potential severity of the wound.

As you move on to your assessment of the patient, do all that you can to preserve the crime scene while providing any needed patient care. Disturb only those materials around the patient that you must move in order to render care. Cut around any bullet or knife holes in clothing and give the clothing to police for use as evidence. If there is ever any doubt about what to do, however, err on the side of providing patient care. (See Volume 5, Chapter 12, "Crime Scene Awareness.") If the victim is obviously dead, employ your jurisdiction's protocols for handling the body, but try to do so without disturbing evidence that may be crucial in determining what happened.

PENETRATING WOUND ASSESSMENT

When assessing the victim of penetrating trauma, try to determine the pathway of the penetrating object and the organs that may have been affected by the wounding process. Anticipate the impact of potential organ injury and use this determination in setting priorities for on-scene care or rapid transport of the victim. Remember, however, that a bullet may not travel in a straight line between entrance and exit wounds. Often, a very small shift in a bullet's pathway may mean the difference between tearing open a large blood vessel or missing critical organs completely. The human body is also a dynamic place. The diaphragm moves the kidneys, pancreas, liver, spleen, and heart during respirations, so whether or not these organs are injured may be somewhat dependent on the phase of respiration in which the injury occurs.

It is often hard to anticipate the severity of a projectile wound. Injuries to the large blood vessels, heart, and brain may be immediately or rapidly fatal, while injuries to solid organs (liver, pancreas, kidneys, or spleen) may also be deadly but take more time in working their effects. Consequently, always suspect the worst with bullet wounds that involve the head, chest, or abdomen. Provide rapid transport in these cases, and treat shock aggressively.

PENETRATING WOUND CARE

Certain penetrating wounds need special attention. These include wounds of the face and chest and those involving impaled objects. Their care is described in the following sections; care for other penetrating injuries and shock is discussed in later chapters.

Facial Wounds

Some facial gunshot wounds destroy many airway landmarks (Figure 3-17 ■). With wounds like these, endotracheal intubation is extremely difficult. You might find it helpful to visualize the larynx with the laryngoscope while another rescuer gently presses on the chest. Look for any bubbling during the chest compression, and try to pass the endotracheal tube through the bubbling tissue. Then, very carefully assure that the endotracheal tube is properly placed in the trachea and that lung ventilation is adequate.

If this approach is not effective, two related techniques may restore the airway, at least for long enough to reach more definitive care. These techniques are the **cricothyrotomy** and the **cricothyrostomy.** These emergency surgical or needle airway procedures perforate the membrane between the thyroid and cricoid cartilages, providing a route for ventilation directly into the lower airway. (These techniques are discussed in detail in Chapter 8, "Head, Facial, and Neck Trauma.")

Chest Wounds

The chest wall is rather thick and resilient. It requires a large wound to create an opening big enough to permit free air movement through the chest wall, an open

Provide rapid transport for patients with bullet wounds to the head, chest, or abdomen and treat aggressively for shock.

If endotracheal intubation cannot be accomplished in a patient whose airway landmarks have been destroyed by a gunshot wound, emergency cricothyrotomy or cricothyrostomy may be necessary to create a route for ventilations.

cricothyrotomy   *a surgical incision into the cricothyroid membrane, usually to provide an emergency airway.*

cricothyrostomy   *the introduction of a needle or other tube into the cricothyroid membrane, usually to provide an emergency airway.*

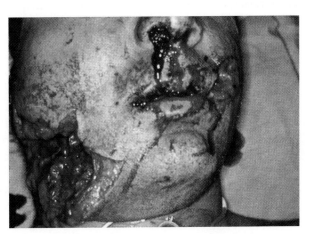

■ Figure 3-17   Facial wounds may distort or destroy airway landmarks. *(Collection of Robert Porter)*

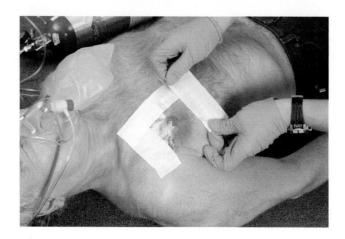

pneumothorax. Wounds caused by small-caliber handguns usually result in no air movement, while wounds caused by shotgun blasts and exiting high-velocity bullets more commonly cause such injuries. If frothy blood is associated with a chest wound, anticipate a developing tension pneumothorax, in which air builds up under pressure within the thorax. Remember, it takes pressure to push air through the wound and froth the blood. If you completely seal the chest wound, you may stop any outward air flow. This can increase both the speed of development of the tension pneumothorax and its severity. Cover any open chest wound with an occlusive dressing sealed on three sides (Figure 3-18 ■). If dyspnea is significant, assess for tension pneumothorax and perform needle decompression as indicated (see Chapter 10, "Thoracic Trauma").

Always consider the possibility of heart and great vessel damage with a penetrating chest wound. These injuries may lead rapidly to severe internal hemorrhage and death. Another serious complication of penetrating chest trauma is pericardial tamponade. This condition occurs when an object or projectile perforates the heart and permits blood to leak into the pericardial sac. As blood accumulates in the sac, the heart no longer fully fills with blood and circulation slows. If pericardial tamponade is uncorrected, the **prognosis** for the patient is very poor. However, a needle introduced into the pericardial space, a procedure available at the emergency department, can quickly alleviate the life threat. Therefore, if you suspect this condition, arrange for rapid transport. The assessment of pericardial tamponade is discussed in Chapter 10, "Thoracic Trauma."

prognosis *the anticipated outcome of a disease or injury.*

Impaled Objects

If an object that causes a low-velocity wound lodges in the body, removal of the object may be dangerous for the patient. If the object bent as it hit a bone upon entry, attempts at removal may cause further injury. If the object is held firmly by soft tissue, it may obstruct blood vessels, thereby restricting blood loss; removal of the object may then increase hemorrhage.

Immobilize impaled objects in place where and as they are found and transport the patient. The only impaled objects that you should remove are those lodged in the cheek or trachea that interfere with the airway or those that you must remove to provide CPR.

Summary

Penetrating injuries, especially those associated with gunshot wounds, are responsible for a high incidence of prehospital trauma and death. Your understanding of the mechanisms of injury that produce these wounds and an understanding of the types of injuries caused by these mechanisms (index of suspicion) can help you rapidly identify serious life threats and assure these patients receive rapid transport to a trauma center. Special prehospital care techniques such as sealing an open pneumothorax and managing a difficult airway can also help you stabilize the patient in the field and help assure that he safely reaches definitive care.

You Make the Call

You are dispatched to a large apartment complex for a "domestic disturbance with injuries." As you pull up to the scene, a bystander states that there were shots fired about 5 minutes ago.
1. What is your first concern?
2. What information is important to gain from your scene size-up?

See Suggested Responses at the back of this book.

Review Questions

1. The tissue displacement caused by the pressure wave that accompanies a bullet as it travels through human tissue is called:
   a. drag.
   b. cavitation.
   c. trajectory.
   d. ballistics.

2. Which of the following would you expect to cause the greatest cavitation?
   a. arrow
   b. ice pick
   c. rifle bullet
   d. handgun bullet

3. Which of the following is considered a high-velocity weapon?
   a. arrow
   b. rifle
   c. shotgun
   d. handgun

4. The characteristics of a bullet determine how much damage it creates as it strikes its target. Which of the following would create the most damage?
   a. a bullet that does not tumble
   b. a bullet that mushrooms when it hits
   c. a small-profile bullet
   d. a full-metal-jacket bullet

5. Which of the following abdominal organs is the most tolerant of the cavitational wave associated with penetrating trauma?
   a. liver
   b. bowel
   c. spleen
   d. kidneys

6. In a puncture wound resulting from a knife or gunshot injury, the paramedic must always examine the patient for:
   a. an exit wound.
   b. epistaxis.
   c. powder burns.
   d. tattooing.

7. Powder burns and crepitus around the entrance generally suggest:
   a. a gun used at close range.
   b. a high-powered rifle.
   c. a handgun.
   d. the use of a black powder.

8. Penetrating trauma is dangerous when it involves the neck because it may cause problems with:
   a. severe hemorrhage.
   b. the airway.
   c. the cervical spine.
   d. all of the above.

9. The path a bullet follows once it is fired is called:
   a. yaw.
   b. drag.
   c. caliber.
   d. trajectory.

10. The forces acting on a bullet to slow it down are called:
    a. yaw.
    b. drag.
    c. profile.
    d. caliber.

See Answers to Review Questions at the back of this book.

Further Reading

Butman, A., S. Martin, R. Vomacka, and N. McSwain. *Comprehensive Guide to Pre-Hospital Skills: A Skills Manual for EMT-Basic, EMT-Intermediate, and EMT-Paramedic.* St. Louis: Mosby, 1996.

Campbell, J., ed. *Basic Trauma Life Support: for Paramedics and Other Advanced Providers.* 5th ed. Upper Saddle River, N.J.: Pearson/Prentice Hall, 2004.

De Lorenzo, Robert A., and Robert S. Porter. *Tactical Emergency Care: Military and Operational Out-of-Hospital Medicine.* Upper Saddle River, N.J.: Pearson/Prentice Hall, 1999.

Di Maio, Vincent, J. *Gunshot Wounds: Practical Aspects of Firearms, Ballistics, and Forensic Techniques.* 2nd ed. New York: CRC Press, 1999.

Ivatury, R.R., and C.G. Cayten. *The Textbook of Penetrating Trauma.* Baltimore: Williams and Wilkins, 1996.

NAEMT (N. McSwain, Jr., S. Frame, and J. Salomone, eds.). *PHTLS: Basic and Advanced Prehospital Trauma Life Support.* 5th ed. St. Louis: Mosby, 2003.

Wilber, Charles G. *Ballistic Science for the Law Enforcement Officer.* Springfield, Ill: Charles C. Thomas, 1977.

On the Web

Visit Brady's Paramedic Website at **www.bradybooks.com/paramedic**.

Hemorrhage and Shock

Objectives

After reading this chapter, you should be able to:

1. Describe the epidemiology, including the morbidity/mortality and prevention strategies, for shock and hemorrhage. (pp. 91–94, 108–113)
2. Discuss the anatomy, physiology, and pathophysiology of the cardiovascular system as they apply to hemorrhage and shock. (pp. 81–84, 101–109)
3. Define shock based on aerobic and anaerobic metabolism. (pp. 101–103)
4. Describe the body's physiological response to changes in blood volume, blood pressure, and perfusion. (pp. 101–113)
5. Describe the effects of decreased perfusion at the capillary level. (pp. 103–105, 108–109)
6. Discuss the cellular ischemic, capillary stagnation, and capillary washout phases related to hemorrhagic shock. (pp. 108–109)
7. Discuss the various types and degrees of shock and hemorrhage. (pp. 91–94, 109–111)
8. Predict shock and hemorrhage based on mechanism of injury. (pp. 94–95, 113)
9. Identify the need for intervention and transport of the patient with hemorrhage or shock. (pp. 94–101, 113–123)
10. Discuss the assessment findings and management of internal and external hemorrhage and shock. (pp. 94–101, 113–123)
11. Differentiate between the administration rate and volume of IV fluid in patients with controlled versus uncontrolled hemorrhage. (pp. 117–119)

12. Relate pulse pressure and orthostatic vital sign changes to perfusion status. (pp. 97–98, 115)

13. Define and differentiate between compensated and decompensated hemorrhagic shock. (pp. 110–111)

14. Discuss the pathophysiological changes, assessment findings, and management associated with compensated and decompensated shock. (pp. 110–111, 113–123)

15. Identify the need for intervention and transport of patients with compensated and decompensated shock. (pp. 113–116)

16. Differentiate among normotensive, hypotensive, or profoundly hypotensive patients. (pp. 113–116)

17. Describe differences in administration of intravenous fluid in the normotensive, hypotensive, or profoundly hypotensive patients. (pp. 117–119)

18. Discuss the physiological changes associated with application and inflation of the pneumatic anti-shock garment (PASG). (pp. 120–121, 122)

19. Discuss the indications and contraindications for the application and inflation of the PASG. (pp. 120–121)

20. Given several preprogrammed and moulaged hemorrhage and shock patients, provide the appropriate scene size-up, initial assessment, rapid trauma or focused physical exam and history, detailed exam, and ongoing assessment and provide appropriate patient care and transportion. (pp. 81–123)

Key Terms

adrenocorticotropic hormone, p. 108
aerobic metabolism, p. 102
afterload, p. 82
aggregate, p. 85
aldosterone, p. 107
anaerobic, p. 89
anaerobic metabolism, p. 102
anaphylactic shock, p. 112
anemia, p. 91
angiotensin, p. 107
antidiuretic hormone (ADH), p. 107
arteries, p. 82
arteriole, p. 83
baroreceptor, p. 106
capillary, p. 83
cardiac output, p. 82
cardioacceleratory center, p. 106
cardiogenic shock, p. 112
cardioinhibitory center, p. 106
catecholamine, p. 92
chemoreceptor, p. 106

citric acid cycle, p. 102
clotting, p. 85
coagulation, p. 85
compensated shock, p. 110
decompensated shock, p. 110
diastolic blood pressure, p. 103
direct pressure, p. 88
distributive shock, p. 111
epistaxis, p. 90
erythrocyte, p. 84
erythropoietin, p. 108
esophageal varices, p. 91
fascia, p. 89
fibrin, p. 86
glucagon, p. 102
glucocorticoids, p. 108
glycogen, p. 107
glycogenolysis, p. 107
glycolysis, p. 102
growth hormone, p. 108
hematochezia, p. 97
hematocrit, p. 84
hematoma, p. 89
hemoglobin, p. 84

hemorrhage, p. 81
histamine, p. 104
homeostasis, p. 81
hydrostatic pressure, p. 109
hypovolemic shock, p. 111
insulin, p. 102
interstitial space, p. 83
irreversible shock, p. 111
ischemia, p. 109
Krebs cycle, p. 102
lactic acid, p. 89
leukocyte, p. 84
melena, p. 91
metabolism, p. 101
microcirculation, p. 104
neurogenic shock, p. 113
obstructive shock, p. 112
orthostatic hypotension, p. 97
overdrive respiration, p. 116
parasympathetic nervous system, p. 81
peripheral vascular resistance, p. 83

Case Study

City Ambulance 1 receives a mutual aid alert. A Basic Life Support ambulance needs assistance in a neighboring community. A bulldozer has overturned, trapping a 39-year-old male.

Upon arrival at the scene, paramedic Dave and his junior partner Ed take a report from the two EMT-Basics about the patient, a man named Ken. They then assess the patient themselves and find him alert and oriented. Ken's airway and breathing appear normal as do the rate and strength of his pulse. His pelvis and lower extremities are pinned under the side of the bulldozer. The rescue team informs the paramedic crew that it will be at least 10 minutes until they can lift and remove the bulldozer. Dave concludes the initial assessment and detects no signs of problems with airway, breathing, or circulation. The EMTs have already administered oxygen at 15 liters per minute, using a nonrebreather mask.

Next, Dave provides a rapid trauma assessment as part of the focused history and physical examination. Ken's breath sounds are good, but he cannot feel his feet. From looking at the positions of the bulldozer and the patient, Dave strongly suspects a pelvic fracture and expects increased hemorrhage to occur when the heavy machine is lifted. Ed reports vital sign findings of blood pressure 110/68, pulse 90, respirations 24, and an oxygen saturation of 99 percent.

Dave then quickly establishes two IVs of normal saline, both infusing at a to-keep-open rate. Ed prepares a backboard and a pelvic sling for the anticipated pelvic injury. As the lifting equipment is readied, the paramedics talk with Ken, explaining the various steps in the operation. Ed rechecks vital signs every 5 minutes, and Dave documents that the vital signs and oxygen saturation remain stable.

The extrication team slowly begins to lift the bulldozer. Dave and Ed rush to position the patient on the prepared backboard. It quickly becomes apparent that Ken has suffered fractures of the pelvis, both femurs, and the left tibia. Very little external hemorrhage is noted. Ed firmly secures the pelvic sling around the unstable pelvis.

Ken reports an increase in pain, becomes restless, and attempts to get up. He then becomes lethargic. The pulse oximeter reveals that oxygen saturation has dropped to 94 percent and then reads erratically. The pulse rate is up to 130 very weak beats per minute, and the systolic blood pressure is now 80 mmHg. Both IVs are set to run wide open to administer a 500-mL fluid bolus. With time, Ken's level of consciousness improves, but his pulse rate remains elevated.

Upon arrival at the hospital, Ken's systolic blood pressure remains around 80 and the heart rate is tachycardic. A repeat fluid bolus is adminstered. The ED team starts type O-negative blood and replaces one of the field IVs. Within 20 minutes, the team transports the patient into surgery.

Ken comes through the surgery well. Because of the multiple fractures, however, his rehabilitation will continue for more than a year.

INTRODUCTION TO HEMORRHAGE AND SHOCK

The loss of the body's most important and dynamic medium, blood, is called **hemorrhage.** Acute and continuing loss of blood adversely impacts the body's ability to provide oxygen and essential nutrients to the cells, while at the same time removing carbon dioxide and other waste products from the body's elemental building blocks, the cells. In the absence of an adequate volume of circulating blood, the cells and the organs begin to function less effectively and can ultimately fail. If allowed to progress untreated, the organism itself may die. The transition between normal function (**homeostasis**) and death is called **shock.** The ability to recognize hemorrhage and shock and to care for these are critical skills for the EMT-Paramedic and are essential to reducing mortality and morbidity in trauma patients. This chapter provides you with an understanding of the cardiovascular system as it relates to hemorrhage and shock and then describes how to recognize and care for these life-threatening assaults on the human body.

hemorrhage *an abnormal internal or external discharge of blood.*

homeostasis *the natural tendency of the body to maintain a steady and normal internal environment.*

shock *a state of inadequate tissue perfusion.*

The EMT-Paramedic must be able to recognize hemorrhage and shock in trauma patients in order to reduce mortality and morbidity.

Hemorrhage is the most common cause of shock and death in trauma patients.

HEMORRHAGE

Hemorrhage is the loss or escape of blood from the vascular space. This loss can be either internal or external and reduces the blood volume within the circulatory system until the heart is no longer able to pump it to the body's cells. Hemorrhage is a frequent consequence of trauma; it is also the most common cause of shock and death in trauma patients. External hemorrhage is, in most cases, easy to recognize and control. Internal hemorrhage, however, may present with only subtle signs and symptoms, and only surgical intervention can halt the blood loss.

THE CIRCULATORY SYSTEM

The circulatory system has three basic components: the heart, the blood vessels, and the blood. Each plays an important role in maintaining the body's cells and in responding to hemorrhage and shock.

The Heart

The heart is a two-sided muscular pump with four valves that define four chambers. It contracts in a coordinated manner as managed by a small system of specialized tissue that constitutes the cardiac conductive system. The heart provides most of the driving force to move the blood through the cardiovascular system. The heart's output of blood, the cardiac output, is determined by the volume of blood ejected with each ventricular contraction (the stroke volume) and the number of contractions per minute (the heart rate). The heart rate is regulated by two divisions of the autonomic nervous system. The **parasympathetic nervous system** slows the rate through stimulation of the vagus nerve. The **sympathetic nervous system** increases the rate through stimulation of the cardiac plexus.

parasympathetic nervous system *division of the autonomic nervous system that is responsible for controlling vegetative functions.*

sympathetic nervous system *division of the autonomic nervous system that prepares the body for stressful situations.*

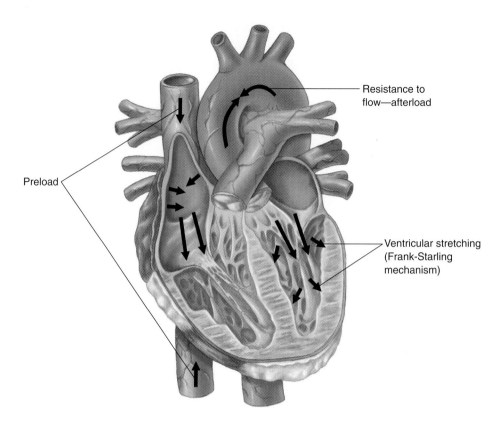

■ **Figure 4-1** Factors affecting cardiac output.

stroke volume *the amount of blood ejected by the heart in one cardiac contraction.*

preload *the pressure within the ventricles at the end of diastole; the volume of blood delivered to the atria prior to ventricular diastole.*

Starling's law of the heart *the law that an increase in cardiac output occurs in proportion to the diastolic stretch of the heart muscle fibers.*

afterload *the resistance a contraction of the heart must overcome in order to eject blood; in cardiac physiology, defined as the tension of cardiac muscle during systole (contraction).*

arteries *vessels that carry blood from the heart to the body tissues.*

cardiac output *the amount of blood pumped by the heart in 1 minute (computed as stroke volume × heart rate).*

Stroke volume, as previously noted, is the amount of blood pumped out of the ventricle with each cardiac contraction. Three elements affect stroke volume: preload, cardiac contractility, and afterload (Figure 4-1 ■). **Preload** is the pressure of returning blood from the venous system. As venous pressure rises, the rate of blood return to the heart increases, stretching the wall of the ventricle as it fills. The more the ventricle is stretched (up to a point), the greater the subsequent myocardial contractility and the strength at which blood is ejected by the ventricle. The increase in cardiac contractility due to myocardial muscle stretching is called **Starling's law of the heart** and results in greater stroke volume. Stroke volume is also affected by arterial tone. The greater the resistance against which the heart pumps—the **afterload**—the slower the flow of blood into the **arteries** and the lower the cardiac output.

The normal heart, at rest, beats about 70 times per minute and moves about 70 mL of blood with each beat. The volume of blood moved by the heart in 1 minute is referred to as **cardiac output.** This volume can be expressed, usually in liters, by the following formula:

$$\text{Stroke Volume} \times \text{Heart Rate} = \text{Cardiac Output}$$
$$70 \text{ mL} \times 70 \text{ bpm} = 4{,}900 \text{ mL } (4.9 \text{ L})$$

The normal cardiac output is about 5 L/minute. This blood is pumped directly into the aorta and distributed by major arteries to the entire body. During physical exercise or stress, the cardiac output may increase six- or sevenfold in a healthy, well-conditioned adult.

The Vascular System

The vascular system is a series of hollow tubes designed to distribute blood to and from body tissues. It consists of three types of vessels—arteries, capillaries, and veins (Figure 4-2 ■).

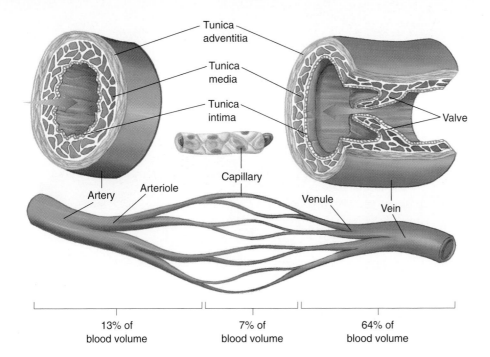

Tunica adventitia

Tunica media

Tunica intima

Valve

Artery Arteriole Capillary Venule Vein

| 13% of blood volume | 7% of blood volume | 64% of blood volume |

■ **Figure 4-2** The vascular system is a network of flexible continuous tubing running from the heart to the body's tissues and back. Arteries distribute oxygenated blood, capillaries are the sites of oxygen-nutrient/waste product exchange, and veins return blood to the heart.

Arteries   Arteries contain about 13 percent of the total blood volume and direct its distribution to the various body organs. They consist of three distinct tissue layers surrounding their internal opening, or lumen. The outer layer is the **tunica adventitia,** a layer of strong, fibrous, nonstretching tissue that forms the artery's outer wall. It determines the artery's maximum diameter. Between the adventitia and the vessel's internal lining is the **tunica media,** a muscular layer. This muscular layer plays a very important role in determining the amount of blood flow through the vessel. When the tunica media constricts, it reduces the arterial lumen and the flow of blood. As the arteries direct blood farther from the heart, their lumens become smaller, the amount of fibrous aventitia decreases, and the proportion of tunica media increases. The smallest of arteries, the **arterioles,** have the greatest ability to vary the size of their internal lumens and thus control blood flow to the organs they supply. In concert, the arteries determine the **peripheral vascular resistance** (also called afterload) against which the heart pumps. The innermost lining of the blood vessel is the **tunica intima.** It is endothelial tissue that provides a smooth inner surface to the blood vessel and prevents any absorption of nutrients from the blood within the vessel's lumen.

Capillaries   The body's capillary network contains 7 percent of the vascular volume and extends to all body cells, assuring blood flow through the tissues. This capillary flow provides essential nutrients and oxygen and removes waste products, including carbon dioxide. The **capillaries** are microscopic vessels only large enough for red blood cells to pass through in single file. This assures a free-flowing nutrient and waste exchange between the bloodstream, the **interstitial spaces,** and the body cells. The capillary walls lack the connective and muscular layers of the arteries and veins. The walls are but one cell thick, allowing efficient diffusion of gases and metabolic substrates.

Veins   Veins are responsible for collecting blood and directing it back to the heart. They are vessels with relatively large lumens, normally twice the diameter of their associated arteries. As a result, the pressure within the vein is much less than that within the artery and, hence, the fluid flow rate is reduced. The vein wall has little musculature and only a modest amount of connective tunica adventitia. This portion of the cardiovascular system contains 64 percent of the total blood volume. Although vein

tunica adventitia   *outer fibrous layer of the blood vessels that maintains their maximum size.*

tunica media   *the middle, muscular layer of the blood vessels that controls the vessel lumen size.*

arteriole   *a small artery.*

peripheral vascular resistance   *the resistance of the vessels to the flow of blood; it increases when the vessels constrict and decreases when the vessels relax.*

tunica intima   *smooth interior layer of the blood vessels that provides for the free flow of blood.*

capillary   *one of the minute blood vessels that connect the ends of arterioles with the beginnings of venules; where oxygen is diffused to body tissue and products of metabolism enter the bloodstream.*

interstitial space   *the space between cells.*

vein   *a blood vessel that carries blood toward the heart.*

■ Figure 4-3   Blood components.

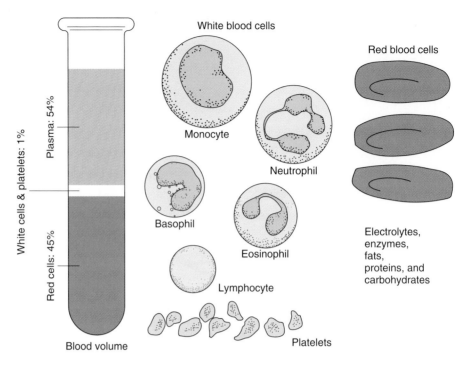

Plasma: 54%

White cells & platelets: 1%

Red cells: 45%

Blood volume

White blood cells

Monocyte

Basophil

Neutrophil

Eosinophil

Lymphocyte

Platelets

Red blood cells

Electrolytes, enzymes, fats, proteins, and carbohydrates

erythrocyte   *peripheral blood cell that contains hemoglobin; responsible for transport of oxygen to the cells.*

hemoglobin   *an iron-based compound found in red blood cells that binds with oxygen and transport it to body cells.*

hematocrit   *the percentage of the blood consisting of the red blood cells, or erythrocytes.*

platelet   *one of the fragments of cytoplasm that circulate in the blood and work with components of the coagulation system to promote blood clotting. Platelets also release serotonin, a vasoconstrictive substance.*

leukocyte   *one of the white blood cells, which play key roles in the body's immune system and inflammatory (infection-fighting) responses.*

 Review

Content

Types of Hemorrhage

Capillary
Venous
Arterial

musculature is limited, if the venous vessels constrict, they return a relatively large blood volume to the active circulation. This constriction can contribute up to 1 liter or about 20 percent of the circulating blood volume to the active circulation. Venous constriction can respond quickly and effectively to small volumes of blood loss. The venous system is also called the capacitance system because it holds and controls such a large portion of the circulating blood volume.

The Blood

Blood is the precious medium circulated by the cardiovascular system that is immediately essential to life. It is a slurry of cells, protein, water, and suspended elements (Figure 4-3 ■). The major blood cell—and the most common—is the red blood cell, or **erythrocyte.** It contains **hemoglobin,** a molecule to which oxygen attaches at the pressures found in the pulmonary tissue and from which it is released at the pressures found in the systemic capillary network. Hence, the red blood cell serves as an efficient transporter of oxygen from the lungs to body cells. It also plays a role in the transport of carbon dioxide from the cells to the lungs. Erythrocytes make up about 45 percent of the total blood volume (**hematocrit**), with the other cells accounting for less than 1 percent. The second most frequent blood cell type is the **platelet,** a small, irregularly shaped cytoplasm fragment important for clotting and the repair of blood vessels. White blood cells, or **leukocytes,** are large cells, varied in structure, that are part of the immune system. They engulf cells recognized as foreign to the human system, then die, killing the invading cells and permitting the body to dispose of such invaders. The blood serum is a watery mixture of proteins, salts, and other necessary components.

HEMORRHAGE CLASSIFICATION

As noted previously, hemorrhage is loss of blood from the closed vascular system because of injury to the blood vessels. Hemorrhage is usually classified based on the injured vessel from which it flows: capillary, venous, or arterial (Figure 4-4 ■).

CAPILLARY	**VENOUS**	**ARTERIAL**

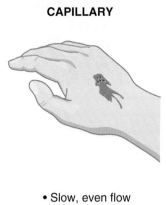 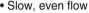 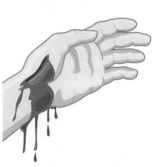 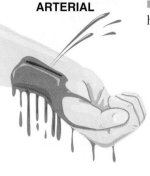

■ Figure 4-4 Types of hemorrhage.

- Slow, even flow
- Bright red color

- Steady, slow flow
- Dark red color

- Spurting blood
- Pulsating flow
- Bright red color

Capillary hemorrhage generally oozes from the wound, normally an abrasion, and clots quickly on its own. The blood is usually bright red because it is well oxygenated.

Venous hemorrhage flows more quickly, though it, too, generally stops in a few minutes. Bleeding associated with venous hemorrhage is generally dark red because the blood has already given up its oxygen as it passed though the capillary beds.

Bleeding associated with arterial hemorrhage flows very rapidly, often spurting from the wound. This blood is well oxygenated and appears bright red as it escapes from the wound. The blood volume lost can be extreme because of the pressure behind arterial bleeding. The spurting nature of arterial hemorrhage results from the variations in the blood pressure driving the blood loss.

While it is convenient to determine the type of hemorrhage, the nature and depth of a wound may make it hard to differentiate between heavy venous and arterial bleeding. Internal hemorrhage cannot be classified by type with the diagnostic techniques available to paramedics providing prehospital care.

CLOTTING

The body's response to local hemorrhage is a complex three-step process called **clotting** (Figure 4-5 ■). As a blood vessel is torn and begins to lose blood, its smooth muscle contracts. This reduces its lumen and the volume and strength of blood flow through it. This is called the **vascular phase.**

At the same time, the vessel's smooth interior lining (the tunica intima) is disrupted, causing a turbulent blood flow. The turbulent blood flow within the vessel attracts platelets. Factors released at the time of hemorrhage make the platelets "sticky," or adherent. Platelets then stick to collagen, a protein fiber found in connective tissue, on the vessel's injured inner surface, and to other injured tissue in the area. The blood vessel walls also become adherent. If they are small enough, like capillaries, they may stick together, further occluding blood flow. As platelets adhere to the vessel walls, they **aggregate,** or collect, other platelets. This is the **platelet phase,** the second step of the clotting process. These events occur almost immediately after injury and effectively halt hemorrhage from capillaries and small venous and arterial vessels. While this is a rapid method of hemorrhage control, the resulting clot is unstable.

As time passes, the wound initiates the third and final step of the process, **coagulation.** In this phase, clotting factors are activated and released into the bloodstream, initiating a complex sequence of events. These clotting factors come from the damaged

It may be hard to differentiate between heavy venous and arterial bleeding in the field; likewise, paramedics cannot classify internal hemorrhage by type when providing prehospital care.

clotting *the body's three-step response to stop the loss of blood.*

vascular phase *step in the clotting process in which smooth blood vessel muscle contracts, reducing the vessel lumen and the flow of blood through it.*

⊘ **Review**

Phases of the Clotting Process

Vascular phase
Platelet phae
Coagulation

aggregate *to cluster or come together.*

platelet phase *second step in the clotting process in which platelets adhere to blood vessel walls and to each other.*

coagulation *the third step in the clotting process, which involves the formation of a protein called fibrin that forms a network around a wound to stop bleeding, ward off infection, and lay a foundation for healing and repair of the wound.*

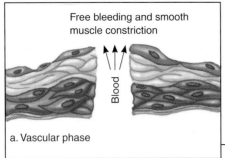

Free bleeding and smooth
muscle constriction

Blood

a. Vascular phase

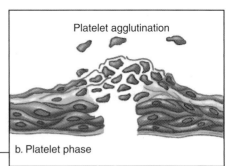

Platelet agglutination

b. Platelet phase

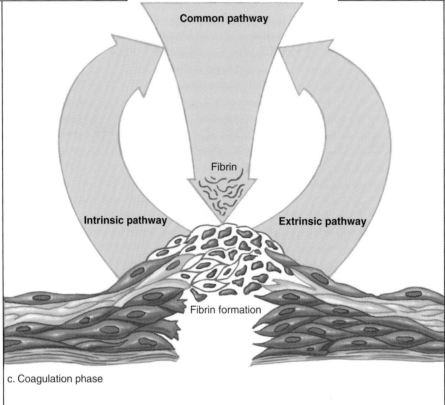

Common pathway

Fibrin

Intrinsic pathway

Extrinsic pathway

Fibrin formation

c. Coagulation phase

■ Figure 4-5   The three steps of the clotting process are the vascular phase, the platelet phase, and coagulation.

fibrin *protein fibers that trap red blood cells as part of the clotting process.*

blood vessel and surrounding tissue (the extrinsic pathway), from the damaged platelets (the intrinsic pathway), or from both. The release of the clotting factors triggers a series of chemical reactions that result in the formation of strong protein fibers, or **fibrin.** These fibers entrap red blood cells and form a stronger, more durable clot. This further collection of cells halts all but the most severe hemorrhage. Coagulation normally takes from 7 to 10 minutes. Over time, the cells trapped in the clot protein matrix slowly contract, drawing the wound and the injured vessel together.

The nature of the wound also affects how rapidly and well the clotting mechanisms respond to hemorrhage (Figure 4-6 ■). If the wound cuts the vessel cleanly in a transverse fashion, the muscles of the vessel wall contract. This retracts the vessel into the surrounding tissues, thickening the now shortened tunica media. This thickening further reduces the vessel's lumen, reduces blood flow, and assists the clotting mechanism. If the blood vessel is lacerated longitudinally rather than transversely, the smooth muscle contraction pulls the vessel open. The vessel does not withdraw and the lumen does

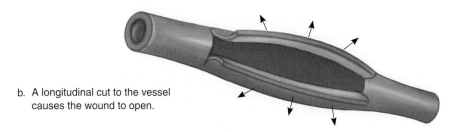

a. A clean lateral cut permits the vessel to retract and thicken its wall.

b. A longitudinal cut to the vessel causes the wound to open.

■ Figure 4-6 The type of blood vessel injury often affects the nature of the hemorrhage.

not constrict. The result is heavy and continued bleeding. Crushing trauma often produces this type of damage. The vessels are not torn cleanly and do not withdraw. The actual hemorrhage site is lost in the disrupted tissue, resulting in severe, hard-to-control bleeding from a large wound area.

If a severe hemorrhage continues, frank hypotension reduces the blood pressure at the hemorrhage site. This limits the flow of blood and enhances the development of clots, thus improving the effectiveness of the clotting mechanism.

FACTORS AFFECTING THE CLOTTING PROCESS

The clotting process can be either helped or hindered by a variety of factors. For example, movement at or around the wound site, as in the manipulation of a fracture, may break the developing clot loose and disrupt the forming fibrin strands. For this reason, immediate wound immobilization (splinting) is beneficial.

Aggressive fluid therapy, which is often provided in cases of severe hemorrhage, may adversely impact the effectiveness of clotting mechanisms. Aggressive fluid resuscitation may increase blood pressure, which in turn increases the pressure pushing against the developing clots. In addition, the water and salts used in fluid therapy dilute the clotting factors and platelets, further inhibiting the clotting process.

The patient's body temperature also has an effect on the clotting process. As the body temperature begins to fall, as it may in shock states, clot formation is neither as rapid nor as effective as when the body temperature is 37° C (98.6° F) degrees. Thus, it is important to keep a patient with severe hemorrhage warm.

Medications may interfere with the body's ability to form a clot and halt both internal and external hemorrhage. Aspirin modifies the enzymes on the surface of platelets that cause them to aggregate after an injury. Aspirin, ibuprofen, and other NSAIDs (nonsteroidal anti-inflammatory drugs) may have a similar but temporary effect. Heparin and warfarin (Coumadin) interfere with the normal generation of protein fibers that produce a stable clot. While these drugs may prevent thrombosis and emboli in patients with heart disease, they may prolong or worsen hemorrhage when

⊘ **Review**

Factors Hindering the Clotting Process

Movement of the wound site
Aggressive fluid therapy
Low body temperature
Medications such as aspirin, heparin, or Coumadin

Immediate immobilization (splinting) of the wound site aids the clotting process.

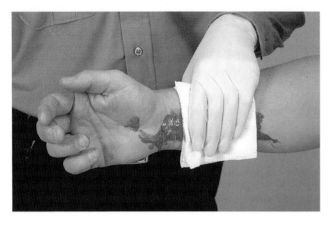

■ **Figure 4-7a** Hemorrhage control: apply direct pressure.

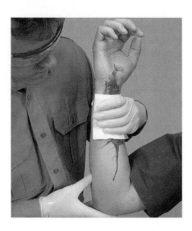

■ **Figure 4-7b** Hemorrhage control: elevate the extremity above the level of the heart.

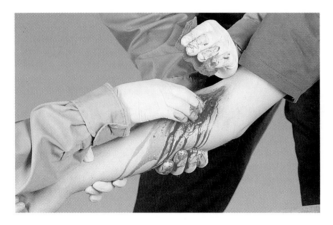

■ **Figure 4-7c** Hemorrhage control: if bleeding does not stop, apply direct fingertip pressure.

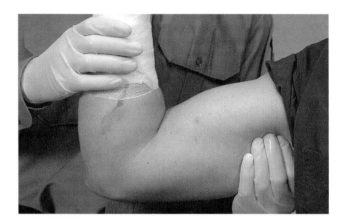

■ **Figure 4-7d** Hemorrhage control: if bleeding continues, apply pressure to a pressure point.

that patient is injured. Try to gather information on whether the patient uses such medications when taking the patient history.

HEMORRHAGE CONTROL

Hemorrhage is either internal or external. While there are a number of steps you can take to control external hemorrhage in the field, prehospital care of internal hemorrhage is more limited.

External Hemorrhage

direct pressure *method of hemorrhage control that relies on the application of pressure to the actual site of the bleeding.*

External hemorrhage is easy to identify and care for. It presents with blood oozing, flowing, or spurting from the wound. Bleeding from capillary and venous wounds is easy to halt because the pressure driving it is limited (Figure 4-7 ■). Usually **direct pressure** on the wound or a combination of direct pressure and elevation work quite well in stopping the bleeding. Bleeding from an arterial wound, however, is powered by the arterial blood pressure and escapes from the blood vessel with significant force. The normal control and clotting mechanisms help reduce blood loss but do not stop it if the injured vessel is large. To stop bleeding from such a wound, pressure on the bleeding site must exceed the arterial pressure. Direct digital pressure on the site of blood loss, maintained by a dressing and pressure bandage, is most effective. Elevation of the wound area and use of pressure points may also be necessary if the bandage cannot apply enough pressure directly to the hemorrhage site.

Be extremely cautious if you consider using a **tourniquet.** Employ the device *only* to halt persistent, life-threatening hemorrhage. If you apply the tourniquet at a pressure less than the arterial pressure, blood continues to flow into the limb, while the tourniquet restricts venous flow out. The limb's arterial and venous pressures then rise, as does the rate of hemorrhage. If the tourniquet meets its objective and halts all blood flow to the limb, blood loss stops, but so does circulation to the distal extremity. During this absence of perfusion, **lactic acid,** potassium, and other **anaerobic** metabolites accumulate in the stagnant blood. When the tourniquet is released, the resumption of blood flow may transport these toxins into the central circulation with devastating results (Figure 4-8 ■). Once you apply the tourniquet, therefore, leave it in place until the patient is in the emergency department or some other facility where the negative effects of reperfusion can be addressed. If you must apply a tourniquet, use a wide cravat or belt or a blood pressure cuff. A thin or narrow constricting device may damage tissue beneath the tourniquet. Despite these hazards, the tourniquet may be essential in halting life-threatening arterial hemorrhage.

Internal Hemorrhage

Internal hemorrhage is associated with almost all serious blunt and penetrating trauma. As with external hemorrhage, internal hemorrhage can involve capillary, venous, or arterial blood loss. The blood can accumulate in the tissue itself, forming a visible or hidden contusion, or it can be forced between **fascia** and form a pocket of blood called a **hematoma.** In most of these cases, the hemorrhage is self-limiting because the pressure within the tissue or fascia controls the blood loss. However, large contusions, massive soft-tissue injuries, and large hematomas, especially those affecting large muscle masses like the thighs or buttocks, can account for moderate blood and body fluid loss. Fractures of the humerus and tibia/fibula may account for 500 to 750 mL of loss, while femur fractures may account for up to 1,500 mL of loss.

In body cavities such as the chest and the abdominal, pelvic, and retroperitoneal spaces, the resistance to continuing blood loss does not develop. With bleeding in these areas, loss continues unabated until the normal clotting process is effective, the blood pressure drops significantly, or surgical intervention is provided. The best indicators of significant internal hemorrhage are the mechanism of injury (MOI), local signs and symptoms of injury, and the early signs and symptoms of blood loss and shock. If a patient has sustained significant trauma to the chest, abdomen, or pelvis, anticipate significant, continuing, and uncontrolled blood loss. Such a patient requires rapid transport to a trauma center or hospital for surgical repair of any damaged vessels or organs. Recent evidence suggests that the mechanism of injury may not be as good a predictor of injury severity as once thought. MOI is best used when coupled with careful evaluation of vital signs and other physical signs of injury.

You can assist the natural internal hemorrhage control mechanisms in the extremities by providing a patient with immobilization and elevation. Continued movement of the injury site, especially if it is associated with a long bone fracture, disrupts the clotting process, causing further soft-tissue, nervous, and vascular damage, and continuing the blood loss. If the patient is a victim of serious or multisystem trauma, however, do not spend time on the scene with aggressive skeletal immobilization. Instead, quickly splint the patient to a long spine board and begin transport. Provide splinting of individual limbs if time permits during transport.

Internal hemorrhage is often associated with injuries to specific organs and can be related either to trauma or to preexisting medical problems. Internal hemorrhage can also present with external signs of injury or disease in addition to the signs and symptoms of blood loss. These signs can help you identify the nature and location of the blood loss.

tourniquet *a constrictor used on an extremity to apply circumferential pressure on all arteries to control bleeding.*

lactic acid *compound produced from pyruvic acid during anaerobic glycolysis.*

anaerobic *able to live without oxygen.*

Use a tourniquet only as a last resort to halt persistent, life-threatening hemorrhage.

fascia *a fibrous membrane that covers, supports, and separates muscles and may also unite the skin with underlying tissue.*

hematoma *collection of blood beneath the skin or trapped within a body compartment.*

Provide a patient with suspected internal bleeding with immobilization and elevation (of extremities) to aid the body's hemorrhage control mechanisms.

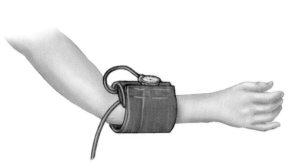

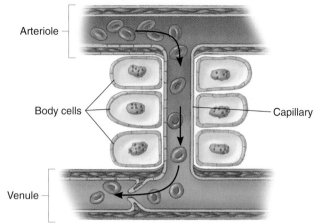

Arteriole

Body cells

Capillary

Venule

a. Blood pressure cuff positioned but not inflated. Normal blood flow.

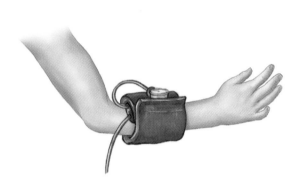

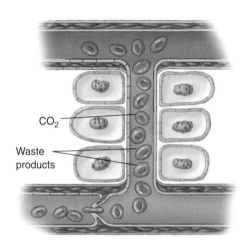

CO_2

Waste products

b. Inflation of B/P cuff as a tourniquet cuts off circulation. Blood flow stagnates and metabolic by-products accumulate

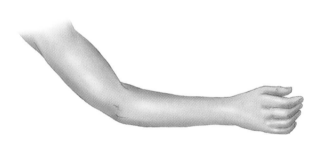

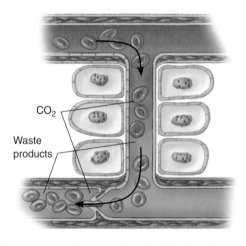

CO_2

Waste products

c. Release of cuff restores circulation. Returning blood flow pushes acidic by-products back into the central circulation.

■ Figure 4-8   Release of a tourniquet may send accumulated toxins into the central circulation with devastating results for the patient.

epistaxis   *bleeding from the nose resulting from injury, disease, or environmental factors; a nosebleed.*

The nasal cavity is lined with a rich supply of capillaries to warm and help humidify incoming air. Hypertension, a strong sneeze, or direct trauma may rupture the vessels supplying these capillary beds and produce the moderate to severe hemorrhage called **epistaxis.** Prolonged epistaxis can result in hypovolemia, while blood flowing down the posterior nasal cavity, down the esophagus, and into the stomach may result

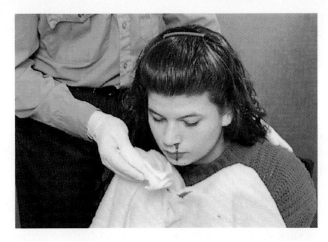

■ **Figure 4-9a** To control nosebleed, have the patient sit leaning forward.

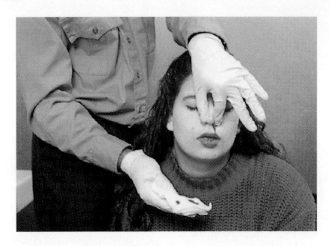

■ **Figure 4-9b** Pinch the fleshy part of the patient's nostrils firmly together.

in nausea, followed by vomiting (Figure 4-9 ■). Trauma to the oral cavity may likewise result in serious hemorrhage, followed by ingestion of blood, nausea, and then emesis.

There are also outward signs that indicate hemorrhage in the lungs and respiratory system. For example, degenerative diseases, such as tuberculosis or cancer, or chest trauma may rupture pulmonary vessels. This leads to the release of blood into the lower airways or alveolar space. The patient may then cough up bright red blood, a sign called hemoptysis.

Trauma, caustic ingestion, degenerative disease (for example, cancer), and ruptur-ing **esophageal varices** may lead to hemorrhage along the esophagus. In these condi-tions, blood is likely to travel, via peristalsis, into the stomach, where it collects. Gastric hemorrhage due to ulceration or trauma may also result in the accumulation of blood in the stomach. A significant collection of blood acts as a gastric irritant, inducing vom-iting. If the blood is evacuated early, it is bright red in color. If blood remains in the stomach for some time, emesis resembles coffee grounds in both color and consistency.

esophageal varices *enlarged and tortuous esophageal veins.*

Hemorrhage in the small or large bowel can be associated with trauma, degenera-tive disease, or diverticulosis (small pouches in the walls of the bowel begin to hemor-rhage). Bowel hemorrhage may present as bleeding from the rectum, or the blood may be digested before release, producing a black and tarry stool called **melena.**

Rectal injury may be caused by pelvic fracture or direct trauma. This presents with bleeding, which may be severe.

melena *black, tar-like feces due to gastrointestinal bleeding.*

Vaginal hemorrhage may be associated with trauma, degenerative disease, men-struation, ectopic pregnancy, placenta previa, and potential or actual miscarriage. Ure-thral hemorrhage is generally minor and may reflect damage to the prostate or urethra. Blood in the urine may indicate injury to the genitourinary tract.

Nontraumatic forms of hemorrhage may be either acute or chronic. Acute hemor-rhage moves the victim rapidly toward shock and is quickly recognizable. Chronic he-morrhage is likely to be rather limited in volume, but it does continue over time. The resulting loss depletes the body of red blood cells and leads to **anemia.** This condition reduces the blood's oxygen-carrying capacity, and the patient experiences fatigue and lethargy. Clotting factors may likewise be depleted, which reduces the blood's ability to coagulate and makes any secondary hemorrhage more difficult to control.

anemia *a reduction in the hemoglobin content in the blood to a point below that required to meet the oxygen requirements of the body.*

STAGES OF HEMORRHAGE

Fluid accounts for about 60 percent of the body's weight and is distributed among the cellular, interstitial, and vascular spaces. The cells contain about 62 percent of the total fluid volume, while the interstitial (nonvascular) space holds 26 percent. Four to five percent of body fluid is found in other spaces such as the ventricles of the brain and meninges (cerebrospinal fluid). The remaining 7 percent of fluid volume resides in the vascular space. This fluid, called plasma, and the blood cells account for 7 percent of the average adult male's body weight (about 6.5 percent in the female). Fluid in the vascular space is distributed among the heart, arteries, veins, and capillaries and accounts for 5 liters (10 units) of blood volume in the healthy 70-kg adult male.

The effects of hemorrhage can be categorized into four progressive stages as blood volume is lost. These stages relate to the volume of blood lost in acute hemorrhage and that result in "classic" signs and symptoms. Remember, however, that each individual's response to blood loss may vary as may the rate and progress of the loss. Use these categories to help determine the relative severity of the loss and the need for intervention. It is also important to identify the following: the length of time elapsed since the incident that caused the trauma; the stage of hemorrhage the victim is in when you arrive at his side; and how quickly the patient is moving from one stage to another (Table 4–1).

Stage 1 Hemorrhage

Stage 1 hemorrhage is a blood loss of up to 15 percent of the circulating blood volume. In the 70-kg male that is approximately 500 to 750 mL of blood, about the amount you might give during a blood drive. The healthy human system can easily compensate for such a blood loss volume by constricting the vascular beds, especially on the venous side. In this stage, the blood pressure remains constant as do the **pulse pressure,** respiratory rate, and urine output. The central venous pressure may drop slightly, but it returns to normal quickly. The pulse rate elevates slightly, and the patient may display some signs of **catecholamine** (epinephrine and norepinephrine) release, notably nervousness and marginally cool skin with a slight pallor.

Stage 2 Hemorrhage

Stage 2 hemorrhage occurs as 15 to 25 percent (750 to 1,250 mL) of the blood volume is lost. The body's first-line compensatory responses can no longer maintain blood pressure, and secondary mechanisms are now employed. Tachycardia becomes very evident, and the pulse strength begins to diminish (the pulse pressure is noticeably narrowed). A strong release of catecholamines increases peripheral vascular resistance. This maintains systolic blood pressure but results in peripheral vasoconstriction and cool, clammy skin. Anxiety increases, and the patient may begin to display restlessness and thirst. Thirst is present as fluid leaves the intracellular and interstitial spaces and the osmotic pressure of the blood changes. Renal output remains normal, but the respiratory rate increases.

Stage 3 Hemorrhage

Stage 3 hemorrhage occurs when blood loss reaches 25 to 35 percent of blood volume (1,250 to 1,750 mL). The body's compensatory mechanisms are unable to cope with the

With hemorrhage patients, determine the relative severity of blood loss, the need for aggressive intervention, the length of time since the incident that caused the trauma, the current stage of hemorrhage, and how quickly the patient is moving from one stage to another.

pulse pressure *difference between the systolic and diastolic blood pressures.*

catecholamine *a hormone, such as epinephrine or norepinephrine, that strongly affects the nervous and cardiovascular systems, metabolic rate, temperature, and smooth muscle.*

Without rapid intervention, survival of a stage 3 hemorrhage patient is unlikely.

Table 4–1		Patient Signs Associated with Stages of Hemorrhage						
Stage	Blood Loss	Vasoconstriction	Pulse Rate	Pulse (Pressure) Strength	Blood Pressure	Respiratory Rate	Respiratory Volume
1	<15%	↑	↑	→	→	→	→
2	15–25%	↑↑	↑↑	↓	→	↑	↑
3	25–35%	↑↑↑	↑↑↑	↓↓	↓	↑↑	↓
4	>35%	↓↓	Variable	↓↓↓	↓↓↓	↓	↓↓

loss, and the classic signs of shock appear. Rapid tachycardia is present as the blood pressure begins to fall. The pulse is barely palpable as the pulse pressure remains very narrow. The patient experiences air hunger and tachypnea. Anxiety, restlessness, and thirst become more severe. The level of responsiveness decreases, and the patient becomes very pale, cool, and diaphoretic. Urinary output declines. Without rapid intervention, this patient's survival is unlikely.

Stage 4 Hemorrhage

Stage 4 hemorrhage occurs with a blood loss of greater than 35 percent of the body's total blood supply. The patient's pulse is barely palpable in the central arteries, if one can be found at all. Respirations are very rapid, shallow, and ineffective. The patient is very lethargic and confused, moving rapidly toward unresponsiveness. The skin is very cool, clammy, and extremely pale. Urinary output ceases. Even with aggressive fluid resuscitation and blood transfusions, patient survival is unlikely.

These descriptions of the stages of hemorrhage presume that the patient is a normally healthy adult. Any preexisting condition may affect the volume of blood loss required for movement from one stage to another as well as the speed at which the patient moves through the stages. The patient's state of hydration, from dehydrated to fluid-rich, may also affect how quickly and to what degree compensation takes place.

The rate of the blood loss also has a profound effect on how quickly a patient moves from stage 1 to stage 4. If the blood loss is very rapid, the compensatory mechanisms may not work as effectively. However, a small wound bleeding uncontrollably but very slowly for days may not move the patient from stage 1 to stage 2, even with a loss much greater than 750 mL.

Certain categories of patients—pregnant women, athletes, obese patients, children, and the elderly—react differently to blood loss. The blood volume of a woman in late pregnancy is 50 percent greater than normal. This patient may lose rather large volumes of blood before progressing through the various stages of hemorrhage. Although the mother in this circumstance appears to be somewhat protected from the effects of serious hemorrhage, the fetus is deprived of good circulation early in the blood loss and is more susceptible to harm.

A well-conditioned athlete often has greater fluid and cardiac reserves than a typical patient. This means that he may move more slowly through the early stages with greater percentages of loss needed to advance from one stage to another.

The obese patient, however, has a blood volume close to 7 percent of ideal body weight, but not actual body weight. Thus, the blood volume as a percentage of actual body weight is lower than 7 percent. This means that what appears to be only a small blood loss may have a more serious effect in such a patient.

In infants and young children, blood volumes approximate 8 to 9 percent of body weight, volumes that are proportionally about 20 percent greater than those of adults. However, compensatory mechanisms in infants and children are neither as well developed nor as effective as those in adults. These young patients may not show early signs and symptoms of compensation as clearly as adults. They may instead move quickly into the later stages of shock. Suspect hemorrhage early with child and infant trauma and treat it aggressively.

The elderly are likewise more adversely affected by blood loss. They have lower volumes of fluid reserves, and their compensatory systems are less responsive to fluid losses. These patients may also be on medications such as beta-blockers that further reduce the body's ability to respond to blood loss and varying blood pressures, or on medications such as aspirin, Coumadin, and heparin that interfere with the body's natural hemorrhage control system. Often, elderly patients do not experience the tachycardia

 Review

Stages of Hemorrhage

Stage 1—blood loss of up to 15 percent; patient may display some nervousness and marginally cool skin with slight pallor

Stage 2—blood loss of 15 to 25 percent; patient displays thirst; anxiety; restlessness; cool, clammy skin; increased respiratory rate

Stage 3—blood loss between 25 and 35 percent; patient experiences air hunger, dyspnea, severe thirst, anxiety, restlessness; survival unlikely without rapid intervention

Stage 4—blood loss greater than 35 percent; pulse barely palpable, respirations ineffective; patient lethargic, confused, moving toward unresponsiveness; survival unlikely

Suspect hemorrhage early in cases of child and infant trauma and treat it aggressively.

Be aware that signs and symptoms of blood loss in elderly patients may be masked by use of medications, bodily changes, reduced perception of pain, and the effects of disease.

The assessment of the hemorrhage patient is directed at identifying the source of the hemorrhage and halting any serious and controllable loss.

Body substance isolation procedures protect the patient as well as the caregiver.

associated with blood loss, and their blood pressures drop before those of healthy adults. Signs of blood loss and shock may be masked by reduced perceptions of pain in the elderly and by lowered levels of mental acuity due to disease. The elderly also do not tolerate periods of inadequate tissue perfusion well because of chronic cardiovascular inefficiency.

HEMORRHAGE ASSESSMENT

The assessment of various types of trauma patients will be the subject of the next few chapters. In these chapters, only the aspects of assessment that are pertinent to those pathologies will be addressed. Please refer to the final chapter of this book—Chapter 12, "Shock Trauma Resuscitation"—for a more complete discussion of the trauma assessment process. You may also wish to refer to Volume 2, "Patient Assessment," in this series.

The assessment of the hemorrhage patient is directed at identifying the source of the hemorrhage and halting any serious and controllable loss. During assessment, you should also examine the circumstances of injury to approximate the volume of blood lost and the rate of past and continuing hemorrhage. This process begins with the scene size-up and continues throughout transport and care.

Scene Size-up

Remember that body substance isolation (BSI) precautions are essential during the assessment of trauma patients. A patient's blood and other body fluids may contain pathogens capable of transmitting HIV, hepatitis, and other diseases to you. Conversely, you may transmit infectious agents to the wounds of the patients you assess and care for. In fact, the risk of your transmitting disease or infection to a patient with open wounds or burns is probably much greater than the risk that he will transmit disease or infection to you. For these reasons, always observe body substance isolation precautions with all trauma patients. These precautions include the use of gloves and a mask when you inspect or palpate any injured area, especially one with open wounds (Figure 4-10 ■). If there is spurting blood, as with arterial hemorrhage; if a patient is combative; or if there is airway trauma with or without bleeding, also wear eye protection and a disposable gown to protect your uniform. Be sure to wash your hands before each ambulance call

■ Figure 4-10   When caring for a hemorrhaging patient, employ appropriate body substance isolation procedures. (© *Eddie Sperling Photography*)

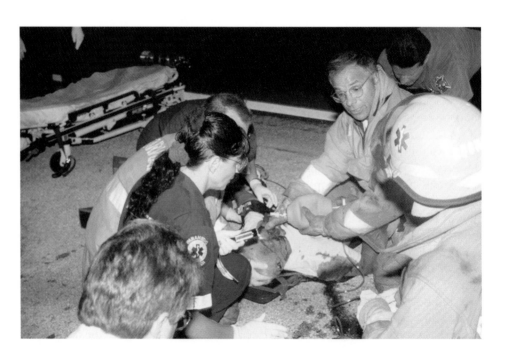

and do so immediately afterward as well. Scrub vigorously when washing to remove as much of the bacterial load as possible.

If your gloves become contaminated with earth, debris, blood, or body fluids while caring for a patient, change them immediately. If you will be assessing or treating multiple patients, consider double gloving. This means that you put on two or more sets of gloves and remove a set each time you complete assessment of one patient and move on to the next. Place any contaminated gloves, clothing, dressings, or other materials in a biohazard bag and assure proper disposal.

The handling of needles presents special problems for prehospital personnel. Once a needle is used, it carries the potential of introducing a patient's blood directly into a caregiver's or bystander's tissues. This greatly increases the likelihood of disease transmission. When dealing with needles, always assure that they are not recapped, but rather placed in a properly marked and secure, puncture-resistant sharps container. Should you be stuck with a needle, continue your care, but document the incident immediately upon arrival at the emergency department. Wash and cover the wound, then report the incident to your service's infection control officer or other designated officer. There are several prophylactic regimens available that may protect against the transmission of some infectious diseases. Even more important, you can guard against some diseases, such as hepatitis, by obtaining immunizations before you begin your career as a care provider.

Patients may see your gloves and then feel uncomfortable about being treated by someone who is "afraid to touch them." Assure those patients that the gloves and other precautions are for their protection as well as yours.

When appropriate BSI precautions have been taken, continue with the scene size-up. Evaluate the mechanism of injury to anticipate sites of both external and internal hemorrhage. Anticipating external hemorrhage sites focuses your subsequent assessment and care, while anticipating internal hemorrhage affects your decision on whether to provide rapid transport.

When evaluating the mechanism of injury (MOI), also attempt to determine the amount of time that has elapsed between the injury and your evaluation of it. Knowing the length of this time period is very important in determining the amount and rate of blood loss. For example, if you arrive on a scene 3 minutes after an injury-producing incident and find a patient losing 150 mL of blood per minute, you can estimate that 450 mL of blood have been lost. You would not expect the patient to display the signs and symptoms of stage 1 hemorrhage. If, however, you arrive 10 minutes after the incident, the same patient, losing blood at the same rate, will have lost 1,500 mL of blood and is likely to have reached stage 3. In both these cases, the patient is suffering serious, life-threatening hemorrhage. Good assessment and recognition assures provision of a proper course of care. However, the earlier you arrive at the patient's side, the harder it is to identify serious hemorrhage. For this reason, you must be aware of and appreciate the progressive effects of blood loss and use both the MOI analysis and the time since an incident to increase your suspicions of a problem. Remember, the sooner the signs of later stages of hemorrhage appear, the greater the rate and volume of blood loss.

Initial Assessment

As you begin the initial assessment, form a general impression of the patient. Be especially alert for any signs and symptoms of internal hemorrhage. These early signs are very subtle and may go unnoticed unless you deliberately look for them. Provide in-line immobilization and correct any immediate life threats if you suspect spinal injury. Assess the patient's initial mental status to determine alertness, orientation, and responsiveness. Be alert for any signs of anxiety, confusion, or combativeness. Any central nervous system deficit may be secondary to hemorrhage, so be suspicious.

Assess both airway and breathing carefully, noting any tachypnea or air hunger. Administer oxygen via nonrebreather mask at a rate of 15 L/minute. When assessing

The sooner the signs of the later stages of hemorrhage appear, the greater the rate and volume of blood loss.

circulation, pay special attention to the pulse strength (the pulse pressure) and rate. Remember that the pulse pressure narrows well before the systolic pressure begins to drop. The pulse rate, too, may suggest developing shock. A fast—and especially a fast, weak (thready)—pulse may be the first noticeable sign of serious internal blood loss. Note also skin color and condition. Pale or mottled skin is an early sign of shock, while cool and clammy skin is also an indicator of potential blood loss and shock.

Complete the initial assessment by establishing patient priorities. Decide, based on your findings to this point, whether the patient is to receive a rapid trauma assessment or a focused history and exam. If any indication, mechanism of injury, sign, or symptom suggests serious internal hemorrhage or uncontrolled external hemorrhage, consider the rapid trauma assessment and then immediate transport for the patient.

Focused History and Physical Exam

Your initial assessment findings and the evaluation of the mechanism of injury determine how you will proceed with the focused history and physical exam. For trauma patients who have a significant MOI, continue spinal immobilization, and perform a rapid trauma assessment. Then obtain baseline vital signs and a patient history.

For trauma patients who have no significant mechanism of injury and who have revealed no critical findings during initial assessment, perform an assessment focused on the area of injury, then obtain baseline vital signs and gather a patient history. Finally, provide care as appropriate and transport.

With both these types of trauma patients, perform ongoing assessments during transport. If time and the patient's condition permit, you may also perform a detailed physical exam. However, you should never delay transport to perform the detailed examination.

Rapid Trauma Assessment   For trauma patients with a significant MOI, you should perform a rapid trauma assessment, inspecting and palpating the patient in an orderly fashion from head to toe. Pay particular attention to areas where critical trauma has occurred and areas where the MOI suggests forces were focused.

Carefully and quickly observe the head for serious bleeding. Internal head injury rarely accounts for the classic signs of shock. However, the scalp bleeds profusely because the vessels there are large and lack the ability to constrict as well as peripheral vessels elsewhere do. If any external bleeding appears serious, halt it immediately.

Next, examine the neck. The carotid arteries and jugular veins are located close to the skin's surface. Injury to them can produce rapid and fatal exsanguination. An added danger is the aspiration of air directly into an open jugular vein. At times, venous pressure, due to deep inspiration, can be less than atmospheric pressure. Air may then be drawn into the vein, traveling to the heart and forming emboli, which then lodge in the pulmonary circulation. Quickly control any serious hemorrhage from neck wounds with sterile occlusive dressings. If spinal injury is suspected, apply a rigid cervical collar when assessment of the neck is complete, but maintain in-line manual immobilization until the patient is immobilized to a spine board.

Visually sweep the chest and abdomen for any serious external hemorrhage, though such bleeding is infrequent there. You are more likely to note signs of blunt or penetrating trauma, suggesting internal injury and hemorrhage within. Look to the abdomen for signs of soft-tissue injury, contusions, abrasions, rigidity, and guarding and tenderness that suggest internal injury.

Quickly examine the pelvic and groin region. Test the integrity of the pelvic ring by pressing gently on the iliac crest. Remember that pelvic fracture can account for blood loss of more than 2,000 mL. Lacerations to the male genitalia may also account for serious external hemorrhage.

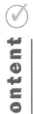 **Review**

Content

Injuries That Can Cause Significant Blood Loss

Fractured pelvis (2,000 mL)
Fractured femur (1,500 mL)
Fractured tibia (750 mL)
Fractured humerus (750 mL)
Large contusion (500 mL)

Assess the extremities and rule out fractures of the femur, tibia/fibula, or humerus. Keep in mind that femur fracture can account for up to 1,500 mL of blood loss, while each tibia/fibula or humerus fracture may contribute an additional 500 to 750 mL of blood loss. Hematomas and large contusions may account for up to 500 mL of blood loss in the larger muscle masses. Quickly check distal pulse strength and muscle tone in the extremities, comparing findings in the opposing extremities.

Finally, visually sweep the body, including the posterior, for any external hemorrhage that may have gone unnoticed in your examination to this point.

At the end of the rapid trauma assessment, assess the patient's vital signs, obtain a patient history if possible, and inventory the injuries that may contribute to shock. Provide rapid transport for any patient with an MOI and physical findings that meet trauma triage criteria (see Chapter 1, "Trauma and Trauma Systems"). Any patient with injuries likely to induce hemorrhage at the level of stage 2 or greater should likewise receive immediate transport. If travel time to the trauma center will exceed 30 minutes, consider requesting air medical transport. Be sure to record the results of your assessment carefully. Compare this information with signs and symptoms you discover during the ongoing assessment to identify trends in the patient's condition.

Perform a detailed physical exam only when all immediate life threats have been addressed. Normally, this would be when you are en route to the hospital or trauma center or when transport has been delayed for some reason.

Focused Physical Exam Employ the focused trauma assessment for patients without a significant MOI; for example, a patient who has lacerated his finger with a knife. In such cases, the hemorrhage can be controlled on the scene and the MOI does not suggest additional problems. With such patients, focus your exam on the area injured, inspecting and palpating the area thoroughly, looking for additional injuries beyond the one that prompted the call. Control the hemorrhage, if you have not already done so. Obtain baseline vital signs and a patient history, and prepare and transport the patient.

In some cases, you may wish to perform a rapid trauma assessment, even though the patient does not have a significant MOI. This would be the case, for example, if you suspect the patient has more injuries than he has complained of or if his condition suddenly begins to deteriorate. With such patients, it may be necessary to perform a rapid head-to-toe examination, inspecting and palpating all body regions.

Additional Assessment Considerations In the trauma patient with a significant MOI or the medical patient showing signs and symptoms of blood loss and shock, it is important to search for evidence of internal hemorrhage. This evidence may be in the form of blood, or material suggestive of blood, flowing from the body orifices. Bright red blood from the mouth, nose, rectum, or other orifice suggests direct bleeding. The vomiting of material that looks like coffee grounds is associated with partially digested blood in the stomach, suggestive of a long-term and slow hemorrhage. A black, tarry stool called melena suggests blood has remained in the bowel for some time. **Hematochezia** is stool with frank blood in it and reflects active bleeding in the colon or rectum.

In the patient with nonspecific complaints—general ill feeling, anxiousness, restlessness—or a lowered level of responsiveness, suspect and look for other signs of internal hemorrhage. Watch for an increasing pulse rate, rising diastolic blood pressure (narrowing blood pressure), and cool and clammy skin.

Also observe for dizziness or syncope when the patient moves from a supine to a sitting or standing position. This condition is called **orthostatic hypotension** and is suggestive of a volume loss, possibly attributable to internal hemorrhage. This phenomenon is the basis of the **tilt test,** which can be employed to determine blood or fluid loss and the body's reduced ability to compensate for normal positional change.

hematochezia *passage of stools containing red blood.*

orthostatic hypotension *a decrease in blood pressure that occurs when a person moves from a supine or sitting to an upright position.*

tilt test *drop in the systolic blood pressure of 20 mmHg or an increase in the pulse rate of 20 beats per minute when a patient is moved from a supine to a sitting position; a finding suggestive of a relative hypovolemia.*

Perform this test only on patients who do not already display signs and symptoms of shock. Prepare for the test by obtaining blood pressure and pulse rates from the patient in a supine or seated position. Then have the supine patient move to a seated position or the seated patient stand up and obtain another set of blood pressure and pulse rates. If the systolic blood pressure drops more than 20 mmHg, the pulse rate rises more than 20 beats per minute, or the patient experiences light-headedness, the test is considered positive, indicating hypovolemia.

Ongoing Assessment

Once you have rendered all appropriate lifesaving care, perform ongoing assessments frequently—at least every 5 minutes with unstable patients and every 15 minutes with stable ones. Reevaluate your general impression, and reassess the patient's mental status, airway, breathing, and circulation, and obtain additional sets of vital signs. Compare each set of findings with earlier ones to determine if the patient's condition is stable, deteriorating, or improving. Pay special attention to the pulse pressure because it is a clear indicator of the body's efforts to compensate for hypovolemia. Also pay particular attention to changes in patient symptoms or mental status, noting any increasing anxiety or restlessness.

HEMORRHAGE MANAGEMENT

The management of hemorrhage is an integral part of care for the trauma patient, one that begins during the initial assessment and is shaped by findings of the rapid trauma assessment or the focused physical exam.

First, assure that the airway is patent, that the patient is breathing adequately, and that you have administered high-flow, high-concentration oxygen. If you have not, establish and maintain the airway and provide the necessary ventilatory support. Be prepared to provide endotracheal intubation if necessary to secure the airway.

Assure that the patient has a pulse. If not, initiate CPR, attach a monitor-defibrillator, and employ advanced cardiac life support measures. Rule out pericardial tamponade and tension pneumothorax as possible causes of cardiac dysfunction. Understand that cardiac arrest in trauma cases due to hypovolemia carries an extremely poor prognosis. When resources are scarce, your efforts may be better utilized caring for other salvageable patients.

During the initial assessment, care for serious (arterial and heavy venous) hemorrhage only after any airway and breathing problems are corrected. Quickly apply a pressure dressing held in place by self-adherent bandage material or a firmly tied cravat. Return to provide better hemorrhage control after you complete the initial and rapid trauma assessments and set priorities for care of the hemorrhages and other trauma you discover. If the patient displays early signs of shock, consider applying a PASG and initiating fluid therapy; do not, however, delay transport in order to carry out these measures.

Once you have completed the focused history and physical exam stage of assessment, begin caring for injuries, including hemorrhage, as you have prioritized them. As you work down your injury priority list and come to a wound, inspect the site to identify the type and exact location of bleeding. This helps you apply pressure—either digitally or with dressings and bandages—most effectively to halt the blood flow. With cases of external hemorrhage, it is important to identify the exact source and type of bleeding and to be sure to look at the wound site.

Document your findings on the prehospital care report. If you document and convey this information clearly to the emergency department staff, you will reduce the need for others to open the wound (thus disrupting the clotting process) to determine and describe its nature.

Direct pressure controls all but the most persistent hemorrhage (Figure 4-11 ■). Although systolic blood pressure drives arterial hemorrhage, you can stop such a hemor-

During the initial assessment, care for serious hemorrhage only after any airway and breathing problems are corrected.

Direct pressure usually controls all but the most persistent hemorrhage.

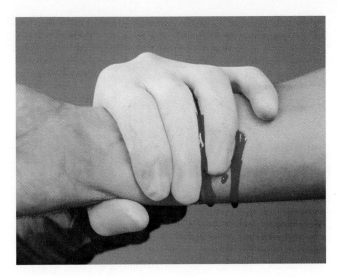

rhage with simple finger pressure properly applied to the source of the bleeding. If a wound looks as though it may pose a problem, insert a wad of dressing material over the site of the heaviest bleeding and apply a bandage over the dressing. This focuses pressure on the site and away from the surrounding area. If bleeding saturates the dressing, cover it with another dressing and apply another bandage to keep pressure on the wound. Removing the soaked bandage and dressing disrupts the clotting process and prolongs the hemorrhage. If, however, the wound continues to bleed through your layers of dressings and bandages, consider removing the dressing materials you have applied, directly visualizing the exact site of bleeding, and then reapplying a wad of dressing and firm direct pressure to the precise hemorrhage site.

If direct pressure alone does not halt the blood flow to an extremity, consider elevation. Elevation reduces the systolic blood pressure because the heart has to push the blood against gravity and up the limb. Employ elevation only when there is an isolated bleeding wound on a limb and movement will not aggravate any other injuries.

If bleeding still persists, find an arterial pulse point proximal to the wound and apply firm pressure there (Figure 4-12 ■). This further reduces the blood pressure within the limb and should reduce the hemorrhaging.

Other techniques that can aid in hemorrhage control include limb splinting and the use of pneumatic splints. Splinting helps maintain the stability of the wound site, thus assisting the mechanisms by which clots develop. Splinting may also protect the site from injuries that might occur if the patient is jostled during extrication and transport or as you assess and care for other wounds. Pneumatic splints can also prevent movement of an injured limb. They may also be helpful in holding dressings in place and in applying direct pressure to a limb circumferentially.

Consider using a tourniquet only as a last resort when hemorrhage is prolonged and persistent. As mentioned earlier, there are hazards associated with tourniquet use. Apply a blood pressure cuff just proximal to the hemorrhage site and inflate it to apply a pressure of 20 to 30 mmHg greater than the systolic blood pressure. Assure there is no continued bleeding after you apply the tourniquet, and mark the patient's forehead with the letters "TQ" and the time of application.

Specific Wound Considerations

Several types of wounds require special attention for hemorrhage control. They include head wounds, neck wounds, large gaping wounds, and crush injuries.

Head injuries raise some special concerns regarding hemorrhage control. Head wounds may be associated with both severe hemorrhage and the loss of skull integrity

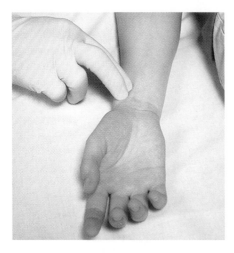

a. Radial artery for hand.

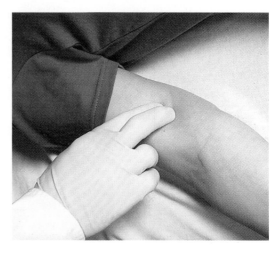

b. Brachial artery for forearm.

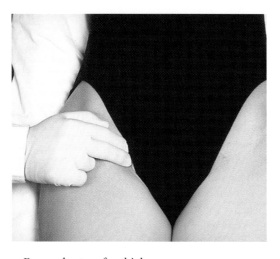

c. Femoral artery for thigh.

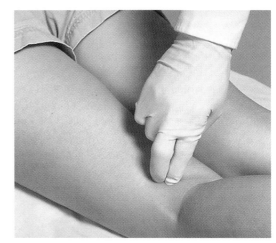

d. Popliteral artery for leg and foot.

■ Figure 4-12   Common pressure points for hemorrhage control.

With head injury patients, do not attempt to stop the flow of blood or fluid from the nose or ear canal, but cover the area with porous dressing to collect the material and bandage loosely.

Cover any open neck wound with an occlusive dressing held firmly in place.

(fracture). Control bleeding with such wounds very carefully, using gentle direct pressure around the wound site and against the stable skull. Fluid drainage from the ears and nose may be secondary to skull fracture. Cerebrospinal fluid, as it escapes the cranial vault, relieves building intracranial pressure. Halting the flow of fluid would end this relief mechanism and compound the increase in pressure. In addition, stopping the flow may provide a pathway for pathogens to enter the meninges and cause serious infection (meningitis). Cerebrospinal fluid quickly regenerates as the injury heals. Thus, if there is hemorrhage from either the nose or ear canal, simply cover the area with a soft, porous dressing and bandage it loosely.

Neck wounds carry the risk of air being drawn into the venous circulation with life-threatening results. Cover any open neck wound with an occlusive dressing held firmly in place. Do not employ circumferential bandages to create direct pressure with neck wounds. Digital pressure controls most, if not all, neck bleeding. It may, however, be necessary to apply and maintain this manual pressure continuously during the patient's prehospital care.

Gaping wounds often present hemorrhage control problems. With such wounds, bleeding originates from many sites and their open nature prevents application of uniform direct pressure. To manage bleeding from such a wound, create a mass of dressing material approximating the volume and shape of the wound. Place the material with the sterile, nonadherent side down on the wound and bandage it firmly in place.

Controlling hemorrhage associated with crush injuries can be particularly challenging. The source of hemorrhage in such cases is frequently difficult to determine, and the vessels are damaged in such a way that the normal hemorrhage control mechanisms may be ineffective. Place a dressing around and over the crushed tissue, place a pneumatic splint over that, and inflate to apply pressure and hold the dressing in place. If bleeding is heavy and persistent, consider using a tourniquet but keep in mind the precautions discussed previously.

Transport Considerations

Consider rapid transport for any patient who experiences serious external hemorrhage that you cannot control and for any patient with suspected serious internal hemorrhage. Be vigilant for any signs of compensation for blood loss and for the early signs of shock. Monitor your patient's mental status, pulse rate, and blood pressure (for narrowing pulse pressure). When in doubt, transport.

Understand that serious hemorrhage can have a significant psychological impact on patients. Stress triggers the "fight-or-flight" response, increases heart rate and blood pressure, increases the body's metabolic demands, works against the body's hemorrhage control mechanisms, and contributes to the development of shock. Do what you can to ease the anxieties of such patients. Communicate freely with them, and explain what care measures you are taking and why. Be especially alert to their comfort needs and address them as appropriate. If possible, keep these patients from seeing their injuries or the serious injuries affecting friends and other accident victims.

Consider rapid transport for any patient who experiences serious external hemorrhage that you cannot control and for any patient with suspected serious internal hemorrhage.

SHOCK

A simple medical definition of shock is "a state of inadequate tissue perfusion." Beyond that simple definition, however, shock is the transitional stage between normal life, called homeostasis, and death. It is the underlying killer of all trauma patients and often presents with only subtle signs and symptoms until the body can no longer compensate. Then the patient moves quickly, and often irreversibly, toward death. Because of this, you, as a paramedic, must understand the process of shock and recognize its earliest signs and symptoms.

Shock is a tissue perfusion problem affecting the individual body cells. There are many causes of shock, though all are commonly manifested by signs and symptoms of cardiovascular system compensation followed by decompensation and, ultimately, collapse. The best way to understand shock and how body systems compensate for it is to look at the cell and its **metabolism** and then to examine how the body provides for the cell's metabolic needs.

Shock is the underlying killer of all trauma patients and often presents with only subtle signs and symptoms.

metabolism *the total changes that take place in an organism during physiological processes.*

CELLULAR METABOLISM

Cells are the microscopic, elemental, structural building blocks of the human body. They make up tissues; tissues make up organs; and organs make up the organism. Cells carry out all the functions performed by the body, but to do so require—primarily—oxygen and essential nutrients such as carbohydrates, lipids, and proteins. The biochemical mechanisms within the cell process these materials, producing energy to do work and perform the functions essential for life. In this process, waste products, including carbon dioxide, water, and other materials, are produced.

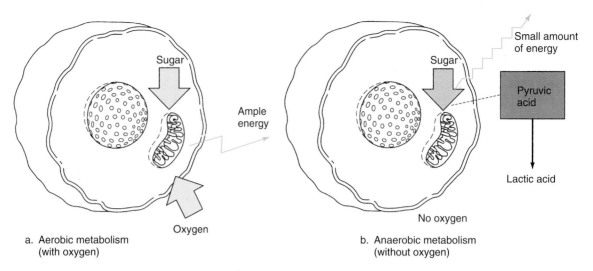

a. Aerobic metabolism
(with oxygen)

b. Anaerobic metabolism
(without oxygen)

■ Figure 4-13   **a.** Aerobic metabolism requires oxygen and is most efficient. **b.** Anaerobic metabolism yields much less energy and toxic byproducts such as lactic acid.

glycolysis   *the first stage of the process in which the cell breaks apart an energy source, commonly glucose, and releases a small amount of energy.*

aerobic metabolism   *the second stage of metabolism, requiring the presence of oxygen, in which the breakdown of glucose (in a process called the Krebs or citric acid cycle) yields a high amount of energy.*

Krebs cycle   *process of aerobic metabolism that uses carbohydrates, proteins, and fats to release energy for the body; also known as the* **citric acid cycle.**

anaerobic metabolism   *the first stage of metabolism, which does not require oxygen, in which the breakdown of glucose (in a process called glycolysis) produces pyruvic acid and yields limited energy.*

portal system   *part of the circulatory system consisting of the veins that drain some of the digestive organs. The portal system delivers blood to the liver.*

glucagon   *hormone that increases the blood glucose level by stimulating the liver to change stored glycogen to glucose.*

insulin   *pancreatic hormone needed to transport simple sugars from the interstitial spaces into the cells.*

The cell breaks down its energy sources, most commonly the carbohydrate molecule glucose, in a two-step process. The first step, called **glycolysis,** requires no oxygen and generates a small amount of energy. The second step, called **aerobic metabolism,** requires oxygen and accounts for 95 percent of the normal cell energy production. This oxygen-dependant energy-generating process involves the **citric acid cycle,** also called the **Krebs cycle.** Without adequate oxygen, cells survive for a time on the inefficient initial glycolysis pathway that generates pyruvic acid as an end product. In the absence of oxygen, pyruvic acid converts to lactic acid. Lactic acid and other by-products of **anaerobic metabolism** build up and create a cellular and interstitial acidosis (Figure 4-13 ■). Without the return of oxygen and the removal of lactic acid and other toxins, the cell soon dies.

The cardiovascular system assures a constant and dependable supply of oxygen and nutrients and the disposal of carbon dioxide and other waste products of metabolism. In turn, many body organs contribute material to, or withdraw material from, the circulation in support of cellular metabolism. All these organs must work properly to assure the blood is in a proper state to support cellular metabolism.

In the lungs, oxygen and carbon dioxide are exchanged with each breath. Oxygen is brought in with inhalation and mixes with alveolar air, providing an oxygen concentration of about 13 percent. Blood returning from the systemic circulation has much less oxygen (5 percent), so it diffuses across the alveolar-capillary membrane and attaches to hemoglobin molecules in the red blood cells. This exchange is very efficient, and oxygen saturates about 99 percent of the hemoglobin leaving the lungs. The carbon dioxide concentration in the returning blood is about 6 percent. This carbon dioxide then diffuses to the alveolar space (at about 4 percent) and is exhaled.

The body's digestive system absorbs carbohydrates and lipids (fats), moving them through the **portal system** (a venous subsystem) to the liver. There they are prepared for the body's use and are released, as needed, into the bloodstream. The pancreas produces two hormones responsible for regulating the amount of circulating glucose, the cell's primary energy source. **Glucagon** enters the circulation, causing the liver to increase glucose production and release it into the bloodstream. The pancreas also releases **insulin,** which circulates directly to the body cells where it helps transport the large glucose molecules across the cell membranes, thus reducing the amount of circulating blood glucose. The kidneys are responsible for regulating the body's fluid/electrolyte balance, excreting excess sodium, potassium, chloride, calcium, bicarbonate, and magnesium, and excreting the waste products of metabolism such as urea and creatinine.

CIRCULATION

While the activities of all organs are essential to proper body function and cell metabolism, the cardiovascular system is responsible for assuring that the necessary materials travel to and from the body's cells. It is also the cardiovascular system that demonstrates the signs and symptoms of problems with cellular metabolism, the signs and symptoms we call shock. Let us look at how the cardiovascular system circulates blood to the organs and cells and then returns it to the heart and lungs.

As discussed earlier in this chapter, cardiac output depends upon three factors: preload, cardiac contractility, and afterload. The blood ejected from the left ventricle is expressed into the aorta and the system of major arteries the aorta feeds. This bolus of blood causes the arterial pressure to increase until the major arteries distribute the blood to the peripheral circulation. This increased pressure is the **systolic blood pressure.** The systolic blood pressure is most indicative of the strength and volume of cardiac output and of the elasticity of the major arterial vessels. As the blood is distributed after systole, the blood pressure decreases. This resulting **diastolic blood pressure** is more indicative of the state of constriction of the arterioles (peripheral vascular resistance) as they direct blood to the various organs and tissues. The diastolic blood pressure is the pressure that allows the body to control blood flow to various organs and tissues. Thus, the major arteries carry out the general distribution of blood, while the arterioles determine the proportion of blood each organ or tissue receives (Figure 4-14 ■).

For the most part, the sympathetic branch of the autonomic nervous system controls constriction of the arterioles. However, reduced sympathetic stimulation, such as that occurring during parasympathetic stimulation, also influences arteriole tone. Arterioles open to permit or close to limit perfusion of organs as needed. Sympathetic stimulation causes the body to be more active, with blood directed to the skeletal muscles, the heart, and the brain. Parasympathetic stimulation causes the body to be more regenerative, directing blood to the bowel and other organs of digestion. During either of these conditions, the blood pressure and, specifically, the peripheral vascular resistance remain stable. However, an abnormal increase in the circulating sympathetic hormones epinephrine and norepinephrine increases cardiac output, the overall peripheral vascular resistance, and both the systolic and diastolic blood pressures.

systolic blood pressure
pressure exerted against the arterial walls during contraction of the left ventricle of the heart.

diastolic blood pressure
pressure exerted against the arterial walls during relaxation of the left ventricle of the heart.

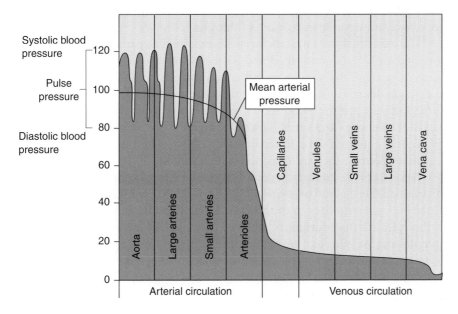

■ Figure 4-14   Vascular distribution and control of circulation.

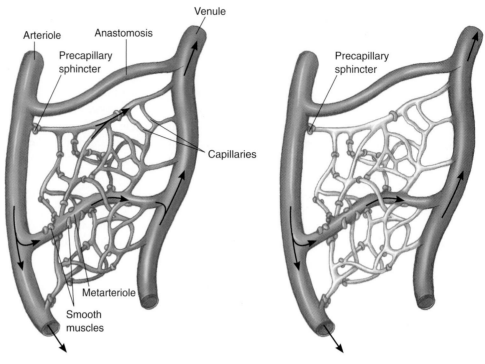

■ Figure 4-15 Blood flow through the microcirculation is controlled by the arterioles and precapillary sphincters.

Venule

Arteriole   Anastomosis

Precapillary
sphincter

Capillaries

Precapillary
sphincter

Metarteriole

Smooth
muscles

a. Blood directed to the tissue.

b. Blood bypassing the tissue.

microcirculation *blood flow in the arterioles, capillaries, and venules.*

histamine *substance released during the degranulation of mast cells and basophils that increases blood flow to the injury site due to vasodilation and increased permeability of capillary walls.*

The arterioles open and close to determine what proportion of the cardiac output circulates through a particular organ or tissue. At the level of the **microcirculation** (the capillary beds), small sphincters that precede and follow each capillary further regulate this circulation (Figure 4-15 ■). When oxygen supplies run low and carbon dioxide begins to build up in the cells, the pH level drops and specialized (mast) cells secrete **histamine.** This short-acting agent causes the sphincters to dilate and permit blood flow through the capillaries. As oxygen returns to the cells and carbon dioxide is removed, the pH returns to normal. Mast cells halt their release of histamine, and the sphincters again close. Tissues that make up most organs, except for the brain, heart, and kidneys, do not need a constant flow of blood; they survive and perform well with blood flowing 5 to 20 percent of the time. This flow permits red blood cells, in single file, to travel through the capillaries, diffusing oxygen and nutrients into, and carbon dioxide and waste products out of, the interstitial space (and fluid). In turn, these agents diffuse or are actively transported into or out of the cells.

The interstitial and intracellular spaces represent 88 percent of the body's fluid volume and are a tremendous fluid and electrolyte reservoir. This fluid can be mobilized when the precapillary sphincters and vessels constrict and the postcapillary sphincters and vessels dilate. Fluid is then drawn from the interstitial spaces and into the vascular space. Conversely, if the body needs to shift fluid away from the vascular space, the postcapillary sphincters and vessels constrict while the precapillary sphincters and vessels dilate, thus pushing fluid into the interstitial space. This mechanism is a rapid way to expand or decrease the cardiovascular system volume.

Blood exits the capillary beds and enters the venous system via the venules. These vessels maintain a blood pressure about one tenth that of the arterial blood pressure as blood begins its trip back to the heart. Valves in the veins of the extremities, especially of the legs, assist the returning blood flow. When skeletal muscles contract, they thicken, compressing the veins that are alongside. This action closes and puts pressure on valves distal to the muscle and opens and pushes blood through the proximal valves. Walking and other activities involving alternating contraction and relaxation of major skeletal muscles are very effective in helping pump blood back toward the heart (Figure 4-16 ■).

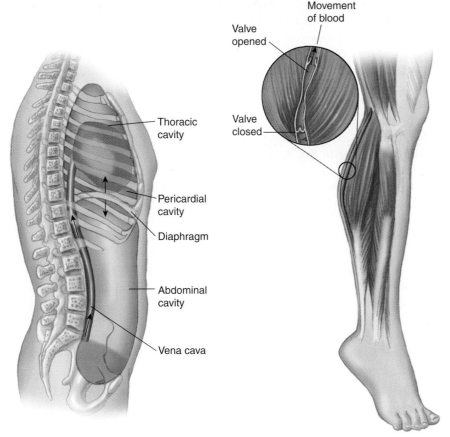

a. Elements of the thoracoabdominal pump.

b. Valves in the leg assist in venous return.

The process of respiration also complements blood return. The changing intrathoracic pressure—alternatively more, then less than the atmospheric pressure—draws blood toward the heart, while the venous valves prevent backflow during periods of higher intrathoracic pressure. This mechanism is called the **thoracoabdominal pump.**

The cardiovascular system of an average adult male contains fluid equal to 7 percent of both the body's weight and fluid volume (with plasma accounting for 4.5 percent of the body's volume and red blood cells for 3.5 percent) with a volume of blood totaling about 5 liters. This blood is distributed in the various vascular vessels. The heart contains about 7 percent of the total blood volume, while another 13 percent is found in the major arteries. The capillaries hold 7 percent, while the venous system contains around 64 percent of the volume. The remaining 9 percent is found in the pulmonary circulation.

Blood completely fills the vascular space, even in states of hypovolemia. The problem in those states, however, is that blood return to the heart is diminished, negatively affecting cardiac output, arterial blood pressure, and, ultimately, the body's ability to direct blood flow to critical organs. This is the point at which the signs and symptoms of shock begin.

thoracoabdominal pump
process by which respirations assist blood return to the heart.

CARDIOVASCULAR SYSTEM REGULATION

The human body is controlled by the autonomic nervous system. This system consists of two opposing subsystems that maintain an equilibrium and help us respond to and recover from the stresses of daily life.

Parasympathetic nervous system stimulation causes decreases in heart rate, strength of contractions, and blood pressure. It decreases respiratory rate, induces bronchoconstriction, and stimulates the activity of the digestive system and kidneys. In general, the parasympathetic system helps the body rest and regenerate energy used in activities induced by the sympathetic nervous system.

The sympathetic nervous system accelerates body activity. It increases heart rate and strength of cardiac contractions, constricts blood vessels supplying the bowel and digestive viscera, dilates vessels supplying the skeletal muscles, increases respiratory rate, causes bronchodilation, and decreases urine production.

These two systems act in balance, with the parasympathetic system inducing sleep and the sympathetic system responding to and controlling normal waking activity. When a stressor such as danger is perceived, the sympathetic nervous system prepares the body either to combat or to physically flee the stressor. This aggressive body response is termed the "fight-or-flight" response and is a deeply ingrained protective reflex. While many sympathetic nervous system activities are aimed at defending the organism, they can be detrimental once injury occurs and shock develops.

A system of receptors, autonomic centers, and nervous and hormonal interventions maintains control over the cardiovascular system (Figure 4-17 ■). **Baroreceptors** in the aortic arch and in the carotid sinuses monitor the arterial blood pressure while chemoreceptors there monitor oxygen and carbon dioxide levels in the blood. (There are additional baroreceptors in the atria and **chemoreceptors** in the brain.) These receptors send impulses to the cardiovascular centers located in the medulla oblongata. Three specific centers help regulate cardiovascular function. They are the cardioacceleratory center, the cardioinhibitory center, and the vasomotor center.

The **cardioacceleratory center** is a sympathetic nervous system center that increases heart rate through stimulation of the cardiac plexus. The **cardioinhibitory center** is a parasympathetic center that decreases heart rate through stimulation of the

baroreceptor *sensory nerve ending, found in the walls of the atria of the heart, vena cava, aortic arch, and carotid sinus, that is stimulated by changes in pressure.*

chemoreceptor *sense organ or sensory nerve ending located outside the central nervous system that is stimulated by and reacts to chemical stimuli.*

cardioacceleratory center *a sympathetic nervous system center in the medulla oblongata, controlling the release of epinephrine and norepinephrine.*

cardioinhibitory center *a parasympathetic center in the medulla oblongata, controlling the vagus nerve.*

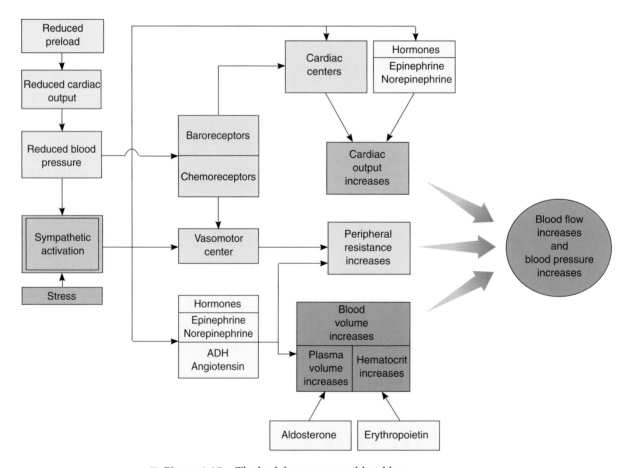

■ Figure 4-17   The body's response to blood loss.

vagus nerve. The **vasomotor center** is a sympathetic nervous center that regulates arterial and, to a lesser degree, venous tone. An increase in blood pressure causes baroreceptor stimulation. This inhibits the cardioacceleratory and vasomotor centers and stimulates the cardioinhibitory center. A slowing cardiac rate, reduction in cardiac contractile force, and a decrease in atrial tone result. This reflex decreases blood pressure. A falling blood pressure inhibits baroreceptor activity, stimulating the cardioacceleratory and vasomotor centers and inhibiting the cardioinhibitory center. The heart rate increases, cardiac contractile force increases, peripheral vascular resistance increases, and the blood pressure rises. These opposing reflex systems respond to changes in the blood pressure to maintain it within a narrow range.

Hormones such as epinephrine, norepinephrine, antidiuretic hormone (ADH), angiotensin II, aldosterone, glucagon, insulin, adrenocorticotropic hormone, and growth hormone, as well as erythropoietin, also influence cardiovascular system function. These agents are released into the bloodstream at the command of the sympathetic nervous system, which is prompted by fluctuations in blood pressure or by changes in perfusion to specific organs like the kidneys.

Epinephrine and norepinephrine are sympathetic agents secreted by the adrenal medulla. They increase peripheral vascular resistance by causing arteriole constriction and by increasing heart rate and contractility. These two hormones, called catecholamines, cause the most rapid hormonal response to hemorrhage and cardiovascular insufficiency. Epinephrine and norepinephrine both have alpha-1 and alpha-2 properties. Alpha-1 receptor stimulation causes vasoconstriction and increases both peripheral vascular resistance and cardiac afterload. Alpha-2 receptor stimulation inhibits the further release of norepinephrine in the sympathetic synapse when norepinephrine levels become too high. Additionally, epinephrine has beta-1 and beta-2 properties. Beta-1 receptor stimulation results in an increase in heart rate (positive chronotrophy), an increase in cardiac contractile strength (positive inotrophy), and an increase in cardiac muscle conductivity (positive dromotrophy). Beta-2 effects include bronchodilation and dilation of smooth muscle in the bowel.

Antidiuretic hormone (ADH), also known as arginine vasopressin (AVP), is released by the posterior pituitary in response either to reduced blood pressure or increased osmotic pressure of the blood (dehydration). ADH induces an increase in peripheral vascular resistance and causes the kidneys to retain water, decreasing urine output. ADH also causes splenic vascular constriction, returning up to 200 mL of free blood into the circulatory system.

Angiotensin is created when the kidneys recognize a lowered blood pressure and decreased perfusion. A chain reaction results when specialized smooth cells in the renal venules release an enzyme, renin. Renin converts angiotensin (an inactive protein) to *angiotensin I*. Angiotensin I is further modified in the lungs by the action of a converting enzyme into *angiotensin II*. This process usually takes about 20 minutes to become fully effective. Angiotensin II is a potent systemic vasoconstrictor that lasts up to an hour. It causes the release of ADH, aldosterone, and epinephrine and also stimulates thirst.

Aldosterone secretion by the adrenal cortex is stimulated by angiotensin II. Aldosterone impacts the cells that maintain ion balance in the kidneys, thereby causing the retention of sodium and water. It also reduces sweating of sodium and water losses through the digestive tract.

Glucagon is a hormone produced by the alpha cells of the pancreas. It controls the amount of available glucose in the bloodstream. When its release is triggered by epinephrine, glucagon enters the bloodstream and causes the liver and skeletal muscles to convert **glycogen,** a form of stored glucose, into glucose (**glycogenolysis**). Glucose is then released into the bloodstream and is available for metabolism. Glucagon also causes some body cells to use alternative energy sources such as lipids and proteins.

Insulin is a hormone, secreted by the beta cells of the pancreas. It facilitates glucose transport across cell membranes. Since glucose is the primary carbohydrate used in

vagus nerve *the 10th cranial nerve that monitors and controls the heart, respiration, and much of the abdominal viscera.*

vasomotor center *center in the medulla oblongata that controls arterial and, to a degree, venous tone.*

antidiuretic hormone (ADH) *hormone released by the posterior pituitary that induces an increase in peripheral vascular resistance and causes the kidneys to retain water, decreasing urine output, and also causes splenic vascular constriction.*

angiotensin *a vasopressor hormone that causes contraction of the smooth muscles of arteries and arterioles, produced when renin is released from the kidneys; angiotensin I is a physiologically inactive form, while angiotensin II is an active form.*

aldosterone *hormone secreted by the adrenal cortex that increases sodium reabsorption by the kidneys; it plays a part in the regulation of blood volume, blood pressure, and blood levels of potassium, chloride, and bicarbonate.*

glycogen *a polysaccharide; one of the forms in which the body stores glucose.*

glycogenolysis *the process by which the body converts glycogen into glucose.*

metabolism, its transport is important. In low volume (hypovolemic) states, increased production and reduced transport of glucose into the cells increases vascular glucose levels. This process may increase the osmotic pressure of the interstitial and vascular fluids and makes glucose available to skeletal muscle and other body cells that may need it.

To further increase the amount of glucose in the bloodstream, the anterior pituitary gland releases **adrenocorticotropic hormone.** This stimulates the release of **glucocorticoids** from the adrenal cortex. These hormones, in turn, increase glucose production and reduce the body's inflammation response, prolonging clotting time, wound healing, and infection control processes.

Growth hormone, also secreted by the anterior pituitary gland, promotes the uptake of glucose and amino acids in the muscle cells. It also stimulates protein synthesis.

Erythropoietin is released by the kidneys in periods of hypoperfusion or hypoxia. This protein increases the production and maturation rates of erythrocytes (red blood cells) in the red bone marrow of the vertebrae, proximal long bones, pelvis, ribs, and sternum. This process can increase red blood cell production by a factor of 10 over time, helping to restore those cells lost through hemorrhage.

These nerve pathways and hormones comprise the sympathetic and parasympathetic nervous systems' chief means of controlling the human body to maintain homeostasis. Minor fluctuations in blood volume are regulated by small changes in peripheral vascular resistance, fluid movement to and from the interstitial space, contraction or dilation of the venous system, and increases or decreases in the heart rate and strength of contractions. The system works very well without our being aware of it until a serious insult to the body produces more intense, then more drastic, responses.

THE BODY'S RESPONSE TO BLOOD LOSS

The sympathetic nervous system and the hormones it releases begin the progressive responses previously described as hemorrhage causes blood to leave the cardiovascular system. As the draw down of the vascular volume reaches the heart, the ventricles do not completely engorge. Cardiac contractility therefore suffers as the ventricular myocardium does not stretch (Starling's law of the heart). The stroke volume drops, and there is an immediate drop in the systolic blood pressure. This reduced pressure reduces the cardiovascular system's ability to drive blood through the capillary beds (tissue perfusion). The carotid and aortic baroreceptors recognize this decrease in blood pressure and signal to the cardiovascular center of the medulla oblongata. The vasomotor center increases peripheral vascular resistance and venous tone while the cardioacceleratory center increases heart rate. With the reduced venous capacitance and an increase in heart rate and peripheral vascular resistance, the blood pressure returns to normal, as does tissue perfusion. These actions normally compensate for small blood losses. If the blood loss stops, the body reconstitutes the volume of loss from the interstitial fluid and replaces the lost red blood cells gradually, without noticeable or ill effects.

Cellular Ischemia

If blood loss continues, the venous system constricts to its limits in order to maintain cardiac preload. However, it becomes more and more difficult for the venous system to compensate because its limited musculature tires and relaxes. Peripheral vascular resistance also continues to increase to maintain the systolic blood pressure. As it does, the diastolic blood pressure rises, the pulse pressure narrows, and the pulse weakens. The constriction of arterioles means that less and less blood is directed to the noncritical organs, and those organs' supply of oxygen is reduced. The skin, the largest of the noncritical organs, receives reduced circulation and becomes cool, pale, and moist. If the hemorrhage continues, some noncritical organ cells begin to starve for oxygen. Anaerobic metabolism is their only energy source, and carbon dioxide and lactic and other

---

adrenocorticotropic hormone *hormone secreted by the anterior lobe of the pituitary gland that is essential to the function of the adrenal cortex, including production of glucocorticoids.*

glucocorticoids *hormones released by the adrenal cortex that increase glucose production and reduce the body's inflammation response.*

growth hormone *hormone secreted by the anterior pituitary gland that promotes the uptake of glucose and amino acids in the muscle cells and stimulates protein synthesis.*

erythropoietin *one of a specialized group of proteins that is produced by the kidneys and spurs production of red blood cells in the bone marrow.*

acids begin to accumulate. Cellular hypoxia begins, followed by **ischemia.** The heart rate increases, but slowly, because the other compensatory mechanisms are still effectively maintaining preload.

As the volume of blood loss increases, more and more body cells are deprived of their oxygen and nutrient supplies, and more and more waste products accumulate. The bloodstream becomes acidic, and the body's chemoreceptors stimulate an increase in depth and rate of respirations. Hypoxia causes alterations in the level of consciousness, and circulating catecholamines cause the patient to become anxious, restless, and possibly combative. Ischemia now affects not only noncritical organs but also the arterioles. These vessels, which also require oxygen, become hypoxic and relax. Meanwhile, the coronary arteries provide a decreasing amount of oxygenated blood to the laboring heart.

If the blood loss stops, the blood draws fluid from within the interstitial space, at a rate of up to 1 L per hour, to restore its volume, and erythropoietin accelerates the production of red blood cells. The kidneys reduce urine output to conserve water and electrolytes, and a period of thirst provides the stimulus for the patient to drink liquids and replace the lost volume on a more permanent basis. Transfusion with whole blood may be required at this point. While some signs of circulatory compromise and fatigue are present, the patient's recovery is probable with a period of rest.

Capillary Microcirculation

If blood loss continues, sympathetic stimulation and reduced perfusion to the kidneys, pancreas, and liver cause the release of hormones. Angiotensin II further increases peripheral vascular resistance and reduces the blood flow to more of the body's tissues. If the blood loss continues, circulation is further limited to only those organs most critical to life. This further decrease in circulation leads to an increase in cellular hypoxia in noncritical tissues, and more cells begin to use anaerobic metabolism for energy in a desperate attempt to survive. The build-up of lactic acid and carbon dioxide relaxes the precapillary sphincters. The circulating blood volume is diminished both by the continued hemorrhage and by fluid loss as the capillary beds engorge. Postcapillary sphincters remain closed, forcing fluids into the interstitial spaces by **hydrostatic pressure.** The circulatory crisis worsens as the compensatory mechanisms begin to fail. Interstitial edema reduces the ability of the capillaries to provide oxygen and nutrients to and remove carbon dioxide and other waste products from the cells. The capillary and cell membranes also begin to break down. Red blood cells begin to clump together, or agglutinate, in the hypoxic and stagnant capillaries forming columns of coagulated cells called **rouleaux.**

Capillary Washout

The building acidosis from the accumulating lactic acid and carbon dioxide (carbonic acid) finally causes relaxation of the postcapillary sphincters. With relaxation, those byproducts along with potassium (released by the cells to maintain a neutral environment in the presence of building acidosis) and the columns of coagulated red blood cells are dumped into the venous circulation. This **washout** causes profound metabolic acidosis and releases microscopic emboli. Cardiac output drops toward zero; peripheral vascular resistance drops toward zero; blood pressure drops toward zero; cellular perfusion, even to the most critical organs, drops toward zero. The body moves quickly and then irreversibly toward death.

STAGES OF SHOCK

The shock process, as previously described, can be divided into three stages based on presenting signs and symptoms. The stages are progressively more serious and include compensated, decompensated, and irreversible shock (Table 4–2).

ischemia   a blockage in the delivery of oxygenated blood to the cells.

hydrostatic pressure   the pressure of liquids in equilibrium; the pressure exerted by or within liquids.

rouleaux   group of red blood cells that are stuck together.

washout   release of accumulated lactic acid, carbon dioxide (carbonic acid), potassium, and rouleaux into the venous circulation.

Table 4-2	The Stages of Shock

Compensated Shock

Initial stage of shock in which the body progressively compensates for continuing blood loss.

- Pulse rate increases
- Pulse strength decreases
- Skin becomes cool and clammy
- Progressing anxiety, restlessness, combativeness
- Thirst, weakness, eventual air hunger

Decompensated Shock

Begins when the body's compensatory mechanisms can no longer maintain preload.

- Pulse becomes unpalpable
- Blood pressure drops precipitously
- Patient becomes unconscious
- Respirations slow or cease

Irreversible Shock

Shortly after the patient enters decompensated shock, the lack of circulation begins to have profound effects on body cells. As they are irreversibly damaged, the cells die, tissues dysfunction, organs dysfunction, and the patient dies.

---

compensated shock
hemodynamic insult to the body in which the body responds effectively. Signs and symptoms are limited, and the human system functions normally.

Compensated shock is the shock stage in which prehospital interventions and rapid transport are most likely to meet with success.

Review

Stages of Shock

Compensated
Decompensated
Irreversible

decompensated shock
continuing hemodynamic insult to the body in which the compensatory mechanisms break down. The signs and symptoms become very pronounced, and the patient moves rapidly toward death.

Compensated Shock

Compensated shock is the initial shock state. In this stage, the body is still capable of meeting its critical metabolic needs through a series of progressive compensating actions (Figure 4-18 ■). This progressive compensation creates a series of signs and symptoms that range from the subtle to the obvious. The compensated shock stage ends with the precipitous drop in blood pressure. Compensated shock is the shock stage in which prehospital interventions and rapid transport are most likely to meet with success.

The body's first recognizable response to serious blood loss is probably an increase in pulse rate. However, a rate increase due to blood loss may be difficult to differentiate from tachycardia due to excitement and the "fight-or-flight" response. The first sign usually attributable to shock is a narrowing pulse pressure and weakening pulse strength (weak and rapid pulse). As the condition becomes more serious, vasoconstriction causes the patient's skin to become pale, cyanotic, or ashen as blood is directed away from the skin and toward the more critical organs. The skin becomes cool and moist (clammy), and capillary refill times begin to exceed 3 seconds. As compensation becomes more acute, the victim becomes anxious, restless, or combative and complains of thirst and weakness. Near the end of the compensated shock stage, the patient may experience air hunger and tachypnea.

Decompensated Shock

Decompensated shock begins as the body's compensatory mechanisms become unable to respond to a continuing blood loss. Mechanisms that initially compensated for blood loss now fail, and the body moves quickly toward complete collapse. Entry into decompensated shock is indicated by a precipitous drop in systolic blood pressure. Despite all compensatory mechanisms, venous return is inadequate, and the heart no longer has enough blood volume to pump. Even extreme tachycardia produces little cardiac output. No amount of vascular resistance can maintain blood pressure and circulation. Even the most critical organs of the body are hypoperfused. The heart, already hypoxic because of poor perfusion and the increased oxygen demands created by tachycardia, begins to fail. This state may be indicated by the presence of a bradycardia. In this stage, the brain is extremely hypoxic. This means that the patient displays a rapidly

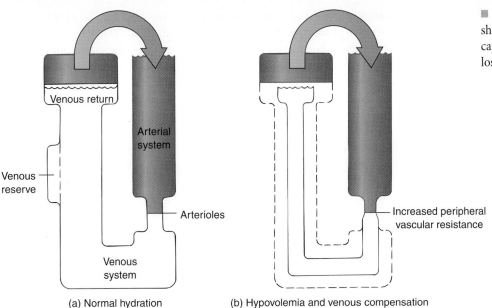

■ Figure 4-18   In compensated shock, the body reduces venous capacitance in response to blood loss.

(a) Normal hydration

(b) Hypovolemia and venous compensation

dropping level of responsiveness. The brain's control over bodily functions, including respiration, ceases, and the body takes on a death-like appearance.

Irreversible Shock

Irreversible shock exists when the body's cells are badly injured and die in such quantities that the organs cannot carry out their normal functions. While aggressive resuscitation may restore blood pressure and pulse, organ failure ultimately results in organism failure. The transition between decompensated and irreversible shock is a clinical one and very difficult to identify in the field. Clearly, the longer a patient is in decompensated shock, the more likely it is that he has moved to irreversible shock.

ETIOLOGY OF SHOCK

The discussion of shock to this point has focused on shock due to blood loss and its effects on the cardiovascular system. Shock can, however, have many causes, and a common way of classifying types of shock is based on its origins: hypovolemic, distributive, obstructive, cardiogenic, respiratory, and neurogenic. Despite the variety of origins, patients suffering from different types of shock present with similar signs and symptoms and suffer similar systemic complications.

Hypovolemic Shock

Hypovolemic shock, which we have discussed in detail, is caused by any significant reduction in the cardiovascular system volume. While hemorrhage is a common cause, fluid loss from other causes can occur. Plasma losses may result from severe and extensive burns or possibly from granulating (seeping) wounds. Fluid and electrolyte losses such as those that occur with protracted vomiting, diarrhea, sweating, and urination also draw down the body's vascular fluids, resulting in hypovolemia. Hypovolemia may also result from "third space" losses such as fluid shifts into various body compartments, like the abdomen in ascites.

Distributive Shock

Distributive shock results from mechanisms that prevent the appropriate distribution of nutrients and removal of metabolic waste products. It may result from increasing capillary permeability, as occurs with anaphylactic shock or septic shock. In

Entry into decompensated shock is indicated by a precipitous drop in systolic blood pressure.

irreversible shock *final stage of shock in which organs and cells are so damaged that recovery is impossible.*

The transition between decompensated and irreversible shock is very difficult to identify in the field.

hypovolemic shock *shock caused by loss of blood or body fluids.*

✓ Review

Types of Shock

Hypovolemic
Distributive
  – Anaphylactic
  – Septic
Obstructive
Cardiogenic
Respiratory
Neurogenic

distributive shock *shock that results from mechanisms that prevent the appropriate distribution of nutrients and removal of metabolic waste products.*

anaphylactic shock *form of distributive shock in which histamine causes general vasodilation, precapillary sphincter dilation, capillary engorgement, and fluid movement into the interstitial compartment.*

septic shock *form of distributive shock caused by massive infection in which toxins compromise the vascular system's ability to control blood vessels and distribute blood.*

anaphylactic shock, histamine causes general vasodilation, precapillary sphincter dilation, capillary engorgement, and fluid movement into the interstitial compartment (see Volume 3, Chapter 5, "Allergies and Anaphylaxis"). **Septic shock** results from massive infection in which the resulting toxins released by the bacteria adversely affect the vascular system's ability to control blood vessels and distribute blood.

Distributive shock may also result from problems with delivery of essential metabolic materials to the cells. Glucose delivery may be disrupted either by a lack of insulin, which restricts transport of glucose into the cells for use, or by a low level of glucose in the blood (hypoglycemia), which again limits its availability for metabolism. When either of these situations occurs, body cells then make use of alternate fuel sources—proteins and lipids. The result is a build-up of substrates that the body has a hard time getting rid of.

Another problem that causes distributive shock occurs when red blood cells are not abundant enough (anemia) or are limited in their ability to carry oxygen, as happens with carbon monoxide poisoning. Distributive shock may also occur when the environment does not contain sufficient oxygen to maintain alveolar oxygen levels. In such cases, the cells lack oxygen despite good circulation and functional hemoglobin.

Obstructive Shock

obstructive shock *shock resulting from interference with the blood flowing through the cardiovascular system.*

Obstructive shock results from interference with the blood flowing through the cardiovascular system. The causes of obstructive shock include tension pneumothorax, cardiac tamponade, and pulmonary emboli. In tension pneumothorax, the intrathoracic pressure builds and reduces the ability of the thoracoabdominal pump to help move blood back toward the heart. The situation is further worsened as the pressure displaces the mediastinum away from the progressing injury. This bends or folds the inferior vena cava as it travels through the diaphragm, further reducing venous return. In cardiac tamponade, the pericardial sac fills with blood or fluid and prevents the ventricles from completely filling. As the fluid accumulates, the filling decreases and cardiac output drops drastically. In obstructive shock involving pulmonary emboli, clots are released from the systemic venous circulation or from the heart and obstruct a significant portion of the pulmonary circulation, restricting oxygenation. This places a great strain on the right heart and reduces preload to the left ventricle.

Cardiogenic Shock

cardiogenic shock *shock resulting from failure to maintain the blood pressure because of inadequate cardiac output.*

Cardiogenic shock results from a problem with the cardiovascular pump, the heart. Due to its absolutely essential function, any problem with the heart has a profound impact on the cardiovascular system and the entire body. If a cardiac artery blockage deprives a portion of the heart muscle of circulation, that portion of the heart becomes hypoxic, then ischemic, and then necrotic, or dead. During the evolution of this infarct, there can be disturbances in the cardiac electrical system, failure of the valves, cardiac rupture, or reduced cardiac pumping action. Any of these problems reduces the cardiac output, which cannot be compensated for by some other body system. If the cardiac output falls below what the body requires, cardiogenic shock ensues. Cardiogenic shock may present with the signs and symptoms of myocardial infarction or pulmonary edema and with the classic signs and symptoms of shock. The prognosis for cardiogenic shock is very poor, with an 80 percent mortality rate.

Respiratory Shock

respiratory shock *shock resulting from failure of the respiratory system to supply oxygen to the alveoli or remove CO_2 from them.*

Respiratory shock occurs when the respiratory system is not able to bring oxygen into the alveoli and remove carbon dioxide from them, as may happen with airway obstruction. Flail chest, respiratory muscle paralysis, pneumothorax, and tension pneumothorax also reduce the respiratory system's ability to maintain alveolar oxygenation. As a result, blood leaves the pulmonary circulation without adequate oxygen and with an excess of carbon dioxide. The cells thus become hypoxic, while the bloodstream becomes acidotic.

Neurogenic Shock

Neurogenic shock results from an interruption in the communication pathway between the central nervous system and the rest of the body. A spinal injury or in some cases a head injury, either temporary or permanent, disrupts nervous (generally, sympathetic nervous) system control over vasculature distal to the injury. The arterioles dilate, the vascular container expands, and fluid is driven into the interstitial space. The body's compensatory mechanisms are often affected, and the tachycardia and rising diastolic blood pressure usually expected with shock states may not occur (see Chapter 9, "Spinal Trauma"). In these cases, the patient's skin below the nervous system injury is warm and pink, while the skin above it displays more classic signs of shock—pallor, coolness, and clamminess.

SHOCK ASSESSMENT

You must be able to recognize shock as early as possible in your patient assessment and begin to provide care just as promptly. You must search out the signs and symptoms of shock in each phase of the assessment process: the scene size-up, the initial assessment, the rapid trauma assessment or focused history and physical exam, and—when appropriate—the detailed physical exam. Further, you must carefully monitor for the development or progression of shock with frequent ongoing assessments during care and transport of the trauma patient.

Scene Size-up

Anticipate shock during the scene size-up. Analyze the forces that caused the trauma and their impacts on your patient for the possibility of both external and internal injury and hemorrhage. Look especially for injury mechanisms that might result in internal chest, abdominal, or pelvic injuries or in external hemorrhage from the head, neck, and extremities. This information will guide your later assessment. Apply trauma triage criteria as early as practical to identify the patients who are most likely to require immediate transport to the trauma center and access to air medical transport, if appropriate. Early planning at the scene of a significant trauma assures that your care is time efficient and medically appropriate.

Initial Assessment

The initial assessment directs your attention to the body systems/patient priorities that present the early signs of shock. Determine the patient's level of consciousness, responsiveness, and orientation. Any mental deficit or restlessness, anxiety, or combativeness may be due to blood loss and hypovolemia. As you assess the airway for patency and breathing for adequacy, apply high-flow, high-concentration oxygen. Watch for tachypnea and air hunger, which are late signs of shock. When assessing circulation, note the heart rate and pulse strength. A heart rate above 100 in an adult (tachycardia) suggests hypovolemia. Baseline rates suggestive of tachycardia are about 160 in the infant, 140 in the preschooler, and 120 in the school-age child. An increase of 20 beats per minute above any of these rates suggests a significant blood loss. The pulse pressure is another indicator of developing circulatory insufficiency. The weaker the pulse, the more the patient is compensating for blood loss.

Carefully observe the patient's body surface and be quick to anticipate potential shock, either as a cause of or a contributing factor to the patient's condition. Look also to the general condition of the skin. It should be warm, pink, and dry. If it is cyanotic, gray, ashen, pale, and cool and moist (clammy), suspect peripheral vasoconstriction, an early sign of shock.

neurogenic shock *type of shock resulting from an interruption in the communication pathway between the central nervous system and the rest of the body leading to decreased peripheral vascular resistance.*

In cases of neurogenic shock, the patient's skin below the nervous injury is warm and pink, while the skin above it displays more classic signs of shock—pallor, coolness, and clamminess.

During assessment, be aware that any mental deficit or restlessness, anxiety, or combativeness may be due to blood loss and hypovolemia.

Watch the pulse oximeter for the saturation value and keep it above 95 percent, if possible. As compensation increases and the pulse strength diminishes, the pulse oximeter readings will become more and more unreliable. If you note erratic or intermittent readings with the device, suspect increasing cardiovascular compensation and progressing shock as the reason.

Capnography can be a valuable assessment tool during the resuscitation of the trauma patient and is rapidly becoming the standard of care. Waveform analysis and evaluation of the end-tidal CO_2 ($ETCO_2$) may assure proper initial and continuing endotracheal tube placement and guide artificial ventilation. The capnograph measures the partial pressures of CO_2 in exhaled air, reflecting the status of both ventilation and circulation. Decreased $ETCO_2$ levels reflect cardiac arrest, shock, pulmonary embolism, or incomplete airway obstruction (bronchospasm, mucus plugging). Increased $ETCO_2$ levels reflect hypoventilation, respiratory depression, or hyperthermia. $ETCO_2$ readings above 40 mmHg suggest the need for increased ventilatory support. Readings below 30 mmHg suggest hyperventilation or the need for cirulatory support. Capnography may not recognize intubation of a mainstem bronchus, so assure breath sounds are equal while an endotracheal tube is in place.

Capnography is especially important in head injury, as an abnormally low alveolar CO_2 level may produce severe cerebral vasoconstriction. Normal expiratory CO_2 levels are between 35 and 40 mmHg and should not drop below 30 mmHg, especially in head trauma patients. An expiratory CO_2 level above 40 mmHg suggests hypoventilation and the need for faster or deeper ventilations.

Conclude the initial assessment by establishing patient priorities. If any indication, MOI, sign, or symptom suggests serious internal hemorrhage or uncontrolled external hemorrhage, consider rapid trauma assessment and expeditious transport. If the patient has minor and isolated injuries, move to the focused history and physical exam.

Focused History, Physical Exam

As noted earlier, the order in which the steps of the focused history and physical exam are performed vary with the patient's MOI. For trauma patients who have no significant mechanism, perform an assessment focused on the area of injury, then obtain baseline vital signs and gather a patient history. For trauma patients who have a significant MOI, continue spinal immobilization and perform a rapid trauma assessment and then obtain baseline vital signs and a patient history. Trauma patients with significant mechanisms of injury are the most likely to suffer from shock, so the discussion of this phase of the assessment process focuses on those patients.

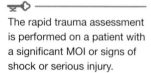

The rapid trauma assessment is performed on a patient with a significant MOI or signs of shock or serious injury.

Rapid Trauma Assessment   When you have a trauma patient with a significant MOI, perform a rapid trauma assessment, inspecting and palpating the patient from head to toe (Figure 4-19 ▪). If you notice any significant hemorrhage, control it immediately. Quickly put a dressing and bandage over the wound and apply direct pressure. Provide more complete hemorrhage control once you attend to the other priorities of care.

Be sure to examine areas of the body where you expect to find serious injury, as suggested by your scene size-up. Pay special attention to the areas most likely to produce serious, life-threatening injury: the head, neck, chest, abdomen, and pelvis. Remember, minor reddening of the skin may be the only sign of a developing contusion and serious internal injury. Also be sure to examine the neck veins. In the supine, normovolemic patient, they should be full. If they are flat, suspect hypovolemia.

During your rapid trauma assessment, rule out the possibility of obstructive shock. Assess the chest to identify any tension pneumothorax. Look for dyspnea, a hy-

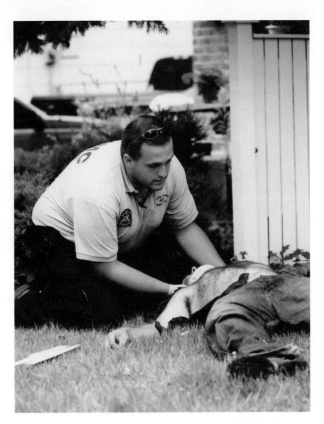

perinflated chest, distended jugular veins, resonant percussion, and diminished or absent breath sounds on the affected side, lower tracheal shift to the opposite side, and any subcutaneous emphysema. Consider pleural decompression if the signs suggest tension pneumothorax (see Chapter 10, "Thoracic Trauma"). Also suspect and search for pericardial tamponade. Look for penetrating injury, distended jugular veins, muffled or distant heart tones, tachycardia, and progressive and extreme hypotension. Pericardial tamponade is treated with IV fluids in the field and requires immediate and rapid transport to a trauma center. If the patient received significant anterior chest trauma, suspect myocardial contusion. Apply an ECG monitor and analyze the cardiac rhythm.

During the assessment, be alert to the possibility that hemorrhagic shock is not the problem or is not the only problem affecting your patient. Conditions such as stroke, epilepsy, or heart attack can lead to auto crashes and other traumatic events. Be careful to rule out cardiogenic shock by questioning the patient about chest pain and looking for pulmonary edema, jugular vein distention, and cardiac dysrhythmias (see Volume 3, Chapter 2, "Cardiology"). Also suspect and check for neurogenic shock (see Chapter 9, "Spinal Trauma"). Ask about neck or back pain and evaluate for tenderness along the spine. Look for the presence of pink and warm skin below the point of nervous system injury, while the skin above the injury is pale, cool, and clammy. Other shock states such as anaphylactic, septic, and diabetic shock are not likely unless the patient history suggests them.

Take a quick set of vital signs, keying in on both the pulse rate and pulse pressure. If the pulse is weak, its rate is elevated, or the pulse pressure is diminished, suspect serious hemorrhage. Gauge your findings against the MOI and the time from the injury to your assessment. The shorter the time and the more pronounced the signs and symptoms, the more rapidly the patient is moving toward decompensation and then irreversible shock.

Complete this step of the assessment process by gathering a patient history. Listen to any patient complaints of weakness, thirst, or nausea, which may be further signs of

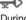

During assessment, be alert to the possibility that hemorrhagic shock is not the problem or is not the only problem affecting your patient.

shock. Be especially alert for patient complaints suggestive of a myocardial infarction. Be prepared to monitor the heart for dysrhythmias.

At the end of the rapid trauma assessment or the focused history and physical exam, inventory your findings. Set the patient's priority for transport, and set priorities for the order in which you will care for injuries. Again, if any indication, MOI, sign, or symptom suggests serious internal hemorrhage or uncontrolled external hemorrhage, consider rapid transport for the patient. Approximate the probable volume of blood lost to fractures, large contusions, and hematomas. Also note the probable locations of internal hemorrhage and attempt to approximate blood loss from them. Identify all significant injuries and assign each a priority for care. While you may not complete care for all the injuries, setting priorities assures that you quickly address those injuries most likely to contribute to the patient's hypovolemia and shock.

Detailed Physical Exam

Consider performing a detailed physical exam on a potential shock patient only after all priorities have been addressed and the patient is either en route to the trauma center or circumstances such as a prolonged extrication prevent immediate transport. If you have the time, assess the patient from head to toe and look for any additional signs of injury. Remember that your early arrival at the patient's side may mean that the ecchymosis (black-and-blue discoloration) associated with injuries has not had time to develop. Therefore, be very careful to look for reddening (erythema) and areas of local warmth, suggestive of trauma.

Ongoing Assessment

After completing the initial assessment and the rapid trauma assessment or focused history and physical exam, perform serial ongoing assessments. Reassess mental status, airway, breathing, and circulation. Reestablish patient priorities and reassess and record the vital signs. This ongoing assessment allows you to identify any trends in the patient's condition. Pay particular attention to the pulse rate and pulse pressure. If the pulse rate is increasing and the difference between the diastolic and systolic pressures is decreasing, suspect increasing compensation and worsening shock. Perform a focused assessment for any changes in symptoms the patient reports. Also, check the adequacy and effectiveness of any interventions you have performed. Provide this ongoing assessment every 5 minutes for the seriously injured patient or for any patient who displays any of the signs or symptoms of shock.

SHOCK MANAGEMENT

Airway and Breathing Management

Management of the shock patient begins with corrective actions taken during the initial assessment. One of the primary principles of shock care is to assure the best possible chance for tissue oxygenation and carbon dioxide offload. Accomplish this by assuring or providing good ventilations with supplemental high-flow, high-concentration oxygen (15 L/min via nonrebreather mask). If the patient is moving air ineffectively (at a breathing rate less than 12/min or with inadequate respiratory volume), provide positive-pressure ventilations.

Positive-pressure ventilation to the breathing patient, called **overdrive respiration,** is coordinated with the patient's breathing attempts, if possible (Figure 4-20). However, assure that the ventilations provide both a good respiratory volume (at least 500 mL) and an adequate respiratory rate (at least 12 to 16 per minute). Overdrive respiration may be indicated in patients with rib fractures, flail chest, spinal injury with di-

A primary principle of shock care is to assure the best possible chance for tissue oxygenation and carbon dioxide offload; do this by providing supplemental high-flow, high-concentration oxygen or positive-pressure ventilation.

overdrive respiration *positive-pressure ventilation supplied to a breathing patient.*

aphragmatic respirations, head injury, or any condition in which the patient, because of bellows system or respiratory control failure, is not breathing adequately on his own.

Two techniques to improve ventilatory efficiency are positive end-expiratory pressure (PEEP) and continuous positive airway pressure (CPAP). PEEP uses a restrictive valve on the endotracheal tube or mask of the bag-valve unit. There it resists exhalation, maintaining a positive pressure and keeping the patient's airway open longer during exhalation. CPAP uses special ventilation equipment that increases pressure during both inspiration and expiration. This keeps the airway open during more of the respiratory cycle.

If necessary, protect the airway with endotracheal intubation. If the patient is unresponsive or somewhat unresponsive and unable to protect his airway, be aggressive in your care. Rapid sequence intubation may be required. Shock patients frequently vomit, and gastric aspiration presents a serious, possibly fatal, consequence. Capnography may help assure proper endotracheal tube placement, help you guide your ventilatory rate and volume, and confirm that the endotracheal tube remains in the trachea.

If there is any sign of tension pneumothorax, confirm it and provide pleural decompression either at the second intercostal space, mid-clavicular line or at the fifth intercostal space, mid-axillary line (see Chapter 10, "Thoracic Trauma"). Continue to monitor the patient, because it is common for the catheter to clog and the tension pneumothorax to reappear. Insert another needle close to the first to relieve any subsequent build-up of pressure.

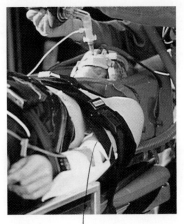

■ Figure 4-20 Assure that the potential shock patient receives adequate ventilation, using overdrive respiration, if necessary.

Hemorrhage Control

Provide rapid control of any significant external hemorrhage. Use direct pressure, direct pressure and elevation where practical, and pressure points as needed. Apply a tourniquet to control serious and continuing hemorrhage only if it is absolutely necessary. Remember, there are serious consequences with both proper and improper use of a tourniquet.

Fluid Resuscitation

The field treatment of choice for significant blood loss in trauma cases is blood. It has red blood cells to carry oxygen, has clotting factors and platelets to assist in hemostasis, and remains in the bloodstream once it is infused. Blood, however, must be refrigerated, typed, and cross-matched. (O-negative blood may be given in emergency circumstances.) Blood also has a short shelf life and is costly for field use. The most practical fluid for prehospital administration, then, is an isotonic crystalloid like lactated Ringer's solution or normal saline.

The most practical choice for prehospital fluid resuscitation is lactated Ringer's solution.

Some hypertonic and synthetic solutions may have some applications for fluid resuscitation. None of these, however, has been identified as superior to isotonic electrolyte solutions for prehospital use. Hypertonic crystalloid solutions can mobilize the interstitial and cellular fluid volumes to replace lost blood volume but, like other crystalloids, they are not able to carry either the oxygen or the clotting factors essential for hemorrhage control. The biggest advantage of hypertonic solutions is their low volume and weight—an advantage in wilderness, remote, and military applications. Synthetic agents are now available that can carry oxygen and may, in the future, assist the clotting process. These agents, however, are expensive, have short shelf lives, and pose some patient compatibility problems.

Another category of new solutions with possible indications for prehospital care are the polyhemoglobins. These solutions are either animal or human hemoglobin that has been processed to exclude antigens and microorganisms that would cause disease or adverse reaction in the recipient. Polyhemoglobins have a prolonged shelf life, are relatively inexpensive, and can effectively carry oxygen from the lungs to the tissues. Prehospital studies are being conducted and, if successful, these agents may be very useful in combating hypovolemia due to hemorrhage.

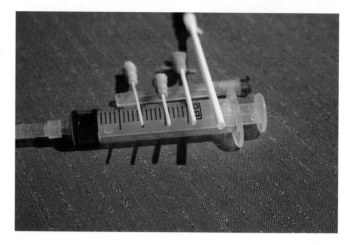

When administering fluids to a trauma patient or to any patient who may need large fluid volumes, consider the internal lumen size of both the catheter and the administration set. Fluid flow is proportional to the fourth power of the internal diameter. This means that if you double the lumen's diameter, the same fluid under the same pressure will flow 16 times more quickly. Hence, use the largest catheter you can introduce into the patient's vein and use a large-bore trauma or blood administration set (Figure 4-21 ■).

Catheter length and fluid pressure also influence fluid flow. The longer the catheter, the greater the resistance to flow. The ideal catheter for the shock patient is relatively short, 1 1/2″ or shorter. An increase in pressure increases fluid flow. This means that the higher you position the bag or the greater the pressure differential between the solution and the venous system, the faster the fluid flow. If you cannot elevate the fluid bag, position it under the patient or place it in a pressure infuser or a blood-pressure cuff inflated to 100 or 200 mmHg.

Electrolyte administration is indicated for the patient with the classic signs and symptoms of shock and isolated external hemorrhage that has been halted. Employ aggressive fluid resuscitation, using lactated Ringer's solution or normal saline via two lines running wide open until the blood pressure returns to 100 mmHg and the level of consciousness increases (Figure 4-22 ■). Use large-bore catheters (14 or 16 gauge) connected to trauma or blood tubing to assure unimpeded flow and a non-flow-restrictive saline lock if your system so requires. This fluid resuscitation approach is also prudent for the patient with continuing (internal or uncontrolled external) hemorrhage with absent peripheral pulses or a systolic BP below 80 mmHg. Run the two lines wide open until 250 to 500 mL of solution is infused. Then evaluate for the return of peripheral pulses or rise of the systolic blood pressure to just under 80 mmHg—sometimes referred to as permissive hypotension. If the patient's condition does not improve, consider repeating the fluid bolus.

Head injury patients (Glasgow Coma Scale [GCS] of 8 or less) may require a slightly higher systolic blood pressure (90 mmHg) to assure cerebral perfusion. Note, however, that prehospital fluid resuscitation is an area of much research and controversy. Consult with your medical director and local protocols to determine your system's parameters for prehospital fluid resuscitation of the shock patient.

In children, infuse 20 mL/kg of body weight rapidly when you see any signs and symptoms of shock. Administer a second fluid bolus if the vital signs do not improve after the first bolus or if, at some later time, the patient again begins to deteriorate. The objective of fluid resuscitation in the field is not the return of normal vital signs but the stabilization of vital signs until the patient reaches the trauma center.

Prehospital fluid resuscitation is an area of much research and controversy. Consult with your medical director and local protocols regarding fluid resuscitation of the shock patient.

Science vs. Dogma For years the principal prehospital treatment of hypotension due to trauma was the administration of large volumes of crystalloid solutions and rapid transport. However, research is starting to show that infusing massive quantities of crystalloids, without correcting the underlying problem, may be detrimental. Consider this: If large quantities of fluid are administered without the injury being repaired, blood loss will continue and the blood will become progressively more diluted. Thus, the number of red blood cells available to carry oxygen will begin to fall. In addition, as blood becomes diluted with IV fluids, the coagulation factors are diluted, and blood clotting becomes slower and less effective. For these reasons, some leading trauma researchers advocate limiting the amount of fluids administered prior to surgery.

Research has also started to demonstrate that hypotension (within certain parameters) following trauma may actually be protective. In fact, some are calling for "permissive hypotension" where the systolic blood pressure is maintained between 70 to 85 mmHg instead of 100 mmHg or more. The theory behind this concept is straightforward. First, several protective mechanisms appear to be activated when the blood pressure is within this range. Second, increasing the blood pressure with fluids, PASG, or similar methods might lead to a more rapid blood loss. Thus, trying to maintain normal blood pressures may actually increase the rate of blood loss and may inhibit clot formation or may cause dislodgement of a clot that formed during periods of hypotension following trauma. This concept is being aggressively studied.

The information in this box is presented to introduce you to controversies and research in the field of trauma care. Despite this information, *always follow the local protocols as established by your system and your medical director*. However, it is important to consider the ongoing research that may affect prehospital practice. EMS in the twenty-first century should be based on scientific evidence—not anecdotes or dogma.

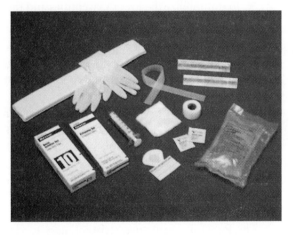

■ Figure 4-22 Supplies for initiating IV therapy.

During fluid resuscitation, cautiously control fluid volume, remembering that your goal is maintaining vital signs, not improving them. Increases in blood pressure can dislodge developing clots and disrupt the normal clotting processes. The result may be further hemorrhage with further dilution of the clotting factors and hemoglobin. Closely monitor your patient's vital signs, and administer lactated Ringer's solution or normal saline to keep the patient's mental status and pulse pressure steady. Maintain the blood pressure at a steady level once it has dropped below 80 mmHg. Do not let the pressure drop below 50 mmHg nor below 90 mmHg for head injury patients with a GCS of 8 or less.

Temperature Control

Trauma and blood loss deal serious blows to the mechanisms that normally adjust the body's core temperature. Reduced body activity reduces heat production to subnormal levels. Cutaneous vasoconstriction decreases the skin's ability to act as part of the body's temperature control system. The result is a patient highly susceptible to fluctuations in body temperature. In cases of trauma, patients commonly lose heat more rapidly than normal and heat production is low. At the same time, the heat-generating reflexes, like shivering, are ineffective and, in fact, are counterproductive to the shock care process.

In all except the warmest environments, help conserve body temperature by covering the patient with a blanket and keeping the patient compartment of the ambulance very warm. If you infuse fluids, assure that they are well above room temperature—ideally at body temperature or slightly above (no more than 104° F). Use fluid warmers or keep IV solutions in a compartment that is warmer than the rest of the ambulance. Be very sensitive to any patient complaints about being cold, and provide whatever assistance you can to assure that heat loss is limited.

Pneumatic Anti-Shock Garment

The **pneumatic anti-shock garment (PASG),** sometimes referred to as the medical anti-shock trouser (MAST), is a device designed to apply firm circumferential pressure around the lower extremities, pelvis, and lower abdomen. The device is intended to compress the vascular space, thereby accomplishing four objectives:

★ To increase peripheral vascular resistance by pressurizing the arteries of the lower abdomen and extremities

★ To reduce the vascular volume by compressing venous vessels

★ To increase the central circulating blood volume with blood returned from areas under the garment

★ To immobilize the lower extremities and the pelvic region

Research has determined that the garment is responsible for a return of about 250 mL of blood to the central circulation and probably reduces the venous capacitance by the same volume. The PASG also does seem to increase the peripheral vascular resistance, although this may be detrimental to patients with uncontrolled internal hemorrhage.

Research has further revealed potential problems with PASG use. The abdominal component of the PASG pressurizes the abdominal cavity, increasing the work associated with breathing and, in some cases, reducing chest excursion. Application of the garment also increases mortality when used in cases of penetrating chest trauma. In light of this information, it is imperative that you understand the limitations of the device and comply with your local protocols and medical direction when considering use of the PASG.

The PASG is a puncture-resistant, easy to clean, three-compartment trouser attached to the patient circumferentially around the lower abdomen and extremities with Velcro closures. The compartments can be inflated either independently or all together with a foot- or electric-powered pump. However, the abdominal segment should be inflated with the leg segments or after them, never before. A PASG may or may not come with pressure gauges, although all models should be equipped with pop-off valves to prevent inflation above 110 mmHg.

Indications for PASG use include shock patients with controlled hemorrhage, patients with pelvic fracture and instability with hypotension, patients with possible neurogenic shock, and any shock patients with uncontrolled hemorrhage below the mid-abdomen. Penetrating chest trauma, pulmonary edema, and cardiogenic shock are contraindications to PASG application and inflation. Use the PASG with caution for patients in late pregnancy, patients with suspected diaphragmatic ruptures, and patients with objects impaled in the abdomen or with abdominal eviscerations. In these cases, do not inflate the abdominal section because doing so increases intraabdominal pressure.

Begin application of the PASG by removing the patient's clothing, although you may leave on the undergarments for patient modesty if they are not bulky (Procedure 4-1). Assess areas of the patient's body that will lie beneath the garment, as these regions will be hidden from view and inaccessible once the PASG is applied. Then move the patient onto a spine board or other patient-carrying device with an opened garment positioned for application. One application technique calls for securing the garment's Velcro attachments at the ends of their travel and having a caregiver at the patient's feet put one arm through each of the garment's leg sections from the foot ends. That caregiver then grasps the patient's toes while another caregiver pulls the garment off the first caregiver's arms, onto the patient's legs, and up to the small of the patient's back. Alternatively, you may slide the device under the patient from the feet with the extra garment and the anterior abdominal segment folded between the legs. Position the PASG so that the upper portion of the abdominal segment is just below the rib margin. Secure the abdominal and leg segments with the Velcro strips, assuring that they hold the segments firmly around the limbs and abdomen. This reduces the air volume necessary to inflate the PASG.

Quickly take baseline vital signs, and be especially alert for breath sounds. If there are no crackles or other suggestions of pulmonary edema, then inflate the PASG slowly. Watch for any change (improvement) in your patient's mental status, skin color, or pulse rate. If you notice such a change, stop the inflation and reassess vital signs and level of responsiveness. The intent of PASG use is to stabilize the patient's condition, not to return the blood pressure and circulation to normal levels. As with too-aggressive fluid resuscitation, inflation of PASG to a point where blood pressure increases can interfere with the clotting process or even increase internal hemorrhage, thus moving the patient more quickly toward decompensation and death. If vital signs and the level of responsiveness deteriorate, continue PASG inflation until you regain the level of your baseline findings. Once the pop-off valves release, stop inflation. Then inflate the garment every few minutes until the pop-off valves release to assure that the PASG maintains its maximum pressure.

Carefully monitor respirations during PASG inflation. The device may put pressure on the diaphragm, thus increasing the work of respiration as well as reducing respiratory excursion. Also listen carefully for breath sounds. The PASG may increase blood pressure and respiratory congestion as well. If you hear any crackles in the chest or if the patient complains of difficulty breathing, halt the PASG inflation.

The PASG should not be deflated in the prehospital setting. The release of circumferential pressure reduces peripheral vascular resistance, expands the size of the vascular space, and removes about 250 mL of blood from the active circulation. This could seriously harm the healthy patient and have devastating effects on one who is compensating for shock.

Pharmacological Intervention

In shock, pharmacological interventions are generally limited, especially in hypovolemic patients. The sympathetic nervous system efficiently compensates for low volume, and no agent has been shown effective in the prehospital setting, other than intravenous fluid and, in some cases, blood and blood products. For cardiogenic shock, fluid challenge, vasopressors like dopamine, and the other cardiac drugs are indicated (see Volume 3, Chapter 2, "Cardiology"). For spinal and obstructive shock, consider intravenous fluids like normal saline and lactated Ringer's solution. For distributive shock, consider IV fluids, dopamine, and use of the PASG.

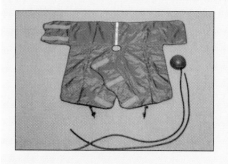

4-1a   Monitor the patient before PASG application.

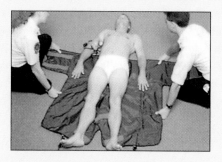

4-1b   Prepare the PASG.

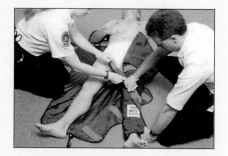

4-1c   Position the patient.

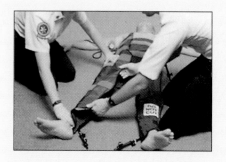

4-1d   Wrap the legs, following the manufacturer's recommendations.

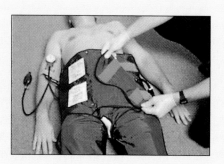

4-1e   Wrap the abdomen last.

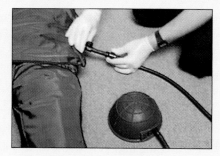

4-1f   Connect the tubing.

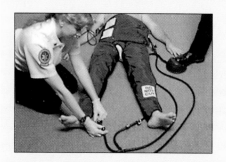

4-1g   Inflate the PASG, both legs first.

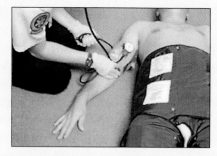

4-1h   Monitor the patient.

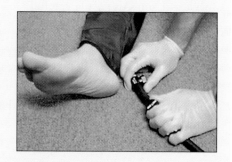

4-1i   Close the stopcock valve.

The PASG should not be deflated in the prehospital setting.

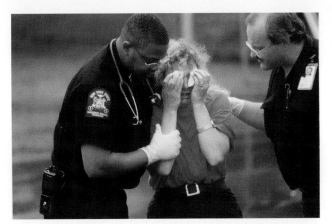

The patient who has experienced trauma sufficient to induce hemorrhage and hypovolemia will be anxious and bewildered. As the care provider at the patient's side, it is your responsibility to be calm and reassuring, thus counteracting the natural "fight-or-flight" response (Figure 4-23 ■). By acting in this manner, you not only help your patient deal with the event's emotional trauma but also combat some of the negative effects of sympathetic stimulation.

Summary

Significant hemorrhage and its serious consequence, shock, are genuine threats to the trauma patient's life. The signs of these threats are often subtle or hidden, especially if bleeding is internal. Only through careful analysis of the mechanism of injury during the scene size-up and careful evaluation of the patient during the assessment process can you recognize and then treat these life-threatening problems. Treatment often involves rapidly bringing the patient to the services of a trauma center and, while doing so, providing aggressive care—supplemental oxygen, positive pressure ventilations, fluid resuscitation, and use of a PASG as necessary—aimed at maintaining vital signs, not necessarily improving them. With this approach, you afford your patient the best chance for survival.

You Make the Call

A teenager working in the high school wood shop slips and runs his forearm into the running blade of a table saw. The blade cuts deeply into an artery, resulting in serious hemorrhage. Upon your arrival, you find the teenager to be very agitated and anxious. Your assessment reveals a blood pressure of 130/86, a pulse of 110, normal respirations at 24 breaths per minute, and skin that is cool and moist.
1. What signs suggest hypovolemia and early shock?
2. Does the blood pressure suggest shock? Why or why not?
3. What progressive steps would you take to control the hemorrhage?
4. What supportive care measures would you employ?

See Suggested Responses at the back of this book.

Review Questions

1. The initial signs of compensated shock accompanying external hemorrhage include all of the following except:
   a. unconsciousness.
   b. thirst.
   c. combativeness.
   d. weakness.

2. You and your crew respond to a motor vehicle collision where a 20-year-old female has received several cuts over her body. You determine that her airway is patent and she is breathing adequately. Her blood pressure is maintaining at a stable level, and you estimate that she has lost approximately 15 percent of her circulating blood volume. She is alert and oriented but seems a bit nervous. From these findings, you determine that your patient is in _____ hemorrhage.
   a. stage 4
   b. stage 1
   c. stage 3
   d. stage 2

3. In a patient with no suspected trauma, and signs and symptoms of shock, you can perform the tilt test. This test is performed to determine:
   a. cardiogenic shock.
   b. septic shock.
   c. orthostatic hypertension.
   d. orthostatic hypotension.

4. The arterial blood pressure is monitored by receptors in the aortic arch and carotid sinuses. These receptors send signals to the medulla oblongata to help maintain a blood pressure that assures adequate perfusion. These receptors are the:
   a. chemoreceptors.
   b. baroreceptors.
   c. cardioinhibitory centers.
   d. cardioacceleratory centers.

5. When the body is working to counteract the effects of hemorrhage and cardiovascular insufficiency, it constricts arterioles and increases the heart rate and contractility. The most rapid hormonal response occurs with the release of:
   a. angiotesin II.
   b. glucocorticoids.
   c. antidiuretic hormone.
   d. catecholamines.

6. You are called to the scene where a man is very nearly unconscious. His vital signs indicate a falling blood pressure and bradycardia as well as cool, clammy skin. Based on these assessment findings, you conclude that the patient is most likely in:
   a. neurogenic shock.
   b. irreversible shock.
   c. decompensated shock.
   d. compensated shock.

7. Rapid transport to a trauma facility is indicated in which of the following patients?
   a. a patient in stage 1 hemorrhage
   b. a patient with suspected serious internal hemorrhage
   c. a patient who is vomiting coffee-ground material
   d. a patient with external hemorrhage that is controlled on the scene

8. The PASG is contraindicated for which of the following types of shock?
   a. neurogenic
   b. respiratory
   c. hypovolemic
   d. cardiogenic

9. Your patient is determined to be in decompensated shock. Fluid therapy is indicated. The most practical fluid for prehospital administration is:
   a. D_5W.
   b. blood plasma.
   c. lactated Ringer's.
   d. D_5W in half normal saline.

10. A patient develops shock secondary to hypovolemia. You understand that the reduced flow of oxygen to the cells leads to a build-up of lactic acid and other byproducts. You further understand that _____ metabolism causes this process to occur.
    a. Krebs
    b. aerobic
    c. glycolysis
    d. anaerobic

See Answers to Review Questions at the back of this book.

Further Reading

Bledsoe, B. E. and D. Clayden. *Prehospital Emergency Pharmacology.* 6th ed. Upper Saddle River, N.J.: Pearson/Prentice Hall, 2005.

Butman, A., S. Martin, R. Vomacka, and N. McSwain, *Comprehensive Guide to Pre-Hospital Skills: A Skills Manual for EMT-Basic, EMT-Intermediate, and EMT-Paramedic.* St. Louis: Mosby, 1996.

Ivatury, R. R, and C. G. Cayten. *The Textbook of Penetrating Trauma.* Baltimore: Williams & Wilkins, 1996.

Martini, Frederic. *Fundamentals of Anatomy and Physiology.* 6th ed. San Francisco: Benjamin Cummings, 2004.

NAEMT (N. McSwain, Jr., S. Frame, and J. Salomone, eds.). *PHTLS: Basic and Advanced Prehospital Trauma Life Support.* 5th ed. St. Louis: Mosby, 2003.

On the Web

Visit Brady's Paramedic Website at **www.bradybooks.com/paramedic**.

Soft-Tissue Trauma

Objectives

After reading this chapter, you should be able to:

1. Describe the incidence, morbidity, and mortality of soft-tissue injuries. (p. 130)
2. Describe the anatomy and physiology of the integumentary system, including:
   a. Epidermis (pp. 130–131)
   b. Dermis (pp. 130, 131–132)
   c. Subcutaneous tissue (pp. 130, 132)
3. Identify the skin tension lines of the body. (p. 134)
4. Predict soft-tissue injuries based on the mechanism of injury. (pp. 135–140, 152–155)
5. Discuss blunt and penetrating trauma. (pp. 135–140)
6. Discuss the pathophysiology of soft-tissue injuries. (pp. 135–150)
7. Differentiate among the following types of soft-tissue injuries:
   a. Closed (pp. 135–136)
      i. Contusion
      ii. Hematoma
      iii. Crush injuries
   b. Open (pp. 136–140)
      i. Abrasions
      ii. Lacerations
      iii. Incisions
      iv. Avulsions
      v. Impaled objects
      vi. Amputations
      vii. Punctures

8. Discuss the assessment and management of open and closed soft-tissue injuries. (pp. 152–172)

9. Discuss the incidence, morbidity, and mortality of crush injuries. (pp. 136, 148–149, 166–169)

10. Define the following conditions:
    a. Crush injury (pp. 136, 148)
    b. Crush syndrome (pp. 148–149, 166–169)
    c. Compartment syndrome (p. 169)

11. Discuss the mechanisms of injury, assessment findings, and management of crush injuries. (pp.136, 148–149, 166–169)

12. Discuss the effects of reperfusion and rhabdomyolysis on the body. (pp. 148–149, 166–169)

13. Discuss the pathophysiology, assessment, and care of hemorrhage associated with soft-tissue injuries, including:
    a. Capillary bleeding (p. 157)
    b. Venous bleeding (p. 157)
    c. Arterial bleeding (pp. 157–160)

14. Describe and identify the indications for and application of the following dressings and bandages: (pp. 150–152)
    a. Sterile/nonsterile dressing
    b. Occlusive/nonocclusive dressing
    c. Adherent/nonadherent dressing
    d. Absorbent/nonabsorbent dressing
    e. Wet/dry dressing
    f. Self-adherent roller bandage
    g. Gauze bandage
    h. Adhesive bandage
    i. Elastic bandage

15. Predict the possible complications of an improperly applied dressing or bandage. (pp. 150–152, 164)

16. Discuss the process of wound healing, including: (pp. 141–143)
    a. Hemostasis
    b. Inflammation
    c. Epithelialization
    d. Neovascularization
    e. Collagen synthesis

17. Discuss the assessment and management of wound healing. (pp. 141–148)

18. Discuss the pathophysiology, assessment, and management of wound infection. (pp. 144–146)

19. Formulate treatment priorities for patients with soft-tissue injuries in conjunction with:
    a. Airway/face/neck trauma (p. 170)
    b. Thoracic trauma (open/closed) (pp. 170–171)
    c. Abdominal trauma (p. 171)

20. Given several preprogrammed and moulaged soft-tissue trauma patients, provide the appropriate scene size-up, initial assessment, rapid trauma or focused physical exam and history, detailed exam, and ongoing assessment and provide appropriate patient care and transportation. (pp. 129–172)

Key Terms

abrasion, p. 136
amputation, p. 140
avulsion, p. 139
chemotactic factors, p. 142
collagen, p. 143
compartment syndrome, p. 146
contusion, p. 135
crush injury, p. 136
crush syndrome, p. 136
degloving injury, p. 139
dermis, p. 131
ecchymosis, p. 135
epidermis, p. 131
epithelialization, p. 143
erythema, p. 135

fibroblasts, p. 143
gangrene, p. 145
granulocytes, p. 143
hematoma, p. 136
hemostasis, p. 141
impaled object, p. 138
incision, p. 138
inflammation, p. 142
integumentary system, p. 129
keloid, p. 147
laceration, p. 137
lumen, p. 132
lymphangitis, p. 144
lymphocyte, p. 132
macrophages, p. 132

muscle, p. 133
necrosis, p. 148
neovascularization, p. 143
phagocytosis, p. 143
puncture, p. 138
remodeling, p. 143
rhabdomyolosis, p. 148
sebaceous glands, p. 131
sebum, p. 131
serous fluid, p. 146
subcutaneous tissue, p. 132
sudoriferous glands, p. 131
tendons, p. 133
tension lines, p. 134

Case Study

Maria and Jon, the paramedics of University Medic 151, respond to an "axe injury." Upon arrival, they find an adult male standing next to a pile of wood, a bloody axe at his feet. The man is holding a blood-soaked rag against his arm. Maria quickly ascertains from the man and several bystanders that the wound is accidental and occurred while he was chopping wood. No other victims are present.

Maria and Jon proceed to help, donning disposable gloves and splash protection as they approach the patient. Initial assessment reveals the patient to be a healthy 42-year-old man, named Walter, who cut his left upper arm when the axe blade slipped during a chopping stroke. Walter states the wound is "deep" and there was "lots of blood" initially, but that he stopped the bleeding fairly easily by putting pressure on it. Walter reports no other injuries or complaints. He is alert and oriented, standing upright, and shows no apparent distress. His airway is obviously open and his breathing is adequate, his skin is slightly pale, and his pulse rate is somewhat rapid.

Because Walter has an isolated injury and no significant mechanism of injury, Maria and Jon proceed with the focused history and physical exam on the scene. They perform a focused trauma assessment of the upper extremity, which reveals an apparently large wound on the middle of the upper arm just over the biceps area. Close inspection of the wound is not yet possible because the patient is holding a folded rag over the wound in an effort to control bleeding. Despite these efforts, a trickle of dark blood continues to flow. A small stain of dark blood is visible on the ground. Distal pulses and capillary refill are both present and equal to the opposite extremity. The patient can move all his fingers and his wrist, but cannot flex his elbow. Sensation appears intact, although Walter reports some vague tingling in the fingers.

To control the bleeding and better visualize the wound, Maria will need to remove the rag and inspect the wound. To prepare for this, she and Jon gather several bulky sterile dressings and have them ready. They then position Walter supine on the stretcher. In a coordinated fashion, they remove the rag (taking care to avoid dislodging clots) and simultaneously replace it with a bulky, sterile dressing. A quick look at the wound indicates that it measures approximately 8 cm long and extends deep into the skin, subcutaneous tissue, and muscle layers. There is no spurting or bright red blood, but a large amount of dark red blood flows from the uncovered wound. The new dressings and direct pressure applied with a bandage easily bring the bleeding under control.

While performing the focused assessment, the paramedics also gather a patient history. Walter reports no significant medical problems and says he takes no medications. He doesn't recall the date of his last tetanus booster. He reports no allergies and that his last meal was a large lunch 2 hours ago.

Following application of the dressings and bandage, distal pulse, motor function, sensation, and capillary refill in the extremity are unchanged. Maria and Jon then take a baseline set of vital signs: respirations—20 per minute and adequate; pulse—92; skin—warm, dry, and slightly pale; pupils—equal and reactive; blood pressure (obtained on the right arm)—134/78 mmHg.

Maria and Jon now transport Walter, with his bleeding under control, uneventfully to the hospital emergency department. In the hospital, the emergency physician examines Walter using local anesthetic and a pneumatic limb tourniquet to obtain a bloodless field. Using a combination of inspection under powerful exam lights and careful palpation with gloved fingers, the physician determines that the wound has not damaged any bones, arteries, nerves, or tendons, and that no foreign bodies have lodged in it. The wound does, however, extend into the muscle layer of the biceps. Using layered closure, the physician sutures the wound, and Walter receives a tetanus booster. The sutures will be removed after 10 to 14 days, by which time Walter should be well on his way to recovery.

INTRODUCTION TO SOFT-TISSUE INJURIES

The skin is one of the largest, most important organs of the human body, comprising 16 percent of total body weight. It provides a protective envelope that keeps invading pathogens out while containing body substances and fluids. It is also a key organ of sensation as well as a radiator of excess body heat in warm weather and a conservator of heat in cold conditions. Even as it accomplishes these various functions, the skin remains a durable, pliable, and accommodating tissue, and one that is very able to repair itself.

Known collectively as the **integumentary system,** the skin is the first tissue of the human body to experience the effects of trauma. Because skin covers the entire body

integumentary system *skin, consisting of the epidermis, dermis, and subcutaneous layers.*

surface, any penetrating injury or the kinetic forces of blunt injury must pass through it before impacting on other vital organs. Often, the signs of this energy transmission can only be observed with very careful examination of the skin. Therefore, the skin is of great significance at all stages of the patient assessment process.

Trauma to the skin may present as open injuries—abrasions, lacerations, incisions, punctures, avulsions, and amputations—or as closed injuries—contusions, hematomas, and crush injuries. Although such injuries only infrequently pose direct threats to life, they may endanger blood vessels, nerves, connective tissue, and other important internal structures. Uncontrolled blood loss may lead to hypovolemia and shock, while the wound may provide a pathway for infection.

EPIDEMIOLOGY

Soft-tissue injuries are by far the most common form of trauma. Over 10 million patients present to emergency departments annually with soft-tissue wounds, many of which require closure. Most, but not all, open wounds require only simple care and limited suturing. A significant minority, however, damage arteries, nerves, or tendons and can lead to permanent disability. Uncontrolled external hemorrhage of an otherwise uncomplicated open wound is a very rare but completely preventable situation that sometimes occurs with this type of injury and can result in death. Of the open wounds presenting to emergency departments, up to 6.5 percent will eventually become infected, resulting in significant morbidity.

Closed wounds share a similar epidemiology, except that they are probably even more common than open injuries. Most minor "bumps and bruises" never reach the paramedic, as most patients elect to self-treat all but the most serious cases. Despite their frequency and usually minor nature, closed injuries *can* result in significant pain, suffering, and morbidity. Infection, however, is not usually a complication with closed wounds.

Risk factors for soft-tissue wounds include age (school-age children and the elderly are most prone), alcohol or drug abuse, and occupation. Laborers, machine operators, and others whose hands and body parts are exposed to heavy objects, machines, or tools are at great risk.

Simple measures can reduce risks and prevent soft-tissue injuries. For example, locating playgrounds on grass, sand, gravel, or other forgiving surfaces and padding the equipment in them can cut injury rates among children. In factories, machine guards, fail-safe switches, and similar engineering controls can reduce injuries. Protective clothing such as steel-toed boots and leather gloves also provide simple methods of reducing the incidence and severity of soft-tissue injuries.

ANATOMY AND PHYSIOLOGY OF SOFT-TISSUE INJURIES

The protective envelope we call the skin is a complex structure. Understanding how it is put together and how it functions will help you appreciate the importance of injuries to it and the value of their proper care.

LAYERS OF THE SKIN

The epidermis, dermis, and subcutaneous tissue layers comprise what is commonly known as the skin (Figure 5-1 ■). Each of these layers performs functions essential to helping the body maintain homeostasis and each plays an important role in the wound repair process.

Soft-tissue injuries are the most common type of trauma.

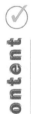

Review

Layers of the Skin

Epidermis
Dermis
Subcutaneous tissue

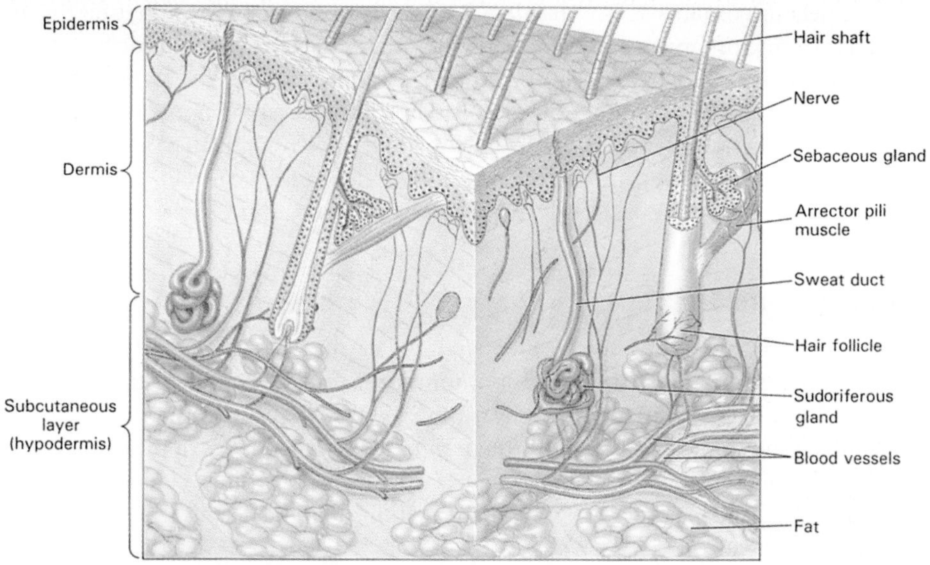

Epidermis
Dermis
Subcutaneous layer (hypodermis)

Hair shaft
Nerve
Sebaceous gland
Arrector pili muscle
Sweat duct
Hair follicle
Sudoriferous gland
Blood vessels
Fat

■ Figure 5-1 Layers and major structures of the skin.

Epidermis

The outermost skin layer is the **epidermis.** It is generated by a layer of cells just above the dermis (stratum germinativum). These cells divide rapidly, generating a movement of cells upward toward the epidermal surface. As the epidermis contains no vasculature, the further these cells are pushed away from the dermis, the less circulation they receive, and they eventually die. As they die, they flatten and interlock, providing a firm and secure barrier around the body (stratum corneum). The outermost cells are eventually abraded or washed away and then replaced, allowing the epidermis to maintain its thickness. It normally takes 2 weeks for a cell to move from the dermal border to the surface of the epidermis and another 2 to 4 weeks until it is abraded away. This outward movement of cells helps the body resist invasion by bacteria.

A waxy substance called **sebum** lubricates the surface of the epidermis. This lubrication acts much like oil on leather. It keeps the outer layers of the skin flexible, strong, and resistant to penetration by water. The epidermis is also responsible for the pigmentation that protects the skin from the harmful effects of ultraviolet radiation. The thickness of the epidermis varies greatly, depending on the amount of abrasion and pressure it receives. On the soles of the feet, it is very thick and strong, while over the eye it is microscopic in thickness and very delicate.

Dermis

Directly beneath the epidermis is the **dermis,** a connective tissue that helps contain the body and supports the functions of the epidermis. The upper layer of the dermis is the papillary layer, consisting of loose connective tissue, capillaries, and nerves supplying the epidermis. The reticular layer is the deeper dermis made up of strong connective tissue that integrates the dermis firmly with the subcutaneous layer below.

The dermis contains blood vessels, nerve endings, glands, and other structures. It is here that **sebaceous glands** produce sebum and secrete it directly onto the surface of the skin or into hair follicles. **Sudoriferous glands** secrete sweat to help move heat out of and away from the body through evaporation. Hair follicles produce hair that helps to reduce surface abrasion and conserve heat. The connective tissue within the dermis bonds it strongly to the subcutaneous tissue beneath and to the epidermis above. This tissue also holds the skin firmly around the body and permits the stretching and flexibility necessary for articulation.

epidermis   *outermost layer of the skin comprised of dead or dying cells.*

sebum   *fatty secretion of the sebaceous gland that helps keep the skin pliable and waterproof.*

dermis   *true skin, also called the corium; it is the layer of tissue producing the epidermis and housing the structures, blood vessels, and nerves normally associated with the skin.*

sebaceous glands   *glands within the dermis secreting sebum.*

sudoriferous glands   *glands within the dermis that secrete sweat.*

The dermis contains several resident body cells responsible for initiating the attack on invading organisms, foreign materials, and damaged cells, and for beginning the repair of damaged tissue. The **macrophages** and **lymphocytes** (types of white blood cells) begin the inflammation response by killing invading bodies and triggering a call for other, similar cells. Mast cells control the microcirculation to tissues and respond to the initial invasion, increasing capillary flow and permeability. Fibroblasts lay down and repair protein strands to strengthen the wound site and begin restoring the skin's integrity.

Subcutaneous Tissue

Subcutaneous tissue is the body layer beneath the dermis. It is rich in fatty or adipose tissue, which helps it absorb the forces of trauma, protecting the tissues and vital organs beneath. Because of its fatty content, heat moves outward through the subcutaneous tissue three times more slowly than through muscles or other layers of the skin; hence, it is of great value in conserving body temperature. The body directs blood below the subcutaneous tissue to conserve heat and above it through the dermis when it is necessary to radiate heat.

BLOOD VESSELS

Blood is an important medium that moves through the skin. It consists of water, electrolytes, proteins, and cells traveling through arteries, arterioles, capillaries, venules, and veins. Any soft-tissue wound can affect this blood flow; therefore, it is important to review the basic structure of the blood vessels and the actions the body takes once they are injured.

All blood vessels, except for the smallest—the capillaries, arterioles, and venules—are made up of three distinct layers: the tunica intima, the tunica media, and the tunica adventitia (Figure 5-2 ■).

The tunica intima is the blood vessel's smooth interior lining. It allows for free blood flow and prevents diffusion of nutrients and oxygen as well as waste products such as carbon dioxide.

The tunica media is the muscular component of the vessel. Its contraction or relaxation, as controlled by the central nervous system, determines the vessel's internal diameter, or **lumen.** The size of the lumen determines the amount of blood flow that passes to a particular organ or extremity. Tunica media muscle fibers are found in two orientations. Most are wrapped around the vessel circumferentially and cause lumen constriction when they contract. Arterioles have the ability to vary their internal diameter by a factor of 5, permitting them to actively regulate blood flow to the tissues they precede. Other muscle fibers run lengthwise with the vessels, and their function is not well understood.

The outer blood vessel layer is the tunica adventitia. It consists of connective tissue defining the maximum vessel lumen when the muscles relax (dilate).

The smallest blood vessels are the capillaries. Their walls are only one cell thick, allowing for the easy diffusion of oxygen, carbon dioxide, nutrients, and waste products among the vascular, interstitial, and intracellular spaces. The capillary wall structure also permits the movement of disease-combating cells into the interstitial space. Capillaries provide oxygenated circulation to virtually every cell of the body.

Not all fluids brought to the body cells are returned directly to the bloodstream. Some fluid is instead returned to the major veins by a system of channels and tissues called the lymphatic system. This system is especially important in carrying the byproducts of pathogen destruction to nodes where macrophages further break the material down. The lymph fluid is then directed to ducts just above the superior vena cavae, where it is mixed with returning venous blood.

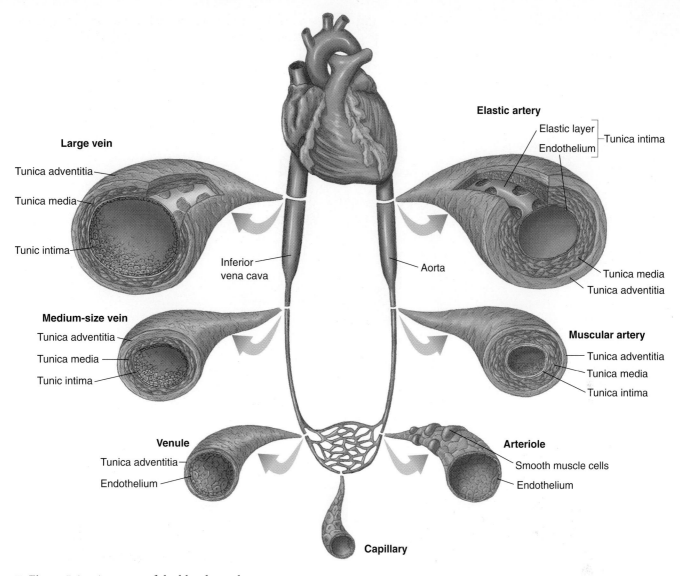

Large vein

Tunica adventitia

Tunica media

Tunic intima

Inferior vena cava

Aorta

Elastic artery

Elastic layer ⎤
Endothelium ⎦ Tunica intima

Tunica media

Tunica adventitia

Medium-size vein

Tunica adventitia

Tunica media

Tunic intima

Muscular artery

Tunica adventitia

Tunica media

Tunica intima

Venule

Tunica adventitia

Endothelium

Arteriole

Smooth muscle cells

Endothelium

Capillary

■ Figure 5-2   Anatomy of the blood vessels.

MUSCLES

Beneath the skin layers are the body's masses of skeletal **muscles.** They provide the power for movement and give the body its shape. They also produce much of the heat necessary to maintain body temperature. The muscles are strong contractile tissue, and their bulk helps protect the vital organs, blood vessels, and nerves underneath. The muscle layer can be quite thick, as in the upper arms, shoulders, thighs and legs, and buttocks; or thin, as in the forehead and hands. The muscles, which are connected to the skeleton by **tendons,** provide the driving force for the system of levers that moves the body and its appendages. Beneath the skeletal muscle layer lies the skeleton (the extremities, chest, and head) or the internal organs (the abdomen).

muscle *contractile tissue organized in large bundles that provides locomotion and movement for the body.*

tendons *long, thin, very strong collagen tissues that connect muscles to bones.*

Fasciae

Fasciae are fibrous sheets that bundle skeletal muscle masses together and segregate them, one from another. The fasciae can be very strong and thick, especially in the leg and upper arm. Within a limb, the fasciae define compartments with relatively fixed capacities and little room for expansion.

Anatomy and Physiology of Soft-Tissue Injuries   **133**

■ Figure 5-3 Tension lines of
the skin.

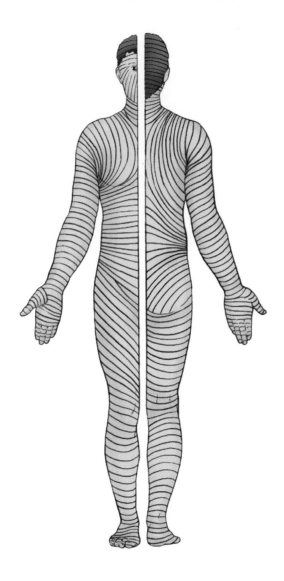

TENSION LINES

The skin does not merely hang on the flesh but rather is spread over the body and attached to fit the contours of the underlying structures. This creates natural stretch or
tension in the skin. The orientation of tension in the skin is revealed in characteristic
patterns called **tension lines** (Figure 5-3 ■). The effects of tension on the skin become
evident when the skin is transected, as with a laceration. Lacerations cutting across the
tension lines have a tendency to be pulled apart and thus spread widely or gape. Lacerations parallel to the tension lines tend to gape very little. Wounds that spread widely
tend to bleed more than those with minimal gaping. Large gaping wounds heal more
slowly and are more likely to leave noticeable scars than wounds that spread less.

   The tension represented by skin tension lines can be either static or dynamic. Static tension is noted in areas with limited movement of the tissue and structures beneath,
as in the anterior abdomen or between joints in the extremities. Dynamic tension lines
occur in areas subject to great movement, as in the skin over joints like the elbow, wrist,
or knee. The increased motion in areas with dynamic skin tension lines means that the
clotting and tissue mending processes in these areas are more frequently interrupted,
disrupting and complicating skin repair.

tension lines *natural patterns
in the surface of the skin revealing
tensions within.*

PATHOPHYSIOLOGY OF SOFT-TISSUE INJURY

Although we often take the skin's functions for granted, soft-tissue injury can seriously affect health, causing severe blood and fluid loss, infection, hypothermia, and other problems. Therefore, as a paramedic, you need to become familiar with the pathophysiology of soft-tissue injuries.

Trauma is a violent transfer of energy that produces an open or closed wound to the skin and possible injury to the structures underneath. Wounds can be either blunt or penetrating (Figure 5-4 ■). While all penetrating wounds are open, blunt trauma can, on occasion, create open wounds. Common soft-tissue injuries include closed wounds—contusions, hematomas, and crush injuries—and open wounds—abrasions, lacerations, incisions, punctures, avulsions, and amputations. Each type of wound is different and deserves special consideration.

CLOSED WOUNDS

Contusions

Contusions are blunt, nonpenetrating injuries that crush and damage small blood vessels (Figure 5-5 ■). Blood is drawn to the inflamed tissue, causing a reddening called **erythema.** Blood also leaks into the surrounding interstitial spaces through damaged vessels. As the hemoglobin within the free blood loses its oxygen, it becomes dark red and then blue, resulting in the black-and-blue discoloration called **ecchymosis.** Because the development of ecchymosis is a progressive process, the discoloration may not be evident during prehospital care.

⊘ Review

Types of Closed Wounds

Contusions
Hematomas
Crush injuries

contusion *closed wound in which the skin is unbroken, although damage has occurred to the tissue immediately beneath.*

erythema *general reddening of the skin due to dilation of the superficial capillaries.*

ecchymosis *blue-black discoloration of the skin due to leakage of blood into the tissues.*

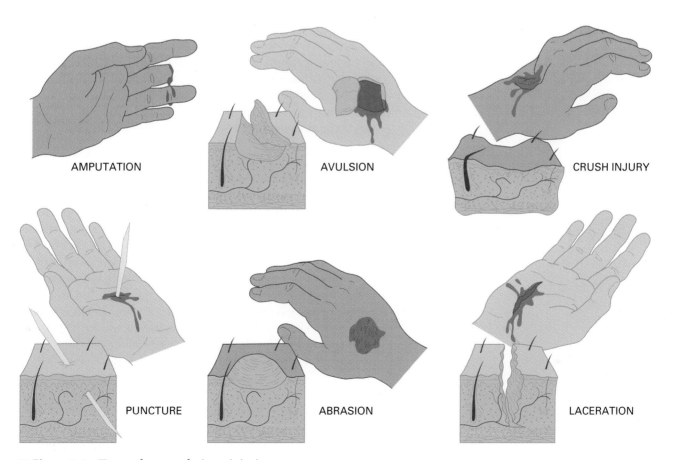

AMPUTATION   AVULSION   CRUSH INJURY

PUNCTURE   ABRASION   LACERATION

■ Figure 5-4   Types of open soft-tissue injuries.

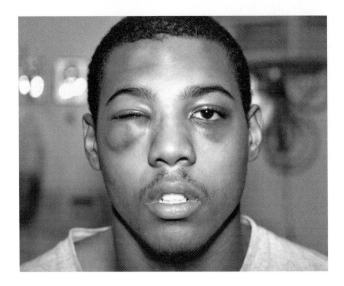

■ Figure 5-5   A contusion. Note that the discoloration of a contusion is a delayed sign. (© *Edward T. Dickinson, MD*)

Contusions are more pronounced in areas where the mechanism causing the injury (for example, a steering wheel) and skeletal structures (such as the ribs or skull) trap the skin. Occasionally, a chest injury displays an erythematous or ecchymotic outline of the ribs and sternum, reflecting an impact with the auto dashboard or some other blunt object. Early signs of such an injury may be difficult to identify, but they will become more evident as time passes and discoloration increases.

Hematomas

hematoma   *collection of blood beneath the skin or trapped within a body compartment.*

Soft-tissue bleeding can occur within the tissue and at times can be quite significant. When the injury involves a larger blood vessel, most commonly an artery, the blood can actually separate tissue and pool in a pocket called a **hematoma.** These injuries are very visible in cases of head trauma because of the unyielding skull underneath. Hematomas tend to be less pronounced in other body areas, even though they can contain significant hemorrhage. Severe hematomas to the thigh, leg, or arm may contribute significantly to hypovolemia. A hematoma in the thigh, for example, can contain over a liter of blood before swelling becomes noticeable.

crush injury   *mechanism of injury in which tissue is locally compressed by high pressure forces.*

crush syndrome   *systemic disorder of severe metabolic disturbances resulting from the crush of a limb or other body part.*

Crush Injuries

The term **crush injury** describes a collection of traumatic insults that includes both crush injury itself and crush syndrome. In crush injury, a body part that is compressed, possibly by a heavy object, sustains deep injury to the muscles, blood vessels, bones, and other internal structures (Figure 5-6 ■). Damage can be massive, despite minimal signs displayed on the skin itself. **Crush syndrome** is the term used to describe the systemic effects of a large crush injury. If the pressure that causes a crush injury remains in place for several hours, the resulting destruction of skeletal muscle cells leads to the accumulation of large quantities of myoglobin (a cell protein), potassium, lactic acid, uric acid, and other toxins. When the pressure is released, these products enter the bloodstream. They circulate, causing a severe metabolic acidosis. These materials are also toxic to the kidneys and heart. Crush syndrome is thus a potentially life-threatening trauma event. It will be discussed in more detail later in this chapter.

 Review

Types of Open Wounds

Abrasions
Lacerations
Incisions
Punctures
Impaled objects
Amputations

OPEN WOUNDS

Abrasions

abrasion   *scraping or abrading away of the superficial layers of the skin; an open soft-tissue injury.*

Abrasions are typically the most minor of injuries that violate the protective envelope of the skin. They involve a scraping or abrasive action that removes layers of the epidermis

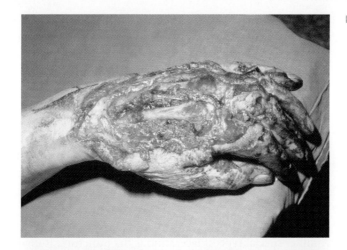

■ Figure 5-6 A crush injury.

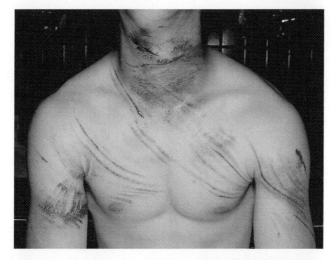

■ Figure 5-7 Abrasions.
(© *Charles Stewart, MD*)

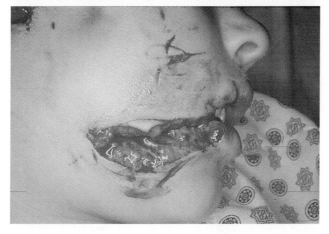

■ Figure 5-8 Lacerations
(secondary to animal bite).

and the upper reaches of the dermis (Figure 5-7 ■). Bleeding can be persistent but is usually limited because the injury involves only superficial capillaries. If the injury compromises a large area of the epidermis, it carries the danger of serious infection.

Lacerations

A **laceration** is an open wound that penetrates more deeply into the dermis than an abrasion (Figure 5-8 ■). A laceration tends to involve a smaller surface area, being limited to the tissue immediately surrounding the penetration. It endangers the deeper and

laceration *an open wound, normally a tear with jagged borders.*

more significant vasculature—arteries, arterioles, venules, and veins—as well as nerves, muscles, tendons, ligaments, and perhaps some underlying organs. As with an abrasion, the injury breaks the skin's protective barrier and provides a pathway for infection. You should note the laceration's orientation to the skin tension lines during your assessment of the patient. If the orientation parallels those lines, the wound may remain closed. If it is perpendicular to them, the wound may gape open.

Incisions

incision *very smooth or surgical laceration, frequently caused by a knife, scalpel, razor blade, or piece of glass.*

An **incision** is a surgically smooth laceration, often caused by a sharp instrument such as a knife, straight razor, or piece of glass. Such a wound tends to bleed freely. In all other ways, it is a laceration.

Punctures

puncture *specific soft-tissue injury involving a deep, narrow wound to the skin and underlying organs that carries an increased danger of infection.*

Another special type of laceration is the **puncture.** It involves a small entrance wound with damage that extends into the body's interior (Figure 5-9 ■). The wound normally seals itself and presents in a way that does not reflect the actual extent of injury. If the puncture penetrates deeply, it may involve not just the skin but underlying muscles, nerves, bones, and organs. A puncture additionally carries an increased danger of infection. A penetrating object introduces bacteria and other pathogens deep into a wound. There, the disrupted tissue and blood vessels, along with a reduced oxygen level, create a warm and moist environment that is ideal for the colonization of bacteria.

Impaled Objects

impaled object *foreign body embedded in a wound.*

An **impaled object** is not a wound itself, but rather a wound complication often associated with a puncture or laceration. Impaled objects are important for the damage they may cause if withdrawn. Frequently, embedded objects are irregular in shape and may become entangled in important structures such as arteries, nerves, or tendons (Figure 5-10 ■). Their removal in the field can result in further damage. Perhaps more critically, the embedded object may have lacerated a large blood vessel and the object's presence temporarily blocks, or tamponades, blood loss. Removal of the object may cause an uncontrollable flow of blood. This situation is particularly dangerous when the object is impaled in the neck or trunk, where the application of effective direct pressure is difficult or impossible.

■ Figure 5-9   A puncture wound.

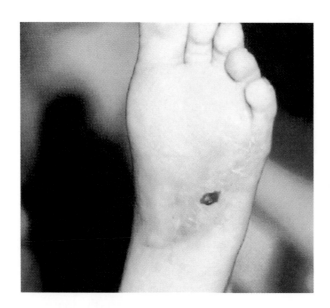

Avulsions

Avulsion occurs when a flap of skin, although torn or cut, is not torn completely loose
from the body (Figure 5-11 ■). Avulsion is frequently seen with blunt trauma to the
skull, where the scalp is torn and folds back. It may also occur with animal bites and machinery accidents. The seriousness of the avulsion depends upon the area involved, the
condition of the circulation to (and distal to) the injury site, and the degree of contamination.

A special type of avulsion is the **degloving injury.** In this wound, the mechanism
of injury tears the skin off the underlying muscle, connective tissue, blood vessels, and
bone. It is a particularly gruesome injury, occurring occasionally with farm and industrial machinery. The device pulls the skin off with great force as the skeletal tissue underneath is held stationary. The wound exposes a large area of tissue and is often
severely contaminated. The injury carries with it a poor prognosis. If, however, the vasculature and innervation remain intact, there may be some hope for future use of the
digit or extremity.

A variation of the degloving process is the ring injury (Figure 5-12 ■). As a person
jumps or falls, the ring is caught, pulling the skin of the finger against the weight of the
victim. The force may tear the upper layers of tissue away from the phalanges, exposing
the tendons, nerves, and blood vessels. Although the ring injury involves a smaller area,
it is otherwise a degloving injury.

avulsion *forceful tearing away
or separation of body tissue; an
avulsion may be partial or
complete.*

degloving injury *avulsion in
which the mechanism of injury
tears the skin off the underlying
muscle, tissue, blood vessels, and
bone.*

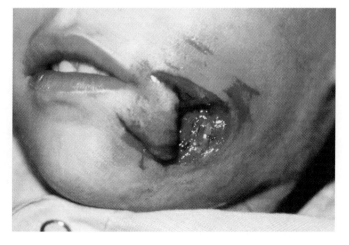

■ Figure 5-11 An avulsion.

■ Figure 5-12 A ring-type degloving injury.

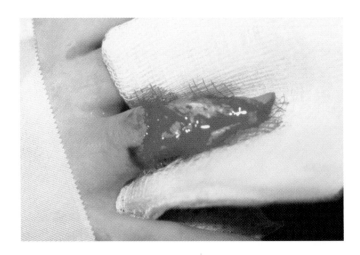

■ Figure 5-12 A ring-type degloving injury.

amputation *severance, removal, or detachment, either partial or complete, of a body part.*

Amputations

The partial or complete severance of a digit or limb is an **amputation** (Figure 5-13 ■). It often results in the complete loss of the limb at the site of severance. The hemorrhage associated with the amputation may be limited if the limb or digit is cut cleanly or may be severe and continuing if the wound is a jagged or crushing one. The surgeon may attempt to replant the amputated part or use its skin for grafting as the remaining limb is repaired. If this skin is unavailable, the surgeon may have to cut the bone and musculature back further to close the wound. This reduces the length of the limb as well as its future usefulness. When amputation is considered, great care is used to assure that the stump will be as functional as possible and suitable for prosthetic devices.

HEMORRHAGE

Soft-tissue injuries frequently cause blood loss, ranging in severity from inconsequential to life threatening. The loss can be arterial, venous, or capillary (Figure 5-14 ■). Bleeding can be easy or almost impossible to control. Hemorrhage is usually dark red with venous injury, red with capillary injury, and bright red with arterial injury. The rate of hemorrhage also varies from oozing capillary, to flowing venous, to pulsing arterial bleeding. In practice, it may be hard to differentiate among the types and origins of hemorrhage. It is important, however, to determine the rate and quantity of blood

🔑 ——————————
During assessment, it is important to determine the rate and quantity of hemorrhage.

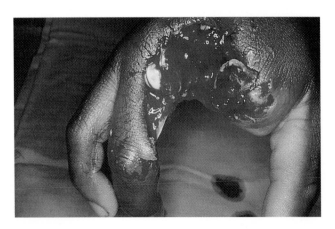
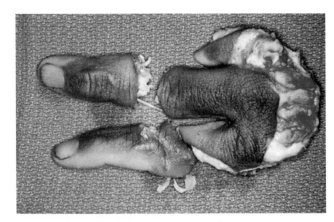

■ Figure 5-13 An amputation of the first two fingers.

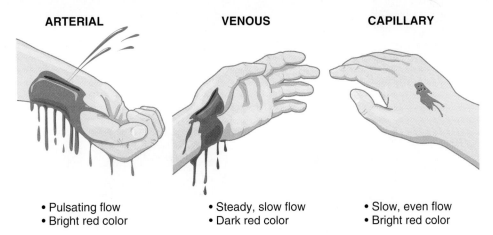

ARTERIAL
- Pulsating flow
- Bright red color

VENOUS
- Steady, slow flow
- Dark red color

CAPILLARY
- Slow, even flow
- Bright red color

■ Figure 5-14 Hemorrhage. Arterial hemorrhage is bright red and flows rapidly from a wound. Venous hemorrhage is darker red and flows slowly. Capillary hemorrhage is also bright red and flows slowly.

loss. This information helps you to decide upon the most effective means of stopping the blood flow and prioritizing the patient for care and transport.

Often the nature of the soft-tissue wound may be more important than the size or type of vessel involved in determining the severity of the blood vessel injury. If a moderately sized vein or artery is cut cleanly, the muscles in the vessel wall will tend to contract. This constricts the vessel's lumen and retracts the severed vessel into the tissue. As the muscle is drawn back from the wound, it thickens and further restricts the lumen. This restricts blood flow, reduces the rate of loss, and assists the clotting mechanisms. Therefore, clean lacerations and amputations generally do not bleed profusely. If, however, the vessel is not severed cleanly but is laid open instead, muscle contraction opens the wound, thereby increasing and prolonging blood loss.

WOUND HEALING

Wound healing is a complex process that begins immediately following injury and can take many months to complete. Wound healing is an essential component of homeostasis, the process whereby the body maintains a uniform environment for itself. Although it is useful to divide the wound healing process into stages or parts, it is important to note that these phases overlap considerably and are intertwined physiologically (Figure 5-15 ■).

Hemostasis

Arguably the most important aspect of wound healing is the body's ability to stop most bleeding on its own. This process is called **hemostasis.** Without hemostasis, even the most trivial nicks and scratches would continue to bleed, leading to life-threatening hemorrhage. Hemostasis has three major components related to the vasculature, the platelets, and the clotting cascade.

Hemostasis begins almost immediately following injury. Arteries, arterioles, and some veins are endowed with a muscular layer that reflexively constricts the vessel in response to local injury. The longitudinal muscles, too, play a role by retracting the cut ends of larger vessels back into the contracted muscle, thus reducing flow. This immediate response usually reduces but does not entirely stop bleeding. Capillaries, which do not have a muscle layer, cannot contract and thus continue to bleed. This explains the continuing but minor bleeding associated with capillary wounds such as paper cuts and minor abrasions.

Platelets begin the clotting process. The damaged vessel wall becomes "sticky," as do the platelets in the turbulent flow of the disrupted vessel. Platelets stick to the vessel wall

Review

Stages of Wound Healing

Hemostasis
Inflammation
Epithelialization
Neovascularization
Collagen synthesis

hemostasis *the body's natural ability to stop bleeding, the ability to clot blood.*

Pathophysiology of Soft-Tissue Injury **141**

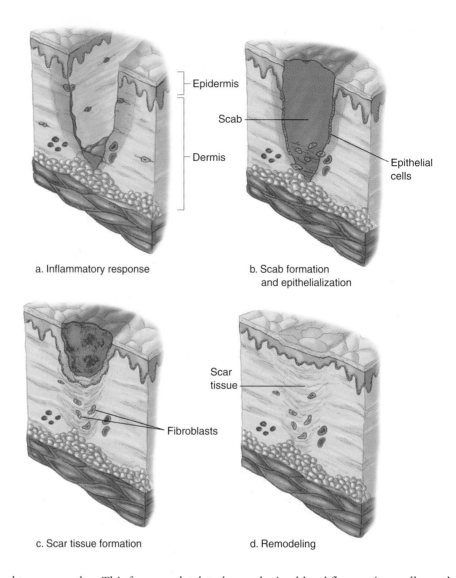

■ **Figure 5-15** The wound healing process.

a. Inflammatory response

b. Scab formation and epithelialization

c. Scar tissue formation

d. Remodeling

and to one another. This forms a platelet plug, reducing blood flow or, in small vessels, stopping it altogether.

When a blood vessel is injured, the disrupted tunica intima exposes collagen and other structural proteins to the blood. These proteins activate a complicated series of enzyme reactions that change certain blood proteins into long fibrin strands. These strands then entrap erythrocytes and produce a gelatinous mass that further occludes the bleeding vessel. This complex process, called coagulation, stops all but the most severe and persistent hemorrhage. With time, the clot shrinks or contracts, bringing the wound margins closer together, further facilitating wound healing. When the clot is no longer needed, it is reabsorbed by the body and any superficial scab merely drops off.

Inflammation

Shortly after hemostasis begins, the body sets in motion a very complex process of healing called **inflammation.** The inflammatory process involves a host of elements including various kinds of white blood cells, proteins involved in immunity, and hormone-like chemicals that signal other cells to mobilize.

Cells damaged by direct trauma or by invading pathogens release a number of proteins and chemicals into the surrounding tissue and blood. These agents, called **chemotactic factors,** recruit cells responsible for consuming cellular debris, invading bacteria, or other foreign or damaged cells and for beginning the inflammatory process. The first

inflammation   *complex process of local cellular and biochemical changes as a consequence of injury or infection; an early stage of healing.*

chemotactic factors   *chemicals released by white blood cells that attract more white blood cells to an area of inflammation.*

cells to arrive are specialized white blood cells called **granulocytes** and macrophages. These cells (also called phagocytes) are capable of engulfing bacteria, debris, and foreign material, digesting them, and then releasing the by-products in a process called **phagocytosis.** Other white blood cells called lymphocytes, in combination with immunoglobulins or immune proteins, are also mobilized. Lymphocytes attack invading pathogens directly or through an antibody response.

granulocytes *white blood cells charged with the primary purpose of neutralizing foreign bacteria.*

phagocytosis *process in which a cell surrounds and absorbs a bacterium or other particle.*

The injury process, the material released from injured cells, and the debris released as the phagocytes destroy invading cells cause mast cells to release histamine. Histamine dilates precapillary blood vessels, increases capillary permeability, and increases blood flow into and through the injured or infected tissue. This brings much-needed oxygen and more phagocytes to the injured area and draws away the by-products of cell destruction and repair. The increasing blood flow and local tissue metabolism also increase tissue temperature, which may in turn denature pathogen membranes. This response produces a swollen (edematous), reddened (erythematous), and warm region, characteristic of inflammation in response to local infection or injury. The result of the inflammation stage is the clearing away of dead and dying tissue, removal of bacteria and other foreign substances, and the preparation of the damaged area for rebuilding.

Epithelialization

Epithelialization is an early stage in wound healing in which epithelial cells migrate over the surface of the wound. The stratum germinativum cells rapidly divide and regenerate, thus restoring a uniform layer of skin cells along the edges of the healing wound. In clean, surgically prepared wounds, complete epithelialization may take place in as little as 48 hours. Except in minor, superficial wounds, the new epithelial layer is not a perfect facsimile of the original, undamaged skin. Instead, the new skin layer may be thinner, pigmented differently, and devoid of normal hair follicles. However, the new skin is usually quite functional and cosmetically similar to the original. If the wound is very large, epithelialization may be incomplete, and collagen will show through as a shiny, pinkish line of tissue called a scar.

epithelialization *early stage of wound healing in which epithelial cells migrate over the surface of the wound.*

Neovascularization

For healing to take place, new tissue must grow and regenerate. That requires blood rich in oxygen and nutrients. The body responds to this increased demand by generating new blood vessels in a process called **neovascularization.** These vessels bud from undamaged capillaries in the wound margins and then grow into the healing tissue. Neovascularized tissue is very fragile and has a tendency to bleed easily. It takes weeks to months for the newly formed blood vessels to become fully resistant to injury and for the surrounding tissue to strengthen enough to protect the new and delicate circulation.

neovascularization *new growth of capillaries in response to healing.*

Collagen Synthesis

Collagen is the body's main structural protein. It is a strong, tough fiber forming part of the hair, bones, and connective tissue. Scar tissue, cartilage, and tendons are almost entirely collagen. Specialized cells called **fibroblasts** are brought to the wound area and synthesize collagen as an important step in rebuilding damaged tissues. Collagen binds the wound margins together and strengthens the healing wound. It is important to note that as the wound heals, it is not "as good as new." Regenerated skin has only about 60 percent of the tensile strength of undamaged skin at 4 months, when the scar is fully mature. This accounts for the occasional re-injury and reopening of wounds weeks or months after healing. The fibroblasts continue to reshape the scar tissue and shrink the wound for months after the scab falls off. This **remodeling** involves reorganizing collagen fibers into neat, parallel bands, strengthening the healing tissue still more. Remodeling can continue for up to 6 to 12 months after the initial injury, so the final cosmetic outcome of the healing process may not be evident until then.

collagen *tough, strong protein that comprises most of the body's connective tissue.*

fibroblasts *specialized cells that form collagen.*

remodeling *stage in the wound healing process in which collagen is broken down and relaid in an orderly fashion.*

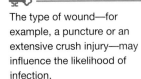
INFECTION

Infection is the most common and, next to hemorrhage, the most serious complication of open wounds. Approximately 1 in 15 wounds seen at the emergency department results in a wound infection. These infections delay healing. They may also spread to adjacent tissues and endanger cosmetic appearances. Occasionally, they cause widespread or systemic infection, called sepsis.

The most common causes of skin and soft-tissue infections are the *Staphylococcus* and *Streptococcus* bacterial families. These bacteria are gram positive (gram staining is a procedure to differentiate between types of bacteria), aerobic, and very common in the environment. *Staphylococcus* bacteria frequently colonize on the surface of normal skin, so it is not surprising to find them driven into wounds by the forces of trauma. Less commonly, wound infections are caused by other bacteria such as gram-negative rods, including *Pseudomonas aeruginosa* (diabetics and foot puncture wounds) and *Pasteurella multocida* (cat and dog bites).

It takes bacteria a few days to grow into numbers sufficient to cause noticeable signs or symptoms of infection. Infections appear at least 2 to 3 days following the initial wound and commonly present with pain, tenderness, erythema, and warmth. Infection earlier than that is very unusual. Pus, a collection of white blood cells, cellular debris, and dead bacteria, may be visible draining from the wound. The pus is usually thick, pale yellowish-to-greenish in color, and has a foul smell. Visible red streaks, or **lymphangitis,** may extend from the wound margins up the affected extremity proximally. These streaks represent inflammation of the lymph channels as a result of the infection. The patient may also complain of fever and malaise, especially if the infection has begun to spread systemically.

lymphangitis   inflammation of the lymph channels, usually as a result of a distal infection.

Infection Risk Factors

Risk factors for wound infections are related to the host's health, the type and location of the wound, any associated contamination, and the treatment provided. Diabetics, the infirm, the elderly, and individuals with serious chronic diseases such as chronic obstructive pulmonary disease are at greater risk for infection and heal more slowly and less efficiently than healthy individuals. Patients with any significant disease or preexisting medical problem such as cancer, anemia, hepatic failure, or cardiovascular disease have difficulty mobilizing the immune and tissue-repair response necessary for good wound healing. HIV and AIDS attack the body's immune system and seriously impair its ability to ward off infection, increasing risk significantly. Smoking constricts blood vessels and robs healing tissues of needed oxygen and nutrients, also increasing infection risk.

Several drugs detract from the body's ability to fight infection. Persons on immunosuppressant medications such as prednisone or cortisone (corticosteroids) are also at increased risk for serious infection. Colchicine, a drug used to treat gout, and nonsteroidal anti-inflammatory drugs (NSAIDs) such as ibuprofen also reduce the body's inflammation response. Neoplastic agents, which are used to combat rapidly reproducing cells in cancer patients, also disrupt cell regeneration at an injury site.

The wound type strongly affects the likelihood of a wound infection. A puncture wound traps contamination deep within tissue where there is a perfect environment for bacterial growth. Avulsion tears away blood vessels and supporting structures, robbing the damaged tissue of its blood supply, a critical factor in preventing or reducing infection. Crush injuries and other wounds that produce large areas of injured or dead (devitalized) tissue provide an excellent environment for bacterial growth and are at great risk for wound infection.

In a similar fashion, wound location influences infection risk. Well-vascularized areas such as the face and scalp are very resistant to infection. Distal extremities, the feet in particular, are at greater risk.

Clean objects, such as uncontaminated sheet metal or a clean knife, usually leave only small amounts of bacteria in a wound and, consequently, do not often cause infections. However, objects contaminated with organic matter and bacteria, such as a nail on a barnyard floor, a knife used to clean raw meat, or a piece of wood, pose much greater risks of infection. The infection risk associated with bites caused by mammals, and carnivores in particular, is very great. Bites by humans, cats, and dogs are among the most common and most serious types of bites.

The type of treatment provided for a wound affects the risk of infection. Use of sterile dressings and clean examination gloves minimizes wound contamination during prehospital treatment. Gloves protect not only the rescuer but also the patient from contaminants on the rescuer's hands. Irrigation of wounds with sterile saline using a pressurized stream device has been shown to reduce bacterial loads and reduce infection rates. Closing wounds (with sutures or staples, for example) increases infection risks as compared to leaving wounds open. However, the risks associated with wound closure are frequently accepted in order to achieve the best possible cosmetic outcome and more rapid healing.

In most cases, routine use of antibiotics with wounds does not help reduce infection rates and, in fact, may increase the likelihood of infection with antibiotic-resistant microorganisms. Antibiotics may be helpful if given within the first hour or so after deep major wounds, such as those from gunshots or stabbings, puncture wounds to the feet, and wounds where retention of a foreign body is suspected.

Infection Management

Despite the potential problems previously noted, the mainstay in treatment for infections is the use of chemical bactericidals, also known as antibiotics. Antibiotics for the treatment of gram-positive infections include the antistaphylococcal penicillins and cephalosporins. Erythromycin (and similar agents) can be used in patients allergic to penicillin. The pharmalogical approach against *Pseudomonas* often requires the use of two drugs, while *Pasteurella* usually can be treated with penicillin.

On occasion, a wound forms a collection of pus called an abscess and requires a minor incision and drainage to correct. Surgical removal of this material helps the body return to normal more quickly.

Gangrene   One of the rarest and most feared wound complications is **gangrene.** Gangrene is a deep space infection usually caused by the anaerobic bacterium *Clostridium perfringens.* These bacteria characteristically produce a gas deep within a wound, causing subcutaneous emphysema and a foul smell whenever the gas escapes. Once they have become established, the bacteria are particularly prolific and can rapidly involve an entire extremity. Left unchecked, gangrene frequently leads to sepsis and death. In the days before antibiotics, amputation was frequently necessary to stop the spread of the disease. Modern treatment with a combination of antibiotics, surgery, and hyperbaric oxygenation effectively arrests most cases of gangrene early in their course.

gangrene *deep space infection usually caused by the anaerobic bacterium* Clostridium perfringens.

Tetanus   Another highly feared but, fortunately, rare complication of wound infections is tetanus, or lockjaw. Tetanus is caused by the bacterium *Clostridium tetani,* and like its cousin *Clostridium perfringens,* it is anaerobic. Tetanus presents with few signs or symptoms at the local wound site, but the bacteria produce a potent toxin that causes widespread, painful, involuntary muscle contractions. Early observers noted mandibular trismus, or jaw-clenching ("lockjaw"). There is an antidote for the tetanus toxin, but it only neutralizes circulating toxin molecules, not those already bound to the motor endplates. Thus, treatment is slow and recovery prolonged.

Fortunately, tetanus is preventable through immunization. Widespread immunization has reduced incidence to a very few cases. The standard immunization is a series of three shots in childhood, with boosters every 10 years thereafter. It is common practice in emergency departments to provide boosters to wound patients if they have not been immunized in the past 5 years. Immigrants from Third World countries often have never completed a tetanus vaccine series. In these cases, it is prudent to administer tetanus immune globulin (TIG) in addition to the tetanus vaccine to prevent development of the disease while the body gears up to make new antibodies.

OTHER WOUND COMPLICATIONS

Several circumstances or conditions can interfere with normal wound healing processes. These conditions include impaired hemostasis, re-bleeding, and delayed healing.

Impaired Hemostasis

Some medications, such as aspirin, warfarin, and heparin, can interfere with the clotting process.

Several medications can interfere with hemostasis and the clotting process. Aspirin is a powerful inhibitor of platelet aggregation, and it is used clinically to help prevent clot formation in the coronary and cerebral arteries of patients at risk for myocardial infarction or stroke. Thus, a side effect of aspirin use is a prolongation of clotting time, an important consideration in a patient who has sustained significant trauma or is undergoing major surgery. Likewise, anticoagulants, such as Coumadin (warfarin) and heparin, and fibrinolytics, such as TPA and streptokinase, interfere with or break down the protein fibers that form clots and are used to prevent or destroy obstructions at critical locations. They also adversely affect clot development in soft-tissue wounds. Penicillins may increase clotting times and interfere with blood cell production. Additionally, abnormalities in proteins involved in the fibrin formation cascade may result in delayed clotting, as is the case in hemophiliacs.

Re-Bleeding

Despite treatment that provides adequate initial control of bleeding, re-bleeding is possible from any wound. Movement of underlying structures, such as muscles or bones, or of the bandage or dressing material may dislodge clots and reinstitute hemorrhage.

Also, hemorrhage that appears to have been stopped may actually be bleeding into an oversized dressing until it saturates the dressing and pushes through it. Monitor your dressings and bandages frequently to assure that blood loss is not continuing.

Partially healed wounds are also at risk for re-bleeding. Postoperative wounds in particular can start bleeding again with life-threatening results. Because patients are discharged from hospitals more quickly today than in the past and return home sooner after surgery, be wary of this potential complication.

Delayed Healing

In some patients, the wound repair process may be delayed or even arrested, resulting in incomplete wound healing. Persons at greatest risk for this complication are diabetics, the elderly, the chronically ill, and the malnourished. Nutrition must be adequate for wound healing to occur. Patients with multiple injuries often require significantly more calories during the healing phase than normal. Seriously or chronically infected wounds and wounds in locations with limited blood flow (distal extremities) are also at risk for incomplete healing. Incompletely healed wounds remain tender and are easily re-injured. A pale yellow or blood-tinged **serous fluid** may drain from them. Out-of-hospital treatment of incompletely healed wounds includes frequent changes of sterile, nonadherent dressings, and protection of the wound.

serous fluid   *a cellular component of blood, similar to plasma.*

compartment syndrome *muscle ischemia that is caused by rising pressures within an anatomical fascial space.*

Compartment Syndrome

Compartment syndrome is a complication of closed and, occasionally, open wounds. In compartment syndrome, an extremity injury causes significant edema and swelling

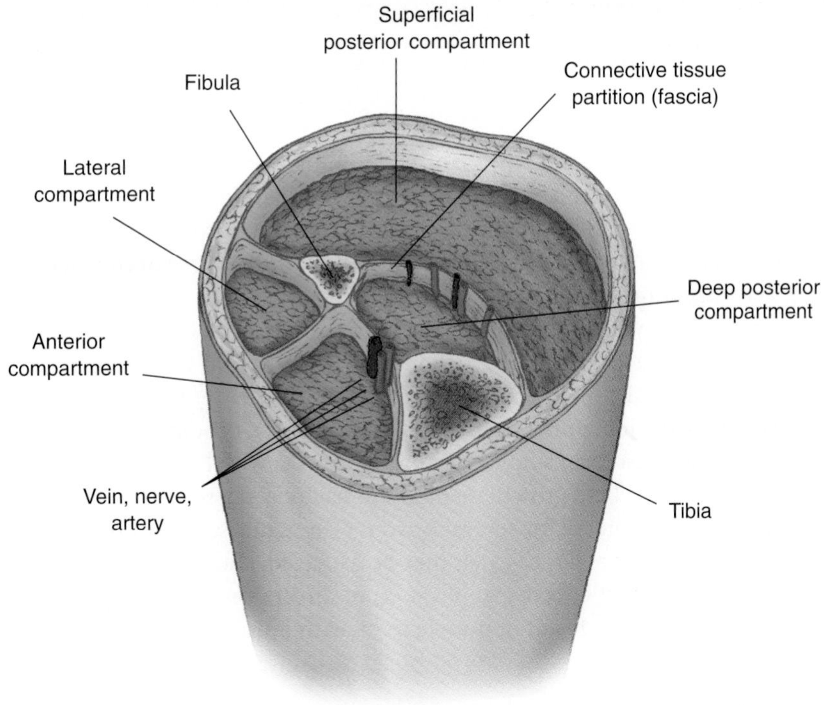
Superficial
posterior compartment
Fibula
Connective tissue
partition (fascia)
Lateral
compartment
Deep posterior
compartment
Anterior
compartment
Vein, nerve,
artery
Tibia

■ Figure 5-16 Musculoskeletal compartments segregated by fascia.

in the deep tissues. Because the extremity muscles are encapsulated in tough, inflexible fasciae, the swollen tissue has "nowhere to go," and the pressure in the compartment rises (Figure 5-16) ■. When the pressure rises above 45 to 60 mmHg, the blood flow to that muscle group or compartment is compromised and ischemia ensues. If the condition continues for more than a few hours, irreversible damage and permanent disability may result. The muscle mass may die and its contribution to limb function may be lost. Frequently, the resulting scar tissue shortens the length of the muscle strand and produces what is called Volkmann's contracture, thus further reducing the usefulness of the limb after compartment syndrome. All extremities may experience compartment syndrome, but the lower extremities, especially the calves, are at greatest risk because of their bulk and fascial anatomy.

Abnormal Scar Formation

During the healing process, scar tissue sometimes develops abnormally. A **keloid** is excessive scar tissue that extends beyond the boundaries of a wound. It develops most commonly in darkly pigmented individuals and develops on the sternum, lower abdomen, upper extremities, and ears. Another healing abnormality is hypertrophic scar formation. This is an excessive accumulation of scar tissue, usually within the injury border, that is often associated with dynamic skin tension lines, like those at flexion joints.

keloid *a formation resulting from overproduction of scar tissue.*

Pressure Injuries

A special type of soft-tissue injury is the pressure injury, which is caused by prolonged compression of the skin and tissues beneath. This may occur in the chronically ill (bedridden) patient, the patient who falls and remains unconscious for hours (due to alcohol intoxication, stroke, or drug overdose), or the patient who is entrapped with no crushing mechanism. The patient's weight against the ground or other surface compresses tissue and induces hypoxic injury. The injury is similar to a crush injury, although the mechanism is more passive and more likely to go unnoticed. Pressure injury may also occur when a long spine board, PASG, air splint, or rigid splint remains on a patient for an extended period of time.

Pressure injuries may occur if a long spine board, splint, or PASG is left on a patient for an extended period.

CRUSH INJURY

Crush injury involves a trauma pattern in which body tissues are subjected to severe compressive forces. A crush injury can be relatively minor—for example, one that involves only a finger or part of an extremity—or it can be massive—one that affects much or all of the body. The mechanisms of injury can be varied. A packing machine might compress a worker's finger or extremity; a collapsed jack might trap a mechanic's leg under a car wheel; the seat and steering column might compress a driver's chest between them in an auto crash; or debris from a building collapse or trench cave-in might bury a construction worker.

A crush injury disrupts the body's tissues—muscles, blood vessels, bone, and, in some cases, internal organs. With such injuries, the skin may remain intact and the limb may appear normal in shape, or the skin may be severely cut and bruised and the extremity mangled and deformed. In both cases, however, the damage within is extensive. The injury often results in a large area of destruction with limited effective circulation, thus creating an excellent growth medium for bacteria. Hemorrhage with crush injuries may be difficult to control for several reasons: The actual source of the bleeding may be hard to identify; several large vessels may be damaged; and the general condition of the limb does not support effective application of direct pressure. The resulting tissue hypoxia and acidosis may result in muscle rigor, with muscles that may feel very hard and "wood-like" on palpation.

Associated Injury

When patients have been subjected to mechanisms that cause crush injuries, those mechanisms or others associated with them often result in additional injuries. For example, patients who have received crush injuries in building collapses or when entrapped by machinery may suffer additional fractures and open or closed soft-tissue injuries. Falling debris can cause direct injury, both blunt and penetrating. Dust and smoke can cause respiratory and eye injuries. Also, entrapment for any length of time leads to dehydration and hypothermia. You should consider all these possibilities when assessing and providing emergency care to victims of crush injury.

Crush Syndrome

Crush syndrome occurs when body parts are entrapped for 4 hours or longer. Shorter periods of entrapment may result in direct body part damage, but they usually do not cause the broad, systemic complications of crush syndrome. The crushed skeletal muscle tissue undergoes **necrosis** and cellular changes with resultant release of metabolic byproducts. This degenerative process, called traumatic **rhabdomyolysis** (skeletal muscle disintegration), releases many toxins. Chief among these by-products of cellular destruction are myoglobin (a muscle protein), phosphate and potassium (from cellular death), lactic acid (from anaerobic metabolism), and uric acid (from protein breakdown). These by-products accumulate in the crushed body part but, because of the entrapment and the resulting minimal circulation through the injured tissue, do not reach the systemic circulation. Once the limb or victim is extricated and the pressure is released, however, the accumulated by-products and toxins flood the central circulation.

High levels of myoglobin can lodge in the filtering tubules of the kidney, especially with patients who are in hypovolemic (shock) states, leading to renal failure, a leading cause of delayed death in crush syndrome. More immediate problems include hypovolemia and shock from the flow of sodium, chloride, and water into the damaged tissue. Increased blood potassium (hyperkalemia) can reduce the cardiac muscle's response to electrical stimuli, induce cardiac dysrhythmias, and lead to sudden death. Rising phosphate levels (hyperphosphatemia) can lead to abnormal calcifications in the

necrosis *tissue death, usually from ischemia.*

rhabdomyolysis *acute pathologic process that involves the destruction of skeletal muscle.*

High-Pressure Tool Injuries Although infrequently encountered, high-pressure tools can cause very serious soft-tissue injuries. High-pressure tools are commonly used in repair shops and often contain fluid or grease (hydraulic fluid or grease guns) or simply air. The most common cause of the injury is accidently discharging the device with the tip in proximity to the skin. This causes a small superficial skin wound. However, tissues below the wound can sustain serious injury from the grease or fluid, the pressure, or a combination of the two. These wounds often cause serious infections and loss of function if not surgically explored and adequately treated. If the injury involves the hand (as is common), the pressure may inject materials into the forearm and even as far as the arm or shoulder. The grease or other foreign substance tends to follow the fascial planes of the hand and forearm and can become embedded within the muscle sheaths. The injury generally presents with a small open wound with some contamination, but its nature is generally far worse than the wound's physical signs and symptoms suggest.

Contaminants introduced deep into the wound exist in an environment with limited air and circulation (anaerobic state). However, the area is warm and moist, providing any bacteria introduced into the wound an ideal environment to proliferate. Hydraulic fluid and grease are toxic to the internal tissues and cause cell injury and death. Because of the depth and extent of contamination, surgical debridement is extremely difficult and may, itself, cause significant and extensive tissue injury. Whenever a patient presents with this type of injury, recognize the likelihood of extensive limb involvement and seek the services of the trauma center.

vasculature and nervous system, compounding problems for the patient. In addition, as oxygenated circulation returns to the cells the aerobic process by which uric acid is produced can operate again, thus increasing cellular acidity and injury.

INJECTION INJURY

A unique type of soft-tissue injury is the injection injury. A bursting high-pressure line, most commonly a hydraulic line, may inject fluid through a patient's skin and into the subcutaneous tissues. If the pressure is strong enough, the fluid may push between tissue layers and travel along the limb (Figure 5-17 ■). The fluid thus injected—for example, a petroleum-based hydraulic fluid—may then chemically damage the

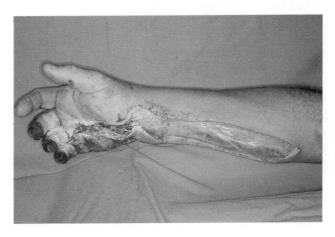

■ Figure 5-17   An injection injury resulting from the pressurized injection of grease.

surrounding tissue. The body's repair mechanisms are unprepared to remove the great quantities of injected material, and the resulting damage is severe. A limb may be lost due to the direct physical damage from the injection process, from the chemical damage done by the injected material, or from infection that develops after the injection.

DRESSING AND BANDAGE MATERIALS

Several types of dressings and bandages are effective in prehospital care. A dressing is the material placed directly on the wound to control bleeding and maintain wound cleanliness (Figure 5-18a ■). A bandage is the material used to hold a dressing in place and to apply direct pressure to control hemorrhage (Figure 5-19 ■). Dressings and bandages have various designs and are used for a variety of purposes in emergency care.

STERILE/NONSTERILE DRESSINGS

Sterile dressings are cotton or other fiber pads that have been specially prepared to be without microorganisms. They are usually packaged individually and remain sterile for as long as the package is intact. Once the packaging is opened, sterile dressings become contaminated by airborne dust and particles that harbor bacteria and other microorganisms. Sterile dressings are designed to be used in direct contact with wounds.

Nonsterile dressings are clean—that is, free of gross contamination—but are not free of microscopic contamination and microorganisms. Nonsterile dressings are not intended to be applied directly to a wound, but rather to be placed over a sterile dressing to add bulk or absorptive power.

OCCLUSIVE/NONOCCLUSIVE DRESSINGS

Some dressings, such as sterilized plastic wrap and petroleum-impregnated gauze, are designed to prevent the movement of fluid and air through them. These dressings are called occlusive and are helpful in preventing air aspiration into chest wounds (open pneumothorax) and open neck wounds (air emboli into the jugular vein). Most dressing material is nonocclusive.

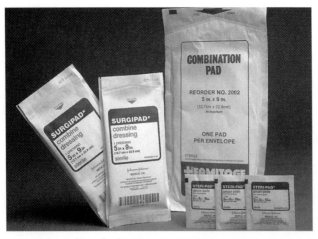

a. A variety of sterile dressings.

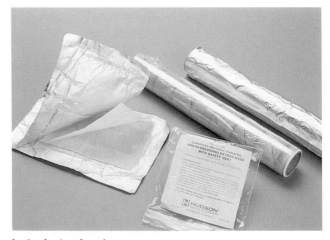

b. Occlusive dressings.

■ Figure 5-18 Assorted dressings used in the care of soft-tissue injuries.

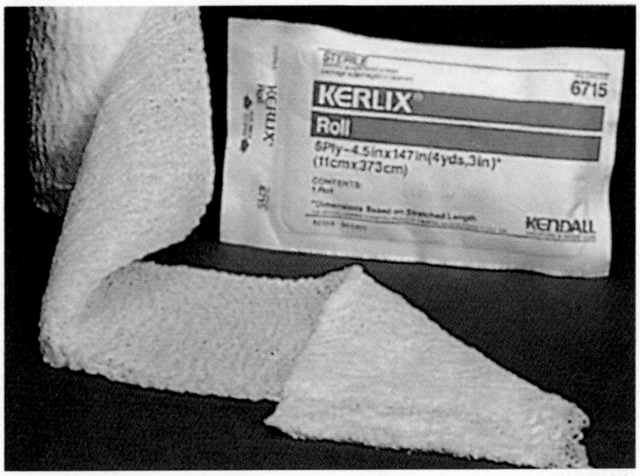

■ Figure 5-19 Kerlix®, a type of self-adherent roller bandage.

ADHERENT/NONADHERENT DRESSINGS

Adherent dressings are untreated cotton or other fiber pads that will stick to drying blood and fluid that has leaked from open wounds. Adherent dressings have the advantage of promoting clot formation and thus reducing hemorrhage, but their removal from wounds can be quite painful. Removal or disturbance of an adherent dressing is also likely to break the clot and cause re-bleeding. Nonadherent dressings are specially treated with chemicals such as polymers to prevent the wound fluids and clotting materials from adhering to the dressing. Nonadherent dressings are preferred for most uncomplicated wounds.

ABSORBENT/NONABSORBENT DRESSINGS

Absorbent dressings readily soak up blood and other fluids, much as a sponge soaks up water. This property is helpful in many bleeding situations. Nonabsorbent dressings absorb little or no fluid and are used when a barrier to leaking is desired. The clear membrane dressings frequently placed over intravenous puncture sites are good examples of nonabsorbent dressings. Most other dressings used in prehospital care are absorbent dressings.

WET/DRY DRESSINGS

Wet dressings are sometimes applied to special types of wounds such as burns. They are also used in the hospital to effect healing in some complicated postoperative wounds. Sterile normal saline is the usual fluid used to wet dressings. Wet dressings provide a medium for the movement of infectious material into wounds, however, and are not commonly used in prehospital care, except with injuries such as abdominal eviscerations or burns involving only a limited body surface area. Dry dressings are the type most often employed for wounds in prehospital care.

SELF-ADHERENT ROLLER BANDAGES

The most common and convenient bandage material is the soft, self-adherent, roller bandage (Kling or Kerlix). It has limited stretch and resists unraveling as it is rolled over itself. It conforms well to body contours and is quick and easy to use. This bandage is most appropriate for injuries located where it can be wrapped circumferentially. It comes in rolls from 1 to 6 inches wide.

GAUZE BANDAGES

Like soft, self-adherent bandages, gauze bandages are a convenient material for securing dressings. They do not stretch, however, and thus do not conform as well to body contours as the self-adherent material, but they are otherwise functional for bandaging. Since gauze bandages do not stretch, they may increase the pressure associated with tissue swelling at injury sites. Gauze usually comes in rolls from 1/2 to 2 inches wide.

ADHESIVE BANDAGES

An adhesive bandage (or adhesive tape) is a strong plastic, paper, or fabric material with adhesive applied to one side. It can effectively secure a small dressing to a location where circumferential wrapping is impractical. When used circumferentially, an adhesive bandage does not allow for any swelling and permits pressure to accumulate in the tissues beneath it. Adhesive bandages usually come in widths that range from 1/4 to 3 inches.

ELASTIC (OR ACE) BANDAGES

Elastic bandages stretch easily and conform to the body contours. Elastic bandages provide stability and support for minor musculoskeletal injuries, but they are not commonly used in prehospital care. When you do use these bandages, however, remember that it is very easy to apply too much pressure with them. Each consecutive wrap applied will contain and add to pressure on the wound site. Swelling associated with the wound may increase the pressure until blood flow through and out of the affected limb is reduced or stopped.

TRIANGULAR BANDAGES

Triangular bandages, or cravats, are large triangles of cotton fabric. They are strong, nonelastic bandages commonly used to make slings and swathes and, in some cases, to affix splints. They can also be used to hold dressings in place, but they do not conform as well to body contours as soft, self-adherent bandages and do not maintain pressure or immobilize wound dressings very well.

ASSESSMENT OF SOFT-TISSUE INJURIES

Wound assessment must be comprehensive to ensure that care of each injury can be assigned an appropriate priority.

Proper evaluation of the skin can tell you more about the body's condition after trauma than any other aspect of patient assessment. Not only is the skin the first body organ to experience the effects of trauma, but it is the first and often the only organ to display them. Therefore, assessment of the skin and its injury must be deliberate, careful, and complete. While the processes that cause soft-tissue injuries and the manifestations of those injuries vary, prehospital assessment is a simple, well-structured process. Follow the assessment process carefully and completely to ensure that you establish the nature and extent of each injury. Doing so enables you to assign soft-tissue injuries, and other injuries associated with them, the appropriate priorities for care.

Assessment of patients with soft-tissue wounds follows the same general progression as the assessment of other trauma patients. First, size up the scene, ruling out potential hazards, identifying the mechanism of injury, and determining the need for additional medical and rescue resources. Next, perform a quick initial assessment and identify and care for any immediately life-threatening injuries. For the patient with a mechanism of injury or signs and symptoms that suggest serious trauma, you will perform a rapid trauma assessment and use trauma triage criteria to determine the need for rapid transport. For a patient with no significant mechanism of injury and no indication from the initial assessment of a serious injury or life threat, perform a focused trauma assessment and gather vital signs and patient history at the scene. Perform a detailed physical exam only if conditions warrant and time permits. Provide serial ongoing assessments to track your patient's response to his injuries and your care.

SCENE SIZE-UP

During the scene size-up, look for evidence that will help you determine the mechanism of injury and anticipate the likely injuries and their severity. While soft-tissue injuries are not usually life threatening, they can suggest other, serious life threats. Remember: No injury mechanism can impact the human body without first traveling through the skin. Identify where injury is likely and be prepared to carefully examine the skin for evidence that suggests internal injury. Consider mechanisms of injury that could cause entrapment and either crush injury or crush syndrome.

Be alert to the fact that the mechanisms that injured the patient may still be present and pose threats to you and other rescuers. Rule out or eliminate any threats to yourself or fellow care providers before entering the scene (Figure 5-20 ■).

Because trauma and injuries that penetrate the skin are likely to expose you to the hazards of contact with a patient's body fluids, don sterile gloves and observe other body substance isolation procedures as you approach the patient. Recognize that arterial bleeding and hemorrhage associated with the airway can cause blood to splatter at the scene. If you suspect these injuries, don splash protection for your eyes and clothing.

> No mechanism of injury can impact the human body without first passing through the skin.

INITIAL ASSESSMENT

Begin your initial assessment by establishing manual cervical in-line immobilization—if you suspect significant head or spine injury—and forming a general impression of the patient. Determine the patient's level of consciousness and assess the airway, breathing, and circulation. Assess perfusion by noting skin color, temperature, and condition and by assessing capillary refill.

During this assessment, pay particular attention to the location and types of visible wounds to gain further understanding of the mechanism of injury and whether it produced blunt or penetrating trauma. If responsive, the patient may be able to give you critical information about how the wound occurred. If the patient is unable to speak, First Responders or bystanders may be able to provide this information. Correct any immediate threats to the patient's life as you discover them.

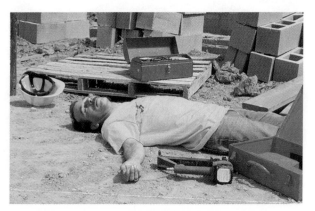

■ Figure 5-20 During the scene size-up, rule out hazards, don gloves, and analyze the mechanism of injury.

FOCUSED HISTORY AND PHYSICAL EXAM

Use the information you have gathered through the initial assessment to determine how to proceed in the assessment process. Patients with serious trauma, suggested by a significant mechanism of injury or the findings of the initial assessment, will receive a rapid trauma assessment. All other patients will receive a focused trauma assessment.

Significant Mechanism of Injury—Rapid Trauma Assessment

In the rapid trauma assessment, you will perform a swift evaluation of the patient's head, neck, chest, abdomen, pelvis, extremities, and posterior body. Examine these areas for signs of internal or life-endangering injuries. Quickly investigate any discolorations, deformities, temperature variations, abnormal muscle tone, or open wounds.

Assure that any wounds that you discover, or the injuries suggested beneath them, do not involve or endanger the airway or breathing or contribute significantly to blood loss. Focus your immediate care during the rapid trauma assessment on continuing to assure the patient's airway and breathing and then on controlling severe blood loss.

Inspect and palpate areas where the mechanism of injury suggests serious injuries may exist. Again, look for discoloration, temperature variation, abnormal muscle tone, and deformity suggestive of trauma (Figure 5-21 ■). If the mechanism of injury suggests open wounds, sweep body areas hidden from sight with gloved hands; this will rule out the possibility of unseen blood loss and pooling. Control moderate to severe hemorrhage immediately. Hemorrhage control need not be definitive, but should stop continuing significant blood loss. Once more serious injuries are cared for, you can return and dress and bandage wounds more carefully.

Survey all bleeding wounds to determine the type of hemorrhage—arterial, venous, or capillary. Attempt to approximate the volume of blood lost since the time of the accident, which suggests the rate of blood loss.

Carry out your exam using the methods described in "Assessment Techniques" later in this chapter. Apply a cervical spinal immobilization collar once you have completed the rapid assessment of the head and neck. Continue to provide manual immobilization, however, until the patient is fully immobilized to a backboard.

When the rapid trauma assessment is complete, obtain a set of baseline vital signs and a patient history. Be sure to maintain manual in-line immobilization while the signs and history are being gathered. If you have enough personnel, the vital signs and history may be obtained simultaneously as the rapid trauma assessment is performed.

■ Figure 5-21   Often the only signs of serious internal injury are external soft-tissue injuries. (© Edward T. Dickinson, MD)

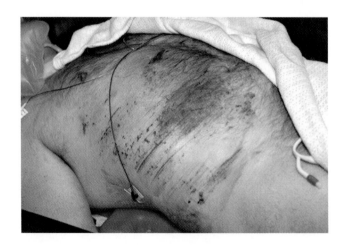

When obtaining the history, be sure to question the patient about medications, especially those that may have some direct relevance to soft-tissue injuries. For example, the patient's tetanus history is important with any penetrating trauma. Determine if the patient has had a tetanus booster and how long ago it was given. Note that a patient's routine use of aspirin or blood thinners—for example, heparin or warfarin for stroke or MI risk—may impact the body's ability to halt even minimal hemorrhage. Ask about the use of anti-inflammatory medications, such as prednisone, because those medications reduce the inflammatory response and slow the normal healing process. Question the patient about any preexisting diseases. Note that certain diseases, especially HIV, AIDS, or anemia, increase the risks of infection and the problems of hemorrhage control.

At the conclusion of the rapid trauma assessment, confirm the decision either to transport the patient immediately with further care provided en route to the hospital or to remain at the scene and complete treatment of non-life-threatening injuries. Consider the rate and volume of any blood loss and any uncontrollable bleeding in this decision.

If your patient's condition merits care at the scene, prioritize the soft-tissue wounds you have identified to establish an order of care to follow. The few moments taken to sort out injuries and to plan the management process save valuable time in the field. They also ensure that you provide early care for injuries with the highest priority.

No Significant Mechanism of Injury—Focused Trauma Assessment

When a patient has a soft-tissue injury but neither a significant mechanism of injury nor an indication of a serious problem from the initial assessment—for example, a cut finger or a knee abrasion from a fall—the sequence of assessment steps is different than for a patient with a significant injury mechanism. Begin this phase of the assessment with a focused trauma assessment, which is an exam directed at the injury site—the finger or the knee in the examples previously noted. A full head-to-toe rapid trauma assessment is not necessary in most such cases.

Direct the focused assessment at the chief complaint and any area of injury suggested by the mechanism of injury. Use the examination techniques of inquiry, inspection, and palpation (described in the following sections) to evaluate the injury and the surrounding area. In the case of a wound to an extremity, be sure to check the distal extremity for pulses, capillary refill, color, and temperature. Then, obtain a set of baseline vital signs and a history from the patient. If any of your findings suggest the patient has more serious injuries, perform a rapid trauma assessment and consider rapid transport.

Depending on the nature of the patient's injury, you may decide to provide transport or to refer/release the patient. If you are treating an isolated injury such as a cut finger, your system's protocols may prescribe whether you may release/refer the patient or transport the patient. More and more often, EMS systems are employing release/referral protocols to increase system efficiency. If you do transport, provide ongoing assessment.

DETAILED PHYSICAL EXAM

Once the rapid or focused trauma assessment has been completed, vital signs and history have been gathered, and necessary emergency care steps have been taken, you may perform a detailed physical exam. Like the rapid trauma assessment, this head-to-toe evaluation of the skin (and the rest of the body) involves the techniques of inquiry, observation, and palpation. The detailed exam should follow a planned and comprehensive process, ideally progressing from head to toe although the order is not critical. The main purpose of the detailed assessment is to pick up any additional information regarding the patient's condition and to search for any unsuspected or subtle injuries.

The detailed head-to-toe examination should be performed at the scene only if significant and life-threatening bleeding can be ruled out.

Manage any additional injuries you discover during the examination. The detailed physical exam is usually performed during transport or on scene if transport has been delayed. Never delay transport to perform it, and only perform it if the patient's condition permits.

ASSESSMENT TECHNIQUES

The assessment techniques that follow can be used during both the rapid trauma assessment and the detailed physical exam.

Inquiry

Question the patient about the mechanism of injury, any pain, pain on touch or movement, and any loss of function or sensation specific to an area. Additionally, attempt to determine the exact nature of the pain or sensory or motor loss by using elements of the OPQRST mnemonic (see Volume 2, Chapter 3, "Patient Assessment in the Field"). Question the patient about signs and symptoms before touching an area.

Inspection

Continue the exam by carefully observing a particular body region. Identify any discolorations, deformities, or open wounds in those regions.

Determine if any discoloration is local, distal, or systemic, reflecting local injury, circulation compromise, or systemic complications such as shock. Contusions, blood vessel injuries, dislocations, and fractures may cause local discoloration, including erythema or ecchymosis. Distal discoloration may present as a pale, cyanotic, or ashen-colored limb distal to the point of circulation loss. You may also notice systemic discoloration, such as pale, ashen, or grayish skin in all limbs, suggestive of hypovolemia and shock.

Examine any deformities you find to determine their cause. Is the deformity due to a developing hematoma, to the normal swelling associated with the inflammatory process, or to underlying injuries?

Inspect any wounds you discover in detail. Study the wound to determine its depth and evaluate its potential for damage to underlying muscles, nerves, blood vessels, organs, or bones. If possible, identify the object that caused the wound and determine the amount of force transmitted by it to the body's interior. Ascertain if there are any foreign bodies, contamination, or impaled objects in the wound. Finally, identify the nature and location of any hemorrhage.

The wound should be observed in such a way that it can later be described to the attending physician.

Observe each wound carefully so you can describe it to the attending physician after you dress and bandage the injury. This information will help the emergency department staff prioritize the patient's injuries. Careful observation will also aid you in preparation of your prehospital care report. Adequate lighting is crucial for evaluating wounds. If necessary, defer this portion of the detailed physical exam until better lighting is available, as in the back of the ambulance.

If a patient's limb or digit has been amputated, have other rescuers conduct a brief but thorough search for the amputated part. If the part cannot be located immediately or remains entrapped, do not delay transport. Instead, leave someone at the scene to continue the search. Ensure that once the body part is retrieved, it is properly handled, packaged, and brought to the same hospital as the patient.

Palpation

In addition to questioning the patient and inspecting the body regions, you should palpate the body's entire surface. Be alert for any deformity, asymmetry, temperature variation, unexpected mass, or localized loss of skin or muscle tone. Gently palpate all apparent closed wounds for evidence of tenderness, swelling, crepitus, and subcutaneous emphysema. Avoid palpating the interior of open wounds, which may introduce contamination and disturb the clotting process. Ascertain the presence or absence of distal pulses and capillary refill time with any extremity injury. Also, check motor and sensory function distal to any extremity wound and compare findings with those from the opposite limb.

ONGOING ASSESSMENT

During transport, provide an ongoing assessment, reassessing the patient's mental status, airway, breathing, and circulation, gathering additional sets of vital signs, and evaluating the sites of the patient's injuries. Also inspect any interventions you have performed. Provide an ongoing assessment at least every 5 minutes with unstable patients and every 15 minutes with stable patients. If you note any change in the patient's condition, modify your priorities for transport and care accordingly.

MANAGEMENT OF SOFT-TISSUE INJURY

Once you complete your patient assessment, take steps to manage the soft-tissue injury, either in the field or en route to the hospital. Control of blood loss, prevention of shock, and decontamination of affected areas take priority. The following sections describe some of the most important of these care steps.

Unless you note extensive bleeding, wound management by dressing and bandaging is a late priority in the care of trauma patients. Dress and bandage wounds whose bleeding does not represent a life threat only after you stabilize your patient by caring for higher priority injuries.

The management of minor wounds is a late priority in the care of the trauma patient, unless extensive bleeding is noted.

OBJECTIVES OF WOUND DRESSING AND BANDAGING

The dressing and bandaging of a wound has three basic objectives. These are to control all hemorrhaging, to keep the wound as clean as possible, and to immobilize the wound (Procedure 5-1). The appearance of the final dressing and bandage is not as critical as the achievement of these three objectives.

The three objectives of bandaging are to control hemorrhage, to keep the wound clean, and to immobilize the wound site.

Hemorrhage Control

The primary method—and the most effective one—of controlling hemorrhage associated with soft-tissue injury is direct pressure. In cases of serious hemorrhage flowing from a wound with some force, place a small dressing directly over the site of the bleeding and apply pressure directly to it with a finger. When the bleeding is the more commonly encountered slow-to-moderate type, use a dressing that has been sized to cover and pad the wound. Then simply wrap the dressing with a soft, self-adherent bandage using moderate pressure to halt the blood loss. Monitor the wound frequently to assure bleeding has stopped.

A combination of techniques for hemorrhage control may be effective when bleeding is resistant to direct pressure.

Elevation can assist in the control of hemorrhage, although it is generally not as effective as direct pressure. Elevation reduces arterial pressure in the extremity and increases venous return. Elevation can thus reduce edema and increase blood flow through the wound and injured extremity. This promotes good oxygenation and wound healing. Do not elevate a limb, however, if doing so will cause any further harm as would be the case if the patient has a suspected spinal or associated musculoskeletal injury or if there is an object impaled in the limb.

Use pressure points to assist with bleeding control and the clotting process when direct pressure and elevation together do not control it. Locate a pulse point immediately

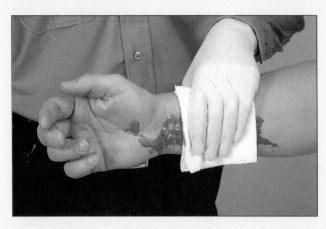

5-1a Apply direct pressure with a dressing to the site of hemorrhage.

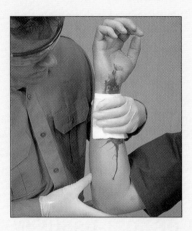

5-1b Elevate the hemorrhage site if there is no serious musculoskeletal injury.

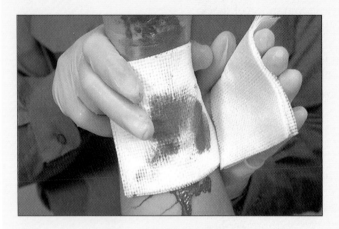

5-1c Apply additional dressings as needed.

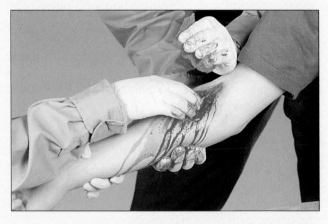

5-1d If serious hemorrhage persists, expose the wound and place digital pressure with a gloved hand on the site of bleeding.

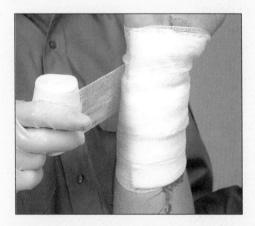

5-1e Bandage the dressing in place, maintaining pressure on the wound.

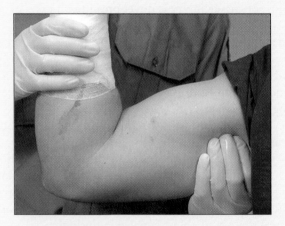

5-1f Apply digital pressure to a proximal artery if the hemorrhage persists.

proximal to the wound and above a bony prominence. Apply firm pressure and maintain it for at least 10 minutes. Assure that the hemorrhage does not continue.

Occasionally, bleeding from a soft-tissue injury can be difficult to control. If the bleeding continues despite the use of direct pressure, elevation, and pressure points, reassess the wound to be sure you have determined the exact site of blood loss. Then reapply direct digital pressure to that precise point. Too often, hemorrhage continues because the bandaging technique distributes pressure over the entire wound site rather than focusing it directly on the source of the bleeding. The force driving the hemorrhage is no greater than the patient's systolic blood pressure, and properly applied digital pressure can thus easily provide a pressure greater than this to compress the vessel and halt any blood loss.

In certain circumstances, the use of direct pressure, elevation, and a pressure point may not control hemorrhage. Crush injuries and amputations are situations in which normal bleeding control measures are often ineffective. With these traumatic injuries, several blood vessels are jaggedly torn, confounding the body's normal hemorrhage control mechanisms and making it difficult to pinpoint the source of bleeding. Even if the source of bleeding can be found, applying firm direct pressure to it may be difficult. In such cases, the application of a tourniquet may be useful. The tourniquet should be considered the last option for controlling hemorrhage. If properly applied, the tourniquet will stop the flow of blood; however, its use has serious associated risks. Keep the following precautions in mind whenever you consider using a tourniquet.

1. If the pressure applied is insufficient, the tourniquet may halt venous return while permitting continued arterial blood flow into the extremity, increasing the rate and volume of blood loss.

2. When the tourniquet is applied properly, the entire limb distal to the device is without circulation. Hypoxia, ischemia, and necrosis may permanently damage the tissue distal to the tourniquet.

3. When circulation is restored, the blood flows and pools in the extremity, adding to any hypovolemia. In addition, any blood that returns to the central circulation is highly hypoxic, acidic, and toxic. This blood can cause shock, lethal dysrhythmias, renal failure, and death. The return of circulation may also restart hemorrhage and introduce emboli into the central circulation.

Do not use a tourniquet unless you cannot control severe bleeding by any other means. Place it just proximal to the wound site, but stay away from the elbow or knee joints (Figure 5-22 ■). Apply the tourniquet in a way that will not injure the tissue beneath. For example, do not use very narrow material, like rope or wire, for a tourniquet; applying great pressure to a limb with such material may cause serious injury in the compressed tissue. Instead, select a 2-inch or wider band for compression.

A readily available, effective, and easily controllable tourniquet is the sphygmomanometer (regular for the upper extremity and thigh for the lower). It is wide, simple to apply, rapid to inflate, and easy to monitor. Inflate it to a pressure 20 to 30 mmHg above the patient's systolic blood pressure and beyond the pressure at which the patient's hemorrhage ceases.

Once you apply a tourniquet, leave it in place until the patient arrives at the emergency department. Monitor the tourniquet during transport to assure that it does not lose pressure, and watch for signs of renewed bleeding. If bleeding starts again, increase the tourniquet pressure. Alert the hospital staff to your use of the tourniquet during transport as well as upon arrival. Mark the patient's forehead clearly with the letters "TQ," and note the time the tourniquet was applied.

Do not release a tourniquet in the field except under exceptional circumstances and then only during consultation with medical direction. Be prepared to provide vigorous

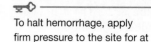

To halt hemorrhage, apply firm pressure to the site for at least 10 minutes.

Do not use a tourniquet unless you cannot control bleeding by any other means.

Once applied, a tourniquet should be left in place until the patient arrives at the emergency department.

■ Figure 5-22   The steps of tourniquet application.

a. Place a bulky dressing over the distal artery.

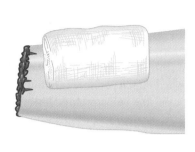

b. Apply a pressure exceeding the systolic pressure.

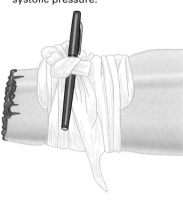

c. Secure the tourniquet and monitor the wound site for continuing hemorrhage.

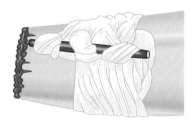

fluid resuscitation, ECG monitoring, dysrhythmia treatment, and rapid transport if a tourniquet release is attempted.

Sterility

Once you halt severe bleeding, keep the wound as sterile as possible. Under field conditions, this may simply mean keeping the wound as clean as reasonably possible. With very small open wounds, like an IV start or a small laceration, you may consider the application of an antibacterial ointment to help with infection control. However, the effectiveness of such ointments on larger wounds is limited, and ointments are not generally applied to these wounds.

Under normal conditions, you need not cleanse the wound. If a wound is grossly contaminated, however, irrigate it with normal saline or lactated Ringer's solution. A 1,000-mL bag of saline, connected to a macrodrip administration set and pressurized by squeezing the bag under your arm, may allow rapid and gentle wound cleansing. Try to move any contamination from the center of the wound outward. You may also carefully remove larger particles—glass, gravel, debris, and so forth—if you can do this swiftly and without inducing further injury.

Apply a bandage to make the dressing appear as neat as time and the conditions under which you are working will allow. Often, this is as easy as covering the entire dressing with wraps of soft, self-adherent roller bandage. The neat appearance calms and reassures the patient, while the bandaging reduces contamination and the chances of post-trauma infection.

Immobilization

The last objective of bandaging is immobilization. The stability of the wound site helps the natural clotting mechanisms operate and reduces the patient's discomfort. Main-

Immobilization is an important, but frequently overlooked, component of hemorrhage control.

taining gentle pressure with the bandage may reduce pain and local swelling. Immobilize the limb with bandaging material to the patient's body or to a rigid surface such as a padded board or ladder splint.

When immobilizing a limb, do not use elastic bandaging material or apply the bandage too tightly. The edema that develops rapidly with an injury puts increasing pressure on underlying tissue. This pressure may quickly reduce or halt circulation.

Frequently monitor any limb that you bandage circumferentially to assure that the distal pulse remains strong and that the distal extremity maintains good color and does not swell. If you cannot locate the distal pulse, monitor capillary refill, skin color, and temperature. If signs or symptoms suggest that the distal circulation is compromised, elevate the extremity, if possible, and check and consider loosening the bandage.

Pain and Edema Control

Treat painful soft-tissue injuries or those likely to cause large debilitating edema with the application of cold packs and moderate-pressure bandages. Cold reduces inflammatory response and local edema. It also dulls the pain associated with serious soft-tissue trauma. Use a commercial cold pack or ice in a plastic bag wrapped in a dry towel and apply it to the wound. Do not use a cold pack directly against the skin as it cools beyond any therapeutic value. Direct application of a cold pack may also cause tissue freezing, especially in areas with reduced circulation.

Some moderate pressure over the wound area may also help reduce pain and wound edema. In cases where the patient reports severe pain, consider use of morphine sulfate, fentanyl, or other analgesics for patient comfort. Administer morphine in 2 mg increments titrated to pain relief every 5 minutes (up to a total of 10 mg). Fentanyl may be administered in a 25–50 mcg dose, followed by 25-mcg doses, titrated to relieve pain.

ANATOMICAL CONSIDERATIONS FOR BANDAGING

Each area of the body has specific anatomical characteristics. Your application of bandages and dressings should take these characteristics into account to provide effective prehospital wound care (Figure 5-23 ■).

Scalp

The scalp has a rich supply of vessels that can bleed heavily when injured. It's commonly said that head wounds rarely account for shock, but scalp hemorrhage can be severe and difficult to control and can lead to the loss of moderate to large volumes of blood.

In scalp hemorrhage uncomplicated by skull fracture, direct pressure against the skull is effective in the control of bleeding. To hold a dressing in place and maintain pressure, wrap a bandage around the head, capturing the occiput or brow or, in some cases, passing the bandage under the chin (while still allowing for jaw movement).

If a head wound is complicated by fracture, be very careful in your application of pressure. Apply gentle digital pressure around the wound and attempt to locate the small scalp arteries that feed it to use as pressure points. Then simply hold a dressing on the wound without much pressure.

Face

Facial wounds are frequently gruesome and bleed heavily. Gentle direct pressure to these wounds can effectively control hemorrhage. You can maintain this pressure by wrapping a bandage around the head. Be careful to assure a clear airway and use your bandaging to splint any facial instability.

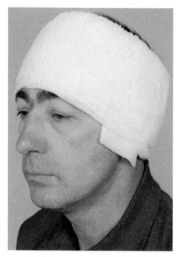

a. Head and/or ear bandage.

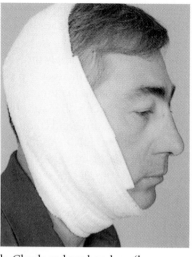

b. Cheek and ear bandage (be sure mouth will open).

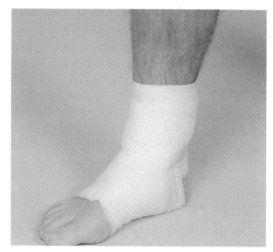

c. Hand bandage.

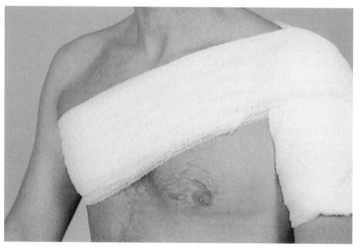

d. Shoulder bandage.

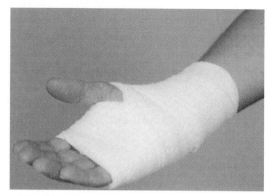

e. Foot and/or ankle bandage.

■ Figure 5-23   Good bandaging uses the natural body curves and the self-adherent characteristics of bandages to hold dressings firmly in place.

Remember, blood is a gastric irritant and swallowed blood may induce emesis. Be ready to provide suctioning in patients with oral or nasal hemorrhage because unexpected emesis may compromise the airway.

Ear or Mastoid

Wounds to the ear region can be easily bandaged by wrapping the head circumferentially. Use open gauze to collect, not stop, any bleeding or fluids flowing from the ear canal. These materials may contain cerebrospinal fluid, and halting their flow may add to any increasing intracranial pressure.

Neck

Minor neck wounds may be lightly wrapped circumferentially with bandages or taped to hold dressings in place. If bleeding is moderate to severe, however, direct manual pressure may be necessary because the amount of pressure applied by circumferential

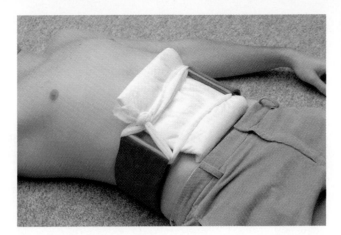

wrapping may compromise both the airway and circulation to and from the head. In cases of large wounds or moderate to severe bleeding, also consider using an occlusive dressing to prevent aspiration of air into a jugular vein.

Shoulder

The shoulder is an easy area to bandage as soft, self-adherent roller bandages readily conform to body contours. Use the axilla, arm, and neck as points of fixation, but be careful not to put pressure on the anterior neck and trachea.

Trunk

For minor trunk wounds, adhesive tape may be sufficient to hold dressings in place. With larger wounds, bandaging can be more difficult because you must wrap the patient's body circumferentially to apply direct pressure to a wound. Applying a bandage in this way may require moving the patient unnecessarily and risk causing or worsening an injury. Consider instead using a ladder splint that is negotiated beneath the patient's torso, folded to the curve of the back, and then folded outward sharply at each end to serve as a bandaging fixation point. You then wrap the bandage between the ends of the ladder splint to hold the dressing in place (Figure 5-24 ■).

Groin and Hip

The groin and the hip are easy places to affix a dressing. Bandage by following the contours of the upper thighs and waist, similar to the technique of bandaging a shoulder. Be careful here, though. Any movement of the patient is likely to affect the tightness of the bandage and the amount of pressure over the dressing. With these injuries, therefore, bandage after the patient is in the final position for transport.

Elbow and Knee

Joints, especially the elbow and knee, are difficult to bandage. Bandage using circumferential wraps and then splint the area to assure that the bandage does not loosen with movement. If possible, place the joint in a position halfway between flexion and extension. This position, called the position of function, relaxes the muscles controlling the joint and the skin tension lines, and is most comfortable for the patient during long transports or periods of immobilization.

Hand and Finger

Hand and finger injuries are easy to bandage by simple circumferential wrapping. Again, consider placing the hand or digit in the position of function, halfway between flexion and extension. Accomplish this by placing a large, bulky dressing in the palm of the patient's hand and then wrapping around it. You may use a malleable finger splint to obtain the position of function and then wrap circumferentially to splint the finger. If possible, before bandaging, carefully remove any jewelry from the wrist and fingers, as swelling may restrict distal circulation and also make it difficult to remove the jewelry later.

Ankle and Foot

Ankle and foot wounds are also easy to bandage by wrapping circumferentially and by using the natural body contours. If strong direct pressure is needed to maintain hemorrhage control, start your wrapping from the toes and work proximally. This assures that the pressure of bandaging does not form a venous tourniquet and compromise circulation to this very distal injury.

COMPLICATIONS OF BANDAGING

Frequently check the pressure beneath a bandage to assure good distal circulation.

Bandaging can lead to some complications, although such occurrences are infrequent. If a bandage—particularly a circumferential bandage—is too tight, the area beneath it may continue to swell, increasing pressure in the area of the wound. This can lead to decreased blood flow and ischemia distal to the bandage. Pressure can build to such an extreme that the bandage acts like a tourniquet. Pain, pallor, tingling, a loss of pulses, and prolonged capillary refill time are typical signs of developing pressure and ischemia. Avoid this complication by making bandages snug but not too tight. A useful technique is to wrap a bandage only so tight that one finger can still be easily slipped beneath it.

Bandages and dressings left on too long can become soaked with blood and body fluids and then serve as incubators for infection. This problem usually takes at least 2 to 3 days to develop and is not a common concern in most prehospital settings.

The size of the dressing is an important consideration in bandaging. An unnecessarily large and bulky dressing can prevent proper inspection of a wound and hide contamination and continued serious bleeding. Too small a dressing can become lost in a wound and become, in effect, a foreign body. This is most frequently a problem with large, gaping wounds and deep wounds that penetrate the thoracic or abdominal body cavities. When dressing a wound, choose a dressing just larger than the wound yet not so small as to become lost in it.

CARE OF SPECIFIC WOUNDS

Some circumstances—amputations, impaled objects, and crush syndrome cases—deserve special attention during the patient management process. These injuries can challenge even the seasoned paramedic to provide the most appropriate care.

Amputations

Current recommendations for managing amputated body parts include dry cooling and rapid transport.

Amputations may bleed either heavily or minimally. Attempt to control hemorrhage with direct pressure by applying a large, bulky dressing to the wound. If this fails to control hemorrhage, consider using a tourniquet just above the point of severance. If there is a crushing wound associated with the limb loss, apply the tourniquet just above the crushed area. Do not delay patient transport while locating or extricating the amputated body part. Transport the patient immediately, and then have other personnel transport the part once it is located or released from entrapment.

Current recommendations for managing separated body parts include dry cooling and rapid transport. Place the amputated part in a plastic bag and immerse the bag in cold water (Figure 5-25 ■). The water may have a few ice cubes in it, but avoid direct contact between the ice and the injured part. Even if the amputated part cannot be totally reattached, skin from it may be used to cover the limb end (Figure 5-26 ■).

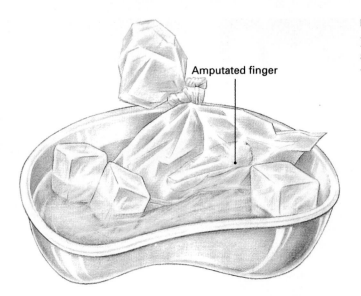

■ Figure 5-25 Amputated parts should be put in a dry bag, sealed, and placed in cool water that contains a few ice cubes.

Amputated finger

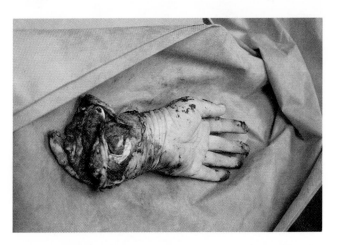

a. An amputated hand.

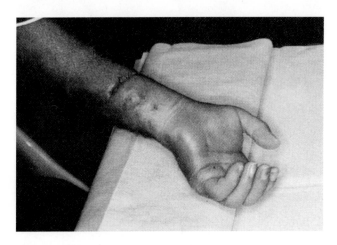

b. A successfully reimplanted hand.

■ Figure 5-26 Amputated parts should be located and transported with the patient to the hospital for possible replantation.

Impaled Objects

When possible, immobilize all impaled objects in place (Figure 5-27). Position bulky dressings around the object to stabilize it, and tape over the dressings to hold them in place. Try to make movement of the patient to the ambulance and transport to the emergency department as smooth and nonjarring as possible. Remember that any movement of the impaled object is likely to cause continued internal bleeding and additional tissue damage.

Do not remove impaled objects because of the risk of serious, uncontrollable bleeding.

If the impaled object is too large to transport or is affixed to something that cannot be moved, such as a reinforcing rod set in concrete, consider cutting it. Use appropriate techniques and tools depending on the circumstances of the impalement. A hand or power saw, an acetylene torch, or bolt cutters might be employed. Whatever tools and techniques are used, be sure to take steps to limit the heat, vibration, or jolting transmitted to the patient. Provide the best possible support for both the object and the patient during the cutting procedure.

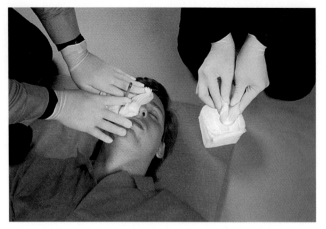

a. Manually stabilize any impaled object.

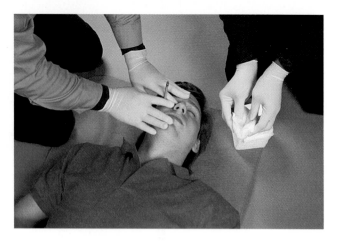

b. Use bulky padding or dressing to immobilize the object.

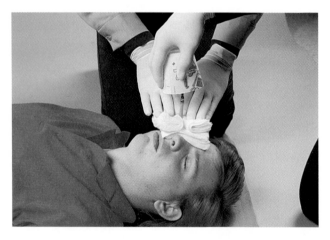

c. If the object protrudes, cover it with a paper cup.

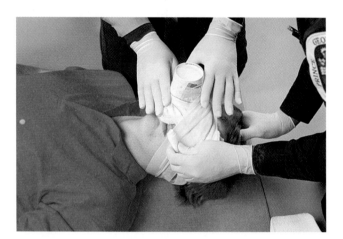

d. Bandage the cup and padding securely in place

■ Figure 5-27 Stabilization of an impaled object.

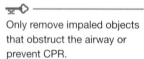

Only remove impaled objects that obstruct the airway or prevent CPR.

There are some special circumstances in which you *should* remove an impaled object. For example, you may remove an object impaled in the cheek if the removal is necessary to maintain a patent airway (Figure 5-28 ■). In this case, be prepared to apply direct pressure to the wound both from inside the cheek (intraorally) and externally.

Another object that would require removal is one impaled in the central chest of a patient who needs CPR. In such a circumstance, the risk associated with not performing resuscitation outweighs the risk of removing the object. Be aware, however, that a trauma patient who needs CPR has a very poor prognosis.

Another complication associated with an impaled object occurs when a patient is impaled on an object that cannot be cut or moved. In such a case, contact medical direction for advice and guidance. If the object is impaled in a limb, bleeding may be controllable. If it has entered the head, neck, chest, or abdomen, it may not be.

Crush Syndrome

The key to successful prehospital management of a crush syndrome patient is anticipation of the problem and prevention of its effects. Since, by definition, all crush syndrome patients are victims of prolonged entrapment, cases can be identified before

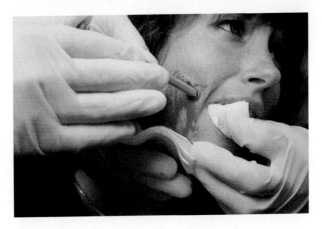

Figure 5-28 Objects impaled in the cheek may be removed because the sites of hemorrhage can be controlled and the object may interfere with airway control.

extrication is complete. The focus of prehospital crush injury care is on rapid transport, adequate fluid resuscitation, diuresis, and—possibly—systemic alkalinization.

The prehospital approach to crush syndrome is similar to that with other trauma patients. Assuring scene safety is particularly important in these cases. Crush syndrome victims are often buried in heavy rubble or other large debris, and access may be difficult (Figure 5-29 ■). You may need to request the assistance of specialized personnel and their equipment—urban search and rescue teams, or trench, heavy, or confined space rescue teams. Never place yourself or other rescuers in unreasonable danger when providing care or attempting a rescue.

Once the scene is safe and you can reach the patient, conduct an initial assessment. Remove debris from around the head, neck, and thorax to minimize airway obstruction and restriction of ventilation. Control any reachable and obvious bleeding. Perform as much of the initial and rapid trauma assessment as possible, keeping in mind that portions of the patient's body will be inaccessible as a result of the entrapment. The dark, dusty, and cramped conditions of many confined space rescues may force you to

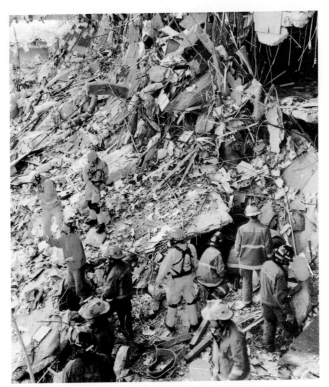

Figure 5-29 Explosion and structural collapse frequently produce crush injury and crush syndrome. *(Pool/Gamma Liaison/Getty Images)*

improvise. Be alert for signs and symptoms of associated injuries such as dust inhalation, dehydration, and hypothermia.

Remember that the greater the body area compressed and the longer the time of entrapment, the greater the risk of crush syndrome. Initially, a trapped patient will usually complain only of entrapment symptoms: pain, lack of motor function, tingling, or loss of sensation in the affected limb. The patient may also experience flaccid paralysis and sensory loss in the limb unrelated to the normal distribution of peripheral nerve control and sensation.

As long as the body part is still trapped and the metabolic by-products of the crush injury are confined to the entrapped part, the patient will not experience the full effects of crush syndrome. With extrication, however, toxic by-products are released into the circulation, and the patient may rapidly develop shock and die. If the patient survives the initial release of the by-products, he remains at great risk of developing renal failure with serious morbidity or delayed death. Note, too, that a crush injury may also induce compartment syndrome (explained later), especially with prolonged entrapment.

Once you have assured the patient's ABCs (airway, breathing, circulation), turn your attention to obtaining IV access. Intravenous fluids and selected medications are important in treating crush syndrome. Initiate two large-bore IVs if possible. Because of the entrapment, it may be necessary to consider alternative IV sites such as the external jugular vein or the veins of a lower extremity. Avoid any site distal to a crush injury.

When you encounter crush syndrome, it is unlikely that your protocols will address it. Contact the trauma center for medical direction and communicate, on-line, with the emergency physician. Expect to provide frequent vital sign and patient updates, and be prepared to administer large fluid volumes and, possibly, alkalizing agents.

Alkalinization of the blood and urine is a consideration for preventing and treating crush syndrome. In combination with fluid resuscitation, alkalinization can correct acidosis, help prevent renal failure, and help correct hyperkalemia. Administer sodium bicarbonate 1 mEq/kg initially, followed by 0.25 mEq/kg/hr thereafter. It is preferable to add the bicarbonate to the normal saline bag rather than administering it as a bolus or IV push.

Diuretics may help keep the kidneys well perfused and more resistant to failure during crush syndrome. Mannitol, an osmotic diuretic, is the drug of choice because it draws interstitial fluid into the vascular space and eliminates it as mannitol is excreted by the kidneys. Furosemide, a loop diuretic, inhibits the reabsorption of both sodium and chloride. Its use is not advisable in hypovolemic states because it may add to the electrolyte imbalance and volume loss.

Consider applying a tourniquet before the entrapping pressure is released if you have been unable to medicate the patient and provide fluid resuscitation. The tourniquet will sequester the toxins and prevent reperfusion injury. Tourniquet use, however, will continue the development of crush syndrome and worsen its effects.

In cases where the entrapping object may not be moved for many hours or days, medical direction may consider field amputation. This operation will likely be performed by a physician responding to the scene but, in dire circumstances, may be performed by a paramedic under the on-line direction of the emergency physician.

Cardiac (ECG) monitoring is important with all crush syndrome patients. Dysrhythmias may develop at any time but are most likely to occur immediately following the release of pressure upon extrication. Sudden cardiac arrest should be treated in the usual fashion with defibrillation and cardiac drugs as appropriate. Consider 500 mg calcium chloride IV push (in addition to the sodium bicarbonate) to counteract life-threatening dysrhythmias induced by hyperkalemia. Watch for the tenting, or peaking, of the T-wave, a prolonged P-R interval, and S-T segment depression. Be sure to flush the IV line between infusions or to use different lines because calcium chloride and sodium bicarbonate precipitate.

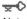

Note: The milliequivalent (mEq) is a means of measuring electrolytes in a standard solution and is based on the molecular weight and valence of the electrolyte in question.

Once the patient is freed from entrapment, be prepared to treat rapidly progressing shock. Continue the normal saline infusions at 30 mL/kg/hr and provide additional boluses of sodium bicarbonate as needed. Rapidly transport the patient to an appropriate hospital (usually a trauma center) for all cases of suspected crush syndrome.

Prehospital care of the crushed limb or body parts requires no special techniques. Cover open wounds and splint fractures, keeping in mind that progressive swelling will necessitate ongoing reassessment, with monitoring of distal circulation and the tightness of bandages, straps, and splints. Handle all crushed limbs gently because the ischemic tissue is prone to injury. Elevation of severely crushed extremities is not indicated in the prehospital setting.

Care at the hospital for crush injury is aggressive and may use techniques such as debridement and hyperbaric oxygenation. During hyperbaric oxygenation, the patient is placed in a chamber with artificially high concentrations of oxygen under several atmospheres of pressure. This drives oxygen into poorly oxygenated tissue to help with the destruction of anaerobic bacteria and to increase tissue oxygenation for repair and regeneration, ultimately reducing tissue necrosis and edema. Hyperbaric oxygenation is most effective when provided early in the course of care.

Hospital care for crush injuries also includes administration of several medications as well as hemodialysis to help salvage the kidneys from the ravages of myoglobin and other toxic agents. Allopurinol, a xanthine oxidase inhibitor, interferes with the production of uric acid, a by-product of skeletal muscle destruction, and may help reperfusion of both the kidneys and the skeletal muscles. It is most effective if administered immediately before release of the compression. Amiloride hydrochloride is a potassium-sparing diuretic that inhibits the sodium/calcium exchange. Mannitol, tetanus toxoid (if needed), and prophylactic antibiotics may also be administered in the hospital to treat crush syndrome.

Once the crush injury patient is freed from entrapment, anticipate the rapid development of shock.

Compartment Syndrome

The most prominent symptom of compartment syndrome is severe pain, often out of proportion to the physical findings. Other signs are often subtle or absent, or they may be overshadowed by the original injury such as a fracture or contusion. Some people suggest using the six Ps—pain, paresthesia, paresis, pressure, passive stretching pain, pulselessness—to identify compartment syndrome, but many of these signs are not dependable or they appear very late in the course of the injury. (Passive stretching pain is pain or an increase in pain noted by a patient as a muscle is extended by a care provider.) Motor and sensory functions are usually normal with compartment syndrome, as are distal pulses. Even capillary refill shows little change. It is important to note that compartment syndrome rarely occurs within the first 4 hours after an acute injury. It is more likely to appear 6 to 8 hours (or as much as a day or more) after the initial injury. Recognition of compartment syndrome can be challenging and requires a healthy suspicion for the problem.

The first step in prehospital treatment for compartment syndrome is care of the underlying injury. Splint and immobilize all suspected fractures, and use traction as appropriate for femur fractures. Apply cold packs to severe contusions. Elevation of the affected extremity is the single most effective prehospital treatment for compartment syndrome. This reduces edema, increases venous return, lowers compartment pressure, and helps prevent ischemia. In the hospital, compartment syndrome is treated surgically, through a procedure that incises the restrictive fascia, a fasciotomy.

The most prominent symptom of compartment syndrome is pain out of proportion with the physical findings.

SPECIAL ANATOMICAL SITES

Several anatomical sites provide challenges to the care of soft-tissue injuries. These include the face and neck, the thorax, and the abdomen.

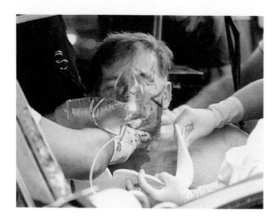

■ **Figure 5-30** Severe facial soft-tissue injuries may interfere with airway control and distort landmarks used for intubation. (© *Eddie Sperling Photography*)

Face and Neck

Soft-tissue injuries to the face and neck present potential challenges owing to the anatomical relationships of the airway and great vessels. Injuries to the face may result in blood and tissue debris in the airway, posing risks of airway obstruction, asphyxia, and aspiration (Figure 5-30 ■). Pooled secretions and tissue edema may add to airway problems. Trauma to the face or neck may also distort the anatomical structures of the upper airway, leading to airway compromise, and complicating attempts at endotracheal intubation.

Emergency treatment of face and neck injuries can be challenging and may tax your skills. First, gain control of the airway. Open the airway using manual maneuvers. If you suspect the possibility of spinal injury, use the jaw-thrust maneuver in conjunction with in-line manual immobilization. Aggressively suction blood, saliva, and debris from the pharynx, but avoid stimulating the gag reflex in the patient or inducing emesis. Insert an oro- or nasopharyngeal airway as needed.

Direct visualization of the endotracheal tube passing through the cords is the gold standard for securing the airway, but achieving it is fraught with complications in cases of face and neck trauma. Secretions and blood may prevent adequate visualization even with aggressive suctioning. Airway edema can distort the anatomy beyond recognition, and even prevent passage of the ET tube. In all cases, meticulous and absolute confirmation of tube placement is mandatory to avoid fatal hypoxia. Continuous waveform capnography can help assure initial and ongoing proper endotracheal tube placement.

In desperate circumstances, needle or surgical cricothyrotomy may be lifesaving. Avoid placing the needle or making the incision through neck hematomas to avoid life-threatening bleeding.

Once you have secured the airway, focus your attention on any serious facial or neck bleeding. Direct pressure is usually successful for bleeding control, but be certain to avoid compressing or occluding the airway. Pressure points and tourniquets should not be used because of the risks they present of cerebral ischemia and strangulation. Open neck wounds also carry the danger of air aspiration and emboli. Cover any open neck wound with an occlusive dressing, which should then be held or bandaged firmly in place. Because of the neck's anatomy, you may have to maintain digital pressure throughout the course of prehospital care to assure effective bleeding control.

Thorax

Superficial soft-tissue injury to the thorax may suggest more serious intrathoracic injuries. The pleural space extends superiorly to the supraclavicular fossa and inferiorly to include the entire rib cage both anteriorly and posteriorly. Trauma to this area is likely to injure both the pleura and lungs. Small "lacerations" may actually be deep, penetrating stab or gunshot wounds with resultant hemothorax, pneumothorax, pericardial tamponade, penetrating heart trauma, or injury to the great vessels, esophagus, bronchi, or diaphragm. A seemingly minor "rib bruise" may be the only visible sign of serious lung or cardiac contusions beneath.

Perform a thorough physical examination to detect any signs of internal bleeding, pulmonary edema, dysrhythmias, or shock. However, never explore a thoracic wound beyond the skin edges. Probing deeper can convert a minor wound to a pneumothorax or a bleeding disaster. Consider all thoracic wounds to be potentially life threatening until evidence proves otherwise. See Chapter 10, "Thoracic Trauma," for detailed care procedures.

Dress all open thoracic wounds with sterile dressings in the usual fashion. Be alert, however, for the presence of air bubbling, subcutaneous emphysema, crepitus, or other hints of open pneumothorax. Be extremely cautious about making an airtight seal on any thoracic wound because doing so can rapidly lead to tension pneumothorax and death. Instead, use an occlusive dressing sealed on three sides and be prepared to assist ventilations. Auscultate the chest and monitor respirations frequently. Watch the occlusive dressing so that it does not seal with blood against the chest wall and convert a simple pneumothorax into a tension pneumothorax.

Never explore a thoracic open wound beyond its edges. Probing may create a pneumothorax or induce serious bleeding.

Watch any patient with an open chest wound for the development of a pneumothorax or tension pneumothorax.

Abdomen

The peritoneal cavity extends approximately from the symphysis pubis inferiorly to the diaphragm superiorly. Since the diaphragm rises and falls with respiration, so too does the border between the abdominal and thoracic cavities. You cannot know the exact position of the diaphragm at the time the injury occurred, so suspect associated injuries to both abdominal and thoracic organs if the soft-tissue injury involves the region between the rib margin and the fifth rib anteriorly, the seventh rib laterally, and the ninth rib posteriorly.

Blunt or penetrating trauma to the abdomen can injure both hollow and solid organs, penetrate or rupture the diaphragm, and cause serious internal bleeding. Anteriorly and just underlying the rib margin are the liver on the right and the spleen on the left. Posteriorly, the kidneys (not true abdominal organs since they lie retroperitoneally) are located in the costovertebral angle region. Hollow organs—the bowel, stomach, and urinary bladder—may rupture. In addition to bleeding copiously, these organs may release their contents and inflame the peritoneum.

Consider any soft-tissue wound in the abdominal region as potentially damaging to the underlying organs. Signs and symptoms of internal damage can be subtle, particularly early on. Eviscerations and other massive injuries are obvious, but other internal injuries that are just as serious may not be apparent. Prehospital treatment is primarily supportive and includes assuring adequate oxygenation, preventing shock, and dressing open wounds (see Chapter 11, "Abdominal Trauma").

WOUNDS REQUIRING TRANSPORT

Transport any patient with a wound that involves a structure beneath the integument for emergency department evaluation. This includes wounds involving, or possibly involving, nerves, blood vessels, ligaments, tendons, or muscles. Also transport any patient with a significantly contaminated wound, a wound involving an impaled object, or a wound that was received in a particularly unclean environment. Also transport any patient with a wound with likely cosmetic implications, such as facial wounds or large gaping wounds.

SOFT-TISSUE TREATMENT AND REFER/RELEASE

In some EMS systems, paramedics are permitted to treat and release patients with minor and superficial soft-tissue injuries or treat and refer them to their personal physicians. This generally occurs under on-line medical direction or according to strict protocols.

In such circumstances, you must evaluate and dress the wound. Then explain to the patient the steps to follow for continuing care of the injury. Tell the patient of the need to change the dressing and to monitor the injury site for further hemorrhage or developing infection. Provide the patient with simple written instructions (approved and/or published by medical direction) explaining wound care, monitoring, protection, dressing change, cleansing, and the signs of problems such as infection or hemorrhage.

Instruct the patient to contact a physician if certain signs and symptoms appear and describe those signs and symptoms thoroughly. Assure that the patient has the means to obtain physician or health care provider follow-up and again stress the circumstances in which such follow-up care should be sought. During any referral or release, if the patient's tetanus immunization history is unclear or it has been longer than 5 years since the last immunization, instruct the patient to obtain a tetanus booster.

Document all refer/release incidents carefully in the prehospital care report. The report should include a description of the nature and extent of the wound and of the care provided for it. Note in the report all instructions and materials provided to the patient and any medical direction you received.

Summary

Soft-tissue injury may compromise the skin—the envelope that protects and contains the human body. Any trauma must penetrate the skin before it can harm the interior organs and threaten life. Any damage to the skin may interfere with its ability to contain water and blood and to prevent damaging agents from entering. For these reasons, the assessment and care of soft-tissue injuries are important parts of prehospital care.

Assess wounds carefully since they may provide the only overt signs of serious internal injury. Realize that discoloration and swelling take time to develop and may not be as apparent in the field as when you present the patient at the emergency department. Look carefully for the early signs of wounds, and use the mechanism of injury to locate potential trauma sites. When caring for soft-tissue injuries, keep in mind the basic goals: controlling hemorrhage, keeping the wound as clean as possible, and immobilizing the injury site. While soft-tissue injuries are not often assigned a high priority in prehospital care, they do account for a large number of patient injuries and are significant to the overall assessment and care of trauma victims.

You Make the Call

You arrive at the scene of a "foot injury" to find a young child lying on the lawn and surrounded by his parents. As you begin to question his father about what happened, he explains, "My son stepped on a board with a nail in it." After donning gloves, you carefully remove the boy's shoe to discover an almost invisible penetration to the sole of the foot. The child is now resting quietly, without much pain.

1. What type of wound is this and what significance does it have for infection?
2. What elements of history and specifically vaccinations will be important in assessing this patient?
3. What direction would you give this patient if his parents do not wish to have him transported to the local emergency department?

See Suggested Responses at the back of this book.

Review Questions

1. How does the integumentary system prevent pathogens from attacking the body?
   a. The skin provides a pathway out of the body for pathogens.
   b. Leukocytes in the skin attack pathogens.
   c. Antibodies in the skin attack and destroy pathogens.
   d. The skin provides a protective barrier against pathogens.

2. Of the open wounds presenting to emergency departments, up to _____ percent will eventually become infected, resulting in significant morbidity.
   a. 8
   b. 6.5
   c. 10
   d. 15

3. Glands within the dermis that secrete sweat are called:
   a. mast cells.
   b. sebaceous glands.
   c. sudoriferous glands.
   d. lymphocyte glands.

4. When an artery is ruptured but the skin is not broken, blood can separate the tissues and pool in a pocket. This pocket of blood is known as a(n):
   a. contusion.
   b. abrasion.
   c. hematoma.
   d. crush injury.

5. _____ are typically the most minor of injuries that violate the protective envelope of the skin.
   a. Incisions
   b. Avulsions
   c. Abrasions
   d. Lacerations

6. Specialized white blood cells capable of engulfing bacteria are called:
   a. granulocytes.
   b. macrophages.
   c. phagocytes.
   d. all of the above.

7. The anaerobic bacterium *Clostridium perfringens* causes a deep space infection called:
   a. gangrene.
   b. tetanus.
   c. collagen.
   d. lockjaw.

8. You have been called to a scene where a patient has caught one of his hands between two pieces of machinery. As the hand is removed from the machinery, there is no visible injury. You should expect the internal injuries to be:
   a. extensive.
   b. unimportant.
   c. life threatening.
   d. minimally significant.

9. Which type of dressing is designed to be placed over a wound without sticking to the fluids or clotting agents?
   a. adherent
   b. nonabsorbent
   c. absorbent
   d. nonadherent

10. As you begin to bandage a soft-tissue injury, you should continue to check distal pulses to ensure proper tissue perfusion. This is primarily because the bandage may fit properly at first but later become too tight and reduce circulation due to the:
    a. shrinking of the bandage.
    b. development of shock.
    c. toxins entering central circulation.
    d. damaged tissue swelling.

11. When bandaging the foot and ankle to create pressure and control bleeding, wrap in a:
    a. distal-to-proximal fashion to avoid forming a venous tourniquet.
    b. proximal-to-distal fashion to avoid forming a venous tourniquet.
    c. proximal-to-distal fashion to help maintain gentle traction.
    d. distal-to-proximal fashion to help maintain gentle traction.

12. When a soft-tissue injury occurs, a process to stop bleeding starts almost immediately; in addition, the vessels constrict, platelets clot, and the blood coagulates. This process is called:
    a. inflammation.
    b. hemostasis.
    c. epithelialization.
    d. neovascularization.

See Answers to Review Questions at the back of this book.

Further Reading

American College of Surgeons, Committee on Trauma. *Advanced Trauma Life Support Course: Student Manual.* Chicago: American College of Surgeons, 2003.

Bates, Barbara, Lynn S. Bickley, and Robert A. Hoekelman. *A Guide to Physical Examination and History Taking.* 8th ed. Philadelphia: J. B. Lippincott, 2003.

Bledsoe, B. E. and D. Clayden. *Prehospital Emergency Pharmacology.* 6th ed. Upper Saddle River, N.J.: Pearson/Prentice Hall, 2005.

Butman, A., S. Martin, R. Vomacka, and N. McSwain. *Comprehensive Guide to Pre-Hospital Skills: A Skills Manual for EMT-Basic, EMT-Intermediate, and EMT-Paramedic.* St. Louis: Mosby, 1996.

Campbell, John E. *Basic Trauma Life Support for Paramedics and Other Advanced Providers.* 5th ed. Upper Saddle River, N.J.: Pearson/Prentice Hall, 2004.

Feliciano, D.V., et al. *Trauma.* 5th ed. New York: McGraw Hill, 2004.

Ivatury R. R., and G. C. Cayten, eds. *Textbook of Penetrating Trauma.* Media, Pa: Williams & Wilkins, 1996.

Martini, Frederic. *Fundamentals of Anatomy and Physiology.* 6th ed. San Francisco: Benjamin Cummings, 2004.

McSwain, N. E. and S. B. Frame, eds. *Prehospital Trauma Life Support.* 5th ed. St. Louis: Mosby, 2003.

Rosen, P., and R. Barkin, eds. *Emergency Medicine: Concepts and Clinical Practice.* 5th ed. St. Louis: Mosby, 2002.

On the Web

Visit Brady's Paramedic Website at **www.bradybooks.com/paramedic**.

Burns

Objectives

After reading this chapter, you should be able to:

1. Describe the anatomy and physiology of the skin and remaining human anatomy as they pertain to thermal burn injuries. (pp. 179–181)
2. Describe the epidemiology, including incidence, mortality, morbidity, and risk factors, for thermal burn injuries as well as strategies to prevent such injuries. (pp. 178–179)
3. Describe the local and systemic complications of a thermal burn injury. (pp. 181–183, 193–195)
4. Identify and describe the depth classifications of burn injuries, including superficial burns, partial thickness burns, and full thickness burns. (pp. 190–192)
5. Describe and apply the "rule of nines" and the "rule of palms" methods for determining the body surface area percentage of a burn injury. (pp. 192–193)
6. Identify and describe the severity of a burn including a minor burn, a moderate burn, and a critical burn. (pp. 198–201)
7. Describe the effects age and preexisting conditions have on burn severity and a patient's prognosis. (pp. 194, 200)
8. Discuss complications of burn injuries caused by trauma, blast injuries, airway compromise, respiratory compromise, and child abuse. (pp. 189–190, 194–195, 204–205)
9. Describe thermal burn management including considerations for airway and ventilation, circulation, pharmacological and nonpharmacological measures, transport decisions, and psychological support/ communication strategies. (pp. 195–205)
10. Describe special considerations for a pediatric patient with a burn injury and describe the criteria for determining pediatric burn severity. (pp. 198–201)

11. Describe the specific epidemiologies, mechanisms of injury, pathophysiologies, and severity assessments for inhalation, chemical, and electrical burn injuries and for radiation exposure. (pp. 206–212)

12. Discuss special considerations that impact the assessment, management, and prognosis of patients with inhalation, chemical, and electrical burn injuries and with exposure to radiation. (pp. 206–212)

13. Differentiate between supraglottic and subglottic inhalation burn injuries. (p. 190)

14. Describe the special considerations for a chemical burn injury to the eye. (pp. 207–210)

15. Given several preprogrammed, simulated thermal, inhalation, electrical, and chemical burn injury and radiation exposure patients, provide the appropriate scene size-up, initial assessment, rapid trauma or focused physical exam and history, detailed exam, and ongoing assessment and provide appropriate patient care and transportation. (pp. 178–212)

Key Terms

alpha radiation, p. 186
ampere, p. 183
beta radiation, p. 186
blepharospasm, p. 209
body surface area (BSA), p. 192
coagulation necrosis, p. 185
current, p. 183
denature, p. 181
emergent phase, p. 182
eschar, p. 193
extravascular space, p. 183
fluid shift phase, p. 183
full thickness burn, p. 191

gamma radiation, p. 186
Gray, p. 188
hypermetabolic phase, p. 183
intravascular space, p. 183
ionization, p. 186
Jackson's theory of thermal wounds, p. 182
Joule's law, p. 183
liquefaction necrosis, p. 185
neutron radiation, p. 186
ohm, p. 183
Ohm's law, p. 183

partial thickness burn, p. 191
rad, p. 188
resistance, p. 183
resolution phase, p. 183
rule of nines, p. 192
rule of palms, p. 193
subglottic, p. 190
superficial burn, p. 191
supraglottic, p. 190
voltage, p. 183
zone of coagulation, p. 182
zone of hyperemia, p. 182
zone of statis, p. 182

Case Study

Ben and Ronny, Fire Rescue paramedics, respond with trucks 23 and 56 to a working structural fire. Upon arrival, they find two fire units already deployed, with firefighters engaging a wood frame home fully engulfed in flames. As Ronny positions their vehicle, the south wall of the structure collapses on a firefighter. Within minutes, other firefighters extinguish the burning wall and free the firefighter.

When the firefighters have secured the scene, Ben and Ronny proceed to the patient and begin their initial assessment. They approach a male who is lying supine, with his turnout gear burned and charred in places, indicating that he has received serious burns.

Because of the wall's collapse on the firefighter, they provide manual in-line cervical immobilization while proceeding with the assessment. The downed firefighter's respirations appear adequate, although the patient is coughing up sooty sputum and is slightly hoarse. The firefighter, who gives his name as Karl, is conscious and alert. His airway seems clear except for the hoarseness. The sooty sputum and hoarseness indicate the possibility of burns to the airway, making Karl a priority for rapid transport.

Ben proceeds to perform the rapid trauma assessment. Upon removal of Karl's turnout gear, Ben exposes relatively painless, dark, discolored burns to his posterior thorax and lower back as well as circumferential burns of the left upper extremity. Despite the burn severity, Karl denies much pain. Ben also finds angulation, false motion, and pain in the right forearm. Vital signs reveal normal breathing in terms of volume and rate and a strong, regular pulse at a rate of about 100. Distal pulses are also strong, and capillary refill is timed at 2 seconds. Karl is fully conscious and oriented and is joking about the incident.

The rescue crew now takes some initial care steps. Ben cuts away Karl's clothing, and then covers the burn site with a dry, sterile sheet and starts an IV line, running normal saline at a wide-open rate. Ronny applies oxygen via a nonrebreather mask and observes an oximetry reading of 97 percent. They package Karl and quickly load him into the ambulance for rapid transport. En route to the hospital, Ben checks Karl's blood pressure (120/88) and respirations (30 and shallow), noting that the patient displays increasing respiratory effort.

While Ronny is splinting the right limb, Karl begins to cough deeply and experiences severe dyspnea. Karl's dyspnea progresses, and his level of consciousness drops. Oxygen saturation falls to 86 percent. Ben begins to provide supplemental oxygen via a bag-valve mask, while Ronny prepares intubation equipment.

Medical direction orders the crew to intubate, and they attempt to do so during transport. The airway is edematous, and visualization of the vocal cords is difficult. After the first attempt, Ronny withdraws the tube when auscultation of breath sounds, failure to obtain chest rise, absent end-tidal CO_2 levels, and a dropping oxygen saturation indicate esophageal placement. Ben hyperventilates Karl, and Ronny attempts another intubation. She is again unsuccessful.

As they withdraw the tube, the ambulance arrives at the emergency department. The ED physician places a large-bore catheter in the cricothyroid membrane and attempts transtracheal jet insufflation. The technique is successful. After an emergency tracheostomy, Karl begins spontaneous respirations and maintains a strong pulse. His level of consciousness does not improve, however, and the hospital staff transfers him to the burn unit for definitive care.

INTRODUCTION TO BURN INJURIES

The incidence of burn injuries in the United States and other developed countries has been declining for several decades. Despite the decline, an estimated 1.25 to 2 million Americans are treated for burns annually and 50,000 are hospitalized. Some 3 to 5 percent of these burns are considered life threatening. Persons at greatest risk for serious burns include the very young and old, the infirm, and workers, such as firefighters, metal smelters, and chemical workers, who are exposed to occupational sources of combustion and chemicals. Burn injuries remain the second leading cause of death in children under 12 years of age and the fourth overall cause of trauma death after vehicular crashes, penetrating trauma, and falls.

Much of the national decline in burn mortality is attributed to improved building codes, safer construction techniques, sprinkler systems, and the use of smoke detectors. Smaller but still important effects are attributed to educational campaigns aimed primarily at schoolchildren. Other simple and inexpensive measures that have helped prevent burns include keeping cigarette lighters and matches away from children and reducing household hot-water temperatures to below scalding levels. Half of all tap-water burns occur in children under 5 years old. Merely adjusting the hot-water temperature to below 48.9° C (120° F) can prevent most scalding burns.

Burns are a specific subset of soft-tissue injuries with a specific pathologic process. While the term "burn" suggests combustion, the actual process that produces burn injuries is much different. The human body is predominantly water and does not support combustion. Instead, body tissues change chemically, evaporating water and denaturing the proteins that make up cell membranes. The result can be widespread damage to the skin, also known as the integumentary system.

To effectively assess and treat burns, you must have a good understanding of the structures and functions of the integumentary system as well as of the pathological processes that affect it. This understanding ensures that you can provide the best possible assessment and care for patients who sustain burn injuries.

ANATOMY AND PHYSIOLOGY OF THE SKIN

The skin is one of the largest, most important, and least appreciated organs of the human body. Covering the entire body, the skin protects it from fluid loss and bacterial invasion. The skin also provides a massive surface for sensation and is a natural radiator for dissipating excess body heat. With all these functions, the skin still remains durable, flexible, and very able to repair itself.

LAYERS OF THE SKIN

The skin comprises three layers of tissue: the epidermis, the dermis, and the subcutaneous tissue (Figure 6-1 ■). Together they form the body's outermost shell.

Epidermis

The first and outermost skin layer is the epidermis. It is an area of dying and dead cells being pushed outward by new cells growing from beneath. As these cells reach the surface, they abrade away during everyday activity. The constant movement outward provides a barrier that is difficult for bacteria and other pathogens to penetrate.

Glands beneath the epidermis secrete an oil called sebum. This oil coats the outer skin layers and makes the epidermis pliable. In addition, sebum provides a barrier to the flow of water through the skin.

Dermis

Directly below the epidermis is the tissue layer called the dermis. It contains many different structures, including blood vessels, glands, and nerve endings. It is in this layer that sebaceous glands produce sebum and secrete it directly onto the skin's surface and into hair follicles. Sudoriferous glands in the dermis secrete sweat and direct it to the skin's surface. As the water in sweat evaporates, passing air carries the vapor and associated heat energy away with it. The change of a fluid to a vapor (evaporation) is

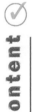

Content

⊘ **Review**

Layers of the Skin

Epidermis—outermost layer
Dermis—layer of tissue
  beneath the epidermis
Subcutaneous tissue—fatty
  layer of tissue beneath the
  dermis

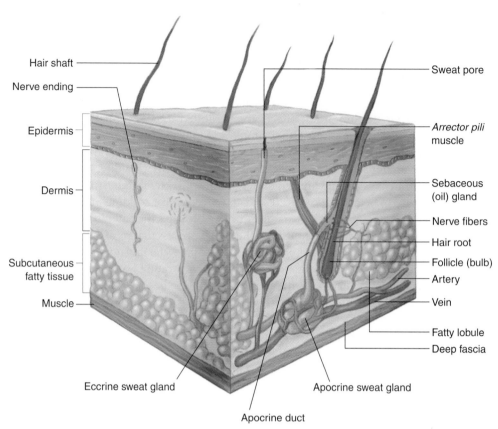

■ **Figure 6-1** The cross-sectional anatomy of the skin.

Hair shaft

Nerve ending

Epidermis

Dermis

Subcutaneous fatty tissue

Muscle

Sweat pore

Arrector pili muscle

Sebaceous (oil) gland

Nerve fibers

Hair root

Follicle (bulb)

Artery

Vein

Fatty lobule

Deep fascia

Eccrine sweat gland

Apocrine sweat gland

Apocrine duct

an efficient method of skin cooling. This process helps the body maintain a normal temperature even when ambient temperatures are greater than 100° F (as long as evaporation is possible). The primary mechanism for maintaining body temperature uses the skin as a radiator of excess body heat. Warm blood from the body's core travels either through blood vessels in the dermis (close to the skin surface) or through the subcutaneous tissues.

Subcutaneous Tissue

Subcutaneous tissue, which is composed of adipose (fat) and connective tissues, serves as a stratum of insulation against both trauma and heat loss. When blood is directed to, and beneath, the subcutaneous tissues, the difference between the skin's temperature and the environment changes. This slows the radiation of heat to the environment and conserves body heat. If warm core blood is directed to the surface above the subcutaneous tissue, heat is transferred to the skin and the skin temperature rises. Accordingly, the temperature difference between the body surface and the environment increases, as does the rate of heat exchange. This causes body cooling.

Underlying Structures

Although they are not part of the integument, it is important to identify the structures underneath the skin. These structures include the muscles and their thick, fibrous capsules of fascia, nerves, tendons, bones, and, of course, the vital organs such as the heart, lungs, and brain. Each of these structures is sensitive to the effects of thermal, chemical, electrical, and radiation injury.

FUNCTIONS OF THE SKIN

The skin varies in thickness from almost a centimeter on the heel of the foot to microscopic dimensions on the surface of the eye. This durable container for the body provides a number of valuable functions:

★ The skin protects the human body from infection by bacteria and other microorganisms.

★ The skin functions as an organ of sensation, perceiving temperature, pressure (touch), and pain.

★ The skin contains vital body fluids and controls their loss to the environment as well as the movement of fluids into the body when it is exposed to water or other fluids.

★ The skin aids in temperature regulation through secretion of sweat and shunting of blood.

★ The skin provides insulation from trauma.

★ The skin is flexible to accommodate free body movement.

Although the skin and its functions are often taken for granted, burn injury can cause severe fluid loss, infection, hypothermia, and other injuries. Therefore, as a paramedic, you need to become familiar with the pathophysiology of burns to the skin.

PATHOPHYSIOLOGY OF BURNS

Burns result from the disruption of proteins in the cell membranes. Burns can be caused by several different mechanisms including thermal, electrical, chemical, or radiation energies, as well as a combination of these. Being able to understand the mechanism of a burn and to determine the degree and area of burn helps you assess the seriousness of the burn and thus guide your care.

TYPES OF BURNS

Soft-tissue burns can occur due to thermal (heat), electrical, chemical, or radiation insults to the body. While the resulting burns are much the same, the damage process differs with the various mechanisms. The following sections describe each of these four types of burns.

Thermal Burns

A thermal burn causes damage by increasing the rate at which the molecules within an object move and collide with each other. We measure the energy of this molecular motion as temperature. At a temperature greater than absolute zero, the molecules of any object move about. As the object's temperature increases, so does the speed of the molecules and the incidences of their collisions with other molecules. These changes in internal energy cause many substances—for example, steel—to expand with increasing temperature. Heat energy may also cause chemical changes. As temperature increases, substances such as gasoline may combine with oxygen. The nature of matter may change as well. Water, for example, may change into ice (with decreasing heat energy) or steam (with increasing heat energy). In addition, the chemical structure of proteins can be affected by heat. An egg changes its nature as the proteins break down, or **denature,** in a hot frying pan. This is why cooked eggs have a rubbery consistency.

Similar changes also take place in burned tissue. As molecular speed increases, the cell components, especially membranes and proteins, begin to break down just like the

Review

Content

Basic Types of Burns

Thermal
Electrical
Chemical
Radiation

denature *alter the usual substance of something.*

Jackson's theory of thermal wounds *explanation of the physical effects of thermal burns.*

 Review

Content

Effects of Heat According to Jackson's Theory of Thermal Wounds

Zone of coagulation—most damaged area nearest heat source; cell membranes rupture and are destroyed, blood coagulates, structural proteins denature

Zone of stasis—adjacent to most damaged region; inflammation present, blood flow decreased

Zone of hyperemia—area farthest from heat source; limited inflammation and changes in blood flow

---

zone of coagulation *area in a burn nearest the heat source that suffers the most damage and is characterized by clotted blood and thrombosed blood vessels.*

zone of stasis *area in a burn surrounding the zone of coagulation that is characterized by decreased blood flow.*

zone of hyperemia *area peripheral to a burn that is characterized by increased blood flow.*

emergent phase *first stage of the burn process that is characterized by a catecholamine release and pain-mediated reaction.*

egg in a frying pan. The result of exposure to extreme heat is progressive injury and cell death.

The extent of burn injury relates to the amount of heat energy transferred to the patient's skin. The amount of that heat energy in turn depends upon three components of the burning agent: its temperature, the concentration of heat energy it possesses, and the length of its contact time with the patient's skin.

Obviously, the greater the temperature of an agent, the greater is the potential for damage. However, it is also important to consider the amount of heat energy possessed by the object or substance. Receiving a blast of heated air from an oven at 350° F is much less damaging than contact with hot cooking oil at the same temperature. In general, water, oils, and other liquids tend to have a high heat energy content. This content is roughly related to the density of the material. In a similar fashion, solids also usually have a high heat content. Gases, however, usually have less capacity to hold heat owing to their less dense nature.

The duration of exposure to the heat source is also obviously important in determining the severity of a burn. A patient's momentary contact with hot oil would result in less damage than if the oil were poured into his shoe with his foot in it.

A burn is a progressive process, and the greater the heat energy transmitted to the body, the deeper the wound. Initially, the burn damages the epidermis through the increase in temperature. As contact with the substance continues, heat energy penetrates further and deeper into the body tissue. Thus, a burn may involve the epidermis, dermis, and subcutaneous tissue as well as muscles, bone, and other internal tissue.

At the level of local tissues, thermal burns cause a number of effects collectively termed **Jackson's theory of thermal wounds.** This theory helps us understand the physical effects of high heat and helps explain a number of clinical effects (Figure 6-2 ■).

With a burn, the skin nearest the heat source suffers the most profound changes. Cell membranes rupture and are destroyed, blood coagulates, and structural proteins denature. This most damaged area is the **zone of coagulation.** If the zone of coagulation penetrates the dermis, the resulting injury is termed a full thickness or third-degree burn. Adjacent to this area is a less damaged yet still inflamed region where blood flow decreases that is called the **zone of stasis.** More distant from the burn source is a broader area where inflammation and changes in blood flow are limited. This is the **zone of hyperemia;** this zone accounts for the erythema (redness) associated with some burns.

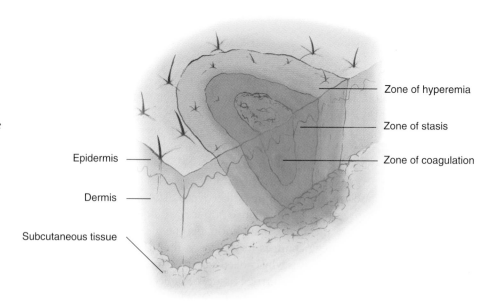

■ Figure 6-2 The zones of injury commonly caused by a thermal burn.

Large burns have profound pathological effects on the body as a whole. In general, these effects are important in any burn that covers more than 15 to 20 percent of the patient's body surface area. To understand these effects and the resulting burn shock, you must first learn a little about the progression of burns.

The body's response to burns occurs over time and can usefully be classified into four stages. The first stage occurs immediately following the burn and is called the **emergent phase.** This is the body's initial reaction to the burn. This phase includes a pain response as well as the outpouring of catecholamines in response to the pain and the physical and emotional stress. During this stage, the patient displays tachycardia, tachypnea, mild hypertension, and mild anxiety.

The **fluid shift phase** follows the initial phase and can last for up to 24 hours. The fluid shift phase begins shortly after the burn and reaches its peak in 6 to 8 hours. You are therefore likely to see the beginning of it in the prehospital setting. In this phase, damaged cells release agents that initiate an inflammatory response in the body. This increases blood flow to the capillaries surrounding the burn and increases the permeability of the capillaries to fluid. The response results in a large shift of fluid away from the **intravascular space** into the **extravascular space** (massive edema). Note that the capillaries leak fluid (water, electrolytes, and some dissolved proteins) and not blood cells. Blood loss from burns uncomplicated by other trauma is usually minimal.

After the fluid shift phase comes the **hypermetabolic phase,** which may last for many days or weeks depending on the burn severity. This phase is characterized by a large increase in the body's demands for nutrients as it begins the long process of repairing damaged tissue. Gradually this phase evolves into the **resolution phase,** in which scar tissue is laid down and remodeled, and the burn patient begins to rehabilitate and return to normal function.

Electrical Burns

Electricity's power is the result of an electron flow from a point of high concentration to one of low concentration. The difference between the two concentrations is called the **voltage.** It is helpful to envision voltage as the "pressure" of the electric flow. The rate or the amount of flow in a given time is termed the **current** and is measured in **amperes.** With direct current, the electrons flow in one direction, while alternating current reverses the flow in short intervals. Standard house current is alternating at 60 cycles per second.

Another factor that affects the flow of electricity is **resistance,** which is measured in **ohms.** Copper electrical wire has very little resistance and allows a free flow of electrons. Tungsten (the filament in a light bulb) is moderately resistant and heats, glows, and emits light as more and more current is applied to it.

The relationship between current (*I*), resistance (*R*), and voltage (*V*) is well known as **Ohm's law:**

$$V = IR \text{ or } I = V/R$$

Like tungsten, the internal parts of the human body are moderately resistant to the flow of electricity. The skin, however, is highly resistant to electrical flow. Moisture or sweat on the skin lowers this resistance. If the human body is subjected to voltage, the body initially resists the flow. If the voltage is strong enough, the current begins to pass into and through the body. As it does, heat energy is created. The heat produced is proportional to the square of the current flow, is related to power, *P*, and increases with exposure time, *t*, as expressed in **Joule's law:**

$$P = I^2Rt$$

fluid shift phase *stage of the burn process in which there is a massive shift of fluid from the intravascular to the extravascular space.*

intravascular space *the volume contained by all the arteries, veins, capillaries, and other components of the circulatory system.*

extravascular space *the volume contained by all the cells (intracellular space) and the spaces between the cells (interstitial space).*

hypermetabolic phase *stage of the burn process in which there is increased body metabolism in an attempt by the body to heal the burn.*

resolution phase *final stage of the burn process in which scar tissue is laid down and the healing process is completed.*

voltage *the difference of electric potential between two points with different concentrations of electrons.*

current *the rate of flow of an electric charge.*

ampere *basic unit for measuring the strength of an electric current.*

resistance *property of a conductor that opposes the passage of an electric current.*

ohm *basic unit for measuring the strength of electrical resistance.*

Ohm's law *the physical law identifying that the current in an electrical circuit is directly proportional to the voltage and inversely proportional to the resistance.*

Joule's law *the physical law stating that the rate of heat production is directly proportional to the resistance of the circuit and to the square of the current.*

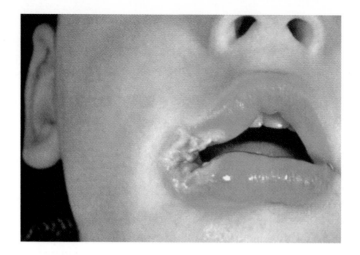

■ **Figure 6-3** Electrical burns to a child's mouth caused by chewing on an electrical cord.

The highest heat occurs at the points of greatest resistance, often at the skin. This accounts for the severe "entry" and "exit" wounds sometimes seen in electrical injuries. Dry, callused skin can have enormous resistance values, ranging from 500,000 to 1,000,000 ohms/cm. Wet skin, particularly the thin skin on the palm side of the arm or on the inner thigh, can have values as low as 300 to 10,000 ohms/cm. Mucous membranes have very low resistance (100 ohms/cm) and allow even small currents to pass. This accounts for the relative ease with which household current can cause lip and oral burns in children who accidentally bite electrical cords (Figure 6-3 ■).

With small currents, the heat energy produced is of little consequence. But if the voltage or current is high, profound body damage can occur. The longer the duration of contact, the greater will be the potential for injury. Electrical burns can be particularly damaging because the burn heats the victim from the inside out, causing great damage to internal organs and structures while possibly leaving little visible damage on the surface, save for the entry and exit wounds (Figure 6-4 ■).

Thermal injury due to electrical current occurs as energy travels from the point of contact to the point of exit. At both these points, the concentration of electricity is great, as is the degree of damage you might expect. The smaller the area of contact, the greater will be the concentration of current flow and the greater the injury. Between the entrance and exit points, the energy spreads out over a larger cross-sectional area and generally causes less injury. Electrical current may follow blood vessels and nerves because they offer less resistance than muscle and bone. This may lead to serious vascular and nervous injury deep within the involved limbs or body cavity.

Electrical contact also interferes with the control of muscle tissue. The passage of current, especially alternating current, severely disrupts the complicated electrochemical reactions that control muscles. If contact with a current as small as 20 to 50 milliamperes (mA) is maintained for a period of time, the muscles of respiration may be

Electrical burns can be particularly damaging because the current burns the victim from the inside out.

■ **Figure 6-4** Injuries due to electrical shock.

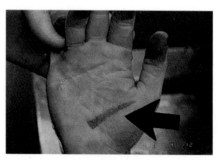

a. Entrance wound

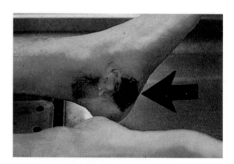

b. Exit wound

immobilized. The result is prolonged respiratory arrest, anoxia, hypoxemia, and—eventually—death. Electrical currents greater than 50 mA may also disrupt the heart's electrical system, causing ventricular fibrillation accompanied by ineffective pumping action. Alternating electrical current such as that found in household current can also cause tetanic convulsions or uncontrolled contractions of muscles. If the victim is holding a wire at such a time, the victim may be unable to let go, thereby prolonging the exposure and increasing the severity of injury. This can occur with as little as 9 mA of current.

Electrical injury may also disrupt muscular and other tissue, leading to its degeneration. As the tissue dies, it releases materials toxic to the human body. These materials may damage the liver and kidneys, leading to failure.

At times, electrical energy may cause flash burns secondary to the heat of current passing through adjacent air. Air is very resistant to the passage of electrical current. If the current is strong enough and the space through which it passes is small, the electricity arcs, producing tremendous heat. If the patient's skin is close by, the heat may severely burn or vaporize tissue. In addition, the heat may ignite articles of clothing or other combustibles and produce thermal burns.

Chemical Burns

Chemical burns denature the biochemical makeup of cell membranes (primarily the proteins) and destroy the cells. Such injuries are not transmitted through the tissue as are thermal injuries. Instead, a chemical burn must destroy the tissue before it can chemically burn any deeper. This fact generally limits the "burn" process unless very strong chemicals are involved (Figure 6-5). Agents that can cause chemical burns are too numerous to mention. However, the most common causes of these burns are either strong acids or alkalis (bases).

Both acids and alkalis burn by disrupting cell membranes and damaging tissues on contact. As they cause damage, acids usually form a thick, insoluble mass, or coagulum, at the point of contact. This process is called **coagulation necrosis** and helps to limit the depth of acid burns. Alkalis, however, do not form a protective coagulum. Instead, the alkali continues to destroy cell membranes, releasing the intercellular and interstitial fluid, destroying tissue in a process called **liquefaction necrosis.** This process allows the alkali to rapidly penetrate the underlying tissue, causing progressively deeper burns. For this reason, alkali burns can be quite serious.

Radiation Injury

Nuclear (ionizing) radiation has bombarded Earth since long before recorded time. It is a daily, natural phenomenon. Radiation becomes a danger when people are exposed

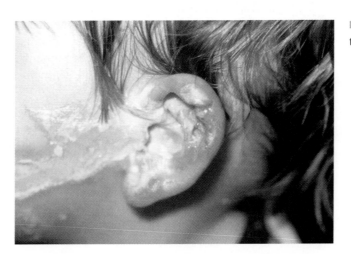

✓ **Review**

Content

Processes of Chemical Burns

Acids—usually form a thick, insoluble mass where they contact tissue through coagulation necrosis, limiting burn damage

Alkalis—usually continue to destroy cell membranes through liquefaction necrosis, allowing them to penetrate underlying tissue and causing deeper burns

coagulation necrosis   *the process in which an acid, while destroying tissue, forms an insoluble layer that limits further damage.*

liquefaction necrosis   *the process in which an alkali dissolves and liquefies tissue.*

■ Figure 6-5   A chemical burn to the ear.

to synthetic sources that greatly increase the intensity of radiation. Medicine and industry use radioactive materials for diagnostic testing and treatment and for energy production. Deaths from exposure to radiation are extremely rare, as are serious injuries, because of the safety measures commonly used with the handling of nuclear materials. However, the possibility of large-scale exposure to radiation from terrorist acts is considered to be increasing. The risk of injury typically comes from accidents associated with improper handling, either in the on-site environment or during transport.

Nuclear radiation causes damage through a process known as **ionization.** A radioactive energy particle travels into a substance and changes an internal atom (Figure 6-6 ■). In the human body, the affected cell either repairs the damage, dies, or goes on to produce damaged cells (cancer). The cells most sensitive to radiation injury are the cells that reproduce most quickly, like those responsible for erythrocyte, leukocyte, and platelet production (bone marrow); cells lining the intestinal tract; and cells involved in human reproduction.

We commonly encounter four types of radiation. These are:

★ *Alpha radiation.* The nucleus of an atom releases **alpha radiation** in the form of a small helium nucleus. Alpha radiation is a very weak energy source and can travel only inches through the air. Paper or clothing can easily stop alpha radiation. This radiation also cannot penetrate the epidermis. On the subatomic scale, however, alpha particles are massive and can cause great damage over the short distance they travel. Alpha radiation is only a significant hazard if the patient inhales or ingests contaminated material, thus bringing the source in proximity to sensitive respiratory and digestive tract tissue.

★ *Beta radiation.* A second type of radiological particle produces **beta radiation.** Its energy is greater than that of alpha radiation. However, the beta particle is relatively lightweight, with the mass of an electron. Beta radiation can travel 6 to 10 feet through air and can penetrate a few layers of clothing. Beta particles can invade the first few millimeters of skin and thus have the potential for causing external as well as internal injury.

★ *Gamma radiation.* **Gamma radiation,** also known as x-rays, is the most powerful type of ionizing radiation. It has the ability to travel through the entire body or ionize any atom within. Its lack of mass or charge (it is pure electromagnetic energy) helps give it great penetrating power. Gamma radiation evokes the greatest concern for external exposure. It is the most dangerous and most feared type of radiation because it is difficult to protect against. Many feet of concrete or many inches of lead are needed to shield against the highest energy gamma rays. Fortunately, exposure to high-energy gamma rays occurs only in individuals who are exposed to nuclear blasts, are near the cores of nuclear reactors, or are very close to highly radioactive materials. More modest amounts of concrete, steel, or lead can provide shielding from the more common and lower energy x-rays and gamma rays.

★ *Neutron radiation.* Neutrons are small, yet moderately massive subatomic particles with no charge. Their small size and lack of charge account for their great penetrating power. Fortunately, strong **neutron radiation** is uncommon outside of nuclear reactors and bombs.

Exposure to radiation and the effects of ionization can occur through two mechanisms. In the first, an unshielded person is directly exposed to a strong radioactive source, for example, an unstable material such as uranium. The second mechanism of

ionization *the process of changing a substance into separate charged particles (ions).*

alpha radiation *low-level form of nuclear radiation; a weak source of energy that is stopped by clothing or the first layers of skin.*

Review

Types of Radiation

Alpha—very weak, stopped by paper, clothing, or the epidermis

Beta—more powerful than alpha; can travel 6 to 10 feet through air; can penetrate some clothing and the first few millimeters of skin

Gamma—most powerful ionizing radiation; great penetrating power; protection requires thick concrete or lead shielding

Neutron—great penetrating power, but uncommon outside nuclear reactors and bombs

beta radiation *medium-strength radiation that is stopped with light clothing or the uppermost layers of skin.*

gamma radiation *powerful electromagnetic radiation emitted by radioactive substances with powerful penetrating properties; it is stronger than alpha and beta radiation.*

neutron radiation *powerful radiation with penetrating properties between that of beta and gamma radiation.*

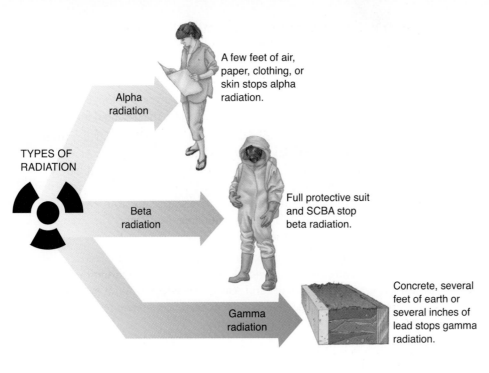

■ Figure 6-6 The injury considerations associated with nuclear radiation.

TYPES OF RADIATION

Alpha radiation — A few feet of air, paper, clothing, or skin stops alpha radiation.

Beta radiation — Full protective suit and SCBA stop beta radiation.

Gamma radiation — Concrete, several feet of earth or several inches of lead stops gamma radiation.

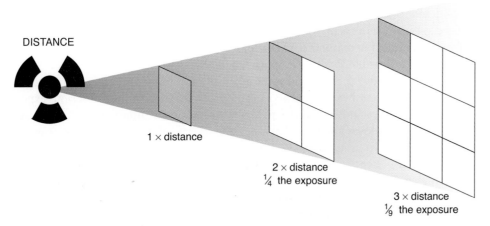

DISTANCE

1 × distance

2 × distance
¼ the exposure

3 × distance
⅑ the exposure

TIME (EXAMPLE SHOWS 300 r/hr)

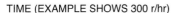

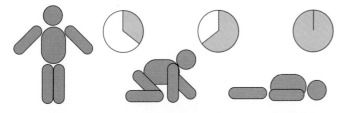

exposure is contamination by dust, debris, or fluids that contain very small particles of radioactive material. These contaminants give off weaker radiation than a direct radioactive source like uranium. However, the proximity of these contaminants to the body and their longer contact times with it may result in greater exposure and contamination. Note that most substances, including human tissue, do not give off radiation. The patient himself is not the danger in a radiological exposure incident. Any danger comes from the radioactive source such as the contaminated material on the patient.

Review

Content

Factors Affecting Exposure to Radiation

Duration of exposure
Distance from the source
Shielding from the source

Three factors are important to keep in mind whenever you are called to incidents of radiation exposure. They include the duration of exposure; the distance from the radioactive source; and the shielding between you, the patient, and the source. Knowledge of these three factors can limit your exposure and potential for injury.

★ *Duration.* Radiation exposure is an accumulative danger. The longer you or the patient remain exposed to the source, the greater the potential for injury.

★ *Distance.* Radiation strength diminishes quickly as you travel farther from the source. The effect is similar to that of a light bulb's intensity. At a few feet, you can easily read by it, while at a few hundred feet the light barely casts a shadow. Mathematically, the relationship is inverse and squared. As you double your distance from the radioactive source, its strength drops to one fourth of the original strength. As you triple the distance, its strength diminishes to one ninth, and so on.

★ *Shielding.* The more material between you and the source, the less radioactive exposure you experience. With alpha and beta radiation, shielding is very easy to provide and reasonably effective. With gamma and neutron sources, dense objects such as earth, concrete, metal, and lead are needed to provide any real protection.

Radiation exposure is measured with a Geiger counter, while cumulative exposure is recorded by a device called a dosimeter (Figure 6-7 ■). They record units of radiation expressed as either the **rad** or the **Gray** (Gy), with 1 Gray equal to 100 rads.

Different tissues are sensitive to different levels of absorbed radiation. As little as 0.2 Gy can cause cataracts in exposed eyes and damage the blood-cell-producing bone marrow (also called hematopoietic) tissue. The radiation dose that is lethal to about 50 percent of exposed individuals is approximately 4.5 Gy.

With whole-body exposure, and as the radiation dose increases, the signs and symptoms of exposure appear earlier and become more severe. The first signs of serious exposure are slight nausea and fatigue, occurring between 4 and 24 hours after exposure. As the radiation dose moves into the lethal range, the severity of the nausea increases and is joined by anorexia, vomiting, diarrhea, and malaise. Erythema of the skin may be present, and fatigue becomes more intense. These signs appear within 2 to 6 hours. With exposure to even higher, fatal doses, the patient displays all the signs of radiation exposure almost immediately and soon thereafter experiences confusion, watery diarrhea, and physical collapse. Note that the signs and symptoms of radiation exposure and the injuries associated with it vary because individual sensitivity to radiation exposure varies greatly.

Prolonged exposure to even small amounts of radiation may produce long-term and delayed problems. Infertility is a potential injury, because the cells producing eggs

rad *basic unit of absorbed radiation dose.*

Gray *a unit of absorbed radiation dose equal to 100 rads.*

■ Figure 6-7   (a) A Geiger counter measures the radiation exposure level *(© Jeff Forster);* (b) a dosimeter records cumulative exposure. *(Courtesy of Ogunquit, Maine Fire-Rescue)*

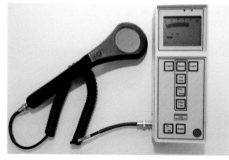

(a)

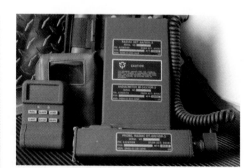

(b)

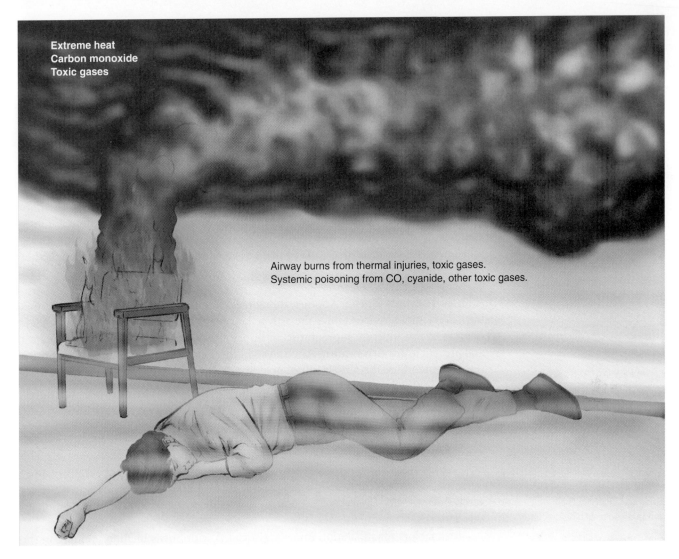

Extreme heat
Carbon monoxide
Toxic gases

Airway burns from thermal injuries, toxic gases.
Systemic poisoning from CO, cyanide, other toxic gases.

■ Figure 6-8   Hazards of fire in an enclosed environment.

and sperm are very susceptible to ionization damage. Cancer is another delayed and severe side effect. It may occur years or even decades after a radiation exposure.

Inhalation Injury

The burn environment frequently produces inhalation injury. This, however, is only true if the patient is trapped or unconscious in an enclosed space. A patient who is unconscious or trapped in a smoke-filled area will eventually inhale gases, heated air, flames, or steam. The inhalation results in airway and respiratory injury.

You can expect to find the following inhalation conditions in a burn environment (Figure 6-8 ■). Keep them in mind as you survey the scene and take the necessary protective measures.

Toxic Inhalation   Modern residential and commercial construction uses synthetic resins and plastics that release toxic gases as they burn. Combustion of these materials can form agents such as cyanide, hydrogen sulfide, and other toxic or caustic substances. If a patient inhales these gases, the gases either react with the lung tissue, causing internal chemical burns, or they diffuse across the alveolar-capillary membrane, enter the bloodstream, and interfere with the delivery to or the cell's use of oxygen. The signs and

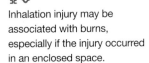

Inhalation injury may be associated with burns, especially if the injury occurred in an enclosed space.

symptoms of these injuries may present immediately following exposure or their onset may be delayed for an hour or two after inhalation. Toxic inhalation injury occurs more frequently than thermal inhalation burns.

Carbon Monoxide Poisoning An additional concern associated with the burn environment is carbon monoxide (CO) poisoning. Suspect it in any patient who has been within an enclosed space during combustion. Carbon monoxide is created during incomplete combustion, like that which may occur with a faulty heating unit or when someone tries to heat a room with an unvented device like a barbecue grill. Poisoning occurs because carbon monoxide has an affinity for hemoglobin more than 200 times greater than oxygen. If your patient inhales carbon monoxide, even in the smallest quantities, the carbon monoxide displaces oxygen in the hemoglobin and remains there for hours. The result is hypoxemia. Hypoxemia, which is difficult to detect, subtly compromises the delivery of oxygen to the patient's vital organs. If carbon monoxide inhalation is associated with airway burns, the respiratory compromise will be further compounded.

Airway Thermal Burn Another, though less frequent, injury is the airway thermal burn. Very moist mucosa lines the airway and helps insulate it against heat damage. Because of this mucosa, **supraglottic,** or upper airway, structures may absorb the heat and prevent lower airway burns. High levels of thermal energy are required to evaporate the fluid and injure the cells. Inspiration of hot air or flame rarely produces enough heat to cause significant thermal burns to the lower airway.

Superheated steam has greater heat content than hot, dry air and can cause **subglottic,** or lower airway, burns. Superheated steam is created under great pressure and can have a temperature well above 212° F. A common hazard to firefighters, superheated steam develops when a stream of water strikes a hot spot and vaporizes explosively. The blast can dislodge the mask of a firefighter's self-contained breathing apparatus, exposing him to superheated steam inhalation. The steam contains enough heat energy to severely burn the upper airway. It also may damage the lower respiratory tract, although this happens less frequently.

Risk factors for inhalation injuries associated with burns include standing in the burn environment (hot gases rise), screaming or yelling there (the open glottis allows toxic gases to enter the lower airway), and being trapped in a closed burn environment.

With any thermal or smoke-related chemical burn injury to the respiratory tract, there is the danger of airway restriction, severe dyspnea, and possible respiratory arrest. The airway is a narrow tube, lined with extremely vascular tissue. If damaged, this tissue swells rapidly, seriously reducing the size of the airway lumen. The patient presents with minor hoarseness, followed precipitously by dyspnea. Stridor or high-pitched "crowing" sounds on inspiration are ominous signs of impending airway obstruction. Other clues leading you to suspect potential airway burns include singed facial and nasal hair, black-tinged (carbonaceous) sputum, and facial burns. The airway injury may be so extensive as to induce complete respiratory obstruction and arrest. Accurate assessment is important because 20 to 35 percent of patients admitted to burn centers and some 60 to 70 percent of burn patients who die have an associated inhalation injury.

DEPTH OF BURN

After you determine the burn source and assess the possibility of associated inhalation injury, you need to assess the burn's severity. One element in determining the severity of a burn is the depth of damage it causes. Depth of burn damage is normally classified into three categories (Figure 6-9 ■).

Suspect carbon monoxide poisoning in any patient who was in an enclosed space during combustion.

supraglottic *referring to the upper airway.*

subglottic *referring to the lower airway.*

Superheated steam is a common cause of airway burns.

 Review

Content

Depth of Burn

Superficial (first degree)—involves only the epidermis; produces pain, minor edema, and erythema (redness)

Partial thickness (second degree)—involves epidermis and dermis; produces pain, edema, erythema, blisters

Full thickness (third degree)—involves all skin layers and possibly structures beneath; painless, but tissue is destroyed; white, brown, or charred, leather-like appearance

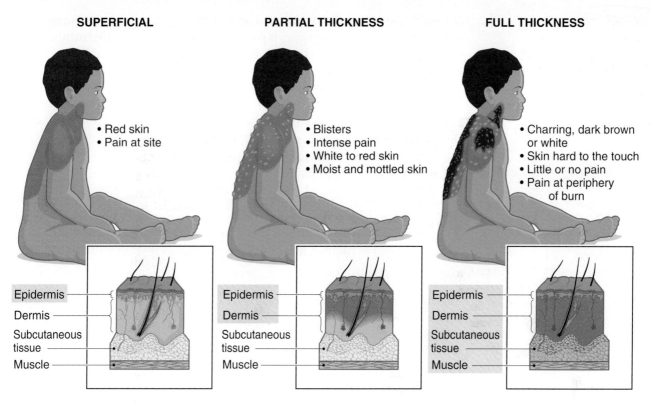

SUPERFICIAL
- Red skin
- Pain at site

Epidermis
Dermis
Subcutaneous tissue
Muscle

PARTIAL THICKNESS
- Blisters
- Intense pain
- White to red skin
- Moist and mottled skin

Epidermis
Dermis
Subcutaneous tissue
Muscle

FULL THICKNESS
- Charring, dark brown or white
- Skin hard to the touch
- Little or no pain
- Pain at periphery of burn

Epidermis
Dermis
Subcutaneous tissue
Muscle

■ Figure 6-9   Classification of burns by depth.

Superficial Burn

The **superficial burn,** also termed a first-degree burn, involves only the epidermis. It is an irritation of the living cells in this region and results in some pain, minor edema, and erythema. It normally heals without complication.

Partial Thickness Burn

The **partial thickness burn,** also termed a second-degree burn, penetrates slightly deeper than a superficial burn and produces blisters. Heat energy travels into the dermis, involving more of the tissue and resulting in greater destruction. The partial thickness burn is similar to a superficial burn in that it is reddened, painful, and edematous. You can differentiate it from the superficial burn only after blisters form. Because there are many nerve endings in the dermis, both superficial and partial thickness burns are often very painful. With both superficial and partial thickness burns, the dermis is still intact and complete skin regeneration is very likely.

The sunburn is a common, but specialized type of burn. Ultraviolet radiation causes the burn rather than normal thermal processes. The radiation penetrates superficially and damages the uppermost layers of the dermis. Sunburn can present as either a superficial or partial thickness burn.

Another similar type of burn occurs as someone watches an arc welder without proper protection. In this injury, called ultraviolet keratitis, the outermost parts of the eye (cornea) trap the ultraviolet radiation, causing injury to the layer. This causes delayed eye pain and, possibly, transient blindness. The injury usually heals completely within 24 hours.

Full Thickness Burn

The **full thickness,** or third-degree, **burn** penetrates both the epidermis and the dermis and extends into the subcutaneous layers or even deeper, into muscles, bones, and

superficial burn *a burn that involves only the epidermis; characterized by reddening of the skin; also called a first-degree burn.*

partial thickness burn *burn in which the epidermis is burned through and the dermis is damaged; characterized by redness and blistering; also called a second-degree burn.*

full thickness burn *burn that damages all layers of the skin; characterized by areas that are white and dry; also called a third-degree burn.*

internal organs. These burns destroy the tissue's regenerative properties and the peripheral nerve endings. The injury is painless because of the nerve destruction, but the margins of the full thickness burn are frequently partial thickness burns, which can be quite painful. The full thickness burn takes on various colorations depending on the nature of the burning agent and the damaged, dying, or dead tissue. They can be white, brown, or a charred color and typically have a dry, leather-like appearance. Because the burn destroys the entire dermis, healing is difficult unless the wound is small or skin grafting is possible.

BODY SURFACE AREA

body surface area (BSA)
amount of a patient's body affected by a burn.

Another factor affecting burn severity is how much of a person's **body surface area (BSA)** the burn involves. There are two approaches to estimating the BSA involved in a burn. The first, the rule of nines, is useful in estimating large burn areas. The second method, the rule of palms, is helpful in assessing smaller wounds more accurately.

Rule of Nines

rule of nines *method of estimating amount of body surface area burned by a division of the body into regions, each of which represents approximately 9 percent of total BSA (plus 1 percent for the genital region).*

The **rule of nines** identifies 11 topographical adult body regions, each of which approximates 9 percent of the patient's BSA (Figure 6-10 ▪). These regions include the entire head and neck; the anterior chest; the anterior abdomen; the posterior chest; the lower back (the posterior abdomen); the anterior surface of each lower extremity; the posterior surface of each lower extremity; and each upper extremity. The genitalia make up the remaining 1 percent of BSA.

Because infant and child anatomy differs significantly from that of adults, you must modify the rule of nines to maintain an accurate approximation of BSA. Divide the head and neck area into the anterior and posterior surface and award 9 percent for each. Reduce the surface area of each lower extremity by 4 1/2 percent to ensure the total body surface area remains at 100 percent. The rule of nines is at best an approximation of the area burned. It is, however, an expedient and useful tool to help measure the burn's extent.

▪ Figure 6-10   The rule of nines.

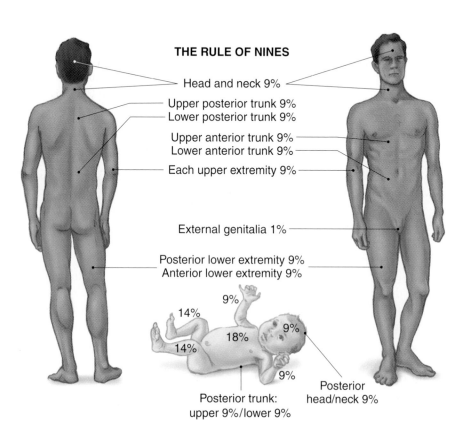

THE RULE OF NINES

Head and neck 9%
Upper posterior trunk 9%
Lower posterior trunk 9%
Upper anterior trunk 9%
Lower anterior trunk 9%
Each upper extremity 9%

External genitalia 1%

Posterior lower extremity 9%
Anterior lower extremity 9%

9%
14%
14%
18%
9%
9%
9%

Posterior trunk:
upper 9%/lower 9%

Posterior
head/neck 9%

Rule of Palms

The **rule of palms,** an alternative system for approximating the extent of a burn, uses the palmar surface as a point of comparison in gauging the size of the affected body area (Figure 6-11 ■). The patient's palm (the hand less the fingers) represents about 1 percent of the BSA, whether the patient is an adult, a child, or an infant. If you can visualize the palmar surface area and apply it to the burn area mentally, you can then obtain an estimate of the total BSA affected.

The rule of palms is easier to use for local burns of up to about 10 percent BSA, while the rule of nines is simpler and more appropriate for larger burns. Many other burn approximation techniques exist that are both more specific to age and, in general, more accurate. However, these techniques are more complicated and time consuming to use. Both the rule of nines and the rule of palms provide reasonable approximations of BSA when used properly in the field.

SYSTEMIC COMPLICATIONS

Burns cause several systemic complications. These can affect the overall severity of a burn. Typical complications include hypothermia, hypovolemia, eschar formation, and infection.

Hypothermia

A burn may disrupt the body's ability to regulate its core temperature. Tissue destruction reduces or eliminates the skin's ability to contain the fluid within. The burn process releases plasma and other fluids, which seep into the wound. There they evaporate and rapidly remove heat energy. The injured skin has increased blood flow, enhancing the heat loss, and the burn injury does not have the reflex vasoconstriction that normally protects against excessive heat loss. If the burn is extensive, uncontrolled body heat loss induces rapid and severe hypothermia.

Hypovolemia

Hypovolemia also may complicate the severe burn. The inability of damaged blood vessels to contain plasma causes a shift of proteins, fluid, and electrolytes into the burned tissue. Additionally, the loss of plasma protein reduces the blood's ability, via osmosis, to draw fluids from the uninjured tissues. This in turn compromises the body's natural response to fluid loss and may produce a profound hypovolemia. Although this is a serious complication of the extensive burn, it takes hours to develop. Modern aggressive fluid resuscitation can effectively counteract this aspect of the burn process.

A related complication is electrolyte imbalance. With the massive shift of fluid to the interstitial space, the body's ability to regulate sodium, potassium, and other electrolytes becomes overwhelmed. In addition, large thermal and electrical burns can lead to massive tissue destruction with a resultant release of breakdown products into the bloodstream. Potassium is one such breakdown product and its oversupply, or hyperkalemia, can lead to life-threatening cardiac dysrhythmias. Careful ECG monitoring and appropriate fluid resuscitation can help prevent hyperkalemic complications.

Eschar

Skin denaturing further complicates full thickness thermal burns. As the burn destroys the dermal cells, they become hard and leathery, producing what is known as an **eschar.** The skin as a whole constricts over the wound site, increasing the pressure of any edema beneath and restricting the flow of blood (Figure 6-12 ■). If the extremity burn is circumferential, the constriction may be severe enough to occlude all blood flow into the distal extremity. In the case of a thoracic burn, eschar may drastically reduce chest excursion and respiratory tidal volume.

rule of palms *method of estimating the amount of body surface area burned that sizes the area burned in comparison to the patient's palmar surface.*

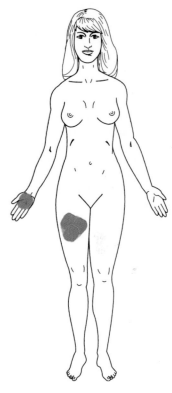

■ Figure 6-11   Using the rule of palms, the surface of the patient's palm represents approximately 1 percent of BSA and is helpful in estimating the area of small burns.

eschar *hard, leathery product of a deep full thickness burn; it consists of dead and denatured skin.*

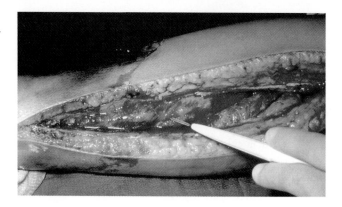

■ Figure 6-12 The constriction created by an eschar can limit chest excursion or cut off blood flow to and from a limb.

It may be acceptable in some systems to cover burns with clean versus sterile dressings. Check with your burn center and medical direction for what is acceptable in your system.

Infection

Although infection is the most persistent killer of burn victims, its effects do not appear for several days following the acute injury. Pathogens invade the wound shortly after the burn occurs and continue to do so until the wound heals. These pathogens pose a hazard to life when they grow to massive numbers, a process that takes days or weeks. To reduce the patient's exposure to infectious pathogens, carefully employ body substance isolation, use sterile dressings and clean equipment, and avoid gross contamination of the burn.

Organ Failure

As previously noted, the burn process releases material from damaged or dying body cells into the bloodstream. Myoglobin from the muscles clogs the tubules of the kidneys and, with hypovolemia, may cause kidney failure. Hypovolemia and the circulating by-products of cellular destruction may also induce liver failure. In addition, the release of cellular potassium into the bloodstream affects the heart's electrical system, causing dysrhythmias and possible cardiac arrest.

Special Factors

Consider any patient with a preexisting illness or disease or any pediatric or geriatric patient as having a more serious burn injury.

Certain factors involving the burn patient's overall health and age will also affect the patient's response to a burn and should influence your field decisions regarding treatment and transport. Geriatric and pediatric patients and patients who are already ill or otherwise injured have greater difficulty coping with burn injuries than do healthy individuals. The pediatric patient has a high body surface area to body weight ratio, which means the fluid reserves needed for dealing with the effects of a burn are low. Geriatric patients have reduced mechanisms for fluid retention and lower fluid reserves. They are also less able to combat infection and more apt to have underlying diseases. Ill patients are already using body energy to fight their diseases; with burns, these patients have additional medical stresses to combat. The fluid loss that accompanies a burn also compounds the effects of blood loss in a trauma patient. This patient now must recover from two injuries.

Physical Abuse

When assessing any burn, particularly in a child or an elderly and infirm adult, be alert for any signs of potential physical abuse. Look for mechanisms of injury that don't make sense, such as stove burns on an infant who cannot yet stand or walk. Certain burn patterns should also give rise to suspicion. Multiple circular burns each about a centimeter in diameter may reflect intentional cigarette burns. Infants who have been dipped in scalding hot water will have characteristic circumferential burns to their buttocks as they raise their feet and legs in an attempt to avoid the burning water (Figure 6-13 ■).

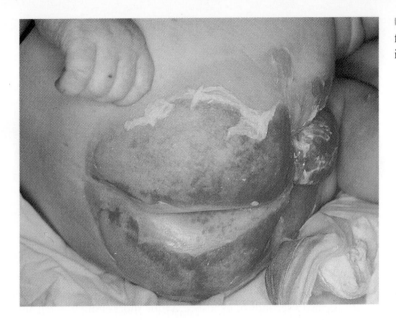

Branding is an unusual form of abuse and is sometimes seen in ritualistic or hazing ceremonies in some organizations. In all cases of suspected abuse, document your findings objectively and accurately, report them to the person assuming patient care in the emergency department, and notify the proper authorities as state and local laws require.

ASSESSMENT OF THERMAL BURNS

Skin evaluation tells more about the body's condition than any other aspect of patient assessment. Not only is the skin the first body organ to experience the effects of burns, but it is the first and often the only organ to display them. Therefore, assessment of the skin and the associated burns must be deliberate, careful, and complete.

While the burn process varies, assessment is simple and well structured. Assess burn patients carefully and completely to assure that you establish the nature and extent of each injury. This helps you to assign burns the appropriate priority for care.

The assessment of thermal burns follows established procedures for performing the scene size-up, the initial assessment, the rapid trauma assessment or focused history and physical exam, the detailed physical exam, and the ongoing assessment.

SCENE SIZE-UP

The safety of your patients, fellow rescuers, and yourself depends upon a complete and thorough scene size-up. Look around carefully as you arrive at the scene to assure there is no continuing danger to you or your patient. Examine the scene to assure it is safe for you to enter. If there is any doubt, do not enter until the scene is made safe by appropriate emergency personnel (Figure 6-14 ■).

On calls involving burn patients, be wary of entering enclosed spaces, such as a bedroom or a garage, if there is recent evidence of a fire. Even small fires can cause intense heat in small, enclosed spaces. This can rapidly lead to a near-explosive process (called flashover) in which the contents of a room rise in temperature to the point of rapid ignition. Flashover is frequently fatal to victims caught in the immediate area.

Another significant hazard at fire-ground scenes is the buildup of toxic gases. Carbon monoxide, cyanide, and hydrogen sulfide are common by-products of combustion

Be wary of entering any enclosed space associated with a fire because of the dangers of flashover and toxic gases.

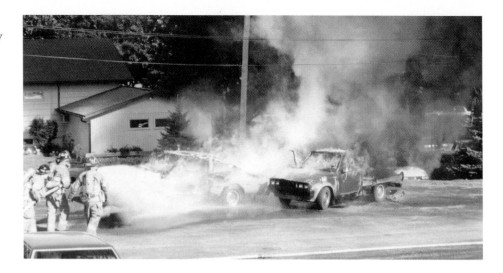

■ Figure 6-14 Never enter a fire scene until it has been safely contained by appropriately trained personnel.

and can be produced in large quantities in some fires. Cyanide, in particular, can kill after as little as 15 seconds of exposure, a time short enough to fell any would-be rescuer without proper protection.

Never enter any potentially hazardous scene. Instead, assure that the fire is thoroughly extinguished or that the patient is brought to you by persons skilled in working in hazardous environments who are using proper personal protective equipment. Assure that the area where you will be caring for the patient is free from dangers such as structural collapse, contamination, electricity, and any other hazards.

Once at the burn patient's side, stop the burning process so it no longer threatens you or the patient. Extinguish any overt flame using copious irrigation, as water is available. As an alternative, a heavy wool or cotton blanket (avoid most synthetics such as nylon or polyester) will smother flames.

Quickly survey the patient for other materials he is wearing that may continue the burn process. Remember that burn patients may be an actual hazard both to themselves and to you. Leather articles, such as shoes, belts, or watchbands, can smolder for hours and continue to induce thermal injury. Watches, rings, and other jewelry may also hold and transmit heat or may restrict swelling tissue and occlude distal circulation. Synthetics (such as a nylon windbreaker) produce great heat as they burn and leave a hot, smoldering residue once the overt flames are out. Remove materials like those previously described as soon as possible. Be careful as you check for and remove these items. They may be hot enough to burn you.

Once the scene is safe and there are no further dangers to you or others, consider the burn mechanism. Ask yourself: "Is there any possibility that the patient was unconscious during the fire or trapped within the building?" If so, be ready to place a special emphasis upon your assessment and management of the patient's airway and breathing. Watch for any signs of airway restriction, and be alert to possible poisoning from carbon monoxide or other toxic gases.

Also consider and examine for other mechanisms of injury associated with the burn. Remember that the victim, in attempting to escape the flames, may have fallen down a flight of stairs or jumped from a second- or third-story window. Anticipate skeletal and internal injuries. In cases of electrical burns, consider the possibility that muscle spasms caused by contact with high voltage may also have caused skeletal fractures. Be aware that trauma injuries will increase the severity of the burn's impact on your patient.

Conclude the scene size-up by considering the need for other resources to manage the scene and treat the patient. Request additional EMS, police, and fire personnel and

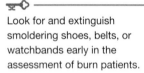

Look for and extinguish smoldering shoes, belts, or watchbands early in the assessment of burn patients.

equipment as necessary. If you suspect serious airway involvement or carbon monoxide poisoning, consider requesting air medical service to reduce transport time to the hospital or burn/trauma center.

INITIAL ASSESSMENT

Start your initial assessment by forming a general impression of the patient. Rule out any danger of associated trauma or the possibility of head and spine injury. Evaluate the patient's level of consciousness, and, if the patient displays an altered state of consciousness, consider toxic inhalation as a cause. Protect the patient from further cervical injury if indicated by the suspected mechanism of injury or by the patient's symptoms.

Next, assure the airway is patent. If it is not, protect it. You must give the airway of a burn patient special consideration. Look for the signs of any thermal or inhalation injury during your initial airway exam (Figure 6-15 ■). Look carefully at the facial and nasal hairs to see if they have been singed. Examine any sputum and the areas around the mouth and nose for carbonaceous residue or any other evidence of inhalation. Listen for airway sounds, such as stridor, hoarseness, or coughing, that indicate irritation or inflammation of the mucosa. Such sounds should alert you to the possibility that the airway has been injured and that progressive swelling of the airway is likely. Stridor, in particular, is a serious finding. Consider a patient with any signs of respiratory involvement as a potential acute emergency, and provide immediate care and transport.

With patients in whom respiratory involvement is suspected, provide high-flow, high-concentration oxygen, and prepare the equipment for endotracheal intubation. High-concentration oxygen (at levels approaching 100 percent) is especially important for burn patients because they may be suffering from carbon monoxide poisoning. Very high oxygen percentages more effectively provide oxygen to body cells and may reduce the half-life of carbon monoxide on the hemoglobin molecule by up to two thirds.

Pulse oximetry is a very useful tool in evaluating respiratory and cardiovascular effectiveness in the burn patient. However, carbon monoxide replaces oxygen in the red blood cell and colors it much as oxygen does. This leads the oximeter to display high saturation readings when the blood actually has greatly reduced oxygen-carrying capacity. Do not rely on pulse oximetry readings alone for the patient who is suspected of suffering carbon monoxide poisoning, who has been burned in an enclosed space, or who has inhaled significant amounts of smoke.

Burn patients may progress rapidly from mild dyspnea to total respiratory arrest. While the intubation of a respiratory burn patient may be difficult in the field, there are

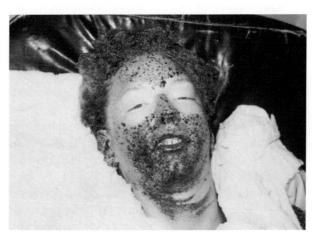

■ Figure 6-15 Facial burns or carbonaceous material around the mouth and nose suggest the potential for chemical and thermal burns to the airway.

distinct advantages to performing it early. The edema is progressive and rapidly reduces the airway lumen. If intubation is delayed until the patient becomes extremely dyspneic or goes into respiratory arrest, the airway may be so edematous that it will be difficult, if not impossible, to intubate.

If you elect field intubation for the burn patient (and medical direction approves), perform it quickly and carefully. The airway is already narrowing, and the normal trauma associated with intubation could make matters worse. Intubation can be more complicated if the patient is conscious and fights the process. Consider using rapid sequence intubation techniques and pharmacological adjuncts including sedatives and paralytics. Use succinylcholine (see Chapter 8, "Head, Facial, and Neck Trauma") cautiously, if at all, since it may worsen the hyperkalemia sometimes associated with severe burns. You may also find nasotracheal intubation useful. In any case, select the crew member with the most experience to assure that intubation is completed quickly and with the least amount of associated airway trauma.

As with all intubation, it is best to maintain an airway using the largest endotracheal tube possible. Be sure, however, to have several tubes smaller than you would normally use ready, because edema may have reduced the size of the airway. Select the largest tube that you think will easily pass through the cords. In extreme cases, creation of a surgical airway by either cricothyrotomy or needle cricothyrostomy may be a lifesaving necessity; in such cases follow local protocols or on-line medical direction. Confirm tube placement with capnography.

Assure that the patient's breathing is adequate in both volume and rate. Carefully assess tidal volume if there are circumferential burns of the chest, because the developing eschar may restrict chest excursion. Ventilate as necessary via bag-valve mask using the reservoir and high-flow, high concentration oxygen.

FOCUSED AND RAPID TRAUMA ASSESSMENT

The focused history and physical exam for the burn patient are much the same as for any other trauma patient, beginning with a rapid trauma assessment or a focused physical exam and proceeding to the taking of baseline vital signs and a patient history. With a burn patient, however, you must also accurately approximate the area of the burn and its depth. This approximation guides your care and helps emergency department personnel prepare for patient arrival.

Except in cases of very localized burns, examine the patient's entire body surface, both anterior and posterior. Remove any clothing that was or could have been involved in the burn. If any of the clothing adheres to the burn or resists removal, cut around it as necessary.

Apply the rule of nines to determine the total body surface area (BSA) burned. Add 9 percent if the burn involves an entire "rule of nines" region. If it only involves a portion, add that proportion of 9 percent. For example, if 1/3 of the upper extremity is burned, the surface area approximation is 3 percent (1/3 of 9 percent = 3 percent). For small burns, use the rule of palms to approximate the affected BSA.

The depth of a burn injury is also an important consideration. Identify areas of painful sensation as partial thickness burns (Figure 6-16 ■). Consider those that present with limited or absent pain as probable full thickness burns (Figure 6-17 ■). This differentiation is difficult because partial thickness injury and its associated pain commonly surrounds the full thickness burn (Figure 6-18 ■). See Table 6–1 for the characteristics of the different types of burns.

A third consideration in determining the severity of a burn is the area of the body affected. The face, hands, feet, joints, genitalia, and circumferential burns deserve particular consideration. Each presents with special problems to patients and their recovery.

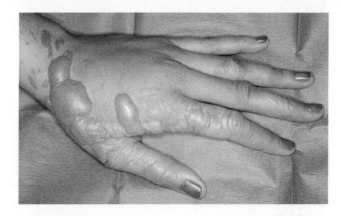

■ Figure 6-16   A partial thickness burn.

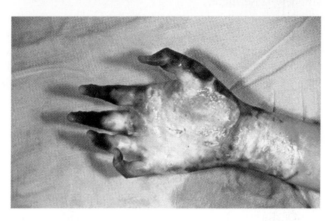

■ Figure 6-17   A deep full thickness burn.

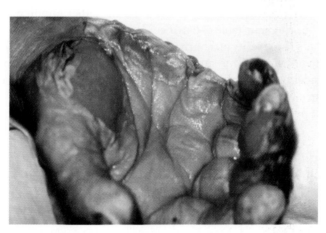

■ Figure 6-18   A hand wound displaying both partial and full thickness burns.

Table 6–1	Characteristics of Various Depths of Burns		
	Superficial (First Degree)	Partial Thickness (Second Degree)	Full Thickness (Third Degree)
Cause	Sun or minor flame	Hot liquids, flame	Chemicals, electricity, hot metals, flame
Skin color	Red	Mottled red	Pearly white and/or charred, translucent, and parchment-like
Skin	Dry with no blister	Blisters with weeping	Dry with thrombosed blood vessels
Sensation	Painful	Painful	Anesthetic
Healing	3–6 days	2–4 weeks	May require skin grafting

You have already assessed the face for burns to eliminate respiratory involvement. But this area also needs special consideration for aesthetic reasons. Facial damage and scarring may be more socially debilitating than a joint or limb burn. Carefully assess and give a high priority to these injuries, even if you do rule out respiratory involvement.

Consider burns involving the feet or the hands as serious. These areas are critical for much of the patient's daily activities. Serious burns and the associated scar tissue make thermal hand or foot injuries very debilitating. Assess these areas and communicate the precise location of the injury and the degree of the burn to the receiving physician. Joint burns can likewise be debilitating for patients. Scar tissue replaces skin, leading to loss of joint flexibility and mobility. Give any burn assessed as full thickness that involves the hands, feet, or joints a higher priority than a burn of equal surface area and depth elsewhere.

Also pay particular attention to burns that completely ring an extremity, the thorax, the abdomen, or the neck. Due to the nature of a full thickness burn, the area underneath the burn may be drastically compressed as an eschar forms. The resulting constriction may hinder respirations, restrict distal blood flow, or cause hypoxia of the tissues beneath. Carefully assess any burn encircling a part of the body for distal circulation or other signs of vascular compromise. Once you note such an injury, perform ongoing assessments to monitor distal circulatory status.

Finally, assign a higher priority to any burns affecting pediatric or geriatric patients or patients who are ill or otherwise injured. Serious burns cause great stress for these patients. The massive fluid and heat loss as well as the infection often associated with burns challenge the ability of body systems to perform adequately. Consider a burn more serious whenever it is accompanied by any other serious patient problem.

Once you determine the depth, extent, and other factors that contribute to burn severity, categorize the patient as having either minor, moderate, or severe burns. Use the criteria in Table 6–2 as a guide.

The severity of a burn should be increased one level with pediatric and geriatric patients and patients suffering from other trauma or acute medical problems. Also consider burns as critical with a patient who shows any signs or symptoms of respiratory involvement. Such patients require immediate transport to a burn (or trauma) center, if possible (Table 6–3).

Table 6–2	Burn Severity
Minor	
Superficial: BSA < 50 percent (sunburns, etc.)	
Partial thickness: BSA < 10 percent	
Moderate	
Superficial: BSA > 50 percent	
Partial thickness: BSA < 30 percent	
Full thickness: BSA > 10 percent	
Critical	
Partial thickness: BSA > 30 percent	
Full thickness: BSA > 10 percent	
Inhalation injury	
Any partial or full thickness burns involving hands, feet, joints, face, or genitalia	

Source: American Burn Association.

what! (handwritten annotation)

Table 6-3	**Injuries That Benefit from Burn Center Care**

Partial thickness (second-degree) burn greater than 10 percent of BSA

Full thickness (third-degree) burn

Significant burns to the face, feet, hands, perineum, or major joints

High-voltage electrical burns

Inhalation injuries

Chemical burns

Associated significant injuries or medical conditions

Source: American Burn Association.

Legal Notes

Transporting a Burn Patient Burn patients require highly specialized care in a facility specifically designed for burn injuries. Burn centers offer a multidisciplinary approach to burn care utilizing plastic surgeons, general surgeons, orthopedic surgeons, rehabilitation specialists, pain management specialists, and others. In addition, burn centers provide nutritional counseling (very important to burn healing), pastoral care, and psychological care. Burn care facilities are expensive to operate and patients tend to remain in them for prolonged periods of time. The American Burn Association (ABA) has published guidelines for determining which patients might benefit from treatment in a burn center.

Most burn centers are regional facilities, and frequently patients must be transported some distance to them. Personnel who routinely transport burn patients should be familiar with burn care including dressings, fluid therapy, and escharotomy (if required). In addition, continued adequate analgesia should be provided according to local protocols and interhospital transfer orders. Burn care should be addressed in any trauma system plan.

The burn center is a hospital with a commitment to providing specialty treatment to burn patients. That commitment includes measures necessary to reduce the risk of infection presented by serious burns. The center must also have the resources to perform delicate skin grafts necessary to replace destroyed skin. Because serious burns leave scar tissue that covers joints and other important areas and affects movement, the center can provide rehabilitation programs requiring prolonged patient stays and intensive nursing care. While immediate transport to a burn center is not as critically time dependant as transport for other seriously injured patients to a trauma center, the burn center's resources can optimize a patient's recovery prospects. Review your local protocols for criteria regarding patient transport to a burn center.

Conclude the focused history and physical exam by prioritizing the patient for transport. Rapidly transport any patient with full thickness burns over a large portion of the BSA. Patients with associated injuries to the face, joints, hands, feet, or genitalia are also candidates for immediate transport. Other cases needing rapid transport include patients who have experienced smoke, steam, or flame inhalation, or any geriatric, pediatric, otherwise ill, or trauma patient. Direct these patients to the nearest burn center as described by your local protocols or by on-line medical direction.

The head-to-toe examination should continue at the scene only if significant and life-threatening burns can be ruled out.

ONGOING ASSESSMENT

Conduct ongoing assessments for all burn patients, every 15 minutes for minor burns and every 5 minutes for moderate or critical burns. Although the burn injury mechanism has been halted, the nature of the burn will continue to affect the patient. In addition to monitoring vital signs, watch for early signs of hypovolemia and airway problems. Also be cautious of aggressive fluid therapy. Monitor for lung sounds and respiratory effort suggestive of pulmonary edema, and slow the fluid resuscitation if any signs develop. Also carefully monitor distal circulation and sensation with any circumferential burn. Finally, monitor the ECG to identify any abnormalities, which may be caused by electrolyte imbalances secondary to fluid movement and tissue destruction.

MANAGEMENT OF THERMAL BURNS

Once you complete your burn patient assessment and correct or address any immediate life threats, you can begin certain burn management steps, either in the field or en route to the hospital. These include the prevention of shock, hypothermia, and any further wound contamination.

Thermal burn management can be divided into two categories: that for local and minor burns and that for moderate to severe burns.

LOCAL AND MINOR BURNS

Use local cooling to treat minor soft-tissue burns involving only a small proportion of the body surface area at a partial thickness. Provide this care only for partial thickness burns that involve less than 15 percent of the BSA or very small full thickness burns (less than 2 percent BSA). Cooling of larger surface areas may subject the patient to the risk of hypothermia. Cold or cool water immersion has some effect in reducing pain and may limit the depth of the burning process if applied immediately (within 1 or 2 minutes) after the burn.

Cool water immersion of minor localized burns may be effective if accomplished in the first few minutes after a burn.

If you have not already done so, remove any article of clothing or jewelry that might possibly act to constrain edema. As body fluids accumulate at the injury site, the site begins to swell. If the swelling encounters any constriction, it increases pressure on other tissue and may, in effect, serve as a tourniquet. This pressure may result in the loss of pulse and circulation distal to the injury. Evaluate distal circulation and sensation frequently during care and transport.

Also provide the burn patient with comfort and support. Even rather minor burns can be very painful. Calm and reassure the patient; in severe cases, consider fentanyl or morphine sulfate.

Standard in-hospital treatment for minor burns includes the application of topical (not systemic) antibiotic ointments such as silver sulfadiazine and bulky sterile dressings. Encourage the patient, as much as possible, to keep the burn elevated. Provide analgesia in either oral or parenteral form as burns can be quite painful. Full thickness burns are open wounds, so any patient without an up-to-date tetanus immunization is given a booster of tetanus-diphtheria toxoid.

MODERATE TO SEVERE BURNS

Cover extensive partial and full thickness burns with dry sterile dressing, keep the patient warm, and initiate fluid resuscitation.

Use dry, sterile dressings to cover partial thickness burns that involve more than 15 percent BSA or full thickness burns involving more than 5 percent of the BSA. Dressings keep air movement past the sensitive partial thickness burn to a minimum, and thereby reduce pain. Bulky sterile dressings also provide padding against minor

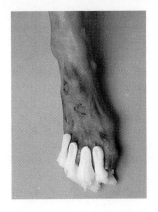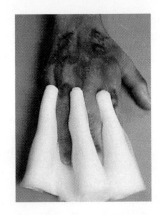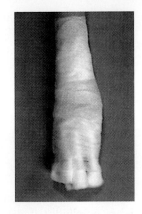

■ Figure 6-19   Separate burned toes and fingers with dry sterile gauze.

bumping and other trauma. In full thickness burns, they provide a barrier to possible contamination.

Keep the patient warm. When burns involve large surface areas, the patient loses the ability to effectively control body temperature. If the burn begins to seep fluid, as in a full thickness burn, evaporative heat loss can be extreme. Cover such an area with dry sterile dressings, cover the patient with a blanket, and maintain a warm environment.

When treating full thickness burns to the fingers, toes, or other locations where burned surfaces may contact each other, place soft, nonadherent bandages between the burned skin areas (Figure 6-19 ■). Without this precaution, the disrupted and wet wounds would stick together and cause further damage when pulled apart for care at the emergency department.

If the surface area of the burn is great, medical direction may ask you to provide aggressive fluid therapy during prehospital care. While hypovolemia is not an early development after a burn, fluid migration into the wound later during the burn cycle eventually leads to serious fluid loss. Early and aggressive fluid therapy can effectively reduce the impact of this fluid loss.

If burns cover all the normal IV access sites, you may place the catheter through tissue with partial thickness burns, proximal to any more serious injury. (Full thickness burns usually damage the blood vessels or coagulate the blood, making intravenous cannulation difficult and possibly impeding effective fluid flow.) Be careful with insertion. The skin may be leathery, but the tissue underneath is very delicate. Adhesive tape may not stick to the burn tissue or may injure the skin when it is removed. Try to secure the intravenous needle and lines by alternate means, when possible.

Establish intravenous routes in any patient with moderate to severe burns. Introduce two large-bore catheters and hang 1,000-mL bags of either normal saline or lactated Ringer's (preferred) solution. Current fluid resuscitation formulas recommend 4 mL of fluid for every kilogram of patient weight multiplied by the percentage of body surface area burned:

$$4 \text{ mL} \times \text{Patient weight in kg} \times \text{BSA burned} = \text{Amount of fluid over 24 hours}$$

Thus, for a 70-kg patient with 30 percent BSA burned, the calculation is

$$4 \times 70 \times 30 = 8{,}400 \text{ mL}$$

The patient needs half this amount of fluid in the first 8 hours after the burn. This particular fluid resuscitation protocol is known as the Parkland formula. Other variations

Use soft, nonadherent dressings between areas of full thickness burns, as between the fingers and toes, to prevent adhesion.

exist and may be in use in your local area. In most prehospital situations where transport time is short (less than 1 hour), an initial fluid bolus of 0.25 mL of fluid for every kilogram of patient weight multiplied by the percentage of BSA burned is reasonable:

$$0.25 \text{ mL} \times \text{Patient weight in kg} \times \text{BSA burned} = \text{Amount of fluid}$$

Thus, for an 80-kg patient with 20 percent BSA burned, the calculation is

$$0.25 \times 80 \times 20 = 400 \text{ mL}$$

You may repeat this infusion once or twice during the first hour or so of care.

Be cautious and conservative when administering fluids to the burn patient if there is any possibility of airway or lung injury. Rapid fluid administration may worsen airway swelling or the edema that accompanies toxic inhalation. Carefully monitor the airway and auscultate for breath sounds frequently whenever you administer fluid to a burn patient.

Burns are quite painful, yet the pain is often paradoxical to the burn severity. Less severe superficial and partial thickness (first- and second-degree) burns are very uncomfortable, while extensive full thickness (third-degree) burns are often almost without pain. Provide patients in severe pain with narcotic analgesia. Fentanyl or morphine should be administered as needed. Consider morphine in 2 mg IV increments every 5 minutes until suffering is relieved. Use morphine with caution as it may depress the respiratory drive and increase any existing hypovolemia. With fentanyl, start with a loading dose of 25 to 50 mcg IV and administer repeat doses of 25 mcg IV as needed.

Infection is another classic and deadly problem associated with extensive soft-tissue burns. This life-threatening condition does not develop until well after prehospital care is concluded. However, proper field care can significantly reduce mortality and morbidity. Providing a clean environment and dressings can lessen the bacterial load for the patient. Avoid prophylactic antibiotics because their early use has been shown to actually worsen outcomes for burn patients.

In dire circumstances medical direction may request you to perform an emergency escharotomy. To do this, you incise the burned tissue through the eschar, perpendicular to the constriction. Be certain to incise about 1 cm deeper than the developing eschar to assure the release of pressure. If adequate respirations or distal pulses do not return after the escharotomy, medical direction may request you to repeat the procedure a short distance from the first incision.

Emergency department personnel will continue fluid resuscitation for serious burn patients according to the Parkland or another suitable formula. They will perform arterial blood gas evaluation to determine oxygen tension, carbon monoxide concentration, and cyanide poisoning levels. Urine output and cardiac monitoring are instituted as well. The staff will assure adequate administration of parenteral narcotic analgesia and provide tetanus immunization if necessary. They will closely evaluate severe circumferential burns for eschar development. If the blood flow in an extremity is impaired, the physician may perform an escharotomy.

INHALATION INJURY

If you suspect thermal (or chemical) airway burns and airway compromise is imminent, intubation can be lifesaving. Once you assure the patient's airway, provide high-flow, high concentration oxygen by nonrebreather mask at 15 lpm. Oxygen not only counters hypoxia but is also therapeutic in carbon monoxide and cyanide poisoning. Consider transport to a center capable of providing hyperbaric oxygen therapy for pa-

Be cautious and conservative when administering fluids to the burn patient with inhalation injury.

Early intubation can be lifesaving for the inhalation injury patient.

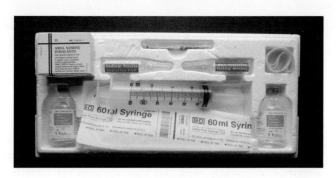

tients with suspected carbon monoxide poisoning. The hyperbaric chamber provides oxygen under the pressure of two or more atmospheres. This pushes oxygen into the patient's bloodstream, carrying it directly to the body's cells. Hyperbaric oxygenation also drives carbon monoxide from the hemoglobin, shortening the time to recovery. If hyperbaric oxygen therapy is available in your area, any smoke inhalation or suspected carbon monoxide poisoning patient should be considered for treatment at the facility.

Suspect cyanide toxicity in patients with severe symptoms such as dyspnea, chest pain, altered mental status, seizures, and unconsciousness. To be effective, antidotal treatment of serious cyanide poisoning must be started early. Vapor exposures are likely to result in severe respiratory distress or apnea in addition to unconsciousness. Rapid airway intervention with endotracheal intubation and ventilatory support with a bag-valve mask are initial priorities. However, a rapid shift to antidotal therapy is essential to save the patient.

Administration of the antidote for cyanide is a two-stage process, first using a nitrite compound, followed by a sulfur-containing compound (Figure 6-20 ■). The nitrite acts by converting the hemoglobin (the primary oxygen-carrying protein in the blood) to methemoglobin. Methemoglobin then binds the cyanide, removing it from the cytochrome$_{a3}$ (an enzyme necessary for oxygen processing by cells). The sulfur-containing antidote then removes the cyanide by forming a nontoxic compound, excreted in the urine. The administration of the cyanide antidote should be reserved for patients with a history of acute cyanide inhalation and frank signs and symptoms of serious exposure. The administration of the nitrites is not without risk because they bind to the hemoglobin molecule and produce an effect similar to carbon monoxide poisoning.

Ambulances serving industrial areas with high cyanide use may carry antidote kits containing amyl nitrite, sodium nitrite, and sodium thiosulfate. If an IV is already established, administer 300 mg sodium nitrite over 2 to 4 minutes for adults. If an IV is not yet established, crush one amyl nitrite ampule for the patient to inhale. If the patient has spontaneous respirations, place the ampule under an oxygen mask with high-flow, high concentration oxygen running. In patients needing ventilatory support, place the ampule in the bag or oxygen reservoir of the bag-valve mask. Do not let the ampule fall into the patient's mouth or down the endotracheal tube. Always follow inhaled amyl nitrite with intravenous sodium nitrite, and do not use amyl nitrite if the patient has already received sodium nitrite. Use care in the administration of sodium nitrite or amyl nitrite as they may induce hypotension. They also bind to the hemoglobin, reducing its ability to carry blood. In addition to antidotal therapy, keep the patient supine and administer high-flow, high-concentration oxygen.

Following administration of IV sodium nitrite, administer 12.5 g of sodium thiosulfate for the adult. Avoid sodium thiosulfate unless the patient has received IV sodium nitrite, as it does not work well by itself. A highly effective and much safer antidote (related to vitamin B$_{12}$) is on the horizon, but is not yet available for general use in the United States.

ASSESSMENT AND MANAGEMENT OF ELECTRICAL, CHEMICAL, AND RADIATION BURNS

ELECTRICAL INJURIES

Until the power is off, no one should be allowed to approach the electrical burn patient.

Be certain that the power has been shut off before you approach the scene of a suspected electrical injury. Until it is, do not allow anyone to approach the patient or the proximity of the electrical source. Remember that an energized power line need not spark or whip around to be deadly; a power line simply lying on the ground can still present a significant danger. Note also that some utility lines have breakers that will try to reestablish power periodically. Establish a safety zone if there is any question about the status of lines that are down. Keep vehicles and personnel at a distance from downed lines or the source pole that is greater than the distance between the power poles. Also be aware that downed power lines may energize metal structures such as buildings, vehicles, or fences.

Once the scene is secure, assess the patient and prepare him for transport. Search for both an entrance and an exit wound. Look specifically for possible contact points with both the ground and the electrical source. In some circumstances, multiple entrance and exit wounds are present. Remember that electrical current passes through the body and therefore may result in significant internal burns, especially to blood vessels and nerves, while the assessment reveals only minimal superficial findings. Rapidly progressive cardiovascular collapse can follow contact with an electrical source. Also, examine the patient for any fractures resulting from forceful muscle contractions caused by the current's passage.

As with thermal burns, look for smoldering shoes, belts, or other items of clothing. Such items may continue the burning process well after the current is shut off. Also remove rings, watches, and any other constrictive items from the fingers, limbs, and the neck.

Monitor the electrical burn patient for abnormalities in the ECG.

Perform ECG monitoring for possible cardiac disturbances in victims of electrical burns. Electrical current may induce dysrhythmias including bradycardias, tachycardias, ventricular fibrillation, and asystole. Assure that emergency department personnel examine any patient who has sustained a significant electrical shock. The damage the current causes may be internal and not apparent to you or your patient during assessment. Consider any significant electrical burn or exposure patient as a high priority for immediate transport.

Lightning strikes to humans occur more than 300 times each year in the United States and result in over 100 deaths. Strikes to people riding tractors, on open water, on golf courses, and under trees are most common, and men are the victims of 75 percent of all strikes. A lightning strike is a high-voltage (up to 100,000 volts), high-current (10,000 amperes), and high-temperature (50,000° F) event that lasts only a fraction of a second. A direct strike will impart this energy to the patient (Figure 6-21 ■). However, the lightning will often strike a nearby object with some current traveling sideways (sideflash) or the current may radiate outward in alternate pathways from the strike point, thus diminishing the voltage (step voltage).

By the time anyone reaches the victim of a lightning strike, the electricity has long since dissipated. (There will be, however, a continued risk of further strikes as long as the storm remains nearby.) There is no danger of electrical shock from touching someone who has been struck by lightning. The person's clothing, however, may continue to smolder, so remove it as necessary. Among other serious effects, lightning can produce a sudden cessation of breathing. Despite being apneic and perhaps pulseless, these patients frequently survive with prompt prehospital intervention.

Treat visible burns ("entrance" and "exit" wounds) just as any thermal burn with cooling, if necessary, followed by the application of dry sterile dressings. Do not focus too much on the visible burns, but instead recognize that the electricity has passed through the body, possibly causing widespread internal effects.

Treat cardiac or respiratory arrest in electrical burn patients with aggressive airway, ventilatory, and circulatory management. Patients in cardiac arrest because of contact with electrical current have a high survival rate if prehospital intervention is prompt. Check immediately for ventricular fibrillation and defibrillate if necessary. Secure the airway with an endotracheal tube and begin ventilations and chest compressions. The usual resuscitative procedures for cases of cardiac arrest apply equally when the cause of the arrest is electrical injury; they might include the use of vasopressors and antidysrhythmics.

For serious electrical burn injuries, initiate at least two large-bore IVs and administer 1,000 mL of fluid per hour in 0.20 mL/kg boluses. Consider the use of sodium bicarbonate and mannitol, usually at the discretion of medical direction, to prevent the complications of rhabdomyolysis (discussed in Chapter 5, "Soft-Tissue Trauma") and hyperkalemia. The usual starting dose is 1 mEq/kg for sodium bicarbonate and 10 g for mannitol.

CHEMICAL BURNS

As you perform the scene size-up, identify the nature of the chemical spill/contamination and, if possible, approach from uphill and upwind. Identify the location of the chemical and assure that it poses no hazard to you, other rescuers, or the public. Be wary of toxic fumes and cross-contamination from the patient and the surrounding environment. If necessary, have hazardous material team members evacuate and decontaminate the victim before you begin assessment and care. Seek out personnel on the scene who are familiar with the agent and consult with them regarding dangers posed by the agent and any specific medical care and patient handling procedures required with it.

During your assessment and care, always wear medical examination (preferably tyvex) gloves, but never presume that they will protect you from the agent. Take appropriate protective action against airborne dust, toxic fumes, and splash exposure for both yourself and the patient (goggles and mask as needed). Wear a disposable gown if there is danger of the agent contacting your clothing. Make certain the agent is isolated and no longer a danger to the patient or others. Have any of the patient's clothing that you suspect may be contaminated removed, and isolate it from accidental

In dealing with a chemical burn, take all precautions to assure that no one else becomes contaminated.

contact. Save the clothing and assure that it is disposed of properly. Identify the type of agent, its exact chemical name, the length of the patient's contact time with it, and the precise areas of the patient's body affected by it.

As you begin your initial assessment, assure that the patient is alert and fully oriented and that airway and breathing are unaffected by the contact. If there is any airway restriction or respiratory involvement, consider early intubation. As airway tissue swells, the obstruction worsens and intubation becomes more difficult. Monitor the patient's heart rate and consider ECG monitoring, because many chemicals (for example, organophosphates) may affect the heart. If the patient is stable, begin the rapid trauma assessment.

Examine any chemical burn carefully to establish the depth, extent, and nature of the injury. If you suspect the involvement of phenol, dry lime, sodium or riot agents, then treat as indicated below.

- ★ *Phenol.* A gelatinous caustic called phenol is used as a powerful industrial cleaner. Phenol is very difficult to remove because it is sticky and insoluble in water. Alcohol, which dissolves it, is frequently available in places where phenol is regularly used. You can use the alcohol to remove the phenol and follow removal with irrigation using large volumes of cool water.

- ★ *Dry lime.* Dry lime is a strong corrosive that reacts with water. It produces heat and subsequent chemical and thermal injuries. Brush dry lime off the patient gently, but as completely as possible. Then rinse the contaminated area with large volumes of cool to cold water. While the water reacts with any remaining lime, it cools the contact area and removes the rest of the chemical. By rinsing with water, you assure the lime reacts with that water rather than with the water contained within the patient's soft tissues.

- ★ *Sodium.* Sodium is an unstable metal that reacts destructively with many substances, including human tissue. It reacts vigorously with water, creating extreme heat, explosive hydrogen gas, and possible ignition. Sodium is normally stored submerged in oil because the metal reacts with moisture in the air. If a patient is contaminated with sodium, decontaminate him quickly by gentle brushing. Then cover the wound with the oil used to store the substance.

- ★ *Riot control agents.* These agents, which include CS, CN (Mace), and oleoresin capsicum (OC, pepper spray), deserve special mention because people are the targets of their intended use and because that use is frequent. These agents cause intense irritation of the eyes, mucous membranes, and respiratory tract. In general, they do not cause permanent damage when properly deployed. Patients who have contacted them typically present with eye pain, tearing, and temporary "blindness." Coughing, gagging, and vomiting are not uncommon. Treatment is supportive and most patients recover spontaneously within 10 to 20 minutes of exposure to fresh air. If necessary, irrigate the patient's eyes with normal saline if you suspect that any riot agent particles remain in the eye.

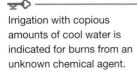

Irrigation with copious amounts of cool water is indicated for burns from an unknown chemical agent.

If it has not been done earlier, decontaminate the patient who has come in contact with any other chemical capable of causing tissue damage. Stop the damage by irrigating the site with large volumes of water (see Figure 6-22 ■). Water rinses away the offending material and dilutes any water-soluble agents. The water also reduces the heat and rate of the chemical reaction and, ultimately, the chemical's effects upon the patient's skin. If the contamination is widespread, douse the patient with large volumes of water. Use a garden hose or low-pressure water from a fire truck. Assure that the water is neither warm nor too cold.

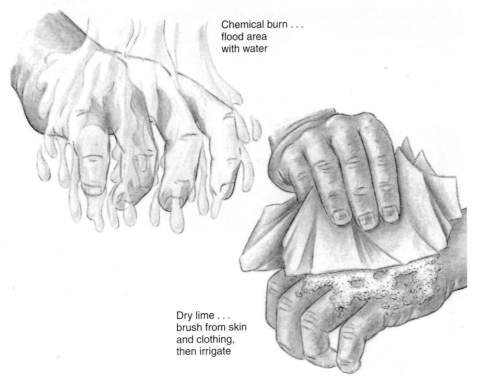

Chemical burn . . .
flood area
with water

Dry lime . . .
brush from skin
and clothing,
then irrigate

■ Figure 6-22 Chemical burns should be flushed with large quantities of water. Dry lime should be first brushed away before applying cool water.

When the patient has been thoroughly rinsed for a few minutes, remove any remaining clothing. Take care that the process does not contaminate rescuers. If the agent is dangerous, save all clothing and contain the rinse water for proper disposal at a later time. Next, gently wash the burn with a mild soap (such as ordinary dish detergent) and a gentle brush or sponge. Be careful not to cause further soft-tissue damage. After washing, gently irrigate the wound with a constant flow of water. While the pain and the burning process may appear to subside, it is important to continue the irrigation until the patient arrives at the emergency department. If practical, transport the label from the corrosive's container or a sample of the agent (safely contained and marked) along with the patient. On arrival at the hospital, be sure to describe to emergency department personnel, and enter in your prehospital care report, any first aid given prior to your arrival.

Do not use any antidote or neutralizing agent. Neutralizing agents often react violently with the contaminants they neutralize. They may ultimately increase the heat of the reaction and induce thermal burns. In some cases, the antidote or neutralizing agent is more damaging to the skin than the contaminant.

With chemical burns, pay particular attention to the patient's eyes. Eyes are very sensitive to chemicals and can easily be damaged, even by weak agents. Prompt treatment of chemical eye injury is critical and can reduce damage and preserve eyesight. Ask the patient about chemical contact with the eyes, eye pain, vision changes, and contact lens use. Examine the eyes for eyelid spasm (**blepharospasm**), conjunctival erythema, discoloration, tearing, and other evidence of burns or irritation.

Irrigate chemical splashes that involve the eye with large volumes of water. Alkali burns are especially damaging and with them you should flush the eye for at least 15 minutes. Irrigate acid burns for at least 5 minutes. Flush splashes of an unknown agent for up to 20 minutes. Do not, however, delay transport while irrigating.

A useful technique for irrigation is to hang a bag of normal saline (lactated Ringer's is an acceptable substitute) and use the flow regulator to control the flow of fluid into the nasal corner of the eye. Turn the patient's head to the side to facilitate drainage and avoid

Do not use any antidote or any neutralizing agent on chemical burns.

blepharospasm *twitching of the eyelids.*

Irrigate all alkali burns to the eye for at least 15 minutes.

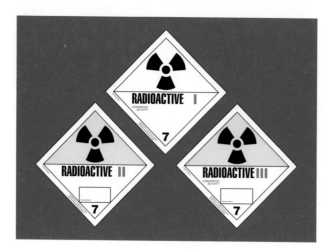

■ Figure 6-23 Warning labels may indicate the presence of radioactive materials.

cross-contaminating the other eye with the waste fluid. Be alert for contact lenses in cases where chemicals are splashed into the eyes. Chemicals may become trapped under the lenses, preventing adequate irrigation. Gently remove the lenses, continuing irrigation.

RADIATION BURNS

An incident involving potential radiation exposure or burns must be a concern during both dispatch and response phases of the emergency call. Because radiation can neither be seen nor felt, it can endanger EMS personnel unless the hazard has been anticipated and proper precautions taken. If you suspect radiation exposure, approach the scene very carefully (Figure 6-23 ■). If the incident occurs at a power generation plant or in an industrial or a medical facility, seek out personnel knowledgeable about the radioactive substance being used. Such persons are always on staff, and frequently on site, at these facilities. Stay a good distance from the scene and assure that bystanders, rescuers, and patients remain remote from the source of the exposure. Remember that distance and the nature of the materials, like concrete or earth, between you and the radiation source reduce potential exposure. If the exposure may be from dust or fire, approach from and remain upwind of the radiation source.

Because radiation can be neither seen nor felt, it can endanger EMS personnel unless proper precautions are taken.

In radiation exposure incidents, assure that personnel trained in radiation hazards isolate the source, contain it, and test the scene for safety. If this is impossible, move the patient to a site remote from the radioactivity source where you can give care without danger either to yourself or the patient. Plan the removal carefully. Use as much shielding as possible and keep exposure times to a minimum. Remember, the dose of radiation received is related to three primary factors: duration, distance, and shielding.

Duration, distance, and shielding are important factors in determining radiation dose exposure.

If you must carry out a patient removal, consider using the oldest rescuers for the evacuation team. This approach is prudent because many of the effects of radiation exposure become evident many years after the exposure. If you use older rescuers, they will more likely be past their reproductive years and have fewer years of life left if and when a problem does surface. This concern is especially important with pregnant females and young adults of both sexes. Remember that radiation damages the reproductive system very easily.

If there is a risk that patients are contaminated, assure that they are properly decontaminated before you begin assessment and care. If available for this task, use persons knowledgeable in decontamination and monitoring techniques who have the appropriate protective gear. If this is not possible, don goggles, a mask, gloves, and a disposable gown. Direct the evacuation team to place the patients in a decontamination area remote from your vehicle and other personnel and where any contamination can be contained. Have the patients disrobe or carefully disrobe them, rinse them with large volumes of water, then wash them with a soft brush and rinse again. Ordinary dish detergent is effective as a cleansing agent. Scrub, or cut off and then scrub, any areas of body hair. As in incidents of chemical contamination, save all clothing and decontamination water and dispose of them safely. Perform decontamination before moving the patients to the ambulance.

Carefully document the circumstances of the radioactive exposure. If possible, identify the source and strength of the agent. Determine the patient's proximity to the source during the exposure as well as the length of exposure.

Once decontaminated, treat a radiation exposure patient as you would any other patient. Because the human body by itself cannot be a source of ionizing radiation, the decontaminated patient poses no threat to you or your crew. Remember, however, that any contaminated material remaining on the patient or any contamination transferred to you does provide a source of radiation exposure and may contaminate you and your vehicle.

The actual assessment of a patient exposed to radiation is quite simple and usually reveals minimal signs or symptoms of injury. Only extreme exposures result in the classical presentation of nausea, vomiting, and malaise. Burns are extremely rare, although they may occur if the exposure is extremely intense. Even though a patient seems well, the delayed consequences of high-dose radiation exposure can be devastating. If you note any early patient complaints, record the findings in the patient's own words and include the time the complaint first was made. This information is helpful in determining the patient's degree of radiation exposure (Table 6–4).

Treat the symptoms of the radiation injury patient, make the patient as comfortable as possible, and offer psychological support. Cover any burns with sterile dressing and, if general symptoms are noticeable, provide oxygen and initiate an IV. Maintain the patient's body temperature and provide transport to the emergency department.

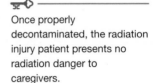

Once properly decontaminated, the radiation injury patient presents no radiation danger to caregivers.

Table 6–4	Dose-Effect Relationships to Ionizing Radiation
Whole Body Exposure Dose (RAD)	**Effect**
5–25	Asymptomatic. Blood studies are normal.
50–75	Asymptomatic. Minor depressions of white blood cells and platelets in a few patients.
75–125	May produce anorexia, nausea, vomiting, and fatigue in approximately 10–20 percent of patients within 2 days.
125–200	Possible nausea and vomiting. Diarrhea, anxiety, tachycardia. Fatal to less than 5 percent of patients.
200–600	Nausea and vomiting. Diarrhea in the first several hours. Weakness, fatigue. Fatal to approximately 50 percent of patients within 6 weeks without prompt medical attention.
600–1,000	"Burning sensation" within minutes. Nausea and vomiting within 10 minutes. Confusion, ataxia, and collapse within 1 hour. Watery diarrhea within 1 to 2 hours. Fatal to 100 percent within short time without prompt medical attention.
Localized Exposure Dose (RAD)	**Effect**
50	Asymptomatic
500	Asymptomatic (usually). May have risk of altered function of exposed area.
2,500	Atrophy, vascular lesion, and altered pigmentation.
5,000	Chronic ulcer, risk of carcinogenesis.

ONGOING ASSESSMENT

Monitor patients with inhalation, chemical, and electrical burns and radiation exposure for signs of increasing complications associated with their burn mechanisms. Also monitor blood pressure, pulse, and respirations and trend any changes. Perform these evaluations every 15 minutes in stable patients and every 5 minutes in unstable patients.

Summary

Burn injuries may compromise the skin—the protective envelope that protects and contains the human body. Burn damage to the skin may interfere with its ability to contain water within the body and to prevent damaging agents from entering. For these reasons, assessment and care of these soft-tissue injuries are important.

Assess the burn to determine its depth and the extent of the body surface area it involves. Be sensitive to any respiratory, joint, hand, foot, or circumferential regions affected by the burn. Give special consideration to pediatric and geriatric burn patients and to burn patients who are also ill or otherwise injured. Consider all these factors in determining the overall severity of a burn. If the patient's condition warrants, institute aggressive care. Anticipate airway compromise and fluid loss. Secure the airway very early in prehospital care. Initiate IV access, and begin fluid administration.

Electrical, chemical, or radiation burns require special care and assessment. An electrical burn requires careful assessment to determine the area and depth of burn involvement and should be followed by wound site dressing and cardiac monitoring. Chemical burns need rapid and effective decontamination. Radiation burns call for extreme care in removing the patient from the radiation source and in providing decontamination and supportive care.

You Make the Call

A young boy scout on a camping trip ignites his coat and shirt sleeve while attempting to light a camp fire. By the time his scout master extinguishes the flames, the arm is seriously burned. Your assessment finds the scout with a relatively painless hand and forearm with some skin discoloration. The upper arm is very painful and reddened with its distal portion just starting to blister.

1. What severity are the burns of the forearm and hand and of the upper arm?
2. What percentage of the body surface area is burned?
3. What level of acuity would you assign this patient?

See Suggested Responses at the back of this book.

Review Questions

1. During the healing process for burns, scar tissue is laid down and remodeled, and the patient begins to rehabilitate and return to normal function. This is called the:
   a. fluid shift phase.
   b. resolution phase.
   c. emergent phase.
   d. hypermetabolic phase.

2. Chemical burns caused by _____ usually continue to destroy cell membranes through liquefaction necrosis, allowing them to penetrate underlying tissue and causing deeper burns.
   a. acids
   b. alkalis
   c. electrical
   d. coagulation

3. The type of radiation that can travel through 6 to 10 feet of air, penetrate a few layers of clothing, and cause both external and internal injuries is:
   a. gamma radiation.
   b. alpha radiation.
   c. beta radiation.
   d. neutron radiation.

4. Airway edema is a major concern when dealing with inhalation injuries. To provide the best protection and prevent patient deterioration, it is important to initiate early:
   a. cardiac monitoring.
   b. endotracheal intubation.
   c. intravenous cannulation.
   d. rapid fluid replacement.

5. To reduce the patient's exposure to infectious pathogens, the paramedic must carefully:
   a. employ body substance isolation.
   b. use sterile dressings and clean equipment.
   c. avoid gross contamination of the burn.
   d. all of the above.

6. For pediatric or geriatric patients and patients suffering from other trauma or medical conditions, always:
   a. increase burn severity one level.
   b. initiate immediate intubation.
   c. reduce administered fluids.
   d. initiate immediate transport.

7. Your patient is experiencing airway compromise due to an inhalation injury. You elect to perform rapid sequence intubation to protect the patient's airway. Which of the following paralytics should you use with caution, if at all, because it may worsen hyperkalemia?
   a. morphine
   b. vecuronium
   c. succinylcholine
   d. pancuronium

8. Which of the following burns would be classified as a moderate burn?
   a. full thickness burns < 2 percent body surface area
   b. superficial burns < 50 percent body surface area
   c. partial thickness burns > 30 percent body surface area
   d. partial thickness burns < 30 percent body surface area

9. Fluid replacement is indicated in the care of patients with moderate to severe burns. The Parkland formula sets up a calculation for determining the amount of fluid to infuse over 24 hours. Which of the following accurately depicts the Parkland formula?
   a. 4 mL × patient weight in kilograms × BSA involved
   b. 4 mL × patient weight in pounds × BSA involved
   c. 6 mL × patient weight in kilograms × BSA involved
   d. 8 mL × patient weight in pounds × BSA involved

10. In general, how should dry lime be removed from the skin?
    a. Flush with vinegar, then with water.
    b. Brush dry lime away and then flush with water.
    c. Apply an oil-based basing soda and a sterile dressing.
    d. Cover the wound as is, flush with water, and transport.

11. Your 45-year-old male patient was working on his roof, came into contact with power lines, and has experienced possible electrocution. The patient has an irregular pulse of 124 BPM and his respiratory rate is 22 and irregular. The patient's blood pressure is 106/76. You note both entrance and exit wounds. You immediately manage the airway and decide to start an IV. You realize that you should administer an initial fluid bolus of:
    a. 20 mL/kg.
    b. 10 mL/kg.
    c. 10 mg/kg.
    d. 20 mg/kg.

12. The burn patient's injured tissue will swell. Therefore, with this knowledge, you realize that it is important to:
    a. start IV therapy early.
    b. remove restrictive jewelry.
    c. administer high-flow, high concentration oxygen.
    d. cover the injury with a burn sheet.

See Answers to Review Questions at the back of this book.

Further Reading

Bledsoe, B. E. and D. Clayden. *Prehospital Emergency Pharmacology*. 6th ed. Upper Saddle River, N.J.: Pearson/Prentice Hall, 2005.

Cooper, M. A. "Electrical and Lightning Injuries," in Rosen, P., and R. Barkin, eds. *Emergency Medicine: Concepts and Clinical Practice*. 5th ed. St. Louis: Mosby, 2002.

De Lorenzo, R. A., and R. S. Porter. *Tactical Emergency Care: Military and Operational Out-of-Hospital Medicine*. Upper Saddle River, N.J.: Pearson/Prentice Hall, 1998.

Edlich, R. F, and J. C. Moghtader. "Chemical Injuries," in Rosen, P., and R. Barkin, eds. *Emergency Medicine: Concepts and Clinical Practice*. 5th ed. St. Louis: Mosby, 2002.

Edlich, R. F., and J. C. Moghtader. "Thermal Burns," in Rosen, P., and R. Barkin, eds. *Emergency Medicine: Concepts and Clinical Practice*. 5th ed. St. Louis: Mosby, 2002.

Markovchick, V. "Radiation Injuries," in Rosen, P., and R. Barkin, eds. *Emergency Medicine: Concepts and Clinical Practice*. 5th ed. St. Louis: Mosby, 2002.

McManus, W. F., and B. A. Pruitt, Jr. "Thermal Injuries," in D. V., Feliciano, E. E. Moore, and K. L. Mattox, eds. *Trauma*. 5th ed. New York: McGraw Hill, 2004.

Monafo, W. W. "Initial Management of Burns." *New England Journal of Medicine335* (1996): 1581–1586.

Uman, Martin A. *All About Lightning*. Mineola, N.Y.: Dover Publications, 1987.

On the Web

Visit Brady's Paramedic Website at **www.bradybooks.com/paramedic**.

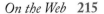

Musculoskeletal Trauma

Objectives

After reading this chapter, you should be able to:

1. Describe the incidence, morbidity, and mortality of musculoskeletal injuries. (pp. 218–219)
2. Discuss the anatomy and physiology of the muscular and skeletal systems. (pp. 219–233)
3. Predict injuries based on the mechanism of injury, including: (pp. 233–239)
   ★ Direct
   ★ Indirect
   ★ Pathological
4. Discuss the types of musculoskeletal injuries, including:
   ★ Fractures (open and closed) (pp. 235–238)
   ★ Dislocations/fractures (p. 235)
   ★ Sprains (p. 235)
   ★ Strains (p. 235)
5. Describe the "six Ps" of musculoskeletal injury assessment. (pp. 243–244)
6. List the primary signs and symptoms of extremity trauma. (pp. 241–245)
7. List other signs and symptoms that can indicate less obvious extremity injury. (pp. 244–246)
8. Discuss the need for assessment of pulses, motor function, and sensation before and after splinting. (p. 249)
9. Identify the circumstances requiring rapid intervention and transport when dealing with musculoskeletal injuries. (pp. 241–242)
10. Discuss the general guidelines for splinting. (pp. 247–253)
11. Explain the benefits of the application of cold and heat for musculoskeletal injuries. (pp. 254, 263)

12. Describe age-associated changes in the bones. (pp. 238–239)

13. Discuss the pathophysiology, assessment findings, and management of open and closed fractures. (pp. 235–238, 241–246, 246–253)

14. Discuss the relationship between the volume of hemorrhage and open or closed fractures. (pp. 242–243, 254–255)

15. Discuss the indications and contraindications for use of the pneumatic anti-shock garment (PASG) in the management of fractures. (p. 255)

16. Describe the special considerations involved in femur fracture management. (pp. 255–256)

17. Discuss the pathophysiology, assessment findings, and management of dislocations. (pp. 235, 253–254, 259–263)

18. Discuss the out-of-hospital management of dislocations/fractures, including splinting and realignment. (pp. 253–263)

19. Explain the importance of manipulating a knee dislocation/fracture with an absent distal pulse. (pp. 247–248, 253, 259–260)

20. Describe the procedure for reduction of a shoulder, finger, or ankle dislocation/fracture. (pp. 260–263)

21. Discuss the pathophysiology, assessment findings, and management of sprains, strains, and tendon injuries. (pp. 235, 263)

22. Differentiate among musculoskeletal injuries based on the assessment findings and history. (pp. 241–246)

23. Given several preprogrammed and moulaged musculoskeletal trauma patients, provide the appropriate scene size-up, initial assessment, rapid trauma or focused physical exam and history, detailed exam, and ongoing assessment and provide appropriate patient care and transportation. (pp. 218–266)

Key Terms

abduction, p. 223
adduction, p. 223
amphiarthroses, p. 222
appendicular skeleton, p. 225
arthritis, p. 240
articular surface, p. 221
axial skeleton, p. 225
bursa, p. 224
bursitis, p. 240
calcaneus, p. 228
callus, p. 240
cancellous, p. 221
carpal bones, p. 227
cartilage, p. 222
circumduction, p. 223
clavicle, p. 226
closed fracture, p. 236
comminuted fracture, p. 238

cramping, p. 234
devascularization, p. 220
diaphysis, p. 220
diarthroses, p. 222
dislocation, p. 235
epiphyseal fracture, p. 238
epiphyseal plate, p. 221
epiphysis, p. 221
fasciculus, p. 229
fatigue, p. 234
fatigue fracture, p. 238
femur, p. 228
fibula, p. 228
gout, p. 241
greenstick fracture, p. 238
hairline fracture, p. 236
haversian canals, p. 220
humerus, p. 226
iliac crest, p. 227
ilium, p. 227

impacted fracture, p. 238
innominate, p. 227
insertion, p. 229
ischial tuberosity, p. 227
ischium, p. 227
joint, p. 222
ligaments, p. 223
malleolus, p. 228
medullary canal, p. 221
metacarpals, p. 227
metaphysis, p. 221
metatarsal, p. 228
oblique fracture, p. 238
olecranon, p. 226
open fracture, p. 236
opposition, p. 229
origin, p. 229
osteoarthritis, p. 240
osteoblast, p. 220
osteoclast, p. 220

Case Study

The dispatch center sends Rescue 201 and the assigned paramedics, Mark and Steffany, to an adult care center for a patient who has fallen down a flight of stairs. Upon arrival, the paramedics find the patient lying on the ground. The resident director explains that Mary Herman, a 91-year-old female resident, tripped and fell down three or four steps while walking out of the building on the way to the cafeteria. Mary complains of moderate pain to her right thigh and lower back. She denies dizziness, nausea, or any other symptoms either now or prior to the fall. She denies striking her head or other injury. Physical assessment by the paramedics reveals pain and tenderness to the right thigh, crepitus, the foot externally rotated, and instability to the hip joint. Both the patient and the nursing staff report that Mrs. Herman has had few medical problems. She has no known allergies, and her medications include a daily vitamin and an aspirin.

Evaluation of vital signs reveals a blood pressure of 120/90, a pulse of 90, and respirations of normal depth at a rate of 22 per minute. Mark, the senior paramedic, applies manual spinal immobilization and places the patient on 12 Lpm of oxygen via nonrebreather mask. The pulse oximeter shows a saturation of 97 percent, and the ECG shows a sinus rhythm at 90.

Next, Mark and Steffany move Mrs. Herman to a spine board via an orthopedic stretcher. They place a folded blanket between her legs, maintain her head slightly off the board, pad under the body spaces, and, gently but firmly, strap her to the spine board. They apply a CID and secure it, along with Mary's head, to the spine board. Once they have loaded the patient into the ambulance, they start an intravenous line, hang a lactated Ringer's drip, and set it to run at a to-keep-open rate. A dextrose stick indicates the patient's glucose to be 110 mg/dL. The paramedics transport her uneventfully to the emergency department. There, x-rays confirm a hip fracture. Due to her age, Mrs. Herman will spend several days in the hospital and then several months in rehabilitation.

INTRODUCTION TO MUSCULOSKELETAL TRAUMA

Incidences of musculoskeletal injury are second in frequency only to soft-tissue injuries in trauma.

In trauma, incidences of musculoskeletal injury are second in frequency only to soft-tissue injuries. They usually result from application of significant direct or transmitted blunt kinetic forces. Skeletal or muscular injuries may also occasionally result from penetrating mechanisms of injury. Millions of Americans sustain musculoskeletal injuries each year from a variety of sources including sports injuries, motor vehicle crashes, falls, and acts of violence. These incidents can cause a variety of injuries to the body's bones, cartilage, ligaments, muscles, or tendons. While injuries to the upper extremities can be painful and sometimes debilitating, they rarely threaten life. Lower extremity injuries, however, are generally associated with a greater magnitude of force and greater secondary blood loss and, thus, more often constitute threats to life or limb. In addition, the same forces responsible for a musculoskeletal injury may damage the spine, internal organs, nerves, and blood vessels, causing serious problems throughout the body. In fact, most patients (up to 80 percent) who suffer multisystem trauma experience significant musculoskeletal injuries.

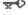

Up to 80 percent of patients who suffer multisystem trauma experience significant musculoskeletal injuries.

PREVENTION STRATEGIES

Stopping injury before it occurs—injury prevention—is the optimal way of dealing with musculoskeletal injuries. Strategies for preventing musculoskeletal injuries include application of modern vehicle and highway designs and safe driving practices, including the use of restraint systems. Auto crashes are the greatest single cause of musculoskeletal injuries, and improved vehicle safety has done much to reduce injury incidence and severity. Workplace safety standards developed by the National Institutes of Safety and Health (NIOSH) and enforced by the Occupational Safety and Health Administration (OSHA) have done much to reduce on-the-job injuries. These standards include criteria for proper footwear, scaffolding, fall protection devices, and the like. Sports injuries, which most commonly affect the musculature, joints, and long bones, account for a significant number of traumas. While protective gear, improved equipment design, and better conditioning of athletes has reduced injuries, the very nature of contact sports means that these activities remain a significant cause of injury. Household accidents and falls also account for many musculoskeletal injuries, and use of good safety practices—for example, proper footwear, well-designed railings, proper use of step ladders—can reduce injury incidence at home.

In musculoskeletal injuries, severe forces are directed to the structures of the body. These forces threaten homeostasis by causing disruption in the tissues responsible for moving the body within the environment and by causing injury in tissues and body systems beyond the muscles and skeleton. To respond properly to musculoskeletal emergencies, you must maintain and build upon the knowledge and skills of the EMT-Basic. In addition to those fundamentals, you need a deeper understanding of the structures and functions of the musculoskeletal system, a fuller knowledge of the progression of the injury process, and a complete grasp of the assessment and care procedures for these injuries.

ANATOMY AND PHYSIOLOGY OF THE MUSCULOSKELETAL SYSTEM

The musculoskeletal system is a complex arrangement of levers and fulcrums, powered by biochemical motors, that provides motion and support for the body. It consists of two distinct subsystems, the skeleton and the muscles. The skeleton is the human body's superstructure, while the muscles supply the power of motion to this superstructure, the organs, and the other body components. These subsystems also produce body heat, store essential salts and energy sources, and create the majority of blood cells for transporting oxygen and combating disease.

The musculoskeletal system is covered by the skin and subcutaneous tissue. These elements protect the skeleton and muscles, as well as other body systems, from trauma, fluid loss, infection, and fluctuations in body temperature. The skin also provides some cushioning for the skeletal components, as on the soles of the feet during walking.

Content

Functions of the Skeleton

Gives the body structural form
Protects vital organs
Allows for efficient movement
Stores salts and other materials for metabolism
Produces red blood cells

Some 20 percent of the total bone mass is replaced each year by the remodeling process.

haversian canals *small perforations of the long bones through which the blood vessels and nerves travel through the bone itself.*

osteocyte *bone-forming cell found in the bone matrix that helps maintain the bone.*

osteoblast *cell that helps in the creation of new bone during growth and bone repair.*

osteoclast *bone cell that absorbs and removes excess bone.*

perforating canals *structures through which blood vessels enter and exit the bone shaft.*

devascularization *loss of blood vessels from a body part.*

diaphysis *hollow shaft found in long bones.*

SKELETAL TISSUE AND STRUCTURE

As the body's living framework, the skeleton has a structure and design that permits it to perform a variety of functions and to repair itself as needed within limits. The skeleton is a complex, living system of cells, salt deposits, protein fibers, and other specialized elements. It serves five important purposes:

★ It gives the body its structural form.
★ It protects the vital organs.
★ It allows for efficient movement despite the forces of gravity.
★ It stores many salts and other materials needed for metabolism.
★ It produces the red blood cells used to transport oxygen.

Although the skeleton is not often thought of as alive, it is exactly that. Its cells live within a matrix of protein fibers and salt deposits. These living cells constantly change the structure and dynamics of the human frame. In fact, 20 percent of the total bone mass (salts, protein fiber, and bone cells) is replaced each year by the remodeling process.

BONE STRUCTURE

The structure of a typical bone consists of numerous aligned cylinders of bone. Minute blood vessels travel lengthwise along the bone through small tubes, called **haversian canals.** These blood vessels are surrounded by layers of salts deposited in collagen fibers. Bone cells called **osteocytes** are trapped within the matrix and maintain the collagen and the calcium, phosphate, carbonate, and other salt crystals. Other bone cells, osteoblasts and osteoclasts, build or dissolve these salt deposits as necessary. **Osteoblasts** lay down new bone in areas of stress during growth and during the bone repair cycle. **Osteoclasts** dissolve bone structures that are not carrying the pressures of articulation and support, or when the body requires more salts for electrolyte balance. These three types of bone cells maintain a dynamic and efficient structure for supporting and moving the body.

A continuous blood supply brings oxygen and nutrients to the bones and removes carbon dioxide and waste products from them. The blood vessels enter and exit the bone shaft through **perforating canals** and distribute blood to both the bone tissue and the structures located within the medullary canal of the shaft and bone ends. As with any other body tissue, bone tissue becomes ischemic and will eventually die if the blood supply is reduced or cut off. The bone does not show evidence of such degeneration for quite some time, and certainly not during prehospital emergency care. However, the long-term effects of **devascularization** may result in loss of bony integrity and failure of the bone to support weight or forces.

The long bones, such as those of the forearm (humerus) and thigh (femur), best demonstrate the organization of bone tissue into structural body elements (Figure 7-1 ■). The major areas and tissues of the long bones include the diaphysis, the epiphysis, the metaphysis, the medullary canal, the periosteum, and the articular cartilage.

The Diaphysis

The **diaphysis** is the central portion or shaft of the long bone. It consists of a very dense and relatively thin layer of compact bone. Because of its tubular structure, the diaphysis efficiently supports weight yet is relatively light. While the design of the bone shaft enables it to carry weight well, lateral forces may cause the shaft to break rather easily.

The Epiphysis

Toward the ends of the long bone, its structure changes. The bone's diameter increases dramatically, and the underlying thin, hard, compact bone of the shaft changes to a net-

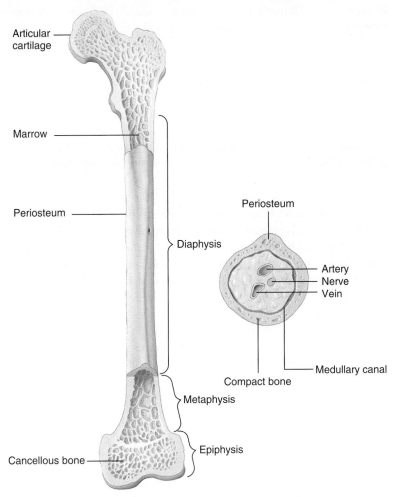

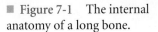

work of skeletal fibers and strands. This network spreads the stresses and pressures of weight bearing over a larger surface. This widened, articular end of the bone is called the **epiphysis.** The tissue within the epiphysis in cross-section resembles a rigid bony sponge and is called spongy or **cancellous** bone. Covering this network of fibers is a very thin layer of compact bone supporting the surface that meets and moves against another bone, the **articular surface.**

The Metaphysis

The **metaphysis** is an intermediate region between the epiphysis and diaphysis. It is where the diaphysis's hollow tube of compact bone makes the transition to the bone-fiber honeycomb of the epiphysis's cancellous bone. In this region is the **epiphyseal plate,** or *growth plate.* During childhood, cartilage is generated here and the plate widens. Osteoblasts from the end of the diaphysis deposit salts within the cartilage's collagen matrix to create new bone tissue. This results in the lengthening of the infant's and then the child's bone. During the growth period, the epiphyseal plate is also weaker than the rest of the bone and associated joints and is thus a frequent site of fractures in pediatric patients.

The Medullary Canal

The chamber formed within the hollow diaphysis and the cancellous bone of the epiphysis is called the **medullary canal.** The central medullary canal is filled with **yellow bone marrow** that stores fat in a semiliquid form. The fat is a readily available energy source the body can use quickly and easily. **Red bone marrow** fills the cancellous bone

epiphysis *end of a long bone, including the epiphyseal, or growth plate, and supporting structures underlying the joint.*

cancellous *having a lattice-work structure, as in the spongy tissue of a bone.*

articular surface *surface of a bone that moves against another bone.*

metaphysis *growth zone of a bone, active during the development stages of youth. It is located between the epiphysis and the diaphysis.*

epiphyseal plate *area of the metaphysis where cartilage is generated during bone growth in childhood. Also called the* growth plate.

medullary canal *cavity within a bone that contains the marrow.*

yellow bone marrow *tissue that stores fat in semiliquid form within the internal cavities of a bone.*

red bone marrow *tissue within the internal cavity of a bone responsible for the manufacture of erythrocytes and other blood cells.*

chambers of the larger long bones, the pelvis, and the sternum. It is responsible for the manufacture of erythrocytes and other blood cells.

The Periosteum

periosteum *the tough exterior covering of a bone.*

A tough fibrous membrane called the **periosteum** covers the exterior of the diaphysis. With extensive vasculature and innervation, it transmits sensations of pain when the bone fractures and then initiates the bone repair cycle. Blood vessels and nerves penetrate both the periosteum and compact bone by traveling through the small perforating canals. Tendons intermingle with the collagen fibers of the periosteum and with the collagen fibers of the bony matrix to form strong attachments.

Cartilage

cartilage *connective tissue providing the articular surfaces of the skeletal system.*

A layer of connective tissue called **cartilage** is a continuous collagen extension of the underlying bone and covers a portion of the epiphyseal surface. It is a smooth, strong, and flexible material that functions as the actual surface of articulation between bones. Cartilage is very slippery and somewhat compressible. It permits relatively friction-free joint movement and absorbs some of the shock associated with activity, such as walking.

Bones are classified according to their general shape.

Bones are classified according to their general shape. Those previously described are considered long bones and include the humerus, radius, ulna, tibia, fibula, metacarpals (hand), metatarsals (foot), and phalanges (fingers and toes). The bones of the wrists and ankles, the carpals and tarsals, are short bones. The bones of the cranium, sternum, ribs, shoulder, and pelvis are classified as flat. Irregularly shaped bones include the bones of the vertebral column and the facial bones. Another special type of bone is the **sesamoid bone,** a bone that grows within tendinous tissue; one example is the kneecap, also called the patella.

sesamoid bone *bone that forms in a tendon.*

joint *area where adjacent bones articulate.*

JOINT STRUCTURE

Bones move at, and are held together by, a relatively sophisticated structure called a **joint.** There are three basic types of joints, which are classified by the amount of movement they permit.

synarthroses *joints that do not permit movement.*

Synarthroses are immovable joints, such as the sutures of the skull or the juncture between the jaw and the teeth (which is called a gomphosis). **Amphiarthroses** are joints that allow some very limited movement. Examples include the joints between the vertebrae and between the sacrum and the ilium of the pelvis. **Diarthroses,** or **synovial joints,** permit relatively free movement. Such joints include the elbow, knee, shoulder, and hip.

amphiarthroses *joints that permit a limited amount of independent motion.*

diarthroses *synovial joints.*

synovial joint *type of joint that permits the greatest degree of independent motion.*

Diarthroses are divided into three categories of joints based on the movements they allow (Figure 7-2 ■). These include:

★ Monaxial joints

Hinge joints permit bending in a single plane. Examples include the knees, elbows, and fingers.

Pivot joints are characterized by the articulation between the atlas (the first cervical vertebrae) and the axis of the spine. They allow the head to rotate through about 180 degrees of motion.

★ Biaxial joints

Condyloid, or gliding, joints provide movement in two directions. They are located at the joints of carpal bones in the wrist and between the clavicle and sternum.

Ellipsoidal joints provide a sliding motion in two planes, as between the wrist and the metacarpals.

Review

Types of Joints

Synarthroses—immovable
Amphiarthroses—very limited movement
Diarthroses (synovial joints)—relatively free movement
  Monaxial
  Biaxial
  Triaxial

Content

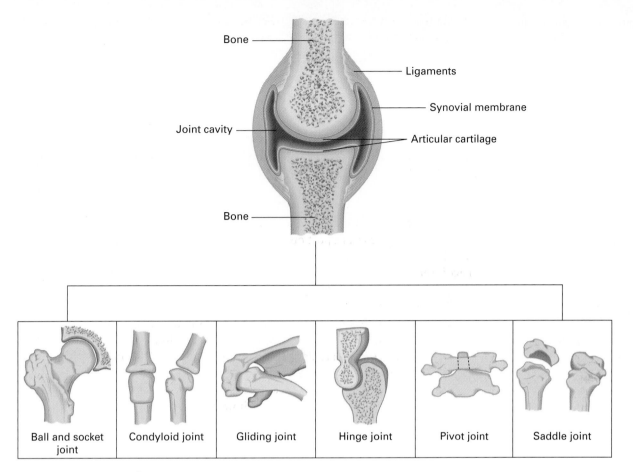

Bone

Ligaments

Synovial membrane

Joint cavity

Articular cartilage

Bone

| Ball and socket joint | Condyloid joint | Gliding joint | Hinge joint | Pivot joint | Saddle joint |

■ Figure 7-2   Types of joints.

Saddle joints allow for movement in two planes at right angles to each other. Examples are the joints at the bases of the thumbs.

★ Triaxial joints

Ball-and-socket joints permit full motion in a cone of about 180 degrees and allow a limb to rotate. Examples include the hip and shoulder.

These joints permit various types of motion. Flexion/extension is the bending motion that reduces/increases the angle between articulating elements. **Adduction/abduction** is the movement of a body part toward/away from the midline. Rotation refers to a turning along the axis of a bone or joint. **Circumduction** refers to movement through an arc of a circle.

Ligaments

Ligaments are bands of connective tissue that hold bones together at joints (Figure 7-3 ■). They stretch and permit motion at the joint while holding the bone ends firmly in position. The ends of the ligaments attach to the joint ends of each of the associated bones. Ligaments surround the articular region and cross it at many oblique angles. This arrangement ensures that the joint is held together firmly but flexibly enough to permit movement through a designed range of motion.

Joint Capsule

The ligaments surrounding a joint form what is known as the synovial, or joint, capsule (Figure 7-4 ■). This chamber holds a small amount of fluid to lubricate the articular

adduction   *movement of a body part toward the midline.*

abduction   *movement of a body part away from the midline.*

circumduction   *movement at a synovial joint where the distal end of a bone describes a circle but the shaft does not rotate.*

ligaments   *bands of connective tissue that connect bone to bone and hold joints together.*

■ Figure 7-3   Ligaments hold bones together at a joint.

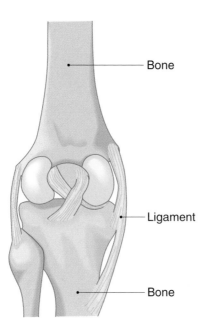

Bone

Ligament

Bone

■ Figure 7-4   Structure of a joint.

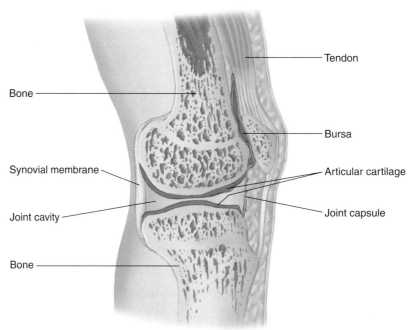

Tendon

Bone

Bursa

Synovial membrane

Articular cartilage

Joint cavity

Joint capsule

Bone

synovial fluid   *substance that lubricates synovial joints.*

bursa   *sac containing synovial fluid that cushions adjacent structures.*

surfaces. This oily, viscous substance, known as **synovial fluid,** assists joint motion by reducing friction. Its lubrication reduces friction to about one fifth that of two pieces of ice sliding together. Small sacs filled with synovial fluid, known as **bursae,** are also located between tendons and ligaments or cartilage in the elbows, knees, and other joints to reduce friction and absorb shock. Synovial fluid flows into and out of the articular cartilage as the joint undergoes pressure and movement. The cartilage acts like a sponge, pushing out fluid as it is compressed and drawing in fluid when it is relaxed. This movement of synovial fluid circulates oxygen, nutrients, and waste products to and from the joint cartilage.

SKELETAL ORGANIZATION

The human skeleton is made up of approximately 206 bones (Figure 7-5 ■). These bones form two major divisions, the axial and the appendicular skeletons.

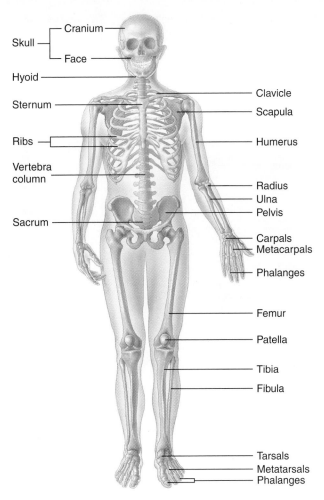

■ Figure 7-5 The human skeleton.

Skull — Cranium
— Face

Hyoid

Sternum

Ribs

Vertebra column

Sacrum

Clavicle

Scapula

Humerus

Radius
Ulna
Pelvis

Carpals
Metacarpals

Phalanges

Femur

Patella

Tibia

Fibula

Tarsals
Metatarsals
Phalanges

The **axial skeleton** consists of the bones of the head, thorax, and spine. These bones form the axis of the body, protect the elements of the central nervous system, and make up the thoracic cage, which is the dynamic housing for respiration. The components of the axial skeleton are discussed in Chapter 8, "Head, Facial, and Neck Trauma"; Chapter 9, "Spinal Trauma"; and Chapter 10, "Thoracic Trauma."

The **appendicular skeleton** consists of the bones of the upper and lower extremities, including both the shoulder girdle and the pelvis, and excepting the sacrum. These bones provide the structure for the extremities and permit the major articulations of the body. Extremity long bones are similar in design and structure. Both upper and lower extremities are affixed to the axial skeleton and articulate with joints supported by several bones. Each of these extremities has a single long bone proximally and paired bones distally. The terminal member, the hand or foot, is made up of numerous bones with differing purposes, yet parallel designs.

Upper Extremity

Each upper extremity (Figure 7-6 ■) consists of a shoulder girdle, arm, forearm, and hand. The shoulder is composed of the clavicle and scapula, which sit high on the posterior and lateral thoracic cage. The **scapula** is a triangular bone buried within the musculature of the upper back. It is basically a flat plate, called the body, with three major irregular outgrowths. The coracoid and acromion processes are protuberances for muscular attachments. The glenoid process provides the glenoid fossa, a shallow socket that accepts the head of the humerus. The scapula moves freely over the posterior thorax,

axial skeleton *bones of the head, thorax, and spine.*

appendicular skeleton *bones of the extremities, shoulder girdle, and pelvis (excepting the sacrum).*

scapula *triangular bone buried within the musculature of the upper back.*

■ Figure 7-6   The upper extremities.

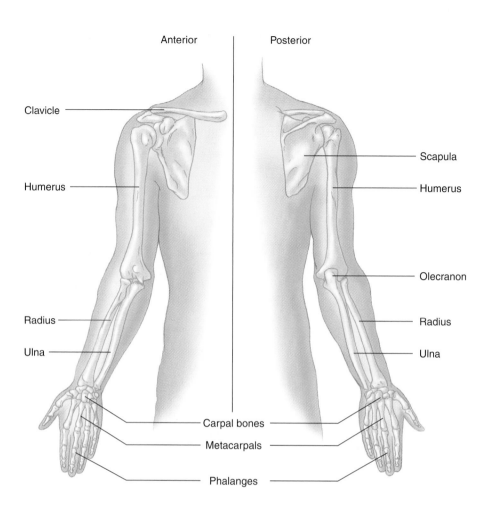

Anterior   Posterior

Clavicle

Humerus

Radius

Ulna

Scapula

Humerus

Olecranon

Radius

Ulna

Carpal bones

Metacarpals

Phalanges

clavicle *bone that holds the scapula and shoulder joint at a fixed distance from the sternum and permits the shoulder to move up and down (shrug).*

humerus *the single bone of the proximal upper extremity.*

radius *bone on the thumb side of the forearm.*

ulna *bone on the little finger side of the forearm.*

olecranon *proximal end of the ulna.*

providing some of the shoulder's large range of motion. The muscular upper back effectively protects the scapula from fracture in all but the most direct and severe trauma.

The **clavicle** articulates with the acromion of the scapula and the manubrium of the sternum. It is not as well protected as the scapula and is, in fact, the most commonly fractured bone of the human body. It holds the scapula and shoulder joint at a fixed distance from the sternum. The clavicle permits the shoulder to move up and down (shrug) while somewhat restricting anterior and posterior motion. The shoulder joint is one of the most mobile in the body. It permits humerus rotation through about 60 degrees and permits circumduction of the limb through 180 degrees.

The **humerus** is the single bone of the proximal upper extremity (the region properly referred to as the arm). Its rounded or surgical head articulates with the glenoid fossa of the scapula proximally. The head is connected to the humeral shaft by the anatomical neck, which also acts as the terminal end of the articular capsule. Two protuberances, the greater and lesser tuberosities, provide places of attachment for tendons and form the superior portion of the humerus. They, and the anatomical neck and surgical head, are connected to the humerus shaft by the surgical neck, a frequent location of fracture. Distally, the humerus shaft widens into the lateral and medial condyles and articulates with the radius and ulna at the elbow.

The **radius** and **ulna** form the forearm. The radius is on the thumb side of the forearm while the ulna is on the little finger side. They move in conjunction with the humerus and with each other. This biaxial articulation allows the distal forearm to rotate palm up (supination) or palm down (pronation). This articulation simultaneously permits the folding of the elbow. The ulna's proximal end forms the bump of the elbow, known as the **olecranon.**

The radius and ulna articulate with the **carpal bones** of the wrist. The carpal bones, in turn, articulate with the long, thin **metacarpals** of the palm. The carpal bones, with their saddle, gliding, and ellipsoidal joints, provide the wrist with a high degree of flexibility.

The metacarpals articulate with the **phalanges** of the fingers. Each of the four fingers consists of three phalanges—the proximal, the middle, and the distal. The thumb has only two—the proximal and distal. The combination of these hinge, saddle, and ellipsoidal joints in the metacarpals and phalanges allows the fine motion and motor control of the hand and fingers.

Lower Extremity

Each lower extremity (Figure 7-7 ■) is similar in structure to the upper extremities and is made up of the pelvis, thigh, leg, and foot. The **pelvis** is a strong skeletal structure where the lower extremities attach to the body. It consists of two symmetrical structures, called the **innominates,** and posterior to and joining them, the sacrum. Each innominate is constructed from one large flat bone, the **ilium,** and two irregular bones, the **ischium** and **pubis,** all fused together. Joined anteriorly at the symphysis pubis, the innominates with the sacrum form the pelvic ring. This rigid ring is very strong and provides the basis for support and movement of the lower extremities as well as forming the bony base of the abdomen. Structural landmarks of the pelvis include the **iliac crests,** the lateral bony ridge that holds the belt, and the **ischial tuberosities,** the bony knobs on which we sit. The pubic bone forms the bony structure at the base of the inguinal area and is divided centrally by the symphysis pubis, the anterior joint between the two innominates. The juncture of the three components of the innominate bones forms the acetabulum, a hollow depression in the lateral pelvis. The acetabulum is the actual articular surface for the femur.

carpal bones *bones of the wrist.*

metacarpals *bones of the palm.*

phalanges *bones of the fingers and toes.*

pelvis *skeletal structure where the lower extremities attach to the body.*

innominate *one of the structures of the pelvis.*

ilium *large, flat innominate bone.*

ischium *irregular innominate bone.*

pubis *irregular innominate bone.*

iliac crest *lateral bony ridge that is a landmark of the pelvis.*

ischial tuberosity *one of the bony knobs of the posterior pelvis.*

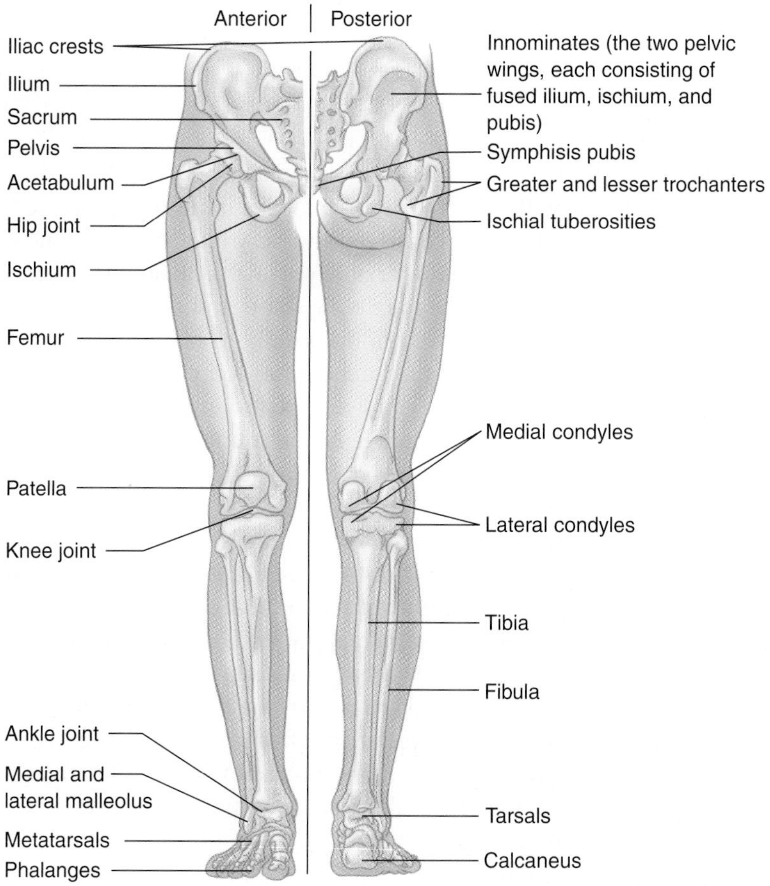

■ Figure 7-7　The lower extremities.

Anterior | Posterior

Iliac crests
Ilium
Sacrum
Pelvis
Acetabulum
Hip joint
Ischium
Femur
Patella
Knee joint
Ankle joint
Medial and lateral malleolus
Metatarsals
Phalanges

Innominates (the two pelvic wings, each consisting of fused ilium, ischium, and pubis)
Symphisis pubis
Greater and lesser trochanters
Ischial tuberosities
Medial condyles
Lateral condyles
Tibia
Fibula
Tarsals
Calcaneus

femur *large bone of the proximal lower extremity.*

The **femur** is the largest and strongest bone in the body. During the normal stress of walking, it often withstands pressures of up to 1,200 pounds per square inch along its diaphysis. Like the humerus, the femur is not a straight long bone. At its superior end, where the head meets the acetabulum, the femur makes an almost 90-degree turn. The head is supported by the surgical neck, a narrow shaft at almost a right angle to the uppermost aspect of the widened femoral shaft. This configuration permits the wide range of motion found in the joint and accounts for the femur's great strength. The greater and lesser trochanters, located at the widening of the femur at its upper end, form attachment points for tendons. The long femoral shaft spreads out for articulation as it meets with the tibia and forms a lateral and medial condyle. The patella, or kneecap, is a free-floating bone within the quadriceps tendon and is located just proximal to the actual knee joint.

tibia *the larger bone of the lower leg that articulates with the femur.*

fibula *the small bone of the lower leg.*

The **tibia** is the only distal bone to articulate with the femur. It pairs with the **fibula,** a smaller and much more delicate bone, just distal to the knee joint. Because of this arrangement, the tibia bears most of the weight supported by the lower extremity. The fibula's primary function is to add control to the placement and motion of the foot during walking. The two bones are held together by a fibrous interosseous membrane, and they articulate, one against the other, to allow the foot to rotate through about 45 degrees of motion.

malleolus *the protuberance of the ankle.*

calcaneus *the largest bone of the foot; the heel.*

metatarsal *one of the bones forming the arch of the foot.*

Both the tibia and fibula join the talus and calcaneus to form the ankle. The tibia forms the medial **malleolus** (protuberance of the ankle), while the fibula forms the lateral malleolus. The **calcaneus** is the largest bone of the foot and forms the heel. The talus articulates with the calcaneus and the tarsals. The tarsals, in turn, articulate with the **metatarsals,** all forming the arch of the foot. There are actually two arches in the foot; one longitudinal and one transverse. This arrangement distributes the stresses of supporting the entire body over all these bones. The metatarsals articulate with the phalanges of the foot, in a configuration parallel to that of the bones of the wrist and hand. The great toe has two phalanges (one proximal and one distal), while the other four toes each have three (proximal, middle, and distal).

BONE AGING

The bones, like all other body tissues, evolve during fetal development and after birth. Bone initially forms in the embryo as loose cartilaginous tissue. Before birth, the skeletal structure is predominantly cartilage, with very little ossified bone evident. This is one reason that infants are highly flexible yet unable to support themselves. Ossified bone begins to appear along the long bone shafts and then extends to the epiphyseal plates. It also develops within the epiphyses and grows outward to form the articular surfaces. Over time, the bone formation becomes complete to the epiphyseal plate, and the epiphysis is fully formed. The epiphyseal plate continues to generate cartilage, with the shaft and epiphyses growing from it. As the young adult reaches full height and the end of skeletal growth, the epiphyseal plates narrow, become bony, and cease to produce cartilage.

Bones of the young child remain flexible and do not reach maximum strength until maturation, which is usually completed by 18 to 20 years of age.

Associated with bone development and aging is the transition from flexible, cartilaginous bone to firm, strong, and fully ossified bone. Bones of the young child remain flexible and do not reach maximum strength until early adulthood. While each bone matures at a different time, almost all maturation is complete by 18 to 20 years of age.

After approximately the age of 40, the body begins to lose the ability to maintain bone structure.

Around the age of 40, the body begins to lose its ability to maintain the bone structure. It is unable to rebuild the collagen matrix and the deposition of salt crystals is reduced from what it was in earlier years. The effects of these changes appear very slowly. They include a very gradual diminution of bone strength, an increase in bone brittleness, a progressive loss of body height, and some curvature of the spine. The incidence of bone fractures also increases, especially at the high stress points of the lumbar spine and the femur's surgical neck.

Age-related changes in the skeletal system also affect other body systems. For example, the cartilage of the costal-condral joints and the costal bones (the ribs) becomes less flexible, which leads to shallower, more energy-consuming respirations. Also, the intravertebral disks lose water content and become less flexible, more prone to herniation, and narrower, thus shortening the trunk.

MUSCULAR TISSUE AND STRUCTURE

More than 600 muscle groups make up the muscular system (Figure 7-8 ■). As you might expect, a large number of EMS calls involve injuries to this extensive system. Injuries to it may result from excessive forces indirectly expressed to the muscles and their attachments or from direct trauma, either blunt or penetrating.

There are three types of muscle tissue within the body—cardiac, smooth, and skeletal (Figure 7-9 ■). Of these, the most specialized is the cardiac muscle comprising the myocardium. It contracts rhythmically on its own (automaticity), emitting an electrical impulse in the process (excitability), and passing that impulse along to the other cells of the myocardium (conductivity). In this way, the heart provides its lifelong rhythmic contraction and pumping. Cardiac muscle can also be classified according to its structure, which combines characteristics of both skeletal and smooth muscle and is thus called smooth-striated. (The particular properties of cardiac muscle tissue and the myocardium are discussed in Volume 3, Chapter 2, "Cardiology.")

The second muscle type is smooth, or involuntary, muscle, which is not under conscious control but functions at the direction of the autonomic nervous system. These muscles are found in the arterial and venous blood vessels, the bronchioles, the bowel, and many other organs. Smooth muscle contracts to reduce (or relaxes to expand) the lumen (diameter) of the vasculature, airways, or digestive tract. Smooth muscles have the ability to contract over a wide lateral distance, enabling them to accommodate great changes in length, such as those that occur during filling and evacuation of the bladder and contraction and dilation of the arterioles.

The final type of muscle tissue is skeletal (also called striated or voluntary). We have conscious control over these muscles, which are associated with the mobility of the extremities and the body in general. Skeletal muscles are also controlled by the nerves of the somatic nervous system. The skeletal muscles are the largest component of the muscular system, comprising between 40 and 50 percent of the body's total weight. They are the type of muscle most commonly traumatized.

Skeletal muscles lie directly beneath a protective layer of skin and subcutaneous fat. Because of their hunger for oxygen during activity, they have a more than ample supply of blood vessels. Individual muscle cells layer together to form a muscle fiber, many fibers layer together to form a muscle **fasciculus,** and fasciculi layer together to form a muscle body, such as the triceps. A muscle body has a strength of about 50 pounds of lift for each square inch of cross-sectional area.

fasciculus *small bundle of muscle fibers.*

Skeletal muscles attach to the bones at a minimum of two locations. These attachment points are called the origin and the insertion, depending upon how the bones move with contraction. The point of attachment that remains stationary as the muscle contracts is the **origin,** while the attachment to the moving bone is the **insertion.**

origin *attachment of a muscle to a bone that does not move (or experiences the least movement) when the muscle contracts.*

Muscles usually pair, one on each side of a joint. This configuration is essential because muscles can actively contract, not lengthen. One muscle moves the extremity in one direction by contraction, while the opposing (and relaxed) muscle stretches. The opposing muscle can then in turn contract, stretching the first muscle and moving the extremity in the opposite direction. This arrangement, called **opposition,** permits the straightening (extension) and then bending (flexion) of the limbs.

insertion *attachment of a muscle to a bone that moves when the muscle contracts.*

With several muscles attached to a joint with different origins and insertions, the body enjoys a wide variety of motions. In the shoulder, for example, the humerus can travel through several types and ranges of motion. These include moving the extremity

opposition *pairing of muscles that permits extension and flexion of limbs.*

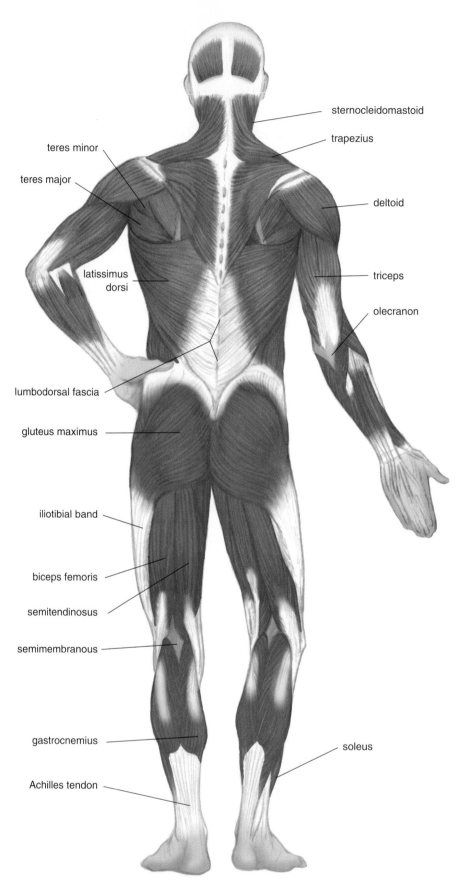

sternocleidomastoid

teres minor

teres major

trapezius

deltoid

latissimus dorsi

triceps

olecranon

lumbodorsal fascia

gluteus maximus

iliotibial band

biceps femoris

semitendinosus

semimembranous

gastrocnemius

soleus

Achilles tendon

■ Figure 7-8 The muscular system (posterior view).

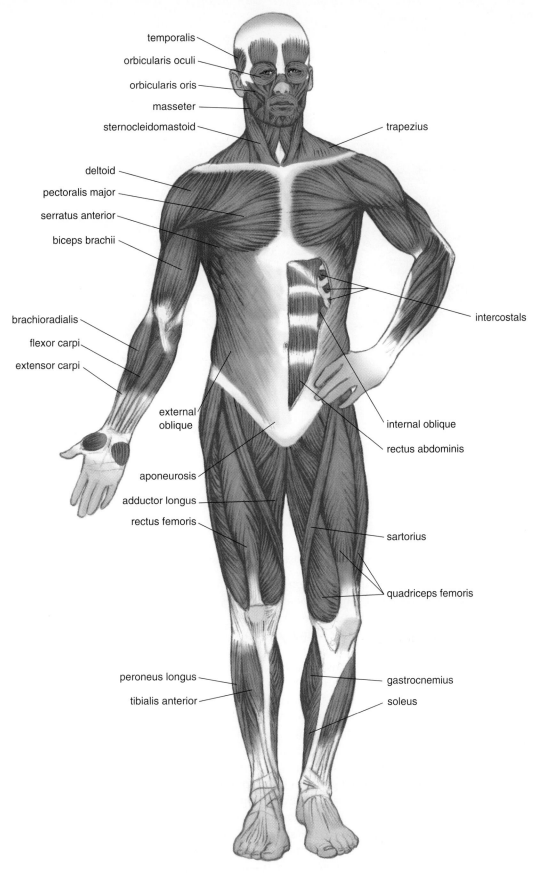

temporalis

orbicularis oculi

orbicularis oris

masseter

sternocleidomastoid

trapezius

deltoid

pectoralis major

serratus anterior

biceps brachii

intercostals

brachioradialis

flexor carpi

extensor carpi

external oblique

internal oblique

rectus abdominis

aponeurosis

adductor longus

rectus femoris

sartorius

quadriceps femoris

peroneus longus

tibialis anterior

gastrocnemius

soleus

■ Figure 7-8 (Continued)   The muscular system (anterior view).

■ Figure 7-9   Three types of
muscle tissue.

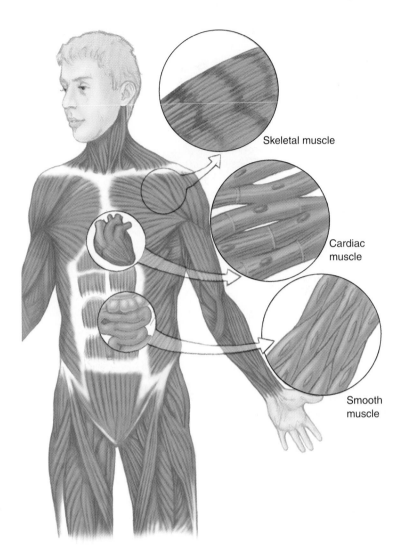

Skeletal muscle

Cardiac
muscle

Smooth
muscle

tendons   *bands of connective
tissue that attach muscle to bone.*

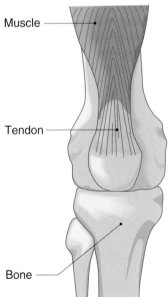

Muscle

Tendon

Bone

■ Figure 7-10   Tendons are the
bands of tissue that connect
muscle to bone.

away from the body (abduction) and toward the body (adduction), turning the
humerus (rotation) through about 60 degrees, and circling the entire extremity (circumduction) through a 180-degree arc.

Tendons are specialized bands of connective tissue that accomplish the attachment
of muscle to bone at the insertion and, in some cases, at the origin (Figure 7-10 ■).
These very fibrous ribbons, actually parts of the muscles, are extremely strong and do
not stretch. They are so strong that in some instances they will break an area of bone
loose rather than tear. The Achilles tendon demonstrates the strength of this particular
tissue. It can be felt as the band posterior to the malleoli of the ankle. This tendon is the
muscle-controlled cord that allows a person to lift the entire body weight when standing on the toes.

The forearm demonstrates the sophistication of the muscle-tendon relationship.
As the muscles controlling finger flexion contract, you can feel them tensing in the dorsal forearm. You can also visualize and palpate tendon movement in the distal forearm
and wrist as the fingers flex and extend. It is easy to appreciate the damage a deep transverse laceration can cause to the underlying connective tissues and their control of distal skeletal structures. Tendons are often classified by the action they perform when the
muscle associated with them contracts—for example, flexor or extensor, abductor or
adductor, and so forth.

The muscle tissue is responsible not only for the body's movement but also for the production of heat energy. A chemical reaction between oxygen and simple sugars produces the energy of motion. Heat, water, and carbon dioxide are by-products of this reaction. More than half the energy created by muscle motion is heat that helps maintain body temperature. The body then excretes water in the urine or sweat, expels carbon dioxide through respiration, and dissipates excess heat through the skin via radiation or convection. The body must constantly meet the requirements of muscle tissues for oxygen and nutrients and eliminate the waste products of those tissues, including heat.

Muscles are found in a condition of slight contraction called **tone.** Even while the body is at rest, the central nervous system sends some limited impulses to the muscle fibers causing a few to contract. These impulses give the muscles firmness and assure that they are ready to contract when the need arises. Muscle tone may be very significant in a well-conditioned athlete or absent (flaccid muscle tone) in someone with peripheral motor nerve disruption.

tone *state of slight contraction of muscles that gives them firmness and keeps them ready to contract.*

PATHOPHYSIOLOGY OF THE MUSCULOSKELETAL SYSTEM

The musculoskeletal injury process is a complicated one, resulting in much more damage than the disruption of an inert structural element of the body. Bone is alive and requires a continuous supply of oxygenated circulation. Bone lies deep within muscle tissue, and major nerves and blood vessels parallel it as they travel to the distal extremity. At points of articulation, there is a complex arrangement of ligaments, cartilage, and synovial fluid that holds the joint together while permitting a wide range of movement. Finally, the muscles attach and direct skeletal movement through the collections of fibers, fasciculi, and muscle bodies connected to the skeletal system by tendons. This complex arrangement of connective, skeletal, vascular, nervous, and muscular tissue is endangered whenever significant kinetic forces are applied to the extremities. If the forces are severe enough, they are likely to cause muscular, joint, or skeletal injury.

Bone is alive and requires a constant supply of oxygenated circulation.

MUSCULAR INJURY

Muscular injuries may result from direct blunt or penetrating trauma, overexertion, or problems with oxygen supply during exertion. These injuries include contusions, comparment syndrome, penetrating injuries, fatigue, strains, cramps, spasms, and strains. Muscular problems usually do not contribute significantly to hypovolemia and shock, with the exceptions of severe contusions with large associated hematomas and penetrating injuries with extensive hemorrhage.

Contusion

Severe trauma frequently crushes muscles between a blunt force and the skeletal structure beneath. This damages both the muscle cells and the blood vessels that supply them. Small blood vessels rupture, leaking blood into the interstitial spaces and causing pain, erythema, and then ecchymosis. Blood in the interstitial spaces and muscle cell damage set off the body's inflammatory response. Capillary beds engorge with blood, and fluid shifts to the interstitial space, leading to tissue edema. The injury may also cause blood to pool beneath tissue layers in a hematoma. In more massive body muscles, like those of the thigh, buttocks, calf, or arm, large volumes of blood may accumulate, contributing significantly to hypovolemia. A large hematoma or significant muscular edema will increase the diameter of the injured limb, especially as compared to the opposing uninjured limb. For the most part, however, signs of muscle injury remain hidden beneath the skin.

Review

Types of Muscular Injuries

Contusion
Compartment syndrome
Penetrating injury
Muscle fatigue
Muscle cramp
Muscle spasm
Muscle strain

Compartment Syndrome

Contusion, crush injury, and fracture may damage the soft tissue of the extremity and cause both internal hemorrhage and swelling. As the swelling and pooling of blood increase, pressure may build within the fascial compartment that contains them. This pressure first restricts capillary blood flow and compresses and damages nerves. If the pressure continues to build, it restricts and then halts venous return through the limb and ultimately stops arterial circulation. The first signs of this developing injury are tension (a feeling like a contracted muscle) within the limb and some loss of distal sensation, especially in the webs of the fingers or toes. The patient may complain of pain and appear more seriously injured than the mechanism of injury or outward signs might suggest. In addition, your moving of the patient's limb (passive extension) may elicit increased pain. Pulse deficit is a late sign of compartment syndrome.

Penetrating Injury

Deep lacerations may penetrate skin and subcutaneous tissues, thus affecting muscle masses and tendons below. Massive wounds involving a large percentage of a muscle body or those injuring or severing a tendon may reduce the distal limb's strength or render muscular control ineffective. When a tendon or muscle is cut, contraction of the opposing muscle moves the limb while the injured muscle/tendon is unable to return the limb toward the neutral position. Such injuries call for surgical intervention to identify and rejoin the damaged tendon or muscle body. These wounds may also introduce infectious agents, damage muscle tissue, and affect the muscle's blood supply. The resulting infection, ischemia, or a combination of the two may result in further tissue injury and poor healing.

Fatigue

fatigue *condition in which a muscle's ability to respond to stimulation is lost or reduced through overactivity.*

Muscle **fatigue** occurs as the muscles reach their limit of performance. Exercise draws down the muscle's oxygen and energy reserves and causes accumulation of metabolic byproducts. The cell environment becomes hypoxic, toxic, and energy deprived. Fewer and fewer muscle fibers are able to contract. The strength of the muscle mass diminishes, and further exertion becomes painful. Until adequate circulation restores oxygen and the muscle cells can replenish energy sources, the muscle fibers and muscle body remain weakened.

Muscle Cramp

cramping *muscle pain resulting from overactivity, lack of oxygen, and accumulation of waste products.*

Cramping is not really an injury, but a painful spasm of the muscle tissue. Muscle pain results when exercise consumes the available oxygen and energy sources and the circulatory system fails to remove metabolic waste products. The pain begins during or immediately after vigorous exercise or after the limb has been left in an unusual position for a period of time (obstructing circulatory flow). Cramping usually presents with a continuous muscle contraction (spasm). Changing the limb's position or massaging it may help return the circulation and reduce the pain. Once rest and adequate circulation restore the metabolic balance, the pain of a muscle cramp usually subsides.

Muscle Spasm

spasm *intermittent or continuous contraction of a muscle.*

In muscle **spasm,** the affected muscle goes into an intermittent (clonic) or continuous (tonic) contraction. The spasm may be firm enough to feel like the deformity associated with a fracture and can confound assessment. (The extreme of muscle spasm is rigor mortis, an anoxic, rigid, whole-body muscle spasm that occurs after death.) As with the cramp, the spasm usually subsides uneventfully with rest.

Strain

A **strain** occurs when muscle fibers are overstretched by forces that exceed the strength of the fibers. The muscle fibers then stretch and tear, causing pain that increases with any use of the muscle. The injury may occur with extreme muscle stress, as during heavy lifting or sprinting, or at times of fatigue, when only a limited number of fibers are in contraction. With a strain, the fibers are damaged without internal bleeding, edema, or discoloration. The site of injury is generally painful to palpation, and patients normally report pain that limits use of the affected muscle.

strain injury resulting from overstretching of muscle fibers.

JOINT INJURY

Joint injuries include sprains, subluxations, and dislocations. The following sections detail the pathologies behind each of these injuries.

Sprain

A **sprain** is a tearing of a joint capsule's connective tissues, specifically a ligament or ligaments. This injury causes acute pain at its site, followed shortly by inflammation and swelling. Ecchymotic discoloration occurs over time, but not usually during prehospital care. The tearing of ligaments weakens the joint. Continued use of the joint may lead to its complete failure. Sprains are classified, or graded, according to their severity, using the following criteria:

* ★ *Grade I.* Minor and incomplete tear. The ligament is painful, and swelling is usually minimal. The joint is stable.
* ★ *Grade II.* Significant but incomplete tear. Swelling and pain range from moderate to severe. The joint is intact but unstable.
* ★ *Grade III.* Complete tear of the ligament. Due to severe pain and spasm, the sprain may present as a fracture. The joint is unstable.

Subluxation

A **subluxation** is a partial displacement of a bone end from its position within a joint capsule. It occurs as the joint separates under stress, stretching the ligaments. The subluxation differs from the sprain in that it more significantly reduces the joint's integrity. The injured joint is painful and swells quickly, its range of motion is limited, and the joint is unstable. Hyperflexion, hyperextension, lateral rotation beyond the normal range of motion, or application of extreme axial force are common causes of subluxations.

Dislocation

A **dislocation** is a complete displacement of bone ends from their normal joint position (Figure 7-11 ■). The joint then fixes in an abnormal position with noticeable deformity. The site is painful, swollen, and immobile. This type of injury carries with it the danger of entrapping, compressing, or tearing blood vessels and nerves. Dislocation occurs when the joint moves beyond its normal range of motion with great force. By its nature, a dislocation has serious associated ligament damage and may involve injury to the joint capsule and articular cartilage.

BONE INJURY

The fracture is an involved process that ultimately disrupts the continuity of the bone. When extreme compressional forces or significant lateral forces exceed the tensile strength of a bone, the bone fractures.

Review

Types of Joint Injury

Sprain
Subluxation
Dislocation

sprain tearing of a joint capsule's connective tissues.

Review

Types of Sprains

Grade I—minor and incomplete capsule tear; painful, but minimal swelling; joint stable
Grade II—significant but incomplete tear; moderate to severe pain, swelling; joint intact but unstable
Grade III—complete tear; severe pain and spasm; joint unstable

subluxation partial displacement of a bone end from its position in a joint capsule.

dislocation complete displacement of a bone end from its position in a joint capsule.

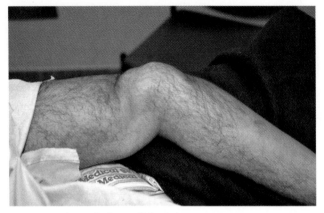

a. Presentation of a knee dislocation.

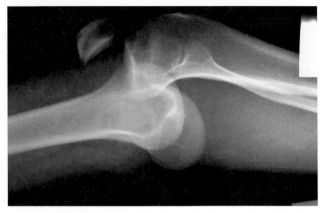

b. X-ray of the dislocation.

■ Figure 7-11   Knee dislocation.

A fracture may be caused by direct injury—for example, an auto bumper impacts a patient's femur or a high-powered rifle bullet slams into a patient's thigh and, then, femur. The cause of the fracture may also be indirect. This might occur when a bike rider is thrown over the handlebars and braces the fall with an outstretched upper extremity. In this case, the energy of impact is transmitted from the hand to the wrist, to the forearm, to the arm, to the shoulder, to the clavicle. The transmitted force fractures the clavicle and may cause internal injury to blood vessels and the upper reaches of the lung. For this reason, always analyze the mechanism of injury carefully, recognizing that kinetic forces may be transmitted and cause injury far from the point of impact. Remember, 80 percent of multisystem trauma cases have associated serious musculoskeletal injury.

As kinetic energy is transmitted to the bone and the bone fractures, the collagen, osteocytes, salt crystals, blood vessels, nerves, and medullary canal of the bone, as well as its periosteum and endosteum (the inner lining of the medullary canal), are disrupted. If the broken bone ends displace, they may further injure surrounding muscles, tendons, ligaments, veins, and arteries. The result is a serious insult to the limb structure.

Vascular damage may restrict blood flow to the distal limb, increasing capillary refill time, diminishing pulse strength and limb temperature, and causing discoloration and paresthesia (a "pins-and-needles" sensation). Nerve injury may result in distal paresthesia, anesthesia (loss of sensation), paresis (weakness), and paralysis (loss of muscle control). Muscle or tendon damage may interfere with the victim's ability to move the limb. If muscle tissue is badly damaged where fasciae firmly contain it, compartment syndrome may develop.

If the bone does not seriously displace and the forces causing fracture do not penetrate, the surrounding skin remains intact and the resulting injury is termed a **closed fracture.** If the sharp bone ends displaced by the forces causing the fracture or other subsequent motion of the limb lacerate through the muscle, subcutaneous tissue, and skin, the result is termed an **open fracture** (Figure 7-12 ■). An open fracture may also occur when a bullet travels through the limb and fractures the bone. Open fractures carry the risk of associated infection within the disrupted soft, bone, and medullary tissues. Such an infection may seriously reduce the bone's ability to heal. Where bones are located very close to the skin, as with the tibia (the shin), an open fracture can occur with relatively minimal bone displacement.

Surprisingly, some fractures may be relatively stable (Figure 7-13 ■). When the bone suffers a small crack that doesn't disrupt its total structure, the injury is termed a **hairline fracture.** This type of injury weakens the bone and is painful, but the bone remains in position, retaining some of its strength. Another type of relatively stable bone

Recognize that kinetic forces may be transmitted through the skeletal system and cause injury remote from the impact site.

closed fracture   *a broken bone in which the bone ends or the forces that caused it do not penetrate the skin.*

open fracture   *a broken bone in which the bone ends or the forces that caused it penetrate the surrounding skin.*

⊘ **Review**

Types of Fractures

Open
Closed
Hairline
Impacted
Transverse
Oblique
Comminuted
Spiral
Greenstick
Epiphyseal

hairline fracture   *small crack in a bone that does not disrupt its total structure.*

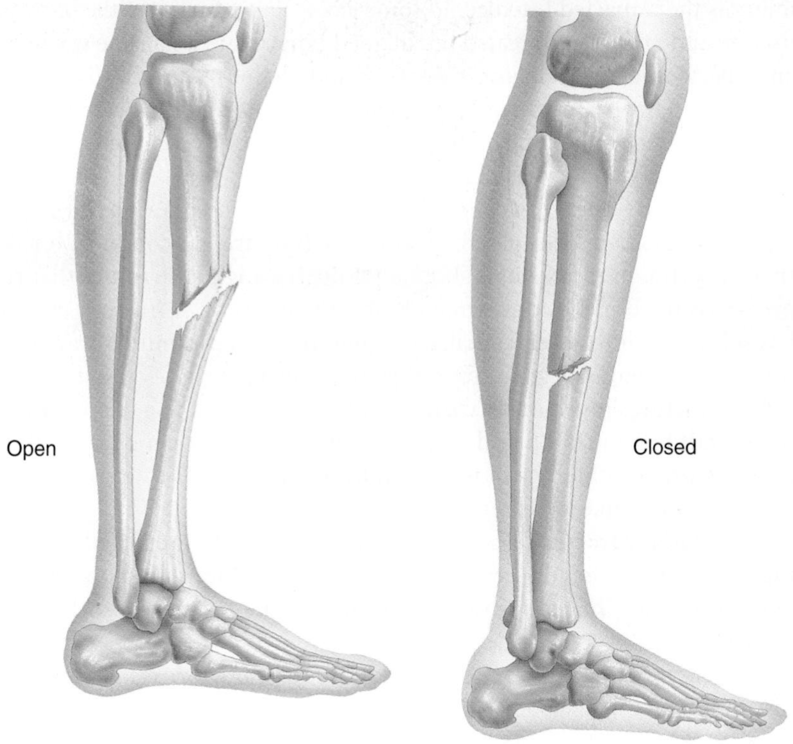

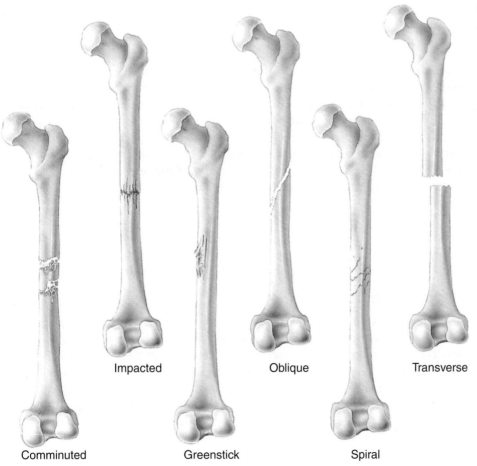

■ Figure 7-12   Open and closed fractures.

Open

Closed

■ Figure 7-13   Types of fractures.

Comminuted

Impacted

Greenstick

Oblique

Spiral

Transverse

impacted fracture *break in a bone in which the bone is compressed on itself.*

transverse fracture *a break that runs across a bone perpendicular to the bone's orientation.*

oblique fracture *break in a bone running across it at an angle other than 90 degrees.*

comminuted fracture *fracture in which a bone is broken into several pieces.*

spiral fracture *a curving break in a bone as may be caused by rotational forces.*

fatigue fracture *break in a bone associated with prolonged or repeated stress.*

greenstick fracture *partial fracture of a child's bone.*

epiphyseal fracture *disruption in the epiphyseal plate of a child's bone.*

osteoporosis *weakening of bone tissue due to loss of essential minerals, especially calcium.*

injury is the **impacted fracture.** In some cases of compression, the bone impacts upon itself resulting in a compressed but aligned bone. As in a hairline fracture, the bone in an impacted fracture remains in position and retains some of its original strength. The danger with both hairline and impacted fractures is that further stress and movement may fracture the remaining bone and displace the bone ends, increasing both the severity of the injury and its healing time.

There are several fracture types whose physical characteristics can be revealed only by x-rays. For example, the **transverse fracture** is a complete break in the bone that runs straight across it at about a 90-degree angle. A fracture that runs at an angle across the bone is considered an **oblique fracture.** A fracture in which the bone has splintered into several smaller fragments is a **comminuted fracture;** this type of fracture is often associated with crushing injuries or the impact of a high-velocity bullet. Fractures involving a twisting motion may result in a curved break around the bone shaft known as a **spiral fracture.** Spiral fractures can occur with twisting motions, as when a child's arm is rotated by an adult or when an adult's limb is pulled into machinery like an auger.

The **fatigue fracture** is associated with prolonged or repeated stress such as walking. The bone generally weakens and fractures without the application of great kinetic force. An example is the metatarsal fatigue fracture, also known as a march fracture.

A very infrequent but serious complication of fracture is fat embolism. The bone's disruption may damage adjacent blood vessels and the medullary canal. The injury may then release fat, stored in a semi-liquid form, into the wound site where it enters the venous system and travels to the heart. The heart distributes the fat to the pulmonary circulation where it becomes pulmonary emboli. Fat embolism is usually associated with severe or crush injuries or post-injury manipulation of larger long bone fractures.

Pediatric Considerations

The bones of infants, young children, and, to a degree, older children contain a greater percentage of cartilage than those of adults and are still growing from the epiphyseal plate. Pediatric patients thus often sustain different types of fractures than adults do.

The flexible nature of pediatric bones is responsible for the **greenstick fracture,** a type of partial fracture. The injury disrupts only one side of the long bone and remains angulated, resisting alignment due to the disrupted bone fibers on the fracture side. During the bone repair process, the injured side experiences more rapid growth than the other side. This results in increasing angulation of the bone as it heals. Surgeons often complete a greenstick fracture by breaking the bone fully, thereby assuring proper healing.

A child's bone grows at the epiphyseal plate, which forms a weak spot in the long bone. In pediatric trauma, this is a common site of the long bone disruption called an **epiphyseal fracture.** If the growth plate is disrupted, the disruption may lead to a reduction or halt in bone growth, a condition most commonly involving the proximal tibia.

Geriatric Considerations

The aging process causes several changes to the musculoskeletal system. A gradual, progressive decrease in bone mass and collagen structure begins at about the age of 40 and results in bones that are less flexible, more brittle, and more easily fractured. The bones also heal more slowly. The aging adult also loses some muscle strength and coordination, increasing the likelihood of skeletal injury. Fractures of the lumbar spine and femoral neck occur because of stress, often without a history of significant trauma.

Another age-related and more significant problem secondary to poor bone remodeling is called **osteoporosis.** Osteoporosis is an accelerated degeneration of bone tissue due to loss of bone minerals, principally calcium. It typically affects women more than men and becomes most serious after menopause. The condition leads to increases in bone structure degeneration, spinal curvature, and incidences of fractures.

Pathological Fractures

Pathological fractures result from disease pathologies that affect bone development or maintenance. Such problems may be caused by tumors of the bone, periosteum, or articular cartilage or by diseases that release agents that increase osteoclast activity and osteoporosis. Other diseases and infections can have the same impact on bone tissue and result in fracture, especially in older patients. Radiation treatment may also kill bone cells, resulting in localized bone degeneration, weakened bones, and fractures. These fractures are not likely to heal well, if they heal at all.

GENERAL CONSIDERATIONS WITH MUSCULOSKELETAL INJURIES

The potential effects of trauma can be better anticipated when the skeletal structure and the musculature are examined together. It is important to note that long bones are smallest through the diaphysis and largest at the epiphyseal area, or joint. However, the external extremity diameter is greatest surrounding the midshaft due to the placement of skeletal muscle. This anatomical relationship is significant when looking at the potential for nervous or vascular injury.

Since there is limited soft tissue surrounding joints, joint fractures, dislocations, and—to a lesser degree—subluxations and sprains may cause severe problems beyond the direct injury. Any swelling, deformity, or displacement may compromise the nerve and vascular supply to the distal extremity. Fractures near a joint are more likely to compress or sever blood vessels or nerves. With shaft fractures, neurovascular injury is less likely, although manipulation of the fracture site or gross deformity may still endanger vessels and nerves running along the bone.

Because there is limited soft tissue surrounding joints, injuries there may cause severe problems beyond the direct injury because blood vessels and nerves may be affected.

Areas around the joints are further endangered because blood vessels supplying the epiphysis enter the long bone through the diaphysis. If a fracture close to the epiphysis displaces the bone ends, it may compromise this blood supply with devastating results. The distal bone tissue may die without adequate circulation, destroying the joint and its function.

Once injury occurs, the stability of the extremity is reduced. Any additional movement can increase pain, damage to soft tissues, and the possibility of vascular or nerve involvement. Even slight manipulation can cause internal trauma. For example, a fractured femur has bone ends that are about the size of a broken broom handle. If, during extrication, splinting, and patient transport, the bone ends move about within the soft tissue, the resulting damage may be much more severe than that which initially occurred with the fracture. Manipulation of the injury site may also increase the likelihood of introducing bone fragments or fat emboli into the venous system, causing pulmonary embolism.

Another complication associated with long bone fracture is muscle spasm induced by pain. In a long bone fracture, pain causes the surrounding muscles to contract. This contraction forces the broken bone ends to override the fracture site. The result, in the case of the femur, is two broom-handle-sized bones driven into the muscles of the thigh, causing a cycle of more pain, more spasm, and more damage.

BONE REPAIR CYCLE

The bone repair cycle is a complex process that results in almost complete healing. When trauma fractures a bone, the periosteum tears, as do local blood vessels, soft tissues, and the endosteum. Blood fills the injured area and congeals, establishing a red blood cell and collagen clot. This hemorrhagic clot is not very stable, but does begin the bone repair process. Osteocytes from the bone ends begin to multiply rapidly and produce osteoblasts. These osteoblasts lay down salt crystals within the collagen clot fibers. This establishes lengthening and widening regions of skeletal tissue from each disrupted bone end. Over time, the two growing ends join and form a large knob of cancellous bone, called the **callus,** that encapsulates the fracture site.

As the process continues, the deposition of salts and the increasing collagen fiber matrix strengthen the callus and stabilize the bone to near-normal strength. Then osteoclasts dissolve salt crystals and collagen in areas where stress is minimal, while osteoblasts lay down new collagen and salts in high-stress areas. Through this process, the bone is remodeled until it looks very much like it did before the injury. If a fracture occurs when a patient is young and the bone ends are well aligned, there may be little evidence to suggest an injury ever occurred. If the bone ends are misaligned or if the bone experiences stress, infection, or movement before it has a chance to heal properly, the injury site may never return to normal and may leave the person with some disability.

INFLAMMATORY AND DEGENERATIVE CONDITIONS

Patients suffering from inflammatory and degenerative conditions may complain of joint pain, tenderness, and fatigue. These patients may also have difficulty walking and moving, may require additional assistance with their normal daily activities, and may be prone to musculoskeletal injuries. Common inflammatory diseases of the musculoskeletal system include bursitis, tendonitis, and arthritis.

Bursitis

Bursitis is an acute or chronic inflammation of the bursae, the small synovial sacs that reduce friction and cushion ligaments and tendons from trauma. Bursitis may result from repeated trauma, gout, infection, and, in some cases, unknown etiologies. A patient with bursitis experiences localized pain, swelling, and tenderness at or near a joint. Commonly affected locations include the olecranon (elbow), the area just above the patella, and the shoulder.

Tendonitis

Tendonitis is characterized by inflammation of a tendon and its protective sheath and has a presentation similar to that of bursitis. Repeated trauma to a particular muscle group is a common cause of the condition, which usually affects the major tendons of the upper and lower extremity.

Arthritis

Arthritis is literally an inflammation of a joint. Three of the most common types of arthritis are osteoarthritis, rheumatoid arthritis, and gout (more formally known as gouty arthritis).

Osteoarthritis, which is also known as degenerative joint disease, is the most common type of connective tissue disorder. It is characterized by a general degeneration, or "wear-and-tear," of articular cartilage that results in irregular bony overgrowths. Signs and symptoms include pain, stiffness, and diminished movement in the joints. Joint enlargement may be visible, especially in the fingers. Predisposing factors for osteoarthritis include trauma, obesity, and aging.

Rheumatoid arthritis is a chronic, systemic, progressive, and debilitating disease resulting in deterioration of peripheral joint connective tissue. It is characterized by inflammation of the synovial joints, which causes immobility, pain, increased pain on movement, and fatigue. The disease occurs two to three times more frequently in

callus *thickened area that forms at the site of a fracture as part of the repair process.*

bursitis *acute or chronic inflammation of the small synovial sacs.*

tendonitis *inflammation of a tendon and/or its protective sheath.*

arthritis *inflammation of a joint.*

osteoarthritis *inflammation of a joint resulting from wearing of the articular cartilage.*

rheumatoid arthritis *chronic disease that causes deterioration of peripheral joint connective tissue.*

women than in men. In extreme cases, flexion contractures may develop due to muscle spasms induced by inflammation.

Gout is an inflammation in joints and connective tissue produced by an accumulation of uric acid crystals. It occurs most frequently in males who often have high concentrations of uric acid in the blood. Uric acid is a metabolism end-product that is not easily dissolved. Signs and symptoms of gout include peripheral joint pain, swelling, and possible deformity.

gout *inflammation of joints and connective tissue due to buildup of uric acid crystals.*

MUSCULOSKELETAL INJURY ASSESSMENT

With the majority of patients, fractures, dislocations, or muscular injuries only infrequently threaten life or seriously contribute to the development of shock. In most circumstances, a patient with an isolated fracture, dislocation, or trauma to muscular or connective tissue will receive complete assessment and management at the scene.

However, serious musculoskeletal injury is common in a patient who presents with other serious injuries. As you read earlier, energy is often transmitted from the point of impact along the skeletal system to the internal organs. Thus, when you discover a skeletal injury, always look for indications of the severity of the trauma forces and the possibility that the forces also caused internal injuries.

As with any trauma patient, the assessment process progresses through the scene size-up, the initial assessment, either the rapid trauma assessment or focused exam and history, the detailed physical examination when appropriate, and serial ongoing assessments. You will usually focus your attention on musculoskeletal injuries during the rapid trauma assessment or focused exam and history and then as part of the detailed physical exam.

When you discover a skeletal injury, always look for indications of the severity of the trauma forces and the possibility that the forces also caused internal injuries.

Any serious musculoskeletal injury suggests kinetic energy forces sufficient to cause spinal injury, so always consider spinal precautions.

SCENE SIZE-UP

Remember to assure scene safety and don the appropriate personal protective equipment before approaching any scene. Gloves are mandatory when dealing with open musculoskeletal wounds, but those wounds, by themselves, do not usually suggest the need for protective eyewear, mask, or gown. Since most musculoskeletal injuries result from trauma, analyze the mechanism of injury to anticipate the nature and severity of those injuries. Enhance your analysis of the mechanism of injury by talking with the patient, family members, and bystanders to identify what happened and how.

Never let the gruesome nature of a musculoskeletal injury distract you from identifying and caring for more subtle, but life-threatening injuries first.

INITIAL ASSESSMENT

It is imperative that assessment of the trauma patient begin with an evaluation of the patient's mental status and ABCs. During this initial assessment, you must also identify the potential for spinal injury and the need for spinal precautions. Remember, any serious musculoskeletal injury suggests kinetic energy forces sufficient to cause spinal injury, so always take spinal precautions with such an injury. Proceed with the initial assessment and assure that any life-threatening injuries are addressed before moving on in the assessment process. Never let the gruesome nature of a musculoskeletal injury distract you from performing a proper initial assessment and identifying and caring for life-threatening injuries first (Figure 7-14 ■).

Patients with musculoskeletal injuries are classified into four categories:

★ Patients with life- and limb-threatening injuries

★ Patients with life-threatening injuries and minor musculoskeletal injuries

★ Patients with non-life-threatening injuries but serious limb-threatening musculoskeletal injuries

✓ Review

Content

Classification of Patients with Musculoskeletal Injuries

Life- and limb-threatening injuries
Life-threatening injuries, minor musculoskeletal injuries
Non-life-threatening injuries, serious limb-threatening injuries
Non-life-threatening injuries, isolated minor musculoskeletal injuries

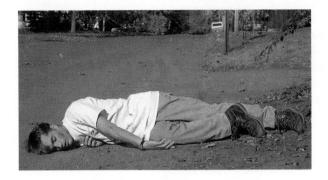

■ **Figure 7-14** As you begin assessment, examine the patient quickly for musculoskeletal injuries, but remember that they are not often life threatening.

★ Patients with non-life-threatening injuries and only isolated minor musculoskeletal injuries

Perform a rapid trauma assessment for those patients with possible life- or limb-threatening injuries. A patient without life threat but with serious musculoskeletal injury may receive the rapid trauma assessment or the focused exam and history, depending upon the mechanism of injury and the information you discover during the initial assessment. Provide patients presenting with isolated and simple musculoskeletal injuries with a focused exam and history, though you must remain watchful for any sign or symptom of more serious injury and the need for both a rapid trauma assessment and rapid patient transport to a trauma center.

RAPID TRAUMA ASSESSMENT

The rapid trauma assessment is performed on any patient with any sign, symptom, or mechanism of injury that suggests serious injury. While musculoskeletal injuries do not often cause life-threatening hemorrhage, remember that 80 percent of patients with serious multisystem trauma have associated musculoskeletal injury. When you have evidence of serious musculoskeletal injury, maintain a high index of suspicion for serious internal injury.

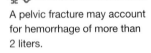

A pelvic fracture may account for hemorrhage of more than 2 liters.

Perform the rapid trauma assessment in a carefully ordered way, progressing through an evaluation of the head, neck, chest, and abdomen, and arriving at the pelvis. Pay particular attention to the possibility of pelvic fracture, because such an injury may account for hemorrhage of more than 2 liters. If no other signs of pelvic fracture exist, check the stability of the pelvic ring by directing firm pressure downward, then inward on the iliac crests, and then directing gentle downward pressure on the symphysis pubis. If the pressure reveals any instability or crepitus or elicits a response of pain from the patient, suspect pelvic fracture. Crepitus is a grating sensation felt as bone ends rub against one another. If you feel crepitus once, presume that bone injury exists and do not attempt to recreate the sensation. Consider the patient a possible candidate for rapid transport and fluid resuscitation.

A femur fracture may account for as much as 1,500 mL of blood loss.

In assessing the thighs, look for signs of tissue swelling and femur fracture. Each femur fracture may account for as much as 1,500 mL of blood loss. Evidence of this loss may be hidden within the tissue and muscle mass of the thigh, so compare one thigh to the other to evaluate swelling. If you find evidence of either pelvic or bilateral femur fracture, apply the pneumatic anti-shock garment (PASG), and inflate all compartments to a pressure that immobilizes the pelvis and the lower extremities. Monitor for the signs that the patient is compensating for blood loss, and consider both rapid transport and fluid resuscitation.

While fractures and muscular injuries of the extremities may not by themselves produce shock, they may significantly contribute to hypovolemia. Consider the effects of these injuries in your decision on whether to provide rapid transport or on-scene care. Further, fractures and dislocations may entrap or damage blood vessels or nerves, thus seriously threatening the future use of a limb. Quickly survey each limb and check the distal pulses, temperature, sensation (if the patient is conscious), motor function, and muscle tone.

Complete the rapid trauma assessment by gathering a patient history and a baseline set of vital signs (which may be done at the same time the physical assessment is being performed). If the rapid trauma assessment reveals a serious threat to life or limb, rapidly transport the patient to the nearest appropriate facility.

FOCUSED HISTORY AND PHYSICAL EXAM

The focused history and physical exam directs your attention to the injuries found or suggested during the initial assessment by the mechanism of injury and the patient's signs and symptoms. This step of the assessment process is performed for patients without life-threatening injuries and permits both assessment and care focused on isolated injuries.

Begin the focused physical exam by observing and inquiring carefully for signs and symptoms of fracture, dislocation, or other musculoskeletal injury in each limb with suspected injury (Figure 7-15 ■). Expose and visualize the entire limb by removing any restrictive clothing or cutting it away carefully. In doing so, avoid manipulation of any potential injury site. Inspect the injury site carefully to locate any deformities (angulation or swelling), discolorations (unlikely in the first minutes after the incident), and indications of soft-tissue wounds that suggest injury beneath. Any unusual limb placement, asymmetry, or inequality in limb length (when compared to the opposing limb) should also arouse suspicion of musculoskeletal injury. Consider the possibility that any open wounds communicate with an associated fracture or dislocation. Observe for any contamination or sign of the bone protruding. Question the patient about pain, pain with attempted movement, discomfort, or unusual feeling or sensation. Also inquire about weakness, paralysis, paresthesia, or anesthesia. It may be helpful to think of the "six Ps" as a way to remember the key elements to be alert for when evaluating an extremity:

★ *Pain.* The patient may report this upon palpation (tenderness) or movement.

★ *Pallor.* The patient's skin may be pale or flushed, and capillary refill may be delayed.

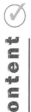

✓ Review

The Six Ps in Evaluating Limb Injury

Pain
Pallor
Paralysis
Paresthesia
Pressure
Pulses

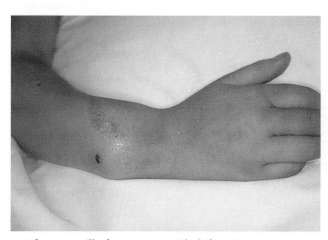

a. A fracture will often present with deformity.

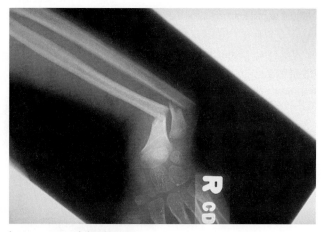

b. An x-ray of the fracture.

■ Figure 7-15 Presentation of a forearm fracture.

★ *Paralysis.* The patient may have inability or difficulty in moving an extremity.

★ *Paresthesia.* The patient may report numbness or tingling in the affected extremity.

★ *Pressure.* The patient reports a feeling of tension within the extremity.

★ *Pulses.* These may be diminished or absent in the extremity.

If you do not identify a specific injury, palpate the extremity for instability, deformity (swelling or angulation), crepitus, unusual motion (joint-like motion where a joint doesn't exist), muscle tone (normal, flaccid, or spasming), or any regions of unusual warmth or coolness. Palpate the entire anterior and posterior surfaces, then the lateral and medial surfaces. Your assessment must be gentle, yet complete. Record any abnormal signs. When assessing the feet, carefully evaluate the distal circulation. Assess pulses for presence and relative strength, and then compare bilaterally. Test the skin for humidity and warmth. Suspect circulatory compromise if capillary refill time is prolonged compared to the uninjured limb. Observe the skin for discoloration, noting any erythema, ecchymosis, or any abnormal hue (pale, ashen, or cyanotic). Approximate the level at which any deficit begins, and note any relation to possible extremity injury.

In a conscious and responsive patient, evaluate sensation and muscle strength distal to the injury (Figure 7-16 ■). Check tactile (touch) response by touching or stroking the bottom of the foot with the blunt end of a bandage scissors or other similar instrument. Ask the patient to describe the feeling. If the patient is responsive and if there is no indication that the limb is injured, ask the patient to push down with the balls of both feet (plantar flexion) against your hands. Then ask the patient to pull upward with the top of the feet (dorsiflexion), again against your hands. If you feel any unilateral or bilateral weakness or the patient reports any pain, document the finding on the prehospital care report and look for the cause. Check abnormal sensation and the patient's ability to wiggle the toes or fingers.

Assess for potential upper extremity injury in a manner similar to your assessment of the lower extremity. Expose, observe, question about, and then palpate the limb as previously described. Determine tactile response by using the back of the patient's hand. Test muscular strength by having the patient squeeze two of your fingers. Compare strength and sensation bilaterally, identify any deficit, and attempt to locate the cause. Evaluate the upper extremity and assure it is uninjured before you use it for blood pressure determination.

When the assessment of an extremity suggests injury, treat the limb as though a fracture or dislocation exists because the only definitive way to rule out these injuries is

---

⚡○ —————

When the assessment of an extremity suggests injury, treat the limb as though a fracture or dislocation exists.

■ Figure 7-16   Evaluate the distal extremity for pulse, temperature, color, sensation, and capillary refill.

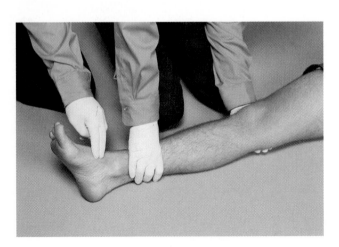

x-ray examination. Also note that splinting protects strains, sprains, and subluxations as well as fractures and dislocations from further injury. Treating a soft-tissue or muscular injury as a fracture or dislocation produces nothing more harmful than slight discomfort for the patient. Failure to immobilize an injury properly, however, may lead to additional soft, skeletal, connective, vascular, or nervous tissue damage and possibly cause permanent harm.

If possible, find the exact site of injury and determine if it involves a joint area or a long bone shaft. Form a clear visual image of the injury site in your mind so that you can describe the injury in the patient care report and to the receiving physician. Remember that the splinting device (e.g., a padded board splint for a wrist fracture) may hide the site from view, leaving the attending physician unable to determine what exists beneath it. A good description of the wound may delay the need to remove the splint to view the injury.

One complication of musculoskeletal injury to the extremities is compartment syndrome. This condition results from bleeding into, or edema within, a muscle mass surrounded by fasciae that do not stretch. The build-up of pressure then compresses capillaries and nerves, leading to local tissue ischemia and then necrosis, with some loss of distal sensation. A pulse deficit may be a very late finding in compartment syndrome. Suspect compartment syndrome in any patient who has any paraesthesia, especially in the webs between the medial toes or fingers; who has an extremity injury with a firm mass or increased skin tension at the injury site; or who has pain out of proportion to the nature of the injury or pain that increases when you move the limb (passive stretching). Also suspect compartment syndrome in any unconscious patient with a swollen limb. Compartment syndrome most often occurs in the forearm or leg.

During the physical exam, question the patient about the symptoms of injury. Assure that your verbal investigation is detailed and complete. Determine the nature and location of pain and tenderness or dysfunction. The patient's description of the fracture or dislocation event may also be helpful. The patient may state that he felt the bone "snap" or the joint "pop out." Determine if the bone snapped, thus causing the fall, or whether the fall caused the fracture. Evaluate for the amount of pain and discomfort the patient is experiencing with the injury. For example, an elderly patient may present with a fractured hip and limited pain, a presentation usually related to a degenerative disease and secondary fracture. These findings may suggest that you adopt a less aggressive approach to care for this patient, focusing upon the patient's comfort rather than upon traction splinting and shock care. Also identify the signs and symptoms of injury as well as pertinent patient allergies, medications, past medical history, last oral intake, and events leading up to the incident.

Compare the findings of your assessment to the index of suspicion for injury you developed during the scene size-up. If you have found less significant injury than you suspected, consider reevaluating the patient to assure that no injury has been overlooked. If you find a more significant injury, suspect other severe injury may have occurred elsewhere and expand your focused exam.

As you conclude the focused history and physical exam, identify all injuries found, prioritize them, and establish the order of care for them. Identify the extent to which each injury may contribute to hemorrhage and shock. Then prioritize the patient for transport. Taking these few moments to sort out what is wrong with the patient and to plan care steps will increase the efficiency of your patient care, reduce on-scene time, and ensure that the patient receives the proper care at the right time.

DETAILED PHYSICAL EXAM

After you have ruled out or addressed potential threats to the patient's life or limbs, attended to any serious problems, and assessed any suspected injuries, you may perform

Form a clear mental picture of the injury site and be able to describe it to the emergency physician.

 Review

Early Indicators of Compartment Syndrome

Feelings of tension within limb

Loss of distal sensation (especially in webs of fingers and toes)

Complaints of pain

Condition more severe than mechanism of injury would indicate

Pain on passive extension of extremity

Pulse deficit (late sign)

At the conclusion of the rapid trauma assessment or the focused exam, identify all injuries and prioritize them for care.

a detailed physical exam. You will most likely perform the detailed physical exam on the patient who is unconscious or has a lowered level of consciousness. The exam may be performed at the scene or, more likely, while en route to the hospital. The detailed physical exam is a search for the signs and symptoms of further injury. It is performed as a head-to-toe evaluation, looking specifically where you have not looked before and with enough care to identify any subtle indications of injury. Be alert for the signs and symptoms of internal or external injury or hemorrhage. Use the same assessment techniques for evaluating musculoskeletal injuries during the detailed physical exam that you employed during the rapid trauma assessment and focused history and physical exam.

ONGOING ASSESSMENT

During the ongoing assessment, be sure to ask about the patient's complaints and description of the musculoskeletal injury, because over time, the patient may display more significant and specific symptoms of injury and complain of other injuries masked earlier by the chief complaint.

The ongoing assessment focuses on serial measurement of the patient's vital signs, level of consciousness, and the signs and symptoms of the major trauma affecting the patient. For patients with musculoskeletal injuries, monitor distal sensation and pulses frequently. Remember to ask about the patient's complaints and description of the musculoskeletal injury, watching for any changes in the responses. As time passes and the effects of the "fight-or-flight" response wear off, the patient may display more significant and specific symptoms of injury. The patient may also begin to complain of other injuries masked earlier by the chief complaint and of other major pain or discomfort. If this occurs, provide a focused assessment on the area of complaint and modify your patient priorities as additional injuries are found.

SPORTS INJURY CONSIDERATIONS

Many of the musculoskeletal injuries you attend as an EMT-Paramedic are associated with sports activities. Activities such as football, basketball, soccer, baseball, in-line skating, skiing, snowboarding, bicycling, wrestling, hiking, and rock climbing often lead to injury for participants. When you are called to the scene of a sports injury, assess the mechanism of injury and determine whether there was a major kinetic force involved, a hyperextension or flexion injury, or a fatigue-type injury. Athletic injuries often affect major body joints like the shoulder, elbow, wrist, knee, and ankle. Injuries in these areas are especially troubling for patients because serious ligament damage might preclude future participation in a sport and limit limb usefulness. It is imperative that any potentially significant sports injury be attended to by an emergency department physician. The competitive natures of players, teammates, coaches, and athletic trainers may lead them to downplay injuries in order to keep an injured athlete in competition. Allowing an injured athlete to keep playing, however, places additional stress on the injury and may result in further, and more debilitating, damage.

Any potentially significant sports injury should be attended to by an emergency department physician.

MUSCULOSKELETAL INJURY MANAGEMENT

Management of musculoskeletal injuries is not normally a high priority in trauma patient care. It usually does not occur until after you have completed the initial assessment; stabilized the airway, breathing, and circulation; and finished the rapid trauma assessment. While the focus of care for the serious trauma patient is the current life threats, some protection for serious musculoskeletal injuries is provided by moving the patient as a unit (with axial alignment) and by packaging the patient for transport using the long spine board (see Chapter 9, "Spinal Trauma"). These techniques help you reduce the risks of aggravating musculoskeletal injuries, increasing hemorrhage, and worsening shock and patient outcome. However, do not let gruesome musculoskeletal injury distract you from the priorities of trauma management.

Fractures of the pelvis and, to a lesser degree, the femur can significantly contribute to hypovolemia and shock. These injuries deserve a high priority in patient care.

Other musculoskeletal injuries that merit a priority for care include those that threaten a limb, such as injuries with loss of distal circulation or sensation (most commonly joint injuries), and those that cause compartment syndrome (most likely leg or forearm injuries). You may prioritize other injuries by the relative size of the bone fractured or the body area involved and by the energy that was required to cause injury. Prioritize the patient's musculoskeletal injuries for care, then proceed with splinting and transport.

GENERAL PRINCIPLES OF MUSCULOSKELETAL INJURY MANAGEMENT

The objectives of musculoskeletal injury care are to reduce the possibility of any further injury during patient care and transport and to reduce the patient's discomfort. Accomplish these goals by protecting open wounds, positioning the extremity properly, immobilizing the injured extremity, and monitoring neurovascular function in the distal limb. In some cases, care involves manipulating the injury to reestablish distal circulation and sensation or simply to restore normal anatomical position for the patient expecting prolonged extrication or transport. In most cases, care for musculoskeletal injuries will also include application of a splinting device.

As you begin to care for a patient with musculoskeletal injuries, talk to him and explain what you are doing, why, and what impact it will have on the patient. Alignment and splinting will likely first cause an increase in pain followed by a significant reduction in it. By telling the patient of this in advance, you will increase confidence in both your intent to help and your ability to provide care.

Protecting Open Wounds

If there is any open wound in proximity to the fracture or dislocation, consider the fracture or dislocation to be an open one. Carefully observe the wound and note any signs of muscle, tendon, ligament, or vascular injury and be prepared to describe the wound in your report and at the emergency department. Cover the wound with a sterile dressing held in place with bandaging or a splint. Frequently, the attempts to align a limb, the splinting process, or the application of traction will draw protruding bones back into the wound. This is an expected consequence of proper care but must be brought to the attention of the attending emergency department physician.

Positioning the Limb

Proper limb positioning is essential to assure patient comfort, to reduce the chances of further limb injury, and to encourage venous drainage. Proper positioning is different with fractures and dislocations, although splinting with the limb in a normal anatomical position, the position of function, is beneficial for both.

Limb alignment is appropriate for any fractures of the midshaft femur, tibia/fibula, humerus, or radius/ulna. Alignment can be maintained by using the air splint, padded rigid splint, PASG, vacuum, or traction splint. Proper alignment of a fracture enhances circulation and reduces the potential for further injury to surrounding tissue. It is also very difficult to immobilize a limb with a fracture in an unaligned, angulated position because the fracture segments are short and buried in soft tissue. Perform any limb alignment with great care so as not to damage the tissue surrounding the fracture site. During the process, the proximal limb should remain in position while you bring the distal limb to the position of alignment using gentle axial traction. Stop the process when you detect any resistance to movement or when the patient reports any significant increase in pain.

Generally, you should not attempt alignment of dislocations and serious injuries within 3 inches of a joint. Only attempt to manipulate such injury sites if the distal circulation is compromised. In such a case, try to move the joint while another care

Review

Basics of Musculoskeletal Injury Care

Protecting open wounds
Proper positioning
Immobilizing the injury
Monitoring of neurovascular function

Stop realignment attempts when you detect any resistance to movement or when the patient reports any significant increase in pain.

Do not attempt alignment of dislocations and serious injuries within 3 inches of a joint.

provider palpates the distal pulse. If the pulse is restored, if you meet significant resistance to movement, or if the patient complains of greatly increased pain, stop the manipulation and splint the injured limb as it is. Be sure to transport the patient quickly, because a loss of circulation can endanger the future usefulness of the limb.

If you suspect a limb will remain dislocated for an extended period, as during lengthy transports or prolonged patient entrapments, consider reducing the dislocation. Apply a firm and progressive traction to the limb, which draws the dislocated ends away from each other and moves the joint toward normal positioning. When (and if) the bone ends "pop" back into position, assure there is a distal pulse and immobilize the limb in the position of function.

Proper positioning of injured limbs is important for maintaining distal circulation and sensation and increasing patient comfort. Deformities and extremes of flexion or extension put pressure on the soft tissues and may compress nerves and blood vessels. These positions also fatigue the surrounding muscles and increase the pain associated with the injury. By placing the uninjured joints of the limb halfway between flexion and extension in what is called the position of function, you place the least stress on the joint ligaments and the muscles and tendons surrounding the injury. Place the limb in the position of function whenever possible (Figure 7-17 ■). Note, however, that some injuries and some splinting devices commonly used for musculoskeletal injuries may preclude this positioning.

When practical, elevate the injured limb. This will assist with venous drainage and reduce the edema associated with musculoskeletal injury.

Immobilizing the Injury

The aim in immobilizing musculoskeletal injuries is to prevent further injury caused by the movement of broken bone ends and bone ends dislodged from a joint and by further stress placed on muscles, ligaments, or tendons already injured by a strain, sprain, subluxation, dislocation, or fracture. This immobilization is usually accomplished through the use of a splinting device.

Since most long bones lie buried deep within the musculature of the extremities, it is very difficult to immobilize them directly. Hence, we immobilize the joint above and the joint below the injury, regardless of whether the injury occurs at a joint or midshaft in a long bone. This assures that no motion is transmitted through the injury site as might occur, for example, with the rotation (supination/pronation) of the radius against the ulna at the elbow when the wrist turns.

Wrap any splinting device or associated bandage from a distal point to a proximal one. This assures that the pressure of bandaging moves any blood into the systemic circulation and does not trap it in the distal limb. This method of wrapping thus assists

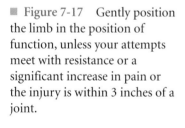

When possible, place injured limbs in the position of function or neutral position.

■ Figure 7-17   Gently position the limb in the position of function, unless your attempts meet with resistance or a significant increase in pain or the injury is within 3 inches of a joint.

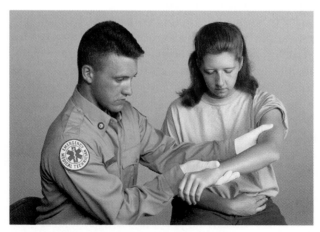

venous drainage and the healing process. Apply firm pressure when wrapping, but be sure you can easily push a finger beneath the wrapping.

Checking Neurovascular Function

It is imperative that you identify the status of the circulation, motor function, and sensation distal to the injury site before, during, and after splinting of all musculoskeletal injuries. The check before splinting identifies a baseline condition and establishes that the initial injury has not disrupted circulation. The check during splinting assures that inadvertent limb movement or circumferential pressure does not compromise distal circulation. The check after splinting identifies any restriction caused by progressive swelling of the injured area against the splinting device. Clearly identify and document these evaluations whenever you apply a splint.

To perform this evaluation, first palpate for a pulse and assure it is equal in strength to that of the opposing limb. If the pulse cannot be located or is weak, check capillary refill and skin temperature, color, and condition. Again compare your findings to the opposing limb. Ask the patient to describe the sensation when you rub or pinch the bottom of the foot or back of the hand and ask him to move the fingers or toes. The patient response establishes your baseline circulation, sensory, and motor findings. Reevaluate pulse, motor function, and sensation frequently during the remaining care and transport. If a care provider is holding the limb while you apply the splint, have him monitor both pulse and skin temperature. That care provider can then immediately note any compromise in circulation.

The pulse oximeter can be used to monitor the distal pulse during the splint process. Affix the probe to a free finger or toe and assure a good reading. Then monitor the oximeter, watching for any change, especially the readings becoming erratic or the device becoming unable to obtain a reading at all. This suggests a compromise in distal circulation (loss of the pulsing necessary to obtain a reading) and the need to reassess the distal pulse, skin temperature, and capillary refill.

Always check pulses, motor function, and sensation in the distal extremity before, during, and after splinting.

SPLINTING DEVICES

An essential part of managing any musculoskeletal system injury is the use of devices to immobilize a limb and permit patient transport without causing further injury. These devices, called splints, are designed to help you reduce or eliminate any movement of the injured extremity. Splints come in several forms that can assist in immobilizing common fractures and dislocations associated with musculoskeletal trauma (Figure 7-18 ■). They include rigid, formable, soft, traction, and other splints.

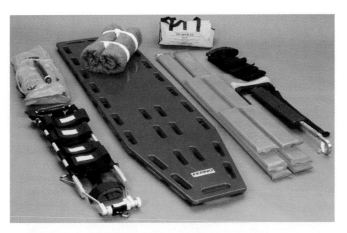

■ Figure 7-18 A variety of splints are available for musculoskeletal injuries.

Rigid Splints

Rigid splints, as the name implies, are firm and durable supports for the injured limb. They can be constructed of cardboard, plastic, metal, synthetic products, or wood. Such devices very effectively immobilize injury sites but require adequate padding to lessen patient discomfort. This padding may be built into the splint or may simply be a bulky dressing affixed to the splint with soft bandaging. Several types of commercially available rigid splints are used in prehospital care. They are usually flat and rigid devices and are about 3 inches wide and from 16 to 48 inches long. The injured limb that is in alignment is immobilized to the splint by circumferential wrapping, while an angulated limb may be held in position by cross-wrapping at two locations.

A special form of rigid splint is the preformed splint. It is usually a stamped metal or preformed plastic or fiberglass device shaped to the contours of the distal limbs. These splints are usually available for the ankles and hands.

Formable Splints

Another type of rigid splint is the formable, or malleable, splint. It is made up of a material that you can easily shape to match the angulation of a limb. You then affix the formed splint to the limb with circumferential bandaging. Formable splints include both the ladder splint, which is a matrix of soft metal wires soldered together, and the metal sheet splint, which is made up of thin aluminum or another easily shaped metal.

Vacuum splints are now available and sized for almost all long-bone fractures. The device is an airtight fabric bag filled with small plastic particles. The splint is applied to the injured limb and formed and secured around it. As the air is withdrawn from the device, the small particles lock in position, creating a firmly fixed form around the limb (Figure 7-19 ■). The splint firmly and comfortably secures the limb in position, although there is a small amount of shrinkage with the evacuation of air.

Soft Splints

Soft splints use padding or air pressure to immobilize an injured limb. Varieties of soft splints include air splints, which include the PASG, pelvic sling, and pillow splints.

The air splint provides immobilization as air pressure fills the splint and compresses the limb. Since the splint is a formed cylinder, and may include shaping for the foot, it immobilizes the limb in an aligned position. Air splints should not be used with long bone injuries at or above the knee or elbow because they cannot prevent movement of hip or shoulder joints and are thus unable to immobilize the proximal joints of the limb. Air splints also apply a pressure that may be helpful in controlling both external and internal hemorrhage. While these devices may limit assessment of the distal extremity, they do permit observation because they are transparent. (Note that the PASG is not transparent, so carefully assess the patient from the rib cage to the feet before applying and inflating it.)

■ Figure 7-19   Suction the air out of a vacuum splint until the device is rigid. Reassess pulse, motor function, and sensation in the extremity after application.

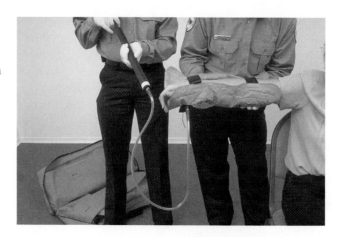

The Traction Splint: Past, Present, and Future The traction splint has been a mainstay of prehospital emergency care ever since J. D. (Deke) Farrington penned the pamphlet entitled "Death in a Ditch" and began what is today's modern EMS system. The traction splint was developed in the late 1800s and its worth was proven during the trench warfare of World War I. The old half-ring splint evolved into the "Hare" and then the "Sager"-style splints we find on almost every ambulance today. And, surely everyone who has been in EMS more than a decade can remember where its application turned a patient writhing in pain into someone with only limited discomfort. However, does the traction splint deserve to be a standard of care in the modern EMS system?

The traction splint is limited in its application to isolated femur fractures. In fractures of the hip or those in the vicinity of the knee, traction risks nervous or vascular complications, and the splint is likewise contraindicated in pelvic fractures or any serious skeletal injury to the distal extremity. It may also be contraindicated in multisystem trauma due to the time required for application and the likelihood of contraindicating injuries. Recent research suggests that the incidence of injury requiring the traction splint is about five times in 10,000 prehospital patients. The study further identifies that 40 percent of patients with indications for the traction splint never had it applied, and an equal number of patients (two) had it applied when contraindications existed.

As we examine past, current, and future prehospital care skills, we must evaluate the traction splints' incidence of use and weigh their benefit against equipment costs and the training time necessary to assure their proper use. As paramedic practitioners, we are aware that we may need to lay aside some mainstays of current prehospital practice as we strive to do the most good for the greatest number of patients.

Monitor air splints carefully with any changes in temperature or atmospheric pressure. Increases in ambient heat or decreases in pressure, as during an ascent in a helicopter, will increase the pressure within the splint. Conversely, decreases in temperature or a descent in a helicopter will decrease pressure in the splint. Constantly monitor the pressure in the air splint and PASG to assure it does not rise or fall during your care.

The pillow splint is a comfortable splint for ankle and foot injuries. The foot is simply placed on the pillow while the outer fabric is drawn around the foot and pillow. The outer fabric is pinned together or wrapped circumferentially with bandage material around the injury site. This device applies gentle and uniform pressure to effectively immobilize the distal extremity. Using a bulky blanket or two and wrapping them firmly may also provide the same type of immobilization.

> Monitor pressure within the air splint or PASG, as it may change with changes in altitude or temperature.

Traction Splints

The traction splint was developed during World War I and used extensively during World War II. This splint dramatically reduced both mortality and limb loss from femur fractures caused by projectile wounds, blast injuries, and other traumas. Today, the traction splint is the mainstay of prehospital care for the isolated traumatic femur fracture.

The traction splint is a frame that applies a pull (traction) on the injured extremity and against the trunk. The application of traction is useful when splinting the femur, which is surrounded by very heavy musculature. Frequently, the pain of fracture initiates muscle spasm that causes the bone ends to override each other causing further pain and muscle spasm and aggravating the original injury. The traction splint prevents overriding of the bone ends, lessens patient pain, and may help relax any muscle spasm.

There are basically two styles of traction splint, the bipolar frame device and the unipolar device (Figure 7-20). The bipolar (Fernotrac or Thomas) traction splint has

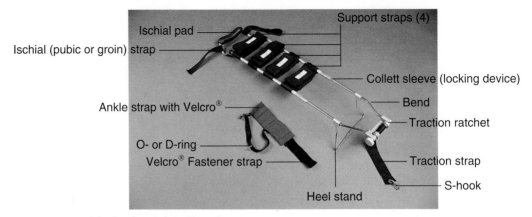

a. A bipolar frame traction splint.

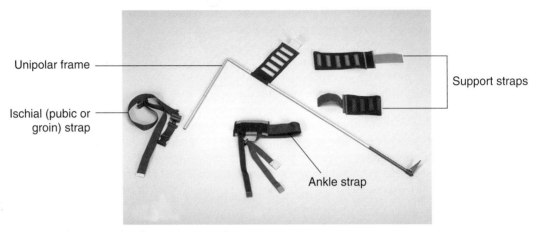

b. A unipolar frame traction splint.

■ Figure 7-20   Traction splints.

a half ring that fits up and against the ischial tuberosity of the pelvis. A distal ratchet connects to a foot harness and pulls traction from the foot and against the pelvis. The frame lifts and supports the limb and a foot stand suspends the injured limb above the ground. This construction helps prevent motion of the limb during movement of the patient, while the elevation supplied by the stand enhances venous drainage. The unipolar (Sager) traction splint uses a single lengthening shaft to pull a foot harness against pressure applied to the pubic bone. The unipolar splint does not elevate or stabilize the extremity, so you must observe greater care whenever you move the patient. You can use the unipolar splint in conjunction with the PASG.

Other Splinting Aids

Cravats or Velcro straps can augment the effectiveness of rigid splints. You can secure the lower extremities, one to the other, to help the patient control the musculoskeletal injury site or you can use a sling and swathe to help immobilize a splinted upper extremity to the chest. Fractures of the humerus are difficult to immobilize because the shoulder is such a large and mobile part of the body. A sling may hold the elbow at a fixed angle, while a swathe secures the limb against the body to limit further shoulder motion. By holding a thumb in the fold of the elbow, the patient can easily reduce any motion of the limb and complement the splinting process.

In some cases of serious musculoskeletal injury, other injuries preclude the splinting of individual fractures and dislocations. In such cases, you may splint the limbs to the body with cravats or bandage material and immobilize the patient to the long spine board. Simply strap the body and limbs to the board and transport the patient as a unit. While this is not definitive splinting, it will provide reasonable protection for musculoskeletal injuries.

FRACTURE CARE

For prehospital care purposes, consider a joint injury to be any muscular or connective tissue injury or dislocation or fracture within 3 inches of a joint. Fractures are then defined as shaft injuries at least 3 inches away from the joint. These definitions are essential because injury near the joint carries a higher incidence of blood vessel and nerve involvement and requires a different approach to positioning and splinting.

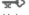

Consider any injury within 3 inches of a joint to be a joint injury.

Begin fracture care by assuring distal pulses, sensation, and motor function. Then align the limb for splinting. Quickly recheck the circulation and motor and sensory function below the injury. If you identify any neurovascular deficit, attempt to correct the problem by gentle repositioning, even if the limb is relatively aligned. If the limb is angulated, proceed with realignment. Remember that most splinting devices are designed to immobilize aligned limbs and that alignment provides the best chance for assuring good neurovascular function distal to the injury.

To move an injured limb from an angulated position into alignment, use gentle distal traction applied manually. Have an assisting EMT immobilize the proximal limb in the position found. Grasp the distal limb firmly and apply traction along the limb's axis, gently moving it from the angulated to an aligned position. Should you feel any resistance to movement or notice a great increase in patient discomfort, stop the alignment attempt and splint the limb as it lies. Once you complete alignment, recheck the distal neurovascular function. If it is adequate, proceed with splinting. If function is inadequate, move the limb around slightly while another care provider monitors for a pulse. If one attempt at gentle manipulation does not reestablish a pulse, splint and transport the patient quickly.

Proceed with splinting by selecting an appropriate device and secure the limb to it in a way that assures you immobilize both the fracture site and the adjacent joints. Have the care provider who is holding the limb apply a gentle traction to stabilize the limb (and monitor the distal pulse) during splinting. If you apply your splint properly, the device may maintain this traction and provide greater stabilization of the limb and greater patient comfort. Secure the limb to the body (upper extremity) or to the opposite limb (lower extremity) to protect it and to give the patient some control over the limb.

JOINT CARE

Joint care, too, begins with assessment for distal neurovascular function. If you find pulse, sensation, and motor function to be adequate, immobilize the joint in the position found. Use a ladder, vacuum, or other malleable splint, shaped to the limb's angle, or cross-wrap with a padded rigid splint to immobilize the joint in place. Assure that your splinting immobilizes the injured joint and both the joint above and the joint below the injury. If not, secure the limb firmly to the body to immobilize these joints.

Unless you identify a neurovascular deficit, immobilize joint injuries as you find them.

If circulation or motor or sensory function is lost below the joint injury, consider moving the limb to reestablish it. While you gently move the limb, have another care provider monitor the circulation and sensation. If you can reestablish neurovascular function quickly, splint the limb in the new position. If not, splint and provide quick transport.

With some joint injuries, you may attempt to return the displaced bone ends to their normal anatomical position. This process is called **reduction** and has both benefits and hazards. An early return to normal position reduces stress on the ligaments and basic joint structure and facilitates better distal circulation and sensation. However, the process creates the risk of trapping blood vessels or nerves as the bone ends return to their normal anatomical position. Attempt reduction of a dislocation only when you

reduction *returning of displaced bone ends to their proper anatomical orientation.*

are sure the injury *is* a dislocation, when you expect the patient's arrival at the emergency department to be delayed (prolonged extrication or long transport time), or when there is a significant neurovascular deficit. Do not attempt a reduction if the dislocation is associated with other serious patient injuries. Consult your protocols and medical direction to determine the criteria for attempting dislocation reduction used in your system.

When performing a joint reduction, you attempt to protect the articular surface while directing the bones back to their normal anatomic position. Begin the process by providing the patient with analgesic therapy to reduce pain associated with the injury and the reduction itself. Then have an assisting care provider hold the proximal extremity in position and provide a countertraction during the reduction. You then apply traction to pull the bone surfaces apart, reducing the pressure between the nonarticular surfaces. Slowly increase traction and direct the displaced limb toward its normal anatomic position. Successful relocation is indicated when you feel the joint "pop" back into position, the patient experiences a lessening of pain, and the joint becomes mobile within at least a few minutes of the procedure. Carefully evaluate the distal circulation, sensation, and motor function after the reduction. If the procedure does not meet with success within a few minutes, splint the limb as it is and provide rapid transport for the patient. If the reduction is successful, splint the limb in the position of function and transport.

MUSCULAR AND CONNECTIVE TISSUE CARE

Injuries to the soft tissues of the musculoskeletal system deserve special care. While such injuries are not usually life threatening, they can be very painful and, in some cases, threaten limbs. For example, compartment syndrome can restrict capillary blood flow, venous blood return, and nerve function beyond the site of the injury. If such an injury is not discovered and relieved, it may produce severe disability. Deep contusions and especially large hematomas can also contribute to blood loss and hypovolemia. Once you care for life threats, fractures, joint injuries, and other limb threats, give injuries to muscular and connective tissues your attention.

To manage these muscle, tendon, and ligament injuries, immobilize the region surrounding them. Doing so will reduce the associated internal hemorrhage and pain. Provide gentle circumferential bandaging (loose enough to let you slide a finger underneath) to further reduce hemorrhage, edema, and pain, but be sure to monitor distal circulation and loosen the bandage further if there are any signs of neurovascular deficit. Application of local cooling will reduce both edema and patient discomfort. Be careful to wrap any cold or ice pack in a dressing to prevent too drastic a cooling and any consequent injury. You may apply heat to the wound after 48 hours to enhance both circulation and healing. If possible, place the limb in the position of function and elevate the extremity to assure good venous return, limit swelling, and reduce patient discomfort. Monitor distal neurovascular function to assure your actions do not compromise circulation, sensation, or motor function.

CARE FOR SPECIFIC FRACTURES
Pelvis

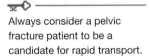

Always consider a pelvic fracture patient to be a candidate for rapid transport.

Pelvic fractures involve either the iliac crest or the pelvic ring. While iliac crest fractures may reflect serious trauma, they do not represent the patient life-threat suggested by ring fractures. Iliac crest fractures are often isolated and stable injuries that you can care for by simple patient immobilization.

Pelvic ring fractures, however, are often serious, life-threatening events. The ring shape of the pelvis provides strength to the structure, but when it breaks, two fracture sites usually result. The kinetic forces necessary to fracture the pelvic ring are significant and are likely to produce fractures and internal injuries elsewhere. In addition, the pelvis is actively involved in blood cell production, has a rich blood supply, and its interior surface is adjacent to major blood vessels serving the lower extremities. Injury to the pelvic ring, therefore, can result in heavy hemorrhage that is likely to empty into the pelvic and retroperitoneal spaces and account for blood loss in excess of 2 liters. Such injury may also result in circulation loss to one or both lower extremities. Pelvic fractures may also be associated with hip dislocations and injuries to the bladder, female reproductive organs, the urethra, the prostate in the male, and the end of the alimentary canal (anus and rectum).

The objectives of pelvic injury care are to stabilize the fractured pelvis, support the patient hemodynamically, and provide rapid transport to a trauma center. Because of the potential for severe blood loss and the difficulty of immobilizing the broken pelvic ring, application of the PASG is sometimes recommended for pelvic fractures (Figure 7-21 ■). Inflate the PASG until it stabilizes the pelvis and hip joint. If the patient is hypotensive, start two large-bore IVs, and hang two 1,000-mL bags of lactated Ringer's solution or normal saline. Set up using trauma tubing, and administer fluid boluses as needed to maintain a systolic blood pressure of at least 80 mmHg. Always consider a pelvic fracture patient to be a candidate for rapid transport.

Another effective technique to immobilize an unstable pelvis is application of a pelvic sling. The sling is a wide band, either commercially available or made from a sheet. To apply, fold a sheet to about 10 inches wide and gently negotiate it under the patient, or move the patient to the spine board with the device in place. The band should engage the pelvis with the band's upper border just below the iliac crests. Secure the commercial device or tie the sheet firmly to immobilize the pelvis with firm but not excessive pressure. Place a folded blanket between the patient's lower extremities and tie them together. If necessary for comfort, place a pillow under the patient's knees. A commercial pelvic sling is now available.

Femur

Femur fractures may be traumatic, resulting from the application of very strong and violent forces, or atraumatic, resulting from degenerative diseases. Patients with disease-induced fractures usually are of advancing age and present with a history of a degenerative disease, a clouded or limited history of trauma, and only moderate discomfort. Care for such patients by immobilizing them as found and then providing gentle transport. Generally, you can provide effective splinting by placing the patient on a long spine board and padding with pillows and blankets for patient comfort. Use of a traction splint is not essential because pain is not inducing the spasms that cause broken bone ends to override.

A patient who has suffered a traumatic femur fracture usually experiences extreme discomfort, and is often writhing in pain. In such a case, providing distal traction immobilizes both bone ends, relieves muscle spasms, and reduces the associated pain. Traction splinting is the best avenue for care of the hemodynamically stable patient with an isolated femur fracture. However, the traction splint is not indicated if the patient has concurrent serious pelvic, knee, tibia, or foot injuries.

Proximal fractures (surgical neck and intertrochanteric fractures) are frequently caused by hip injuries, transmitted forces, or the degenerative effects of aging. Midshaft fractures often result from high-energy, lateral traumas and are associated with significant blood loss. Injuries to the distal femur (condylar and epicondylar fractures) can be extensive and are likely to involve blood vessels, nerves, and connective tissue. The energy necessary to fracture the femur may be sufficient to dislocate the hip and cause serious internal injuries elsewhere in the body.

If the femur fracture is accompanied by a severe pelvic fracture, you may best achieve limb immobilization and hemodynamic stability by using the PASG alone or by simply immobilizing the patient on a backboard, pelvic sling, vacuum splint, or vacuum mattress. If

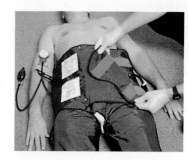

■ Figure 7-21   The PASG is an effective splint for traumatic pelvic fractures and helps control internal hemorrhage.

Atraumatic femur fractures may be splinted by gently placing the patient on a long spine board.

a pelvic fracture is suspected, do *not* apply a traction splint, which may apply pressure to the fractured pelvis, thereby causing further bone displacement and hemorrhage. Also, if the early signs of shock are present or if the history suggests that the patient has sustained trauma severe enough to induce shock, the PASG may be a better choice because it effectively splints the entire region and contributes to hemodynamic stability.

You may find it difficult to differentiate between proximal fractures of the femur (hip fractures) and anterior hip dislocations. Generally, a femur fracture presents with the foot externally rotated (turned outward) and the injured limb shortened when compared to the other. This difference may be slight and may be unnoticeable if the patient's legs are not straight and parallel. An anterior dislocation presents similarly to the femur fracture, but with the head of the femur protruding in the inguinal region. In either case, treat as a dislocation. Traction splints should not be used if a joint injury (hip or knee) is suspected.

If you suspect femur fracture, align the limb, determine the status of circulation and sensory and motor function, and apply the traction splint (Figure 7-22 ■). (If you use manual traction to align the femur, maintain it until the splint is applied and continues the traction.) Adjust the length of the splint to the uninjured extremity, position the device against the pelvis, and secure it in position with the inguinal strap. With a bipolar splint, apply the ankle hitch, provide gentle traction, and elevate the distal limb to place the splint's ring against the ischial tuberosity. With a unipolar splint, position the T-shaped support against the pubic bone and simply apply the ankle hitch. Assure that hitch and splint hold the foot and limb in an anatomic position as you apply firm traction. Position and secure the limb to the splint with straps, then gently move the patient and splint to the long spine board. Firmly secure the patient and limb for transport.

Guide your application of traction by the patient's response. Ask the patient how the limb feels as you initiate and increase the amount of traction. Stop the application of traction when the limb is immobilized and patient discomfort decreases. Remember, as the traction splint prevents the overriding of bone ends, the pain of injury decreases. This reduces the strength of muscle spasm and lets the limb return toward its initial length. This, in turn, reduces the traction provided by the splint, which means that the bone ends will no longer be as well immobilized. Check the amount of traction frequently to assure that it does not lessen during your care. If the patient reports increasing pain, consider increasing traction gradually until some reduction in pain is noted.

When the need for rapid transport or other patient injuries preclude the use of the traction splint, consider using the long spine board for immobilizing and transporting the femur fracture patient. Use long padded rigid splints, one medial and one lateral, to quickly splint the injured limb, and then tie that limb to the uninjured one. Use an orthopedic stretcher or another device or movement technique to transfer the patient to a long spine board and secure the patient firmly on it.

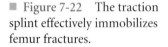 Figure 7-22   The traction splint effectively immobilizes femur fractures.

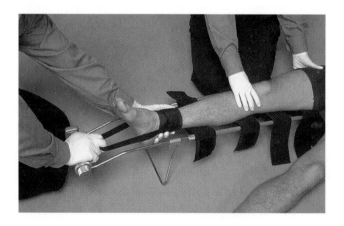

Tibia/Fibula

Fractures of the leg bones, the tibia and the fibula, can occur separately or together. The tibia is the most commonly fractured leg bone and may be broken by direct force, crushing injury, or twisting forces. Tibial fracture is likely to cause an open wound. Fibular fractures are often associated with damage to the knee or ankle. If the tibia is fractured and the fibula is intact, the extremity may not angulate, but it is not able to bear weight. If only the fibula is broken, the limb may be relatively stable. Injuries to either bone may result in compartment syndrome. Direct trauma suffered during an auto crash or athletic impact frequently causes these tibia and fibula injuries.

Fibular fractures are relatively stable, while tibial fractures are not.

Align the injured limb; assess circulation, sensation, and motor function; and then immobilize the limb with gentle traction. A full-leg air splint (one that accommodates the foot), vacuum, or lateral or medial padded rigid splint will provide effective immobilization (Figure 7-23 ■). You may also use a cardboard splint as long as it accommodates the full limb and is rigid enough to maintain immobilization. After you splint the injured limb, secure it to the uninjured leg. This affords some protection against uncontrolled movement and may reassure the patient that he still has some control over the extremity.

Clavicle

The clavicle is the most frequently fractured bone in the human body. Fractures to it usually result from transmitted forces directed along the upper extremity that cause relatively minor skeletal injury. The clavicle, however, is located adjacent to both the upper reaches of the lung and the vasculature that serves the upper extremity and head. Hence, an injury to the clavicle has the potential to cause serious internal injury, especially if very powerful mechanisms of injury are involved. The clavicular fracture patient often presents with pain and the shoulder shifted forward with palpable deformity along the clavicle. Accomplish splinting either by immobilizing the affected limb in a sling and swathe or by wrapping a figure-eight bandage around the shoulders, drawing the shoulders back, and then securing the bandage tension. Monitor the patient carefully for any sign of internal hemorrhage or respiratory compromise.

Humerus

A fractured humerus is very difficult to immobilize at its proximal end. The proximal humerus is buried within the shoulder muscles, and the shoulder joint is very mobile atop the thoracic cage. The axillary artery runs through the axilla, making it difficult to apply any mechanical traction to the limb without compromising circulation. Hence, the most effective techniques for splinting this fracture are to apply a sling and swathe to immobilize the bent limb against the chest or to tie the extended and splinted limb to the body.

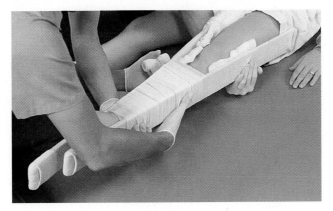

■ Figure 7-23 Placement of long padded board splints laterally and medially can effectively splint tibia/fibula fractures.

The preferred technique is to use the sling and swathe. Apply a short padded rigid splint to the lateral surface of the arm to distribute the pressure of the swathing and better immobilize the arm. Sling the forearm with a cravat, catching just the wrist region and not the elbow. This permits some gravitational traction in the seated patient and prevents inadvertent application of pressure by the sling, which could push the limb together. Then use several cravats to gently swathe the arm and forearm to the chest. If the patient is conscious, have him place the thumb of the uninjured extremity in the fold of the elbow to help control the injured limb's motion. This gives the patient control over the limb, decreases limb movement, and increases patient comfort.

You may also immobilize the limb by using a long padded rigid splint affixed to the extended limb. Place the splint along the medial aspect of the upper extremity and assure that it does not apply pressure to the axilla. Such pressure disrupts axillary artery blood flow to the limb and is uncomfortable for the patient. Secure the splint firmly to the limb, wrapping from the distal end toward the proximal end. Then secure the splint to the supine patient's body, and move the patient and splint to a long spine board.

Radius/Ulna

The forearm may fracture anywhere along its length and the fracture may involve the radius, the ulna, or both. Most commonly, fracture occurs at the distal end of the radius, just above the articular surface. This is known as Colles' fracture, and it presents with the wrist turned up at an unusual angle. Another term for this injury is the "silver fork deformity" because it is contoured like a fork and the distal limb often becomes ashen. As with most joint fractures, the major concern here is for distal circulation and innervation. If you find a neurovascular injury, use only slight adjustments to restore nervous or circulatory function because movement in this area is likely to cause further injury.

Splint forearm fractures with a short, padded rigid splint affixed to the forearm and hand. Secure the hand in the position of function by placing a large wad of dressing material in the palm to maintain a position like that of holding a large ball. Place the rigid splint along the medial forearm surface and wrap circumferentially from the fingers to the elbow. Leave at least one digit exposed to permit checking for capillary refill. Bend the elbow across the chest and use a sling and swathe to hold the limb in position. This provides relative elevation and improved venous drainage in both seated and supine patients.

The air splint or long padded rigid splint, tied firmly to the body, may also adequately immobilize forearm fractures (Figure 7-24 ■). When using these devices, remember to place the hand in the position of function to increase patient comfort.

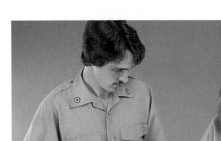
When possible, leave a distal digit exposed to evaluate capillary refill and skin color and temperature.

■ Figure 7-24 A full-arm air splint can effectively splint fractures of the radius and/or ulna.

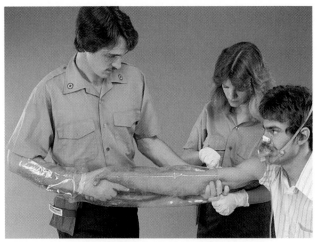

CARE FOR SPECIFIC JOINT INJURIES
Hip

The hip may dislocate in two directions, anteriorly and posteriorly. The anterior dislocation presents with the foot turned outward and the head of the femur palpable in the inguinal area. The posterior dislocation is most common and presents with the knee flexed and the foot rotated internally. The displaced head of the femur is buried in the muscle of the buttocks. Immobilize a patient with either type of dislocation on a long spine board using pillows and blankets as padding to maintain the patient's position and provide comfort. If distal circulation, sensation, or motor function is severely compromised, consider one attempt at reduction of a posterior dislocation. (Consult local protocols and medical direction to identify criteria for reduction attempts.) However, do not attempt reduction if there are other serious injuries, like a pelvic fracture, associated with the hip dislocation. Anterior dislocations in general cannot be managed by reduction in the prehospital setting.

For reduction of a posterior hip dislocation, have a care provider hold the pelvis firmly against the long spine board or other firm surface by placing downward pressure on the iliac crests. Flex both the patient's hip and knee at 90 degrees and apply a firm, slowly increasing traction along the axis of the femur. Gently rotate the femur externally. It takes some time for the muscles to relax, but when they do the head of the femur will "pop" back into position. If you feel this "pop" or if the patient reports a sudden relief of pain and is able to extend the leg easily, the reduction has likely been a success. Immobilize the patient in a comfortable position, either in flexion (not to exceed 90 degrees) or fully supine with the hip and leg in full extension. Reevaluate sensation, motor function, and circulation. If the femur head does not move into the acetabulum after a few minutes of your attempted reduction, immobilize the patient as found and consider rapid transport.

Knee

Knee injuries may include fractures of the femur, the tibia, or both; patellar dislocations; or frank dislocations of the knee. Because the knee is such a large joint and bears such a great amount of weight, an injury to it is serious and threatens the patient's future ability to walk. Another concern with knee injury is possible injury to the major blood vessel traversing the area, the popliteal artery. This artery is less mobile than blood vessels in other joints, which leaves it more subject to injury and distal vascular compromise.

Immobilize knee joint fractures and patellar dislocations in the position found unless distal circulation, sensation, or motor function is disrupted. If the limb is flexed, splint it with two medium rigid splints, placing one medially and one laterally (Figure 7-25 ▪). Cross-wrap with bandage material to secure the limb in position. You may also

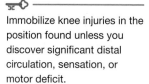

Immobilize knee injuries in the position found unless you discover significant distal circulation, sensation, or motor deficit.

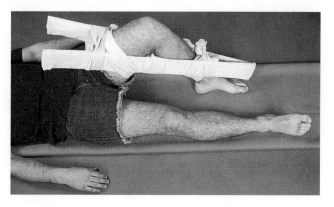

▪ Figure 7-25 Angulated knee dislocations can be immobilized with two padded rigid splints.

use ladder or malleable splints, conformed to the angle of the limb and placed anteriorly and posteriorly, or a vacuum splint to immobilize the knee. If the limb is extended, simply apply two padded rigid splints or a full-leg air splint.

Dislocation of the patella is more common than dislocation of the knee joint and usually leaves the knee in a flexed position with a lateral displacement of the patella. The injured knee appears significantly deformed, though patellar dislocation has a lower incidence of associated vascular injury than does knee dislocation.

Anterior dislocations of the knee produce an extended limb contour that lifts at the knee (moving from proximal to distal) while posterior dislocations produce a limb that drops at the knee. (Assure that the injury is not a patellar dislocation.) If there is neurovascular compromise, have another care provider immobilize the femur. You should then grasp the limb just above the ankle and at the calf muscle and apply a firm and progressive traction, first along the axis of the tibia and then pulling the limb toward alignment with the femur. With posterior dislocations, a third care provider may provide moderate downward pressure on the distal femur and upward pressure on the proximal tibia to facilitate the reduction. As with most dislocations, success is measured by feeling the bone end "pop" back into place, hearing the patient report a dramatic reduction in pain, and noting a freer movement of the limb at the knee joint. Once you reduce the knee dislocation, immobilize the joint in the position of function and transport the patient. If you cannot reduce the dislocation with a few minutes of distal traction, immobilize the extremity in the position found and transport quickly. Perform a knee dislocation reduction even if the patient has good distal circulation and nervous function when the time to definitive care will exceed 2 hours.

Ankle

Ankle injuries often produce a distal lower limb that is grossly deformed, either due to malleolar fracture, dislocation, or both. Sprains are also injuries of concern, although with them the limb remains in anatomical position. Splint sprains or nondisplaced fractures with an air splint (shaped to accommodate the foot) or with long rigid splints positioned on either side of the limb, padded liberally, and wrapped firmly. You may also use a pillow splint, especially if there is any ankle deformity (Figure 7-26 ■). Apply local cooling to ease the pain and reduce swelling.

Ankle dislocation may occur in any of three directions: anteriorly, posteriorly, or laterally. The anterior dislocation presents with a dorsiflexed (upward pointing) foot that appears shortened. The posterior dislocation appears to lengthen the plantar flexed (downward-pointing) foot. The lateral dislocation is most common and presents with a foot turned outward with respect to the ankle. If distal neurovascular compromise indicates the need for reduction, have a care provider grasp the calf,

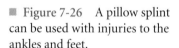
■ Figure 7-26   A pillow splint can be used with injuries to the ankles and feet.

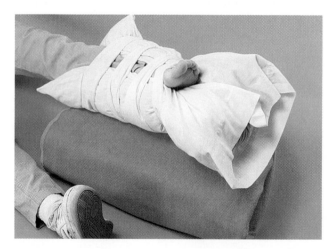

hold it in position, and pull against the traction you apply. You then grasp the heel with one hand and the metatarsal arch with the other. Pull a distal traction to disengage the bone ends and protect the articular cartilage during the relocation. For anterior dislocations, move the foot posteriorly with respect to the ankle; with lateral dislocations, rotate the foot medially; with posterior dislocations, pull the heel toward you and the foot toward you, then away. The joint should return to the normal position with a "pop," a reduction in patient pain, and an increase in the mobility of the joint. Apply local cooling and immobilize the limb. If the procedure does not result in joint reduction within a few minutes, splint the joint as found and provide rapid transport.

Foot

Injuries to the foot include dislocations and fractures to the calcanei (heel bones), metatarsals, and phalanges. Injuries to the calcanei generally result from falls and can cause significant pain and swelling. Injuries to the metatarsals and phalanges can result from penetrating or blunt trauma or the typical "stubbing" of a toe. Fatigue fractures of the metatarsal bones, or "march fractures," are relatively common. These injuries are reasonably stable, even though the extremity cannot bear weight. When foot or ankle injury is suspected, anticipate both bilateral foot injuries and lumbar spinal injury.

Immobilize foot injuries in much the same way you do with ankle injuries. Use pillow, vacuum, ladder, or air splints (with foot accommodation). If possible, leave some portion of the foot accessible so you can monitor distal capillary refill or, at least, skin temperature and color.

Shoulder

Fractures to the shoulder most commonly involve the proximal humerus, lateral scapula, and distal clavicle. Dislocations can include anterior, posterior, and inferior displacement of the humoral head. Anterior dislocations displace the humoral head forward, resulting in a shoulder that appears "hollow" or "squared-off," with the patient holding the arm close to the chest and forward of the mid-axillary line. Posterior dislocations rotate the arm internally, and the patient presents with the elbow and forearm held away from the chest. Inferior dislocations displace the humoral head downward, with the result that the patient's arm is often locked above the head.

You should immobilize shoulder injuries, like all joint injuries, as found, unless pulse, sensation, or motor function distal to the injury is absent. Immobilize anterior and posterior dislocations with a sling and swathe and, if needed, place a pillow under the arm and forearm. Immobilization of any inferior dislocation (with the upper extremity fixed above the head) will call for ingenuity on your part in splinting. In such cases, immobilize the extended arm in the position found. Using cravats, tie a long, padded splint to the torso, shoulder girdle, arm, and forearm to immobilize the arm above the head. Gently move the patient to the long spine board and secure both splint and patient to the spine board.

Begin reduction of anterior and posterior shoulder dislocations by placing a strap across the patient's chest, under the affected shoulder (through the axilla) and across the back. Have a care provider prepared to pull countertraction across the chest and superiorly using the strap. You, meanwhile, should flex the patient's elbow, drawing the arm somewhat away from the body (abduction) and pull firm traction along the axis of the humerus. Some slight internal and external rotation of the humerus may facilitate reduction. For reduction of inferior dislocations, have one care provider hold the thorax while you flex the elbow. Gradually apply firm traction along the axis of the humerus and gently rotate the arm externally. If the joint does not relocate in a few minutes, immobilize it as it lies and transport the patient. If reduction is successful, immobilize the upper extremity in the normal anatomical position with a sling and swathe.

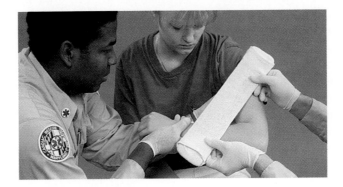

■ Figure 7-27 Use a padded board splint to immobilize angulated fractures or dislocations of the elbow.

Elbow

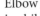
Elbow dislocations should not be reduced in the prehospital setting.

Elbow injuries display a high incidence of nervous and vascular involvement, especially in children. As in the knee, the blood vessels running through the elbow region are held firmly in place. The probability is good, therefore, that any fracture or dislocation will involve the brachial artery and the medial, ulnar, and radial nerves. Assess the distal neurovascular function and, if you detect a deficit, move the joint very carefully and minimally to restore distal circulation. Then splint the elbow with a single padded rigid splint, providing cross-strapping as necessary, or use a ladder splint bent to conform to the angle of the limb (Figure 7-27 ■). Keeping the wrist slightly elevated above the elbow, secure the limb to the chest using a sling and swathe. This position increases venous return and reduces the swelling and pain associated with the injury.

Wrist/Hand

Fractures of the hand and wrist are commonly associated with direct trauma. They present with very noticeable deformity and significant pain reported by the patient. These fractures are of serious concern to the patient. Since the hand and wrist bones are small, any fracture is close to a joint. Exercise concern when you care for these injuries because of the possibility of vascular and neural involvement.

When splinting the distal upper extremity, place padding in the palm of the hand to maintain the position of function.

You can effectively immobilize musculoskeletal injuries of the forearm, wrist, hand, or fingers with a padded rigid, vacuum, or air splint. Place a roll of bandaging, a wad of dressing material, or some similar object in the patient's hand to maintain the position of function. Then secure the extremity to the padded board or inflate the air splint. Be sure to leave some portion of the distal extremity accessible so that you can monitor the adequacy of perfusion and sensation. Place the wrist above the elbow to assist venous return and reduce distal swelling.

Hand and wrist injuries are very common, particularly among athletes and children. A particular type of wrist fracture is Colles' fracture in which the wrist has a "silver fork" appearance. Fortunately, such injuries are seldom serious and can be managed in the prehospital setting quite easily.

Finger

Forces may displace the phalanges from their joints, resulting in deformity and pain. Displacement usually occurs between the phalanges or between the proximal phalanx and the metacarpal and causes the bone to be moved either anteriorly or posteriorly. (Amputations are multisystem injuries that severely damage the musculoskeletal system. They are addressed in depth in Chapter 5, "Soft-Tissue Trauma.")

Splint finger fractures using tongue blades or small, malleable splints designed for the purpose that you shape to the contour of the injured finger. The finger may also be taped to the adjoining fingers to limit additional motion. The hand is then placed in the position of function and further immobilized.

Finger dislocations usually involve the proximal joint (and sometimes the distal joint) with the digit commonly displacing posteriorly. If reduction is indicated, grasp the distal finger and apply a firm distal traction. Then direct the digit toward the normal anatomic position by moving its proximal end. You should feel the finger "pop" into place, and the digit should resume its normal alignment when compared to the uninjured finger on the other hand. Splint the finger with a slight bend (10 to 15 degrees) and immobilize the hand in the position of function.

SOFT AND CONNECTIVE TISSUE INJURIES

Tendon, ligament, and muscle injuries are rarely, if ever, life threatening. Massive muscular contusions and hematomas can, however, contribute to hypovolemia, while ligament and tendon injuries can endanger the future function of a limb. Be careful about permitting the patient to put further stress on a limb, especially with higher grades of sprains. The weakened ligaments may fail completely, resulting in dislocation or complete joint instability. For the purpose of care, treat these injuries as you would dislocations and immobilize the adjacent joints. Monitor distal neurovascular function because tissue swelling within the circumferential wrapping of a splint may compress blood vessels and nerves. Care for muscular injuries with immobilization, gentle compression with snug (but not overly tight) dressings, and local cooling to suppress edema and pain using cold packs or ice wrapped in dressing material. Be watchful for signs of compartment syndrome, especially in the calf and forearm regions.

Open wounds involving the muscles, tendons, and ligaments can be severe and debilitating. Carefully evaluate such wounds for signs of connective tissue involvement. Be especially watchful with deep open injuries close to the joints. With such wounds, the likelihood of tendon and ligament disruption is great and may affect the use of the joint, the muscles controlling the joint, or the muscles controlling joint movement distal to the injury. Carefully evaluate for circulation, sensation, and motor function below these injuries.

Injury to a muscle or tendon may limit its ability to either extend or flex the limb. The opposing muscle moves the limb, while the injured muscle cannot return it to the normal position. With limb injuries, note any unusual limb position, especially if the patient is unable to return the limb to a neutral position. At any sign of pain or dysfunction, splint the limb.

Tendon, ligament, and muscle injuries are rarely life threatening.

Care for muscular injuries with immobilization, gentle compression with snug dressings, and local cooling to suppress edema and pain.

MEDICATIONS

Medications are frequently administered to the patient with musculoskeletal injury to relieve pain and to premedicate before the relocation of a dislocation. Medications used include nitrous oxide, diazepam, morphine, fentanyl, and nalbuphine.

Sedatives/Analgesics

Nitrous Oxide   Nitrous oxide (Nitronox) is a nitrogen and oxygen compound in a gas state. It is administered in the prehospital setting for its anesthetic properties, specifically to reduce the perception of pain in cases of musculoskeletal injuries. For prehospital care, it is administered in a 50 percent nitrous oxide and 50 percent oxygen mixture via a special regulator and a self-administration mask. Self-administration of nitrous oxide prevents overmedication because the patient will drop the mask when too heavily sedated.

Nitrous oxide is nonexplosive, and its analgesic effects dissipate within 2 to 5 minutes of discontinuing administration. High concentrations of nitrous oxide may lead to hypoxia and may cause respiratory depression and vomiting. These side effects are minimized, however, because the gas is premixed with oxygen by the administration set during prehospital delivery.

The chief concern with the use of nitrous oxide is that it diffuses easily into air-filled spaces in the body, increasing the pressure within them. This diffusion is especially dangerous in patients with pneumothorax or tension pneumothorax, bowel obstruction, and middle ear obstruction. Rule out COPD and these pathologies before you administer nitrous oxide in the prehospital setting.

The nitrous oxide administration device consists of two cylinders of equal size, one holding oxygen (green) and the other, nitrous oxide (blue). The gases are mixed in a special blender/regulator and distributed to the patient when his inspiration generates a less-than-atmospheric pressure. (In other countries, both gases are premixed in one cylinder, reducing the weight and size of the administration device.) The patient must hold the administration mask firmly to the face to trigger administration, thus preventing administration in a patient who is heavily sedated. Nitrous oxide is a controlled substance and its use is carefully monitored for provider abuse.

Diazepam Diazepam (Valium) is a benzodiazepine with both anti-anxiety and skeletal muscle relaxant qualities. Although it does not have any pain-relieving properties, diazepam does reduce the patient's perception and memory of pain. It is used with musculoskeletal injuries and to premedicate patients before painful procedures such as cardioversion and dislocation reduction. It is administered in a slow IV bolus of 5 to 15 mg, not to exceed 5 mg/minute, into a large vein. Diazepam is rather fast acting, with IV effects occurring almost immediately and reaching peak effectiveness in 15 minutes. Its duration of effectiveness is from 15 to 60 minutes. Do not mix diazepam with any other drugs, and flush the IV line before and after administration. Administer diazepam as close to the IV catheter as possible, and do not inject it into a plastic IV bag. Diazepam is readily absorbed by plastic, which quickly reduces its concentration.

Diazepam is usually supplied in single-use vials or preloaded syringes containing 2 mL of a 5 mg/mL solution (10 mg). Administer 5 to 15 mg IV and repeat in 10 to 15 minutes if necessary.

The effects of diazepam may be reversed by the administration of flumazenil. Usually, 2 mL of a 0.1 mg/mL solution is given IV (over 15 seconds) with a second dose repeated at 60 seconds.

Morphine Morphine sulfate (Duramorph, Astramorph) is an opium alkaloid used to relieve pain (narcotic analgesic), to sedate, and to reduce anxiety. It is used with musculoskeletal injuries for its ability to reduce pain perception. Morphine may reduce vascular volume and cardiac preload by increasing venous capacitance and may thus decrease blood pressure in the hypovolemic patient. It should not be administered to a patient with hypovolemia or hypotension. Its major side effects are respiratory depression and possible nausea and vomiting.

Morphine is available in 10-mL single-use vials or Tubex units of a 1 mg/mL solution or as 1 mL of a 10 mg/mL solution vial for dilution with 9 mL normal saline. Administer a 2-mg bolus slowly IV, repeating as necessary every few minutes to effect.

Naloxone hydrochloride (Narcan) is a narcotic antagonist that can quickly reverse the effects of narcotics (morphine, fentanyl, and nalbuphine) and should be available anytime you use any of these drugs. Naloxone is administered as an IV bolus of 0.4 to 2 mg, repeated every 2 to 3 minutes until effective. Naloxone is a shorter acting drug than morphine, so repeat doses may be necessary.

Fentanyl Fentanyl is an opiate narcotic, chemically unrelated to morphine, that provides immediate and effective pain control. Fentanyl's onset of action is more rapid than morphine's and it is considerably more potent, thus requiring lower doses. Fentanyl does not cause hypotension to the same degree as does morphine, which makes it an ideal agent for trauma.

Fentanyl is supplied in various doses. The typical starting dose is 25 to 50 mcg IV. Repeat doses of 25 mcg IV can be provided as needed. As with all opiates, continuously monitor the patient's vital signs.

Nalbuphine Nalbuphine hydrochloride (Nubain) is a synthetic narcotic analgesic with properties much like those of morphine. It is equivalent on a milligram-to-milligram basis to morphine, although it antagonizes some of the actions of that drug. Recent studies have questioned the effectiveness of nalbuphine as a prehospital analgesic, and it has fallen into relative disuse. Nalbuphine does not generally decrease blood pressure, although it may produce respiratory depression and bradycardia. Unlike morphine and meperidine, it is not a controlled substance. It is a rapid acting—within 2 to 3 minutes—drug with a long duration of effectiveness—3 to 6 hours.

Nalbuphine is supplied in ampules or preloaded syringes containing 1 mL of a 10 or 20 mg/mL solution. It is administered IV in a dose of 5 mg, then 2 mg repeated as needed up to 20 mg. Narcan will reverse its effects.

OTHER MUSCULOSKELETAL INJURY CONSIDERATIONS

Other areas for special consideration with musculoskeletal injuries include pediatric injuries, athletic injuries, patient refusals and referrals, and the psychological support for the patient with musculoskeletal injury.

Pediatric Musculoskeletal Injury

Children are at higher risk than adults for musculoskeletal injuries due to their activity levels and incompletely developed coordination. Special injuries affecting them include greenstick fractures and epiphyseal fractures.

The incomplete nature of the greenstick fracture produces a stable but angulated limb in the young child. The injured limb is painful and will not bear weight. In these cases, do not attempt to realign the limb and understand that the orthopedic specialist will probably complete the fracture to permit proper healing.

Epiphyseal fractures disrupt the child's growth plate and endanger future bone growth. This injury is likely with fractures within a few inches of the joint because the epiphyseal plate is a point of skeletal weakness. Treat these fractures as you would for an adult, but recognize that they are potentially limb-threatening injuries.

Athletic Musculoskeletal Injuries

Athletes, especially those involved in contact sports like football, soccer, basketball, and wrestling, have a higher incidence of musculoskeletal injuries than the general public. Injuries to the joints, often serious knee and ankle sprains, are common reasons for calls to EMS. Such injuries are especially important because they occur in individuals who are at least moderately well conditioned and result from the application of significant kinetic forces. When you are called to the side of an injured athlete, be especially sensitive to the potential for residual disability caused by these injuries and be predisposed to transport instead of permitting the patient to remain at the scene.

Knowing the athletic trainers in your area may help your on-scene operations run more smoothly and efficiently. In many cases, the athletic trainer works under the supervision of a local physician much as you work under medical direction. It is important for trainers to understand that, once you are called to the scene, the injured athlete becomes a patient of the EMS system and will be treated under the system's medical direction and protocols. Also, as the representative of that system, you are likely to assume responsibility for decisions about care and transport of the patient. Assuring that trainers understand these facts may eliminate confrontations over care of injured athletes.

Athletic trainers use the acronym RICE to identify the recommended treatment for sprains, strains, and other soft-tissue injuries. RICE stands for: *R*est the extremity, *I*ce for the first 48 hours, *C*ompression with an elastic bandage, and *E*levation for venous drainage. This is consistent with standard emergency care for sprains and strains. (Note, however, that the application of the elastic bandage in this case is to strengthen the limb for further activity and is not recommended for prehospital care.)

Knowing the athletic trainers in your area may help your on-scene operations run more smoothly and efficiently.

Review

Content

RICE Procedure for Strains, Sprains, and Soft-Tissue Injuries

*R*est the extremity
*I*ce for first 48 hours
*C*ompress with elastic bandage
*E*levate extremity

Contact medical direction and follow local protocols with patient refusals and referrals. Document such cases thoroughly.

Patient Refusals and Referral

In some situations, you may encounter a patient suffering from an isolated sprain or strain with no significant mechanism of injury and no other signs, symptoms, or complaints. This patient may refuse your assistance or be a candidate for on-scene treatment and referral for follow-up medical care. Evaluate the need for immobilization and x-rays and determine if the patient should seek immediate care in an emergency department or see a personal physician. Any referral to a personal physician must be done in conjunction with medical direction and following local protocol.

Psychological Support for the Musculoskeletal Injury Patient

Psychological support provided by the paramedic can have a significant impact on a patient's emotional response to trauma.

Regardless of the specific type of injury sustained, patients need psychological as well as physiological support. Too often, we concentrate all efforts on the patient's injuries, forgetting the emotional impact that the incident and the emergency care measures employed have on the patient. Keep in mind that patients are not frequently exposed to injuries. They do not know what effects injuries will have on their lives or what to expect from medical care in the prehospital, emergency department, or in-hospital settings. Remember that you can have a significant impact on a patient's emotional response to trauma. Displaying a concerned attitude and a professional demeanor and communicating frequently and compassionately with patients will go far to calm and reassure them. Simple attention paid to the patient may make the experience with prehospital emergency medical service one that is remembered positively.

Summary

Injuries to the bones, ligaments, tendons, and muscles of the extremities rarely threaten your patient's life. Major exceptions to this statement are pelvic and serious or bilateral femur fractures, in which associated hemorrhage can contribute significantly to hypovolemia and shock. In addition, serious musculoskeletal trauma suggests the possibility of other, life-threatening trauma and, in fact, occurs in about 80 percent of cases of major multisystem trauma. The presence of serious musculoskeletal trauma should increase your index of suspicion for other serious internal injuries.

Care for isolated musculoskeletal trauma is usually delayed until the ABCs and other patient life threats are stabilized. The goals of the care are to protect any open wounds, position affected limbs properly, immobilize the area of injury, and carefully monitor distal extremities to assure neurovascular function.

Pelvic and bilateral femur fractures are immobilized through application of the PASG. This device both provides splinting for the pelvis and upper portion of the lower extremity and helps control internal blood loss in the region. Manage other fractures by aligning the extremity with gentle traction and immobilizing it by splinting. In cases where you discover a loss of distal neurovascular function, move the extremity slightly to restore distal neurovascular function and then splint.

Joint injuries carry a greater risk of damage to distal circulation, sensation, and motor function. Splint these injuries as you find them unless there is distal neurovascular compromise. If that is the case, employ gentle manipulation to restore circulation, motor function, or sensation. If gentle manipulation is unsuccessful and transport is to be delayed, attempt reduction of dislocations for the hip, knee, ankle, shoulder, or finger as permitted by local protocol.

Care for injuries to connective and muscular tissues by immobilizing the area of injury in the position of function. Evaluate distal extremities for pulse, capillary refill, color, temperature, sensation, and motor function before, during, and after any immobilization or movement of a limb and provide frequent monitoring thereafter.

You Make the Call

You and your partner are called to 1616 Hampton Avenue for a patient who has tripped in the yard and injured his ankle. Dispatch reports that the patient is a 16-year-old male who is conscious, alert, and breathing; there is no bleeding present. Bystanders are on the scene performing first aid.

Upon arrival at the scene, you find the patient, Hank Tomlin, leaning against a tree in the front yard of his mother's home. As you interview Hank and bystanders, you discover that he is complaining of pain, swelling, and deformity to his right ankle. Hank tells you that he was running after his dog when his foot twisted in the grass and he fell to the ground. You suspect that the patient has probably dislocated or fractured his ankle.

While your partner continues to obtain a patient history and vital signs, you assess the site of the injury. A third off-duty paramedic is also on the scene to assist.

1. When assessing the injury site, what signs of fracture will you be evaluating?
2. What are the three main factors to consider when evaluating distal neurovascular status?
3. What steps should you take if you determine the patient is suffering from distal neurovascular impairment and choose to realign the injury?
4. How many attempts are permitted when realigning an injury?
5. How would you splint this injury once realignment has taken place?

See Suggested Responses at the back of this book.

Review Questions

1. The skeleton gives the body its structural form and it also:
   a. protects the vital organs.
   b. allows for efficient movement despite the forces of gravity.
   c. stores salts and other materials needed for metabolism.
   d. all of the above.

2. Bones are classified according to their:
   a. size.
   b. shape.
   c. weight.
   d. diameter.

3. Minute blood vessels, surrounded by layers of salts deposited in collagen fibers, travel lengthwise along the bone through small tubes known as:
   a. osteocytic pores.
   b. osteoblastic pores.
   c. perforating canals.
   d. haversian canals.

4. There are approximately 206 bones in the human body. Many are arranged in a contiguous fashion into jointed systems. The connective tissue(s) holding these bones together at a joint is/are:
   a. tendons.
   b. cartilage.
   c. bursal tissue.
   d. ligaments.

5. Biaxial joints allow movement in two planes. An example from this category of joints would be the:
   a. knee.
   b. shoulder.
   c. thumb bases.
   d. fingers.

6. Age-related changes in the skeletal system begin to occur as early as 40 years of age. These changes include:
   a. calcium retention.
   b. progression in body height.
   c. loss of ability to maintain bone structure.
   d. an increase in flexibility of costal-condral joints.

7. Skeletal muscles provide the ability for voluntary movement associated with the mobility of the body and its extremities. These muscles are controlled by the _____ nervous system.
   a. somatic
   b. autonomic
   c. sympathetic
   d. musculoskeletal

8. More than half of the energy created by muscle motion is:
   a. heat energy.
   b. chemical energy.
   c. electrical energy.
   d. mechanical energy.

9. Joints can move beyond their normal range of motion with a great enough applied force. This movement causes a complete displacement of bone ends from their normal position and is known as a(n) _____, and is characterized by_____.
   a. oblique fracture; pain, edema, and possibly bleeding
   b. dislocation; pain, edema, and immobility
   c. grade III sprain; severe pain and spasm without joint instability
   d. subluxation; pain, rapid edema, and an unlimited range of motion

10. Red marrow is found within the cancellous bone chambers of the long bones, sternum, and pelvis. The function of the marrow in these sites is:
    a. destruction and recycling of old and fragile blood cells.
    b. manufacturing of erythrocytes and other blood cells.
    c. storage of essential salts and minerals for bone aggregation.
    d. storage of a readily available source of energy generation.

11. A grade _____ sprain may present as a fracture.
    a. I
    b. II
    c. III
    d. IV

12. A small crack in a bone that does not disrupt its total structure is called a(n) _____ fracture.
    a. open
    b. closed
    c. impacted
    d. hairline

13. A common disintegration of the articular joints often associated with the aging process describes degenerative joint disease. Another disorder, characterized by inflammation of the synovial joints and causing immobility, pain, and fatigue, is known as:

    a. osteoarthritis.

    b. costrochondritis.

    c. inflammatory gout.

    d. rheumatoid arthritis.

14. A femur fracture may account for as much as _____ mL of blood loss.

    a. 1,000

    b. 1,500

    c. 2,000

    d. 2,500

15. Your patient has been involved in a motor vehicle collision. You suspect concurrent femur and pelvic fractures. Treatment of this patient would best be provided by:

    a. traction device, long board, transport to trauma center.

    b. long board, one IV line, transport to emergency department.

    c. traction device, PASG, transport to trauma center.

    d. PASG, supportive oxygen and fluid therapies, transport to trauma center.

See Answers to Review Questions at the back of this book.

Further Reading

American College of Surgeons, Committee on Trauma. *Advanced Trauma Life Support Course: Student Manual.* Chicago: American College of Surgeons, 2003.

Bates, Barbara, Lynn S. Bickley, and Robert A. Hoekelman. *A Guide to Physical Examination and History Taking.* 8th ed. Philadelphia: J. B. Lippincott, 2003.

Bledsoe, B. E. and D. Clayden. *Prehospital Emergency Pharmacology.* 6th ed. Upper Saddle River, N.J.: Pearson/Prentice Hall, 2005.

Butman, A., S. Martin, R. Vomacka, and N. McSwain. *Comprehensive Guide to Pre-Hospital Skills: A Skills Manual for EMT-Basic, EMT-Intermediate, and EMT-Paramedic.* St. Louis: Mosby, 1996.

Butman, Alexander M., and James L. Paturas. *Pre-Hospital Trauma Life Support.* Akron, Ohio: Emergency Training, 1999.

Campbell, John E. *Basic Trauma Life Support for Paramedics and Other Advanced Providers.* 5th ed. Upper Saddle River, N.J.: Pearson/Prentice Hall, 2004.

Jastremski, M. E., M. Dumas, and L. Penalver. *Emergency Procedures.* Philadelphia: W. B. Saunders, 1992.

Martini, Frederic. *Fundamentals of Anatomy and Physiology.* 6th ed. San Francisco: Benjamin Cummings, 2004.

Rosen, P., and R. Barkin, eds. *Emergency Medicine: Concepts and Clinical Practice.* 5th ed. St. Louis: Mosby, 2002.

On the Web

Visit Brady's Paramedic Website at **www.bradybooks.com/paramedic.**

Head, Facial, and Neck Trauma

Objectives

After reading this chapter, you should be able to:

1. Describe the incidence, morbidity, and mortality of head, facial, and neck injuries. (p. 273)
2. Explain head and facial anatomy and physiology as they relate to head and facial injuries. (pp. 273–285)
3. Predict head, facial, and other related injuries based on the mechanism of injury. (pp. 286–287)
4. Differentiate between the following types of facial injuries, highlighting the defining characteristics of each:
   a. Eye (pp. 302–303)
   b. Ear (p. 302)
   c. Nose (pp. 301–302)
   d. Throat (pp. 304–305)
   e. Mouth (pp. 300–301)
5. Differentiate between facial injuries based on the assessment and history. (p. 309)
6. Explain the pathophysiology, assessment, and management for patients with eye, ear, nose, throat, and mouth injuries. (pp. 300–305, 312–327)
7. Explain the anatomy and relate the physiology of the CNS to head injuries. (pp. 274–280, 287–299)
8. Distinguish between facial, head, and brain injury. (pp. 287–303)
9. Explain the pathophysiology of head/brain injuries. (pp. 287–299)
10. Explain the concept of increasing intracranial pressure (ICP). (pp. 295–296)
11. Explain the effect of increased and decreased carbon dioxide on ICP. (pp. 295–296)
12. Define and explain the process involved with each of the levels of increasing ICP. (pp. 295–296)

13. Relate assessment findings associated with head/brain injuries to the pathophysiological process. (pp. 296–299)

14. Classify head injuries (mild, moderate, severe) according to assessment findings. (pp. 310–311)

15. Identify the need for rapid intervention and transport of the patient with a head/brain injury. (pp. 305–311, 325)

16. Describe and explain the general management of the head/brain injury patient, including pharmacological and nonpharmacological treatment. (pp. 313–327)

17. Analyze the relationship between carbon dioxide concentration in the blood and management of the airway in the head/brain-injured patient. (pp. 295–296)

18. Explain the pathophysiology, assessment, and management of a patient with:
    a. Scalp injury (pp. 287–288, 308–309, 325–326)
    b. Skull fracture (pp. 288–291, 308–309)
    c. Cerebral contusion (pp. 292, 294, 296–299)
    d. Intracranial hemorrhage (including epidural, subdural, subarachnoid, and intracerebral hemorrhage) (pp. 292–294, 296–299)
    e. Axonal injury (including concussion and moderate and severe diffuse axonal injury) (p. 294)
    f. Facial injury (pp. 299–303, 309, 326–327)
    g. Neck injury (pp. 304–305, 309–310)

19. Develop a management plan for the removal of a helmet for a head-injured patient. (p. 306)

20. Differentiate between the types of head/brain injuries based on the assessment and history. (pp. 296–299, 305–313)

21. Given several preprogrammed and moulaged head, face, and neck trauma patients, provide the appropriate scene size-up, initial assessment, rapid trauma or focused physical exam and history, detailed exam, and ongoing assessment and provide appropriate patient care and transportation. (pp. 273–327)

Key Terms

acute retinal artery occlusion, p. 303
anterograde amnesia, p. 297
aqueous humor, p. 283
arachnoid membrane, p. 276
ascending reticular activating system, p. 278
autoregulation, p. 279
bilateral periorbital ecchymosis, p. 288
brainstem, p. 277
cerebellum, p. 277
cerebral perfusion pressure, p. 278

cerebrospinal fluid, p. 276
cerebrum, p. 276
Cheyne-Stokes respirations, p. 297
concussion, p. 294
conjunctiva, p. 283
consensual reactivity, p. 309
contrecoup injury, p. 292
cornea, p. 283
coup injury, p. 292
cranium, p. 274
Cushing's reflex, p. 297
Cushing's triad, p. 297
diffuse axonal injury, p. 294
diplopia, p. 300

dura mater, p. 275
epidural hematoma, p. 293
fasciculations, p. 322
galea aponeurotica, p. 274
Glasgow Coma Scale, p. 299
hyphema, p. 303
hypothalamus, p. 277
intracerebral hemorrhage, p. 294
intracranial pressure (ICP), p. 274
iris, p. 283
lacrimal fluid, p. 283
Le Fort criteria, p. 300
mandible, p. 280

Case Study

Unit 765 responds to a report of a one-car crash with a single victim. Arriving at the scene, the two paramedics, Jan and Steve, observe an automobile against a tree. The frontal impact has greatly deformed the vehicle and severely bent the frame. The driver's side windshield is broken in a "spider web" configuration, and the driver's door is ajar. No wires are down, there does not appear to be any leaking gas or an ignition source, and the vehicle does not have air bags. Police at the scene have already controlled traffic. A police officer reports that the sole patient was initially unconscious, but awakened a few minutes ago.

When Jan and Steve approach the vehicle, they discover a conscious 31-year-old male sitting in the car. He states his name is John, but he is disoriented to time and event and doesn't know what day it is or what happened. He repeatedly asks where he is and what happened. Even after being reoriented, he repeats the same questions. Jan manually stabilizes his head, while Steve continues his initial assessment. Steve notes a contusion on John's left forehead. He also notes that John complains of moderate chest pain that varies with respiration. John doesn't remember any pain prior to the crash and denies any history of heart or other significant preexisting medical problems. John's motor and eye opening responses are normal.

Since John complains of chest pain, Steve palpates the thorax and feels some crepitus with respiratory movement. Lung sounds are clear and the monitor shows a sinus rhythm at a rate of 70 per minute. Vital signs include a blood pressure of 124/88, a distal pulse of 70, rapid capillary refill, deep respirations at a rate of 20, and a pulse oximeter reading of 99 percent. The patient's pupils are equal and briskly reactive to light changes. The Glasgow Coma Scale score is 14. During further questioning, John denies using any prescribed medications or having a history of allergies.

As assessment continues, John becomes agitated and then progressively more combative. Steve and Jan apply oxygen, but the patient's condition worsens. John becomes unresponsive and his left pupil dilates noticeably. He now only responds to deep pain and then with ineffective motion. Steve quickly applies a cervical collar and then he and Jan move John rapidly to a long spine board and begin transport.

En route to the hospital, Jan starts an IV with normal saline running at a to-keep-open rate. She calls for medical direction, gives a short report, and receives orders from the on-line physician to intubate the patient and divert the ambulance to the regional neurocenter. Steve intubates the patient orally, while Jan firmly immobilizes the head. Because John's respirations are now very shallow and rapid, they ventilate the patient at 10 full breaths per minute with high-flow, high-concentration oxygen. Reassessment of vital signs reveals that John's blood pressure is now 142/92, and his pulse is 62. The pulse oximeter reading is 96 percent, the capnography is 40 mmHg, and the Glasgow Coma Scale score is 5.

At the receiving hospital, the staff quickly assesses John and sends him off for X-rays and a CT scan. Although they find no cervical spine injury, they do note an expanding epidural hematoma. They rush John into surgery, where a neurosurgeon successfully evacuates blood from the epidural space. When the EMS crew does a 24-hour follow-up, they find John is conscious and confused but otherwise doing well.

INTRODUCTION TO HEAD, FACIAL, AND NECK INJURIES

Head, facial, and neck injuries are common with major trauma. Approximately 4 million people experience a significant head impact each year, with 1 in 10 requiring hospitalization. While most of these hospitalizations are due to relatively minor injuries, severe head injury is the most frequent cause of trauma death. It is especially lethal in auto crashes and frequently produces significant long-term disability in patients who survive them. Gunshot wounds that penetrate the cranium result in a mortality of about 75 to 80 percent. Injuries to the face and neck threaten critical airway structures as well as the significant vasculature found in these regions.

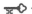

Severe head injury is the most frequent cause of trauma death.

The populations most at risk for serious head injury are males between the years of 15 and 24, infants and young children, and the elderly. Education programs promoting safe practices in many different fields and the use of head protection, seat belts, and air bags have had major effects on reducing head injury mortality and morbidity. The use of helmets for bicycling, rollerblading, and motorcycling and in contact sports such as football has also significantly reduced the incidence of serious head injury. In motorcycle crashes, for example, helmet use reduces serious head injury by more than 50 percent. Once a head injury occurs, however, time becomes a critical consideration. Intracranial hemorrhage and progressing edema can increase the intracranial pressure, hypoxia, and the internal and permanent damage done.

Despite the dangers posed by these injuries, the severity of head, facial, and neck injuries is often difficult to recognize in the prehospital setting. As a result, subtle and unforeseen problems associated with injuries to these regions too often cause a patient to quietly deteriorate while caregivers direct attention toward more apparent and gruesome injuries that are not as critical. Even if a life-threatening injury is recognized, you as a paramedic can provide little definitive field care. To lessen the chances of death and disability, you must learn to recognize the signs and symptoms of head, facial, and neck injury early in your assessment, maintain a clear airway and adequate respirations, maintain the patient's blood pressure, and provide rapid transport to a facility that can administer proper care.

ANATOMY AND PHYSIOLOGY OF THE HEAD, FACE, AND NECK

This chapter will consider injuries to three areas: the head, which contains the brain; the facial region, which contains the beginning of the airway, the beginning of the alimentary canal, and sense organs of sight, taste, hearing, and smell; and the neck, which contains the blood vessels, the midportion of the airway, and other vital structures that link the head and torso. Let us begin by looking at the relevant anatomy and physiology of these three areas.

ANATOMY AND PHYSIOLOGY OF THE HEAD

The head is made up of three structures that cover the brain: the scalp, the cranium, and the meninges. Each of these structures provides essential protection from the environment and from trauma.

The Scalp

The scalp is a strong and flexible mass of skin, fascia (bands of connective tissue), and muscular tissue that is able to withstand and absorb tremendous kinetic energy. The scalp is also extremely vascular in order to help maintain the brain at the body's core temperature. Scalp hair further insulates the brain from environmental temperatures and, to a lesser degree, from trauma.

The scalp is only loosely attached to the skull and is made up of the overlying skin and a number of thin layers of muscle and connective tissue underneath. Directly beneath the skin and covering the most superior surface of the head is a fibrous connective tissue sheet called the **galea aponeurotica.** Connected anteriorly to it and covering the forehead is a flat sheet of muscle, the frontal muscle. Connected posteriorly and covering the posterior skull surface is the occipitalis muscle. Laterally, the auricularis muscles cover the areas above the ears and between the lateral brow ridge and the occiput. A layer of loose connective tissue beneath these muscles and the galea and just above the periosteum is called the areolar tissue. It contains emissary veins that permit venous blood to flow from the dural sinuses into the venous vessels of the scalp. These emissary veins also exist in the upper reaches of the nasal cavity. These veins become potential routes for infection in scalp wounds or nasal injuries. A helpful way to remember the layers of skin protecting the scalp is the mnemonic SCALP: S—skin; C—connective tissue; A—aponeurotica; L—layer of subaponeurotica (areolar) tissue; P—the periosteum of the skull (the pericranium).

The Cranium

The bony structure supporting the head and face is the skull. It can be subdivided into two components: the vault for the brain, called the **cranium,** and the facial bones that form the skeletal base for the face (Figure 8-1 ▮). The cranium actually consists of several bones fused together at pseudojoints called **sutures.** These bony plates are constructed of two narrow layers of hard compact bone, separated by a layer of spongy cancellous bone. The plates form a strong, light, rigid, and spherical container for the brain. The cranium is, therefore, quite effective in protecting its contents from the direct effects of trauma. This cranial vault, however, provides very little space for internal swelling or hemorrhage. Any expanding lesion within the cranium results in an increase in **intracranial pressure (ICP).** This reduces cerebral perfusion and can severely damage the delicate brain tissue.

The cranial bones form regions that are helpful in describing the cerebral structures beneath. The anterior or frontal bone begins at the brow ridge and covers the upper and anterior surface of the brain. The parietal bones, one on either side, begin just behind the lateral brow ridge and form the skull above the external portions (pinnae) of the ears. The occipital bone forms the posterior and inferior aspect of the cranium, extending to and forming the foramen magnum. The temporal bones form the lateral cranial surfaces anterior to the ears, while the ethmoid and sphenoid bones, which are very irregular in shape, form the portion of the cranium concealed and protected by the facial bones.

The base of the skull consists of portions of the occipital, temporal, sphenoid, and ethmoid bones. This area is important in cases of trauma because the openings, or foramina,

galea aponeurotica *connective tissue sheet covering the superior aspect of the cranium.*

cranium *vaultlike portion of the skull encasing the brain.*

sutures *pseudojoints that join the various bones of the skull to form the cranium.*

intracranial pressure (ICP) *pressure exerted on the brain by the blood and cerebrospinal fluid.*

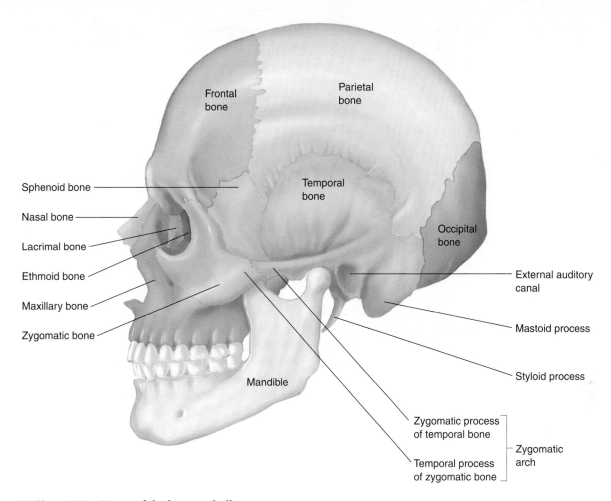

Labels on figure:

Frontal bone

Parietal bone

Temporal bone

Sphenoid bone

Nasal bone

Lacrimal bone

Ethmoid bone

Maxillary bone

Zygomatic bone

Occipital bone

External auditory canal

Mastoid process

Styloid process

Zygomatic process of temporal bone

Temporal process of zygomatic bone

Zygomatic arch

Mandible

■ Figure 8-1 Bones of the human skull.

for blood vessels, the spinal cord, the auditory canal, and the cranial nerves pass through it. These openings weaken the area, leaving it prone to fracture with serious trauma.

Other anatomical points of interest within the cranium are the cribiform plate and the foramen magnum. The cribiform plate is an irregular portion of the ethmoid bone and a portion of the base of the cranium. It and the remainder of the base of the cranium have rough surfaces against which the brain may abrade, lacerate, or contuse during severe deceleration. The foramen magnum is the largest opening in the skull. It is located at the base of the skull where it meets the spinal column and is where the spinal cord exits the cranium.

The Meninges

The final protective mechanisms for the brain and the spinal cord are the **meninges** (Figure 8-2 ■). They are three layers of tissue that lie between the cranium and the brain and also between the spinal column and the spinal cord. The outermost layer is the **dura mater** (meaning, literally, "tough mother"), which consists of a tough connective tissue. The dura mater is actually two layers. The outer layer is the cranium's inner periosteum. The dural layer is made up of tough, continuous connective tissue that extends into the cranial cavity where it forms partial structural divisions (the falx cerebri and the tentorium cerebelli). Above the dura mater lie some of the larger arteries that provide blood flow to the surface of the brain. Between the dural layers lie the dural sinuses, major venous drains for the brain.

The meningeal layer closest to the brain and spinal cord is the **pia mater** (meaning "tender mother"). It is a delicate tissue that covers all the convolutions of the brain and spinal cord. Although delicate when compared to the dura mater, the pia mater is still

meninges *three membranes that surround and protect the brain and spinal cord. They are the dura mater, pia mater, and arachnoid membrane.*

dura mater *tough layer of the meninges firmly attached to the interior of the skull and interior of the spinal column.*

pia mater *inner and most delicate layer of the meninges. It covers the convolutions of the brain and spinal cord.*

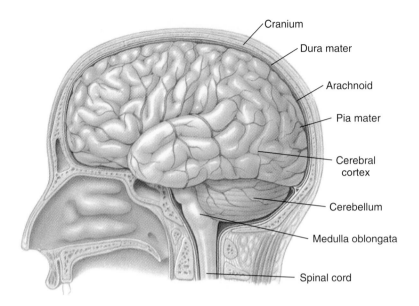

■ **Figure 8-2**   The meninges and skull.

Cranium
Dura mater
Arachnoid
Pia mater
Cerebral cortex
Cerebellum
Medulla oblongata
Spinal cord

arachnoid membrane   *middle layer of the meninges.*

cerebrospinal fluid   *fluid surrounding and bathing the brain and spinal cord (the elements of the central nervous system).*

cerebrum   *largest part of the brain. It consists of two hemispheres separated by a deep longitudinal fissure. It is the seat of consciousness and the center of the higher mental functions such as memory, learning, reasoning, judgment, intelligence, and emotions.*

more substantial than brain and spinal cord tissue. The pia mater is a highly vascular tissue with large vessels that supply the superficial areas of the brain.

Separating the two layers of mater is a stratum of connective tissue called the **arachnoid membrane.** It covers the inner dura mater and suspends the brain in the cranial cavity with collagen and elastin fibers. The arachnoid membrane gets its name from its weblike appearance (arachnoid meaning "spiderlike"). Beneath the arachnoid membrane is the subarachnoid space, which is filled with cerebrospinal fluid. This region provides cushioning for the brain when the head is subjected to strong forces of acceleration or deceleration.

Cerebrospinal Fluid

Cerebrospinal fluid is a clear, colorless solution of water, proteins, and salts that surrounds the central nervous system and absorbs the shock of minor acceleration and deceleration. The brain constantly generates cerebrospinal fluid in the largest two of four spaces (or ventricles) within the substance of the brain. The fluid circulates through the ventricles, then through the subarachnoid space, where it is returned to the venous circulation through the dural sinuses. The cerebrospinal fluid provides buoyancy for the brain and actually floats it in a near-weightless environment within the cranial cavity. This fluid also is a medium through which nutrients and waste products such as oxygen, proteins, salts, and carbon dioxide are diffused into and out of the brain tissue.

The Brain

The brain occupies about 80 percent of the interior of the cranium. It is made up of three major structures essential to human function—the cerebrum, the cerebellum, and the brainstem.

The **cerebrum** is the largest element of the nervous system and occupies most of the cranial cavity. It consists of an exterior cortex of gray matter (cell bodies) and is the highest functional portion of the brain. The central portion of the cerebrum is predominantly white matter, mostly communication pathways (axons). The cerebrum is the center of conscious thought, personality, speech, motor control, and of visual, auditory, and tactile (touch) perception. The cerebrum is regionalized into lobes roughly lying beneath the bones of the cranium (and given the same names). The frontal region is anterior and determines personality. The parietal region, which is superior and posterior, directs motor and sensory activities as well as memory and emotions. The occipital region, which is posterior and inferior, is responsible for sight. Laterally, the temporal regions are the centers for long-term memory, hearing, speech, taste, and smell.

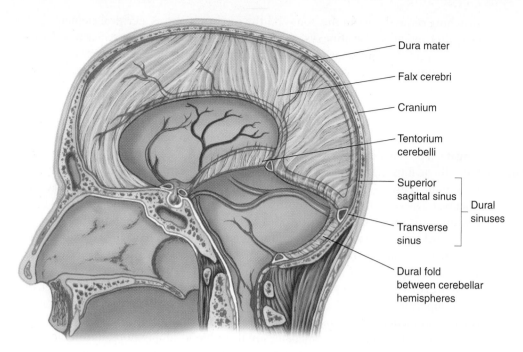

The following labels appear on the figure:

- Dura mater
- Falx cerebri
- Cranium
- Tentorium cerebelli
- Superior sagittal sinus
- Transverse sinus
- Dural sinuses
- Dural fold between cerebellar hemispheres

■ **Figure 8-3**   The partitions extending into the skull, the falx cerebri, and tentorium cerebellum.

A structure called the falx cerebri divides the cerebrum into right and left hemispheres. A dural partition, the falx cerebri extends into the cranial cavity from the interior and superior surface of the cranium (Figure 8-3 ■). Corresponding to the falx cerebri is a fissure in the cerebrum called the central sulcus. This fissure physically splits the cerebrum into the left and right hemispheres, each of which controls (for the most part) the activities of the opposite side of the body. The crossing of nerve impulses (from one side to the other) takes place just below the medulla oblongata. The tentorium cerebelli is a similar fibrous sheet within the occipital region, running at right angles to the falx cerebri. It separates the cerebrum from the cerebellum. The brainstem perforates the tentorium through an opening called the tentorium incisura.

The oculomotor nerve (CN-III), which controls pupil size, travels along the tentorium. It is likely to be compressed as intracranial pressure rises or the brain is displaced due to edema, a growing mass, or hemorrhage. This compression causes pupillary disturbances that manifest most commonly on the same side as the problem. If the pressure is great enough, it may affect both sides and both pupils may dilate and fix.

The left cerebral hemisphere is identified as the dominant hemisphere in most of the population, excepting a few left-handed individuals. It is responsible for mathematical computations (occipital region) and writing (parietal region) and is the center for language interpretation (occipital region) and speech (frontal region). The right, nondominant cerebral hemisphere processes nonverbal imagery (occipital region).

The **cerebellum** is located directly under the tentorium. It lies posterior and inferior to the cerebrum. The cerebellum "fine tunes" motor control and allows the body to move smoothly from one position to another. Additionally, it is responsible for balance and maintenance of muscle tone.

The **brainstem** is an important central processing center and the communication junction among the cerebrum, spinal cord, cranial nerves, and cerebellum. It includes the midbrain, the pons, and the medulla oblongata. The **midbrain** makes up the upper portion of the brainstem and consists of the hypothalamus, thalamus, and associated structures. The **hypothalamus** controls much of the endocrine function, the vomiting reflex, hunger, thirst, kidney function, body temperature, and emotions. The **thalamus** is the

The crossing of nerve impulses from one side of the body to the other takes place just below the medulla oblongata.

cerebellum   *portion of the brain located dorsally to the pons and medulla oblongata. It plays an important role in the fine control of voluntary muscular movements.*

brainstem   *the part of the brain connecting the cerebral hemispheres with the spinal cord. It is comprised of the medulla oblongata, the pons, and the midbrain.*

midbrain   *portion of the brain connecting the pons and cerebellum with the cerebral hemispheres.*

hypothalamus   *portion of the brain important for controlling certain metabolic activities, including regulation of body temperature.*

thalamus   *switching station between the pons and the cerebrum in the brain.*

ascending reticular activating system *a series of nervous tissues keeping the human system in a state of consciousness.*

pons *process of tissue responsible for the communication interchange between the cerebellum, the cerebrum, the midbrain, and the spinal cord.*

medulla oblongata *lower portion of the brainstem containing the respiratory, cardiac, and vasomotor centers.*

Though the brain accounts for only 2 percent of the body's total weight, it consumes about 20 percent of the body's oxygen.

switching center between the pons and the cerebrum and is a critical element in the **ascending reticular activating system,** the system that establishes consciousness. This region also provides the major tracts, or pathways, for the optic and olfactory nerves.

The **pons** acts as the communication interchange between the various components of the central nervous system—the cerebellum, the cerebrum, midbrain, and the spinal cord. It is a bulb-shaped structure directly above the medulla oblongata and appears to be responsible for the sleep component of the reticular activating system.

The last nervous system structure still within the cranial vault is the **medulla oblongata.** It is recognizable as a bulge in the very top of the spinal cord. The medulla contains three important centers—the respiratory center, the cardiac center, and the vasomotor center. The cardiac center regulates the rate and strength of cardiac contractions. The vasomotor center controls the distribution of blood and maintains blood pressure. The respiratory center controls respiratory depth, rate, and rhythm.

In order to maintain its advanced functioning, the brain has a high metabolic rate. Though the brain accounts for only 2 percent of the body's total weight, it receives about 15 percent of the cardiac output and consumes about 20 percent of the body's oxygen. It requires this circulation whether it is at rest or engaged in active thought. Further, this blood supply must be constant because the brain has no stored energy sources. It needs constant availability of glucose, thiamine (to help metabolize glucose), and oxygen and relies almost solely on aerobic metabolism. If the blood supply stops, unconsciousness follows within 10 seconds, and brain death will ensue within 4 to 6 minutes.

CNS Circulation

Four major arterial vessels provide blood flow to the brain. The first two are the internal carotid arteries. These vessels divide from the common carotid at the carotid sinus and then enter the cranium through its base. The two posterior vessels, the vertebral arteries, ascend along and through the vertebral column. They then enter the base of the skull, where they join and form a single basilar artery.

The internal carotid and basilar arteries interconnect through the circle of Willis in the base of the brain. This structure is an arterial circle that assures good circulation to the brain, even if one of the large feeder vessels is obstructed. Various arteries branch out from the circle of Willis and supply the substance of the brain itself.

Venous drainage occurs initially through bridging veins that drain the surface of the cerebrum. They "bridge" with the dural sinuses (large, thin-walled veins). These ultimately drain into the internal jugular veins and then into the superior vena cava.

Blood–Brain Barrier

The capillaries of the brain are special in that their walls are thicker and not as permeable as those found elsewhere in the body. They do not permit the interstitial flow of proteins and other materials as freely as do other body capillaries. This assures that many substances found in the circulatory system, such as some hormones, do not affect the central nervous system cells. Lymphatic circulation is also lacking in the brain and is replaced by the cerebrospinal fluid flow system. This results in a very special and protected environment for central nervous system cells. If frank blood seeps into the central nervous system tissue, it acts as an irritant, initiating an inflammatory response, resulting in edema.

Cerebral Perfusion Pressure

cerebral perfusion pressure *(CPP) the pressure moving blood through the brain.*

Cerebral perfusion is exceptionally critical and depends on many factors. Primarily, the pressure within the cranium (intracranial pressure or ICP) resists blood flow and limits perfusion to the central nervous system tissue. Usually the pressure is less than 10 mmHg and does not significantly impede blood flow as long as the mean arterial blood pressure (MAP is the diastolic blood pressure plus one third the pulse pressure) is at least 50 mmHg. The pressure moving blood through the cranium is the **cerebral perfusion pressure** (CPP). This is calculated as the mean arterial pressure (MAP) minus the intracranial pressure (ICP). Changes in ICP are met with compensatory changes in blood pressure to assure adequate cerebral perfusion pressure and cerebral blood flow. This compensating reflex is called **autoregulation.**

Since the cranium is a fixed vault for the structures of the brain, its volume and the pressure within are shared by the occupants. Any expanding mass (tumor), hemorrhage, or edema within the cranium will displace some other occupant, particularly the cerebrospinal fluid or blood, since they are the only readily movable media. This displacement maintains the intracranial pressure very effectively, up to a point. When the volumes of cerebrospinal fluid and venous blood are reduced to their limits, however, the intracranial pressure begins to rise. Autoregulation then raises the blood pressure to assure there is enough differential (CPP) to provide good cerebral perfusion. However, this increase in blood pressure causes the intracranial pressure to rise still higher and cerebral blood perfusion to diminish even more. As this cycle of increasing intracranial pressure and increasing blood pressure continues, brain injury and death are close at hand.

autoregulation *process that controls blood flow to brain tissue by causing alterations in the blood pressure.*

CPP = MAP − ICP

Cranial Nerves

The cranial nerves are nerve roots originating within the cranium and along the brainstem. They comprise 12 distinct pathways that account for some of the more important senses, innervate the facial area, and control significant body functions (see Table 8–1 and Figure 8-4 ■).

Ascending Reticular Activating System

The ascending reticular activating system is a tract of neurons within the upper brainstem, the pons, and the midbrain that is responsible for the sleep-wake cycle. It is a complex control system that monitors the amount of stimulation the body receives and

Table 8–1	Cranial Nerves	
Nerve	**Nerve Name**	**Nerve Function**
CN-I	Olfactory	Responsible for the sense of smell and actually branches from the cerebrum.
CN-II	Optic	Responsible for image transmission from the retina to the brain.
CN-III	Oculomotor	Controls four of the six oculomotor muscles and is responsible for most eyeball motion, iris constriction, and the movement of the upper eyelid. Due to its pathway within the skull, the third cranial nerve may be compressed, causing pupillary dilation and limiting eye movement.
CN-IV	Trochlear	In conjunction with the oculomotor and abducens nerves, this nerve results in conjugate gaze (the eyes looking in the same direction and moving together).
CN-V	Trigeminal	Innervates and receives sensation from the facial region and the gums, teeth, and palate and controls the muscles of chewing.
CN-VI	Abducens	Responsible for moving the eyeball downward.
CN-VII	Facial	Controls the muscles responsible for facial expression and receives sensation from the anterior tongue.
CN-VIII	Acoustic	Innervates the cochlea and vestibule of the ear and is responsible for hearing as well as positional sense, motion sensation, and balance.
CN-IX	Glossopharyngeal	Innervates the posterior tongue and pharynx and is important in swallowing; also monitors the baro- and chemoreceptors within the major blood vessels.
CN-X	Vagus	Major nerve of the parasympathetic nervous system that monitors and controls the heart, respiration, and much of the abdominal viscera.
CN-XI	Spinal Accessory	Controls the major muscles of the neck, as well as some of the muscles associated with swallowing, and the vocal cords.
CN-XII	Hypoglossal	Exercises voluntary muscular control over the tongue.

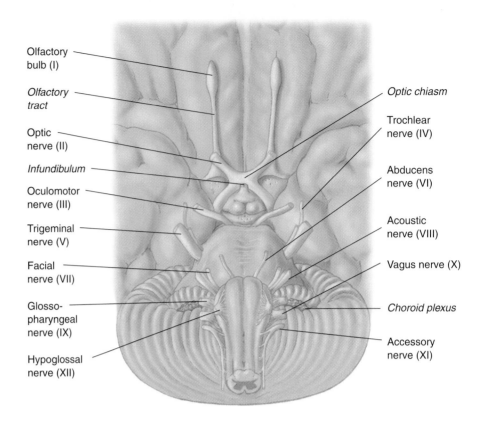

■ Figure 8-4 The cranial nerves as they exit the base of the brain.

Olfactory bulb (I)

Olfactory tract

Optic nerve (II)

Infundibulum

Oculomotor nerve (III)

Trigeminal nerve (V)

Facial nerve (VII)

Glosso-pharyngeal nerve (IX)

Hypoglossal nerve (XII)

Optic chiasm

Trochlear nerve (IV)

Abducens nerve (VI)

Acoustic nerve (VIII)

Vagus nerve (X)

Choroid plexus

Accessory nerve (XI)

regulates important bodily functions such as respiration, heart rate, and peripheral vascular resistance. Injury to the midbrain may result in unconsciousness or coma, while injury to the pons may result in a protracted waking state.

ANATOMY AND PHYSIOLOGY OF THE FACE

Facial bones make up the anterior and inferior structures of the head and include the zygoma, maxilla, mandible, and nasal bones (Figure 8-5 ■). The **zygoma** is the prominent bone of the cheek. It protects the eyes and the muscles controlling eye and jaw movement. The **maxilla** comprises the upper jaw, supports the nasal bone, and provides the lower border of the orbit. The nasal bone is the attachment for the nasal cartilage as it forms the shape of the nose. The last of the facial bones is the **mandible,** or jawbone. It resembles two horizontal "L's," which join anteriorly and hinge underneath the posterior zygomatic arch. Besides forming the beginning of the airway and the alimentary canal, the facial bones form supporting and protective structures for several sense organs, including the tongue (taste), eye (sight), and olfactory nerve (smell).

The facial region, like most other areas of the body, is covered with skin that serves to protect the tissue underneath from trauma and against adverse environmental effects. In the facial region, the skin is very flexible and relatively thin. It also has a very good vascular supply and hemorrhages freely when injured. Beneath the skin is a minimal layer of subcutaneous tissue; beneath that, there are many small muscles that control facial expression and the movements of the mouth, eyes, and eyelids.

Circulation for the facial area is provided by the external carotid artery as it branches into the facial, temporal, and maxillary arteries. The facial artery crosses the mandible, then travels up and along the nasal bone. The maxillary artery runs under the mandible and zygoma, then provides circulation to the cheek area. The temporal artery runs anterior to the ear just posterior to the zygoma. Each major artery has an associated vein paralleling its path.

zygoma   *the cheekbone.*

maxilla   *bone of the upper jaw.*

mandible   *the jawbone.*

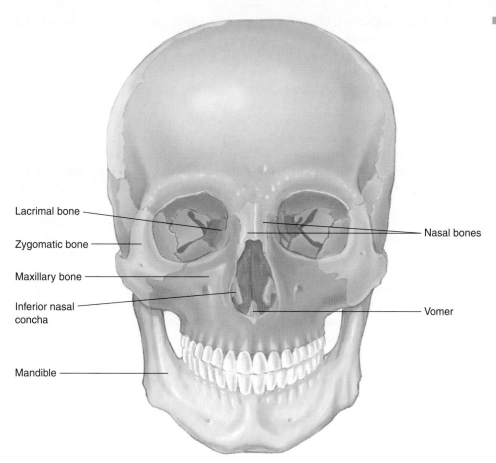

■ Figure 8-5   The facial bones.

Lacrimal bone

Zygomatic bone

Maxillary bone

Inferior nasal concha

Mandible

Nasal bones

Vomer

The most important cranial nerves traversing this area are the trigeminal (CN-V) and the facial (CN-VII). The trigeminal nerve provides sensation for the face and some motor control over eye movement as well as enabling the chewing process. The facial nerve provides motor control to the facial muscles and contributes to the sensation of taste.

The nasal cavity is formed by the juncture of the ethmoid, nasal, and maxillary bones. It is a channel running posteriorly with a bony septum dividing it into left and right chambers and plates protruding medially from the lateral sides. These plates, called turbinates, form support for the vascular mucous membranes that serve to warm, humidify, and collect particulate matter from the incoming air. The lower border of the nasal cavity is formed by the bony hard palate and then, posteriorly, by the more flexible cartilaginous soft palate. The soft palate moves upward to close off the opening of the posterior nasal cavity during swallowing. The nasal bone lies anterior and inferior to the eyes and provides a base for the nasal cartilage. The nasal cartilage defines the shape of the nose and divides the nostrils and their openings, which are called the **nares.**

nares   *the openings of the nostrils.*

The oral cavity is formed by the concave shape of the maxillary bone, the palate, and the upper teeth meeting the mandible and the lower teeth. The floor of the chamber consists of musculature and connective tissue that span the mandible and support the tongue. The tongue is a large muscle that occupies much of the oral cavity, provides the taste sensation, and moves food between the teeth during chewing (mastication) and propels the chewed food posteriorly, then inferiorly during swallowing. The tongue connects with the hyoid bone, a free floating U-shaped bone located inferiorly and posteriorly to the mandible. The mandible articulates with the temporal bone at the temporomandibular joint, under the posterior zygoma, and is moved by the masseter

Anatomy and Physiology of the Head, Face, and Neck   **281**

muscles. The lip muscles (obicularis oris) are responsible for sealing the mouth during chewing and swallowing.

Special structures are found in and around the oral cavity. Salivary glands provide saliva, the first of the digestive juices. These glands are located just anterior and inferior to the ear, under the tongue, and just inside the inferior mandible. Specialized lymphoid nodules, the tonsils, are located in the posterior wall of the pharynx.

Prominent cranial nerves serving the oral area include the hypoglossal, the glossopharyngeal, the trigeminal, and the facial nerves. The hypoglossal nerve (CN-XII) directs swallowing and tongue movement. The glossopharyngeal nerve (CN-IX) controls saliva production and taste. The trigeminal nerve (CN-V) carries sensations from the facial region and assists in chewing control. The facial nerve (CN-VII) controls the muscles of facial expression and taste.

Posterior and inferior to the oral cavity is a collection of soft tissue called the pharynx. The process of swallowing begins in the pharynx once the bolus of food has been propelled back and down by the tongue. The epiglottis moves downward while the larynx moves up, sealing the lower airway opening. The food or liquid moves into the esophagus where a peristaltic wave begins its trip to the stomach. This area is of great importance because it maintains the critical segregation of materials between the digestive tract and the airway.

Sinuses are hollow spaces within the bones of the cranium and face that lighten the head, protect the eyes and nasal cavity, and help produce the resonant tones of the voice. They also strengthen this region against the forces of trauma.

The Ear

pinna *outer, visible portion of the ear.*

The outer, visible portion of the ear is termed the **pinna.** It is composed of cartilage and has a poor blood supply. It connects to the external auditory canal, which leads to the eardrum. The external auditory canal contains glands that secrete wax (cerumen) for protection. The ear's important structures are interior and exceptionally well protected from nearly all trauma (Figure 8-6 ■). Only trauma involving great pressure differentials (e.g., blast and diving injuries) or basilar skull fractures are likely to damage this area.

The ear provides the body with two very useful functions, hearing and positional sense. The middle and inner ear contain the structures needed for hearing. Hearing occurs when sound waves cause the tympanic membrane (eardrum) to vibrate. The eardrum transmits the vibrations through three very small bones (the ossicles) to the cochlea, the organ of hearing. These vibrations stimulate the auditory nerve, which in turn transmits the signal to the brain.

semicircular canals *the three rings of the inner ear. They sense the motion of the head and provide positional sense for the body.*

The **semicircular canals** are responsible for sensing position and motion. They are three hollow, fluid-filled rings set at different angles. When the head moves, fluid in these rings shifts. Small cells with hairlike projections sense the motion and signal the brain to help maintain balance. This positional sense is present even when the eyes are closed. If injury or illness disturbs this area, it transmits excess signals to the brain. Patients then experience a continuous moving sensation known as vertigo.

The Eye

orbit *the eye socket.*

The eyes provide much of the input we use to interact with our environment. Although they are placed prominently on the face, the eyes are well protected from trauma by a series of facial bones. The frontal bones project above the globe of the eye, while the nasal bones and cartilage protect medially. The bone of the cheek, or zygoma, completes the physical protection both laterally and inferiorly. These bones collectively form the eye socket or **orbit.** The soft tissue of the eyelid and the eyelashes give additional protection to the critical ocular surface.

The eye is a spherical globe, filled with liquid (Figure 8-7 ■). Its major compartment (the posterior chamber) contains a crystal-clear gelatinous fluid called

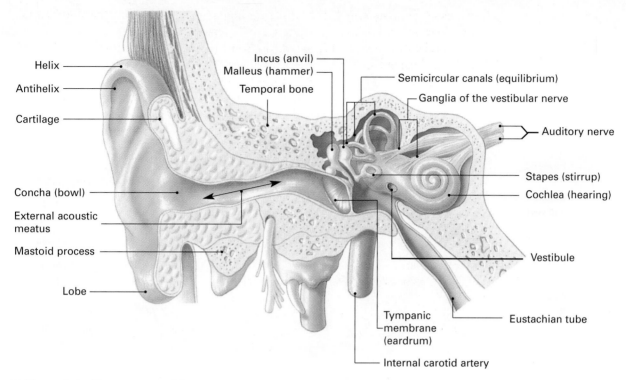

Figure 8-6 The anatomy of the ear.

vitreous humor. Lining the posterior of the compartment is a light- and color-sensing tissue known as the **retina.** Images focused on the retina are transmitted to the brain via the optic nerve. The lens separates the posterior and anterior chambers. The lens is responsible for focusing light and images on the retina by the action of small muscles that change its thickness. A fluid called **aqueous humor,** which is similar to vitreous humor, fills the anterior chamber. The anterior chamber also contains the **iris,** the muscular and colored portion of the eye that regulates the amount of light reaching the retina. Light enters the eye through the dark opening in the center of the iris called the **pupil.**

By examining the eye, you can easily identify several of its components such as the colored iris and the central black pupil. Bordering the iris is the **sclera,** the white and vascular area that forms the remaining, underlying surface of the exposed eye. The **cornea,** a very thin, clear, and delicate layer, covers both the pupil and iris. Contiguous with the cornea and extending out to the eyelid's interior surface is the **conjunctiva,** another delicate, smooth layer that slides over itself and the cornea when the eye closes or blinks.

The eye is bathed in **lacrimal fluid,** which is produced by almond-shaped lacrimal glands located along the brow ridge just lateral and superior to the eyeball. Lacrimal fluid flows through lacrimal ducts and then over the cornea. Because the cornea does not have blood vessels, the fluid provides crucial lubrication, oxygen, and nutrients. If injury or some other mechanism—for example, a contact lens left in an unconscious patient's eye—prevents this fluid from reaching the cornea, the surface of the eye may be damaged. The lacrimal fluid is drained from the eye into the lacrimal sac, located along the medial orbit, and empties then into the nose.

The last major functional elements of the eye are the muscles that move them and their controlling cranial nerves. These small muscles are attached to the eyeball in the region of the conjunctival fold and are hidden within the eye socket and under the zygomatic arch. The oculomotor (CN-III), trochlear (CN-IV), and abducens (CN-VI) nerves control these muscles, which in turn control the eye's motion. The oculomotor nerve controls pupil dilation, conjugate movement (movement of the eyes together), and most of the eye's travel

vitreous humor *clear watery fluid filling the posterior chamber of the eye. It is responsible for giving the eye its spherical shape.*

retina *light- and color-sensing tissue lining the posterior chamber of the eye.*

aqueous humor *clear fluid filling the anterior chamber of the eye.*

iris *pigmented portion of the eye. It is the muscular area that constricts or dilates to change the size of the pupil.*

pupil *dark opening in the center of the iris through which light enters the eye.*

sclera *the "white" of the eye.*

cornea *thin, delicate layer covering the pupil and the iris.*

conjuctiva *mucous membrane that lines the eyelids.*

lacrimal fluid *liquid that lubricates the eye.*

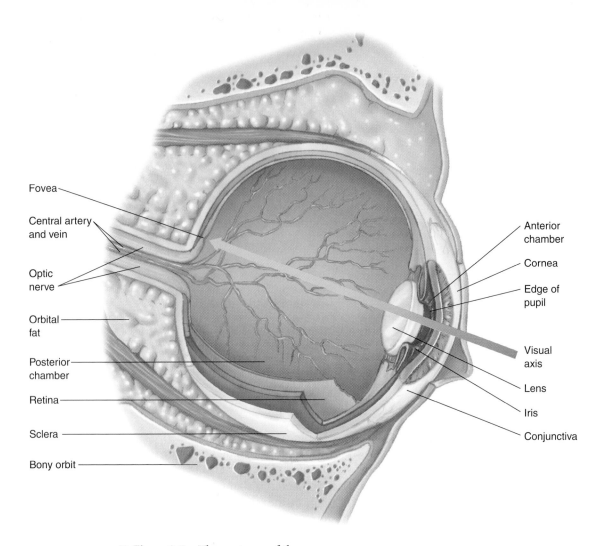

Fovea

Central artery
and vein

Optic
nerve

Orbital
fat

Posterior
chamber

Retina

Sclera

Bony orbit

Anterior
chamber

Cornea

Edge of
pupil

Visual
axis

Lens

Iris

Conjunctiva

■ Figure 8-7   The anatomy of the eye.

through its normal range of motion. The trochlear nerve moves the eye downward and inward, while the abducens nerve is responsible for eye abduction (outward gaze).

ANATOMY AND PHYSIOLOGY OF THE NECK

The neck is the region that links the head to the rest of the body. Traveling through this anatomical area are blood for the facial region and brain, air for respiration, food for digestion, and neural communications to sense the body and its environment and to control both the voluntary and involuntary muscles and glands of the body. The neck also contains some of the important muscles used to provide head and shoulder movement as well as the thyroid and parathyroid glands of the endocrine system.

Vasculature of the Neck

The major blood vessels traversing the neck are the carotid arteries and the jugular veins. The carotid arteries arise from the brachiocephalic artery on the right and the aorta on the left. They travel upward and medially along the trachea and split into internal and external carotid arteries at about the level of the larynx's upper border. At this split are the carotid bodies and carotid sinuses, which are responsible for monitoring carbon dioxide and oxygen levels in the blood and the blood pressure, respectively. The jugular veins are paired on each side of the neck. The internal jugular vein runs in a sheath with the carotid artery and vagus nerve, while the external jugular vein runs superficially just lateral to the trachea. The jugular veins join the brachiocephalic veins just beneath the clavicles.

Airway Structures

The airway structures of the neck begin with the larynx. It is a prominent hollow cylindrical column made up of the thyroid and cricoid cartilages, atop the trachea. The thyroid opening is covered during swallowing by a cartilaginous and soft-tissue flap, the epiglottis. The vocal cords, two folds of connective tissue sitting atop the opening of the larynx, further protect the airway. These cords vibrate with air passage and form sounds; they may also close in spasm to prevent foreign bodies from entering the lower airway. The cricoid cartilage is a circular ring between the thyroid cartilage and the trachea. The trachea is a series of C-shaped cartilages that maintain the tracheal opening. The posterior trachea shares a common border with the anterior surface of the esophagus. The trachea extends inferiorly to just below the sternum, where it bifurcates into the left and right mainstem bronchi at the carina.

Other Structures of the Neck

The cervical portion of the spinal column traverses the neck and provides the skeletal support for both the head and neck. It is also an attachment point for the ligaments that hold the column together and give it its strength and for the tendons that support and move the head and shoulders.

The cervical spine also contains the spinal cord. The spinal cord is the critical conduit for nervous signals between the brain and the body, and injury to it can be serious, even life threatening. From the spinal cord and between each vertebral junction, the peripheral nerve roots branch out. These structures direct signals to and receive signals from the limbs, internal organs, and sensory structures of the body. (The anatomy of the cervical spine is addressed in detail in Chapter 9, "Spinal Trauma.")

Other structures within the neck include the esophagus, cranial nerves, thoracic duct, thyroid and parathyroid glands, and brachial plexus. The esophagus is a smooth muscle tube located behind the trachea that carries food and liquid to the stomach. Its anterior border is continuous with the posterior border of the trachea. Some cranial nerves, including the glossopharyngeal (CN-IX) and the vagus (CN-X), traverse the neck. The vagus nerve is essential for many parasympathetic activities including speech, swallowing, and cardiac, respiratory, and visceral function. The glossopharyngeal nerve innervates the carotid bodies and carotid sinuses, monitoring blood oxygen levels and blood pressure. The right and left thoracic ducts deliver lymph to the venous system at the juncture of the jugular and subclavian veins. The thyroid gland sits over the trachea just below the cricoid cartilage and controls the rate of cellular metabolism as well as the systemic levels of calcium. The brachial plexus is a network of nerves in the lower neck and shoulder responsible for lower arm and hand function. Lastly, numerous muscles (including the sternocleidomastoid, platysma, and upper trapezius), fascia, and soft tissues are found in the neck. The neck muscles, like those of the extremities, are contained within fascial compartments. In the presence of soft-tissue injury, rapid swelling may increase pressure within a compartment and restrict blood flow.

PATHOPHYSIOLOGY OF HEAD, FACIAL, AND NECK INJURY

Head, facial, and neck injuries are difficult to assess in the prehospital setting, yet they commonly threaten life or may expose victims to lifelong disability. A clearer appreciation of the anatomy of these regions, of the various mechanisms of injury affecting them, and of the specific pathological processes related to head, facial, and neck injury can help you better anticipate, assess, and then manage these injuries and their effects on the human system.

MECHANISMS OF INJURY

Injuries to the head, neck, and face are divided by mechanisms of injury into blunt (closed) and penetrating (open).

Blunt Injury

The structures of the head, face, and neck protect very well against most blunt trauma. At times, however, the forces producing blunt trauma are of such magnitude as to compromise the body's well-designed protective mechanisms. For example, head injuries most frequently result from auto and motorcycle crashes and account for more than half of vehicle crash deaths. Sports-related impacts, falling objects, falls, and acts of violence, like assault with a club, are less common, but still significant mechanisms of head injury (Figure 8-8 ■).

The face is another area frequently subjected to blunt trauma. Significant facial injury occurs less frequently than head injury in auto impacts because the head's frontal or parietal regions are more likely to impact the windshield than the face. The same holds true for falls, as the arms, chest, or head absorb energy as the conscious victim tries to protect the facial area from injury. Intentional violence is less likely to spare the facial region. The face is often the target of blows from a fist or from impact-enhancing objects like sticks or clubs. The middle and inner ears and the eyes are very well protected against most blunt trauma, though ear injury may be caused by compressional forces associated with diving or explosions. The eyes may occasionally be injured by impacts from smaller blunt objects like a racquetball, baseball, or tennis ball.

The neck is anatomically well protected from most blunt trauma because the head and chest protrude more anteriorly. Laterally, the neck is protected as the shoulders protrude a significant distance from the neck. The neck is, however, a point of impact in special situations. For example, during an auto crash the neck may strike the steering wheel or be injured by a shoulder strap that is worn without a lap belt. The region may also be impacted by objects during fights or traumatically constricted or distracted during an attempted suicide by hanging.

■ Figure 8-8   Blunt injury to the facial region can produce hemorrhage, soft-tissue injuries, internal fractures, and brain injuries.

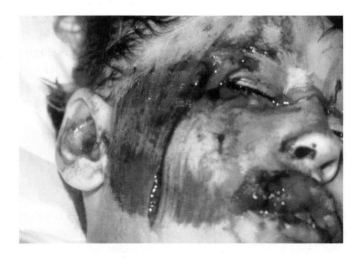

Penetrating Injury

Penetrating injuries to the head, face, and neck are not as common as those resulting from blunt trauma, but they can be just as severe and potentially life threatening. In addition, a penetrating injury to the head suggests the meninges have been opened, producing a route for potentially serious infection.

Penetrating injuries to the head, face, and neck usually result from either gunshots or stabbings. Gunshot wounds are most common and especially hideous because bullets release tremendous energy as they slow during collision with skeletal and central nervous tissue. Similarly, explosions propel projectiles, either intrinsic to the explosive device or from debris produced by the blast, that may penetrate and damage this region. Knife wounds to the head and face tend to be superficial because of the region's extensive skeletal components. The anterior and lateral neck, however, are not as well protected, and wounds there may compromise both the airway and major blood vessels, quickly threatening the patient's life.

There are many other types of penetrating injuries that may involve the head, face, and neck. Some examples include the "clothesline" impact with a wire fence while a victim is riding an all-terrain vehicle or snowmobile; bites from humans, dogs, and other animals; or a tongue bitten when the victim traps it between the teeth during an impact. Infrequently, a fall may impale a person on a fixed object such as a concrete reinforcing bar, producing a penetrating injury.

Blunt and penetrating injury mechanisms have different impacts depending on the structures they involve. The following sections discuss the pathological processes of injuries as they affect the head, face, and neck.

HEAD INJURY

Head injury is defined as a traumatic insult to the cranial region that may result in injury to soft tissues, bony structures, and the brain. Let us look at head injury as it progresses from the exterior to the interior, examining scalp, cranial, and brain injuries.

Scalp Injury

The most superficial head injuries involve the scalp (Figure 8-9 ■). A scalp injury may also be the only overt indication of deeper, more serious injury beneath. The scalp overlies the firm cranium and is very vascular. Its blood vessels lack the ability to constrict as effectively as those elsewhere in the body; hence, scalp wounds tend to bleed heavily. Some people believe that head injuries do not result in shock. This, however, assumes that the hemorrhage they cause is easy to control. In fact, any serious blood loss from scalp wounds can contribute to shock and, if left uncontrolled, may itself cause hypovolemia and shock. Scalp wounds further provide a route for infection because emissary veins drain from the dural sinuses, through the cranium, and into the superficial venous circulation. Because of rich circulation to the area, scalp wounds tend to heal well.

Scalp wounds may present in a manner that confounds assessment (Figure 8-10 ■). Usually, blunt trauma creates a contusion that, because of the firm skull underneath, expands outwardly in a very rapid and noticeable way. However, blunt trauma may also tear underlying fascia and areolar tissue, causing it to separate. This can leave an elevated border surrounding a depression, mimicking the contour of a depressed skull fracture. However, the scalp's blood vessels may bleed into a depressed skull fracture, fill any depression, and conceal the injury's true nature.

A common and special type of scalp wound is the avulsion. Areolar tissue is only loosely attached to the skull, and glancing blows can create a shearing force against the scalp's border. Such blows frequently tear a flap of scalp loose and fold it back against

The presentation of scalp wounds may make them difficult to assess.

■ **Figure 8-9** Scalp wounds can bleed heavily.

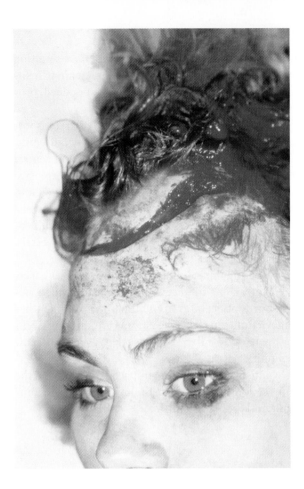

the uninjured scalp, exposing a portion of the cranium. The mechanism of injury may also seriously contaminate the wound and may cause moderate hemorrhage unless the avulsed tissue folds back sharply, compressing the blood vessels.

Cranial Injury

Because of its spherical shape and skeletal design, the skull does not fracture unless trauma is extreme. Such fractures may present as linear, depressed, comminuted, or basilar in nature (Figure 8-11 ■). Linear fractures are small cracks in the cranium and represent about 80 percent of all skull fractures. The temporal bone is one of the thinnest and most frequently fractured cranial bones. If there are no associated intracranial injuries, a linear fracture poses very little danger to the patient. In contrast, a depressed fracture represents an inward displacement of the skull's surface and results in a greater likelihood of intracranial damage. Comminuted fractures involve multiple skull fragments that may penetrate the meninges and cause physical harm to the structures beneath.

A common type of skull fracture involves the base of the skull. This area is permeated with foramina (openings) for the spinal cord, cranial nerves, and various blood vessels. The basilar skull also has hollow or open structures such as the sinuses, the orbits of the eye, the nasal cavities, the external auditory canals, and the middle and inner ears. These spaces weaken the skull and leave the basilar area prone to fracture.

The signs of basilar skull fracture vary with the injury's location (Figure 8-12 ■). If the fracture involves the auditory canal and the lower lateral areas of the skull, hemorrhage may migrate to the mastoid region (just posterior and slightly inferior to the ear). This causes a characteristic discoloration called **retroauricular ecchymosis** or "Battle's sign." Another classic sign of basilar skull fracture is **bilateral periorbital ecchymosis,**

The temporal bone is one of the thinnest and most frequently fractured cranial bones.

retroauricular ecchymosis *black-and-blue discoloration over the mastoid process (just behind the ear) that is characteristic of a basilar skull fracture. (Also called Battle's sign.)*

bilateral periorbital ecchymosis *black-and-blue discoloration of the area surrounding the eyes. It is usually associated with basilar skull fracture. (Also called raccoon eyes.)*

Scalp/Head Injury Presentations

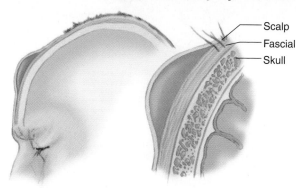

- Scalp
- Fascial
- Skull

Hematoma The blow disrupts blood vessels, resulting in accumulating blood and a hematoma.

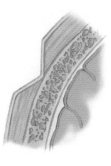

Depression The blow may tear fascial layers under the scalp and result in a depression, with or without a depressed skull fracture.

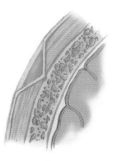

Normal Scalp Contour Blood may fill the space vacated by the torn fascial layers, or...

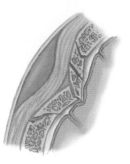

Blood may fill the area vacated by a depressed skull fracture.

■ Figure 8-10   Scalp/head injuries can present as a raised hematoma, a depression, or be disguised by a normal scalp contour.

sometimes referred to as "raccoon eyes." This is a dramatic discoloration around the eyes associated with orbital fractures and hemorrhage into the surrounding tissue. Both retroauricular ecchymosis and bilateral periorbital ecchymosis take time to develop; neither is likely to develop during the period after an injury when the patient is under paramedic care.

Basilar skull fracture can tear the dura mater, opening a wound between the brain and the body's exterior. Such a wound may permit cerebrospinal fluid to seep out through a nasal cavity or an external auditory canal and also provide a possible route for infection to enter the meninges.

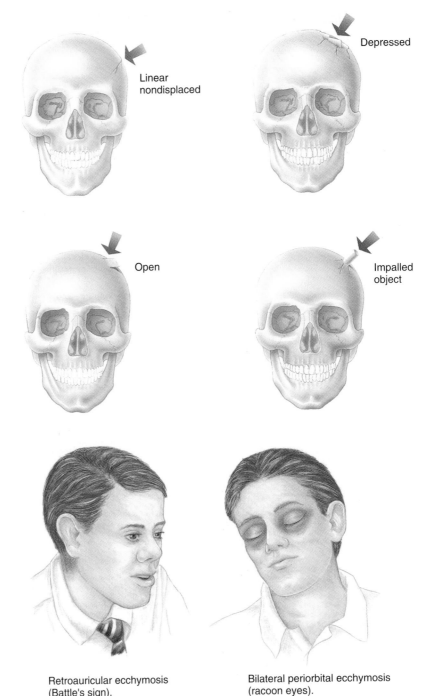

■ Figure 8-11 Various types of skull fractures.

Linear nondisplaced

Depressed

Open

Impalled object

■ Figure 8-12 Retroauricular or periorbital ecchymosis may indicate a basilar skull fracture.

Retroauricular ecchymosis (Battle's sign).

Bilateral periorbital ecchymosis (racoon eyes).

The "halo" sign is most reliable when associated with fluid leaking from the ear.

The glucose level of CSF is normally half that of the blood. If you are unsure whether a clear fluid is water or CSF, check the glucose level of the fluid and compare it to the patient's blood glucose level.

This type of wound may also provide an escape for cerebrospinal fluid in the presence of increasing intracranial pressure. Escaping cerebrospinal fluid may mediate the rise in ICP and somewhat limit damage to the brain. (While cerebrospinal fluid is an important medium, the body can regenerate it quite rapidly.) Blood mixed with cerebrospinal fluid and flowing from the nose, mouth, or ears will demonstrate the target or "halo" sign (a dark red circle surrounded by a lighter yellowish one) when dropped on a pillow or towel (Figure 8-13 ■). Normal blood demonstrates a narrow concentric ring of yellowish coloration surrounding the red circle produced by the less mobile erythrocytes. If cerebrospinal fluid is mixed with the blood, this outer ring is much larger. Be aware, however, that other fluids, like lacrimal or nasal fluids or saliva, may cause a

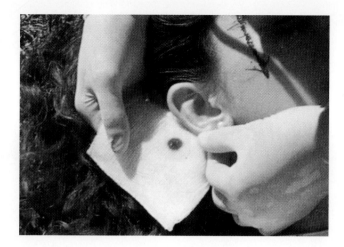

similar response. Hence, the halo sign is most reliable when associated with fluid leaking from the ear.

Bullet impacts induce specific types of cranial fracture. The entrance wound often produces a comminuted fracture and sends bone fragments into the brain. Often the bullet's kinetic energy is sufficient to permit the bullet to exit from the cranium and cause a second fracture. This exit wound site is blown outward and is often more severe in appearance than the entrance wound.

In many cases, the energy of the projectile's passage through the cranium causes a cavitational wave of extreme pressure, which is contained and enhanced by the rigid container of the skull. The result is extreme damage to the cranial contents, and, if the transmitted kinetic energy is strong enough, the skull may fracture and "explode" outward.

Another type of wound occurs when a bullet enters the cranium at an angle, is deflected within, and continues to move along the cranium's interior until its energy is completely exhausted. This process does devastating damage to the cerebral cortex and is rarely survivable.

A special type of cranial injury involves an impaled object. As is the case with objects impaled in most other regions of the body, any further motion of the object may cause additional hemorrhage and tissue damage. When the object is impaled in the cranium, the situation is especially serious. Brain tissue is much more delicate than other body tissue, does not immobilize the object as well, and is easily injured by the object's motion. As with objects impaled elsewhere, removal of the impaled object from the cranium may cause further injury and increase blood accumulation.

Note that a cranial fracture, by itself, is a skeletal injury that will heal with time; it does not, by itself, threaten the brain. Rather, it is the possibility of injury beneath and suggested by the skull fracture that is of greatest concern. The forces necessary to fracture the cranium are extreme and likely to cause injury within.

A cranial fracture, by itself, is a skeletal injury that will heal with time. However, the forces necessary to fracture the skull are often sufficient to induce brain injury.

Brain Injury

Brain injury is defined by the National Head Injury Foundation as "a traumatic insult to the brain capable of producing physical, intellectual, emotional, social, and vocational changes." It is classified as a direct or indirect injury to the tissue of the cerebrum, cerebellum, or brainstem.

Direct Injury Direct (or primary) injury is caused by the forces of trauma and can be associated with a variety of mechanisms. Rapid acceleration (or deceleration) or penetrating injury can cause mechanical injury to nervous system cells and impair their function. The forces causing direct injury can also disrupt blood vessels, both restricting blood flow through the injured area and causing irritation of nervous tissue

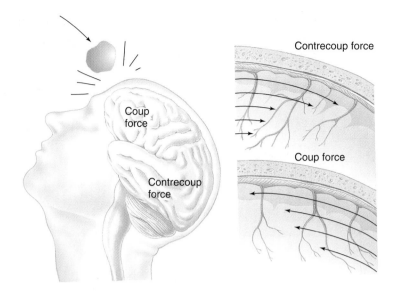

■ Figure 8-14   Coup and contrecoup movement of the brain.

Contrecoup force

Coup force

Coup force

Contrecoup force

Coup force

as blood flows into it. Remember that the brain is specially protected from contact with some of the blood's content by the blood–brain barrier. Injury disrupts this barrier. Lastly, serious jarring may damage capillary walls, affect their permeability, and cause a fluid shift to the interstitial space, or tissue edema. Most frequently, there is a mixture of these mechanisms associated with direct brain injury.

Two specific types of direct brain injury are coup and contrecoup injury (Figure 8-14 ■). **Coup injuries** are tissue disruptions that occur directly at the point of impact. These injuries are inflicted as the brain displaces toward the impact surface and collides with the interior of the cranium. They are most common in the frontal region because its interior surface is rough and irregular. In contrast, the occipital areas are smooth and coup injuries occur there less frequently. Coup injury may also occur as the brain slides along the rough contours at the base of the skull.

Contrecoup injuries produce tissue damage away from the impact point as the brain, floating in cerebrospinal fluid inside the cranium, "sloshes" toward the impact, then away from it, again impacting the interior of the skull. For example, a blow to the forehead might result in injury to the occipital region (visual center) and produce visual disturbances (seeing stars). Contrecoup injury to the frontal region of the brain is most common (from an impact to the occipital region) again because the frontal bones have an irregular inner surface.

Direct brain injuries can be further assigned to one of two specific categories—focal or diffuse.

Focal Injuries   Focal injuries occur at a specific location in the brain and include contusions and intracranial hemorrhages.

Cerebral Contusion   A cerebral contusion is caused by blunt trauma to local brain tissue that produces capillary bleeding into the substance of the brain. The contusion is relatively common with blunt head injuries and often produces prolonged confusion or other types of neurologic deficit. This pathology may result from a coup or contrecoup mechanism and may occur at one or several sites in the brain. The localized form of the injury manifests with dysfunctions related to the site of the injury. For example, a patient who suffers a contusion of the frontal lobe after trauma to the forehead may experience personality changes. (Remember, the frontal lobe is the most commonly injured lobe.)

Intracranial Hemorrhage   Bleeding can occur at several locations within the brain, each presenting with a different pathologic process. These injuries—proceeding

coup injury   *an injury to the brain occurring on the same side as the site of impact.*

contrecoup injury   *occurring on the opposite side; an injury to the brain opposite the site of impact.*

 Review

Types of Direct Brain Injury

Focal
Cerebral contusion
Intracranial hemorrhage
Epidural hematoma
Subdural hematoma
Intracerebral hemorrhage
Diffuse
Concussion (mild to
   moderate diffuse axonal
   injury)
Moderate diffuse axonal
   injury
Severe diffuse axonal injury
   (formerly, brainstem injury)

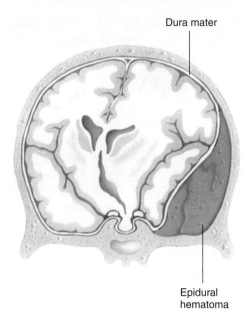

Dura mater

Epidural
hematoma

■ Figure 8-15   Epidural hematoma.

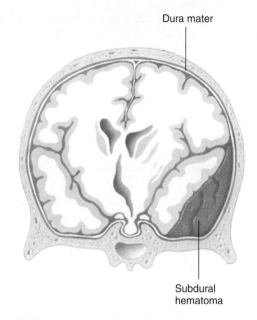

Dura mater

Subdural
hematoma

■ Figure 8-16   Subdural hematoma.

from the most superficial to the deepest—are epidural, subdural, and intracerebral hemorrhages. In contrast to patients with concussions and contusions, expect the intracranial hemorrhage patient to deteriorate during your assessment and care because of associated indirect injury such as increasing intracranial pressure.

Bleeding between the dura mater and the skull's interior surface is called **epidural hematoma** (Figure 8-15 ■). It usually involves arterial vessels, often the middle meningeal artery in the temporal region. Because the bleeding is from a relatively high-pressure vessel, intracranial pressure builds rapidly, compressing the cerebrum and increasing the pressure within the skull. As pressure builds, the patient moves quickly toward unresponsiveness. The hemorrhage-induced increase in intracranial pressure reduces oxygenated circulation to the nerve cells (indirect injury). Bleeding may be so extensive that it displaces the brain away from the injury site, pushing it toward the foramen magnum. Although the progression is both rapid and life threatening, immediate surgery can frequently reverse it.

epidural hematoma
accumulation of blood between the dura mater and the cranium.

Bleeding within the meninges, specifically beneath the dura mater and within the subarachnoid space, is called **subdural hematoma** (Figure 8-16 ■). This type of bleeding occurs very slowly and may have a subtle presentation because blood loss is usually due to rupture of a small venous vessel, often one of those bridging to the dural sinuses. The vessel most commonly involved is the superior sagittal sinus. Because the subdural hemorrhage occurs above the pia mater, it does not cause the cerebral irritation associated with intracerebral hemorrhage. The free blood in the cerebrospinal fluid may clog the structures responsible for the fluid's reabsorption, which can result in an increasing intracranial pressure. The patient usually does not show overt signs and symptoms until hours or even days after the injury. Because of this delay, subdural hemorrhage is difficult to detect in the prehospital setting.

subdural hematoma
collection of blood directly beneath the dura mater.

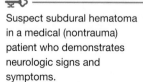

Suspect subdural hematoma in a medical (nontrauma) patient who demonstrates neurologic signs and symptoms. Careful history taking may uncover a recent mechanism of injury, such as a fall, that could cause this presentation. You occasionally encounter such pathologies with the elderly or with chronic alcoholics. Because both the aging process and chronic alcoholism reduce the size of the brain, head impact causes greater and less controlled motion of the brain within the cranium. This increases the likelihood of injury and, specifically, the subdural hematoma.

Suspect subdural hematoma in a medical (nontrauma) patient who demonstrates neurologic signs and symptoms.

intracerebral hemorrhage
bleeding directly into the tissue of the brain.

Intracerebral hemorrhage results from a ruptured blood vessel within the substance of the brain. Although blood loss is generally minimal, it is particularly damaging. Tissue edema results because free blood, outside the blood vessels, irritates the nervous tissue. Intracerebral hemorrhage often presents much like a stroke with the manifestations occurring very quickly. The particular presentation relates to the area of the brain involved. Normally, the signs and symptoms will progressively worsen with time.

Diffuse Injuries   Diffuse injuries involve a more general scenario of injury than do focal injuries. They include mild (concussions), moderate, and severe axonal disruptions. During head impact, a shearing, tearing, or stretching force is applied to the nerve fibers and causes damage to the axons, the long communication pathways of the nerve cells. This pathology is frequently distributed throughout the brain and thus is called **diffuse axonal injury (DAI).** Diffuse axonal injuries are common among vehicle occupants involved in collisions and in pedestrians struck by vehicles because of the severe acceleration/deceleration mechanisms. DAIs can range from the mild (a concussion) to the severe and life threatening (a brainstem injury).

diffuse axonal injury *type of brain injury characterized by shearing, stretching, or tearing of nerve fibers with subsequent axonal damage.*

concussion *a transient period of unconsciousness. In most cases, the unconsciousness will be followed by a complete return of function.*

Concussion   A **concussion** is a mild to moderate form of DAI and is the most common outcome of blunt head trauma. It represents nerve dysfunction without substantial anatomical damage (i.e., a normal head CT scan). Concussion results in a transient episode of neuronal dysfunction (confusion, disorientation, event amnesia), followed by a rapid return to normal neurologic activity. Prehospital management of concussion consists of frequent neurologic assessments with attention to the airway, to respiratory effort, and to subtle changes in the level of consciousness. Most patients survive with no neurologic impairment.

A concussion, contusion, intracerebral hemorrhage, subdural hematoma, and epidural hematoma may occur alone or in combination with one another. For example, an injury may cause a patient to sustain a concussion and an epidural hematoma concurrently. The concussion results in immediate unconsciousness, which resolves after only a few minutes. The patient becomes conscious and alert, but then later exhibits a deteriorating level of consciousness. This interim period of consciousness, called a lucid interval, occurs while the epidural hematoma expands.

A concussion disrupts the electrical activities of the brain without causing detectable injury to the brain itself.

Moderate Diffuse Axonal Injury   Here again, shearing, stretching, or tearing of the axons occurs, but now there is minute bruising of brain tissue. This type of injury is often referred to as the "classic concussion." If the cerebral cortex or reticular activating system of the brainstem is involved, the patient may be rendered unconscious. This type of injury is more severe than a mild concussion, occurs in 20 percent of all severe head injuries, and comprises 45 percent of all DAI cases. Moderate DAI is commonly associated with basilar skull fracture. Although most patients survive this injury, some degree of residual neurological impairment is common.

Short- and long-term signs and symptoms associated with moderate DAI include immediate unconsciousness, followed by persistent confusion, inability to concentrate, disorientation, and retrograde and anterograde amnesia. The victim may also complain of headache, focal neurologic deficits, light sensitivity (photophobia), and disturbances in smell and other senses. Anxiety may be present, and the patient may experience significant mood swings.

Severe Diffuse Axonal Injury   Severe DAI (previously known as brainstem injury) is a significant mechanical disruption of many axons in both cerebral hemispheres with extension into the brainstem. Approximately 16 percent of all severe head injuries and 36 percent of all cases of DAI are classified as severe. Many patients do not survive this type of injury; those that do have some degree of permanent neurologic impairment. The patient experiencing severe DAI is unconscious for a prolonged period of time and displays the signs of increased ICP (Cushing response) and decerebrate or decorticate posturing.

Indirect Injury   Indirect (or secondary) injuries are the result of factors that occur because of, though after, the initial (or primary) injury. These processes are progressive and cause the patient deterioration often associated with serious head injuries. The indirect injuries may be as or more damaging than the initial injury because of the unique design of the skull and the especially delicate nature of central nervous system tissue.

Indirect injuries are caused by two distinct pathological processes. The first process is a diminishing circulation to brain tissue (intracranial perfusion) due to an increasing intracranial pressure and possibly exacerbated by hypoxia, hypercarbia, and systemic hypotension. The second process is progressive pressure against, or physical displacement of, brain tissue secondary to an expanding mass within the cranium. Both these pathologies continue and expand the nervous tissue injury and cause some of the specific and progressive signs and symptoms associated with head injury.

Intracranial Perfusion   The brain is one of the body's most perfusion-sensitive organs. Any injury that affects perfusion has a rapid and devastating effect on the brain and its control of body systems. Cerebral, cerebellar, and brainstem perfusion may be disrupted both by increasing intracranial pressure and by low systemic blood pressure (hypotension).

As mentioned earlier, the cranial volume is fixed and does not vary. The cerebrum, cerebellum, and brainstem account for 80 percent (1,200 mL) of this volume. Venous, capillary, and arterial blood account for most of the remaining space, or about 12 percent (150 mL), while cerebrospinal fluid accounts for roughly the remaining 8 percent (90 mL). Any increase in the size of one internal component must be matched by a similar reduction in another component. If it is not, the intracranial pressure will rise.

As a mass expands within the cranium, the first means of compensating for the expansion is compression of the venous blood vessels. If the mass continues to expand, the next intracranial volume affected is the cerebrospinal fluid, which is pushed out of the cranium and into the spinal cord. These mechanisms respond very quickly and maintain an ICP very close to normal. However, once they reach their compensatory limits, the intracranial pressure rises quickly and begins to restrict arterial blood flow. The reduction in cerebral blood flow triggers a rise in the systemic blood pressure in an attempt to assure adequate cerebral perfusion, a process known as autoregulation. The greater the pressure of arterial blood flow, the greater the ICP. This increase in ICP further increases the resistance to cerebral blood flow, producing more hypoxia and hypercarbia. The resulting additional increase in systolic blood pressure, and then ICP, leads to a worsening, eventually deadly, cycle (Figure 8-17). If the mass, injury (edema), or hemorrhage continues to expand, the ICP becomes so high that cerebral circulation all but stops.

Another factor affecting ICP and circulation through the brain is the level of carbon dioxide in the cerebrospinal fluid. As the carbon dioxide level rises, the cerebral arteries dilate to encourage greater blood flow and reduce the hypercarbia. In the presence of an already high ICP, this process can have devastating results. The brain's response to high carbon dioxide concentrations and the increasing ICP causes the classical hyperventilation and hypertension associated with head injury. Low levels of carbon dioxide, however, can also have dire effects, triggering cerebral arterial constriction. In extreme cases, the resulting constriction can all but stop circulation through the brain. This is the reason that capnography is a valuable tool in the ongoing assessment of head injury patients, especially if you are ventilating them.

Two systemic problems frequently associated with trauma and sometimes related to brain injury are low blood pressure and poor ventilation. These problems seriously compound any existing head injury through a tertiary injury mechanism.

Hypotension, especially in the brain-injured patient with increasing ICP, may contribute to poor cerebral perfusion pressure. In turn, diminished cerebral circulation causes increasing acidosis (retained carbon dioxide) and anaerobic metabolism. This

Remember:
CPP = MAP − ICP

Low blood pressure and poor respiratory exchange seriously compound any existing head injury.

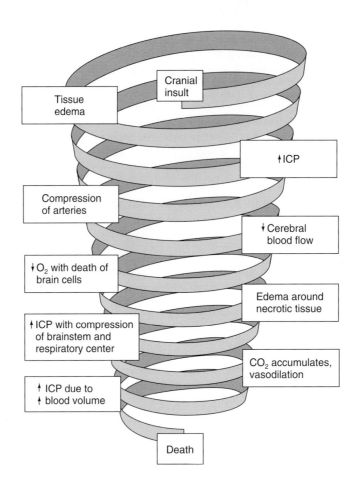

■ Figure 8-17 Pathway of deterioration following central nervous system insult.

induces further neural cell injury due to hypoxia and acidosis. At the same time, vasodilation (in response to increasing acidosis and carbon dioxide levels) elevates any existing intracranial pressure.

Hypoxia, secondary to shock or respiratory injury, increases the severity of any head injury. The reduced blood oxygen levels increase the cellular hypoxia at and around the injury site. Since central nervous tissue is extremely dependent upon good cellular oxygenation, neural cell damage becomes more severe.

Pressure and Structural Displacement As hemorrhage accumulates or edema increases in a region of the brain, this expansion pushes uninjured tissue away from the injury site. Even in the absence of increased ICP, such expansion puts pressure on adjacent brain tissue, most commonly along the brainstem. As the mass continues to increase in size, it may physically compress brainstem components. With further expansion, it may push the brain tissue against and around the falx cerebri and the tentorium cerebelli. Because these are basically immobile structures within the skull, the displacement results in a process called herniation. With herniation, a portion of a brain structure is pushed into and through an opening, physically disrupting the structure and compromising its blood supply. If the displacement affects the upper brainstem by pushing it through the tentorium incisura, it causes vomiting, changes in the level of consciousness, and pupillary dilation. If the displacement affects the medulla oblongata by pushing it into the foramen magnum, it results in disturbances in breathing, blood pressure, and heart rate.

Signs and Symptoms of Brain Injury

Direct injury, increasing intracranial pressure, and compression and displacement of brain tissue produce an altered level of orientation and of consciousness as well as spe-

 Review

Signs and Symptoms of Brain Injury

Altered level of
  consciousness
Altered level of orientation
Alterations in personality
Amnesia
  Retrograde
  Anterograde
Cushing's triad
  Increasing blood pressure
  Slowing pulse rate
  Irregular respirations
Vomiting (often without
  nausea)
Body temperature changes
Changes in reactivity of
  pupils
Decorticate posturing

Edema Edema (swelling) is the accumulation of fluid in the interstitial space. It can be localized or generalized. Local swelling may appear at the site of an injury (e.g., damaged airway structures or a sprained ankle) or within a certain organ system such as the lungs (pulmonary edema), heart (pericardial effusion), abdomen (ascites), or brain (cerebral edema).

Edema not only is a sign of an underlying disease or problem, but it also causes problems. It interferes with the movement of nutrients and wastes between tissues and capillaries. It may diminish capillary blood flow, depriving tissues of oxygen. In turn, this may slow the healing of wounds, promote infection, and facilitate formation of pressure sores. Edema affecting organs such as the brain, lung, heart, or larynx may be life threatening. Body water that is retained in the interstitial spaces is body water not available for metabolic processes in the cells. Therefore, even if the total body water is normal, edema can cause a relative condition of dehydration. Damage to the airway, where development of edema is life threatening, requires that the patient be intubated before the swelling develops to the point of airway obstruction.

Edema that occurs with injury to the brain is especially dangerous. Because the brain is confined within the bony skull, there is no room for expansion, so edema places pressure on the brain tissues, especially the brainstem. As the edema progresses, it causes herniation, in which brain tissues are pushed out through the foramen magnum, the opening through which the spinal cord connects to the brain.

---

cific signs and symptoms related to the central nervous system structure(s) affected. The actual process of brain injury can be mapped as the pressure increases and the injury moves from the cortical surface and down the brainstem.

As a portion of the cerebral cortex is disrupted by injury, the specific activity it controls is affected. For example, if the frontal lobe is injured, the patient will likely present with alterations in personality. If the occipital region is affected, visual disturbances are expected. A large region of cortical disruption may reduce the patient's level of awareness. The patient may become unaware of the circumstances leading up to the incident (**retrograde amnesia**) or following it (**anterograde amnesia**) or become disoriented (to time, place, and person), confused, or combative. Focal deficits, like hemiplegia or weakness, or seizures may also result. When intracranial injury extends to components of the ascending reticular activating system in the brainstem, the patient may display an altered level of arousal, including lethargy, somnolence, or coma.

If the compression results from a building mass along the central region of the cerebrum, pressure is first directed to the midbrain, then the pons, and finally to the medulla oblongata. The signs and symptoms of this progressive pressure and structural displacement are somewhat predictable and are known as the central syndrome.

In this syndrome, upper brainstem compression produces an increase in blood pressure to maintain cerebral perfusion pressure (called **Cushing's reflex**) and a reflex decrease in heart rate in response to vagus nerve (parasympathetic) stimulation of the SA node and AV junction (Figure 8-18 ■). The patient may also exhibit a characteristic cyclic breathing pattern called **Cheyne-Stokes respirations.** This consists of increasing, then decreasing respiratory volumes, followed by a period of apnea. The combination of an increasing blood pressure, slowing pulse, and irregular respirations is a classical sign of brainstem pressure or injury called **Cushing's triad.** If the brain injury involves the hypothalamus, the patient may experience vomiting, frequently without nausea, and body temperature changes. The pupils remain small and reactive. Decorticate posturing (body extension with arm flexion) in response to painful stimuli may occur as the neural pathways through the upper brainstem are disrupted.

retrograde amnesia *inability to remember events that occurred before the trauma that caused the condition.*

anterograde amnesia *inability to remember events that occurred after the trauma that caused the condition.*

Cushing's reflex *response due to cerebral ischemia that causes an increase in systemic blood pressure, which maintains cerebral perfusion during increased intracranial pressure.*

Cheyne-Stokes respirations *respiratory pattern of alternating periods of apnea and tachypnea.*

Cushing's triad *the combination of increasing blood pressure, slowing pulse, and irregular respirations in response to increased intracranial pressure.*

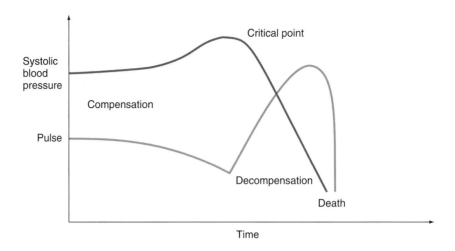

■ Figure 8-18 How systolic blood pressure and pulse rate respond to increasing intracranial pressure.

As the middle brainstem becomes involved the pulse pressure widens and the heart rate becomes bradycardic. Respirations now may be deep and rapid (central neurologic hyperventilation). Increasing intracranial pressure may also induce pupil sluggishness or nonreactivity (bilaterally since the pathology involves compression from above) as the oculomotor nerve (CN-III) is compressed. The patient develops extension (decerebrate) posturing. Few patients ever function normally again once they have reached this ICP level.

Finally, as the pressure reaches the lower brainstem the pupils become fully dilated and unreactive. Respirations become ataxic (erratic with no characteristic rhythm) or may even cease altogether. The pulse rate is often very irregular with great swings in rate. ECG conduction disturbances become apparent, including QRS complex, S-T segment, and T-wave changes. As control over blood pressure is disrupted, the patient becomes hypotensive. The patient no longer responds to painful stimuli, and the skeletal muscles become flaccid. Patients rarely survive once the ICP rises to this level.

If the mass causing the compression is located more laterally than in the central syndrome just described, the signs and symptoms occur in a less predictable sequence. The pupillary responses, sluggishness, nonreactivity, and dilation are usually ipsilateral (on the same side) to the expanding mass.

Recognition of Herniation

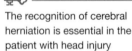

The recognition of cerebral herniation is essential in the patient with head injury because it directs your care.

The recognition of cerebral herniation is essential in the patient with head injury because it directs your care. The patient with herniation has a history of head trauma and is likely to display an increasing blood pressure, decreasing pulse rate, and respirations that become irregular (Cushing's triad). They also may have a lowering level of consciousness (Glasgow Coma Scale <9 and dropping), singular or bilaterally dilated and fixed pupils, and posturing (decerebrate or decorticate) or no movement with noxious stimuli.

Pediatric Head Trauma

Pediatric head trauma has a very different pathology than that in the older patient. The skull is not fully formed at birth and is still rather cartilaginous. It will distort more easily with the force of an impact and transmit that force more directly to the delicate central nervous tissue. However, the incomplete formation of the skull with its "soft spots" (the anterior and posterior fontanelles) permits some intracranial expansion. The fontanelles bulge outward with increasing intracranial pressure. Generally, then, this softer skeletal structure increases the direct injury associated with head trauma in the very young pediatric patient but slows the progression of increasing intracranial pressure.

As noted earlier, the blood and cerebrospinal fluid represent about 20 percent of the total volume of the adult cranium (about 240 mL). A blood loss into the cranium cannot account for a significant component of hypovolemia in the adult. A pediatric patient, however, has a proportionally larger head, the ability to accommodate increased fluids because of the fontanelles, and a much smaller total body fluid volume and reserves. In the pediatric patient, therefore, intracranial hemorrhage may significantly contribute to hypovolemia.

When treating an infant with head, face, or neck injury, pay particular attention to the airway. Infants are obligate nasal breathers and must have a patent nasal passage and pharynx to assure a clear airway. Hyperextension of the head will obstruct the airway as the tongue pushes the soft pallet closed. Assure proper head positioning, and ventilate using both the mouth and nose.

In the pediatric patient, intracranial hemorrhage may significantly contribute to hypovolemia.

Glasgow Coma Scale

The **Glasgow Coma Scale** (GCS) is a standardized evaluation method used to measure a patient's level of consciousness. The scale assesses the best eye opening, verbal, and motor response and awards points for the various responses. Responses must be determined for both sides of the patient and any side-to-side differences noted. (A more detailed discussion of the scale is found later in this chapter.)

Glasgow Coma Scale scoring system for monitoring the neurologic status of patients with head injuries.

Eye Signs

Pay close attention to the eyes when evaluating a patient with possible head trauma. The eyes are a very specialized body tissue (like central nervous system tissue) and a very visible special sense organ. The eyes can give indications of problems with cranial nerves CN-II, III, IV, and VI and with perfusion associated with cerebral blood flow. The surface of the eye is very dependent on good perfusion and lacrimal fluid flow. If perfusion is diminished, the eyes lose their luster quickly. The eyes also give quick, highly visible signs of the patient's demeanor—anxiety, fear, anger, and so forth.

Evaluation of the eyes is very important in patients with suspected head injury.

Pupil size and reactivity also give clues to underlying conditions. Depressant drugs or cerebral hypoxia will reduce pupillary responsiveness, while extreme hypoxia causes them to dilate and fix. An expanding cranial lesion places progressive pressure on the oculomotor nerve (CN-III), causing the ipsilateral (same side) pupil to become sluggish, then dilated, then fixed. This occurs because the outer oculomotor nerve contains parasympathetic fibers. As increasing pressure interferes with these nerve fibers, the pupil dilates and is unable to constrict. If one pupil is fixed yet shows some response to consensual stimulation (light variations in the other eye), the problem most likely lies with the oculomotor nerve.

FACIAL INJURY

Facial injury is a serious trauma complication, not only because of the cosmetic importance people place on facial appearance, but also because of the region's vasculature and the location of the initial airway and alimentary canal structures and the organs of sight, smell, taste, and hearing present there. Remember, too, that serious facial injuries suggest associated head and spinal injuries.

Facial Soft-Tissue Injury

Facial soft-tissue injury is common and can threaten both the patient's airway and physical appearance. Because of the ample supply of arterial and venous vessels, injuries in the region may bleed heavily, contributing to hypovolemia. Facial injuries are often the result of violence, from, for instance, bullet or knife wounds. Superficial injuries and hemorrhage rarely affect the airway. With deep lacerations, however, blood may accumulate and endanger the airway or enter the digestive tract and induce vomiting.

Patients with serious facial
soft-tissue injuries are likely to
have associated injury,
especially basilar skull
fractures and spine injuries.

Serious blunt or penetrating injury to the soft tissues and skeletal structures supporting the pharynx may reduce the patient's ability to control the airway, increasing the likelihood of foreign body or fluid aspiration and airway compromise. Hypoxia caused by aspiration is more likely caused by blood than by other fluids or physical obstruction.

Remember, the process of inspiration creates a less-than-atmospheric pressure in the lungs to draw air in. This reduction in pressure may collapse damaged structures along the airway that are normally held open by bony or cartilaginous formations. Soft-tissue swelling may also rapidly restrict the airway or close it completely. Swelling and deformity from trauma may distort the facial region so landmarks are hard to recognize, making airway control even more difficult. In serious facial soft-tissue injury, always consider the likelihood of associated injury, especially basilar skull fracture and spine injury.

Facial Dislocations and Fractures

Trauma may result in open or closed facial fractures with significant associated pain, swelling, deformity, crepitus, and hemorrhage. Common injuries include mandibular, maxillary, nasal, and orbital fractures and dislocations.

Mandibular dislocation occurs as the condylar process displaces from the temporomandibular joint, just anterior to the ear. This dislocation may result in the malocclusion of the mouth, misalignment of teeth, deformity of the facial region at or around the joint, immobility of the jaw, and pain. The patient's ability to control the airway may be decreased, but dislocation is not usually a significant airway or breathing threat.

Fractures of the mandible are painful, present with deformity along the jaw's surface, and may result in the loosening of a few teeth. An open mandibular fracture may produce a blood-stained saliva. Mandibular fracture may represent a serious life threat if the patient is placed supine. With such a fracture, the tongue is no longer supported at its base and may displace posteriorly, blocking the airway even in a conscious patient. Always look for a second fracture site when you encounter a patient with a mandibular fracture.

Maxillary fractures are classified according to **Le Fort criteria** (Figure 8-19 ■). A slight instability involving the maxilla alone usually presents with no associated displacement and is classified as a Le Fort I fracture. A Le Fort II fracture results in fractures of both the maxilla and nasal bones. Le Fort III fractures characteristically involve the entire facial region below the brow ridge, including the zygoma, nasal bone, and maxilla. The Le Fort II and III fractures usually result in cerebrospinal fluid leakage and may endanger the patency of the nasal and oral portions of the airway.

Le Fort criteria *classification system for fractures involving the maxilla.*

With a Le Fort II injury, the
midface and zygoma move
concurrently. This results in
the "dish-face" description
often given to this injury.

Dental injury is commonly associated with serious blunt facial trauma. Teeth may chip, break, loosen, or dislodge from the mandible or maxilla. They may then become foreign objects drawn (aspirated) into the airway. Note that a dislodged tooth may be reimplanted if fully intact and handled properly during prehospital care.

Orbital (blowout) fractures most commonly involve the zygoma or maxilla of the inferior shelf. Zygomatic arch fractures are painful and present with a unilateral depression over the prominence of one cheek. The fracture may entrap the extraocular muscles, reducing the eye's range of motion and can cause blurred or double vision (**diplopia**). Zygomatic fracture may also entrap the masseter muscle and limit jaw movement. With maxillary bone fracture, the patient often experiences significant swelling and pain in the maxillary sinus region. Although these injuries are not life threatening, they warrant evaluation by emergency department staff.

A special type of facial injury is that associated with a suicide attempt using a rifle or shotgun. The victim places the barrel under the chin but in an effort to push the trigger, stretches and tilts the head back. The gunshot blast is directed under the chin and at the facial region but may be deflected from entering the cranium. The result is a very

Review

Le Fort Facial Fractures

I—slight instability to maxilla; no displacement
II—fracture of both maxilla and nasal bones
III—fracture involving entire face below brow ridge (zygoma, nasal bone, maxilla)

diplopia *double vision.*

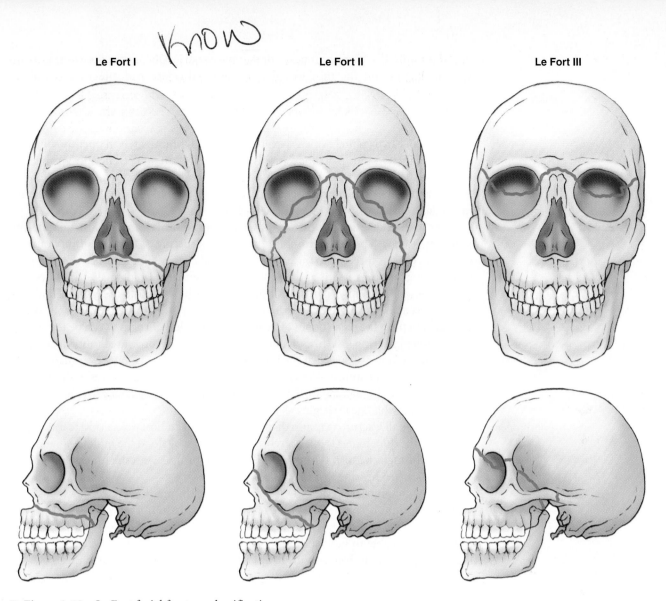

Le Fort I   Le Fort II   Le Fort III

■ Figure 8-19   Le Fort facial fracture classification.

disrupted facial region with most of the structures of, and supporting, the airway destroyed. The patient may still be conscious, there is usually heavy bleeding, and the remains of the airway are hard to locate. With such a patient, the airway is in serious danger of obstruction and attempts to secure it are very challenging.

Nasal Injury

Nasal injuries are painful and often create a grossly deformed appearance, but they are not usually life threatening. While dislocation or fracture of the cartilage and nasal bone may interfere with nasal air movement, the swelling and associated hemorrhage are more likely threats to the airway. However, the conscious and alert patient is usually very able to control the airway.

Epistaxis (nosebleed) is a common nasal problem. Bleeding can be spontaneous as well as traumatic and can be further classified as either anterior or posterior. Anterior hemorrhage comes from the septum and is usually due to bleeding from a network of vessels called Kisselbach's plexus. Such hemorrhage bleeds slowly and is usually self-limiting. Posterior hemorrhage may be severe and cause blood to drain down the back of the patient's throat. In epistaxis secondary to severe head trauma with likely basilar skull fracture, the integrity of the nasal cavity's posterior wall may be compromised. Attempts at nasal airway, nasogastric tube, or nasotracheal tube insertion may permit the tube to enter the cerebral cavity and directly damage the brain.

Ear Injury

The external ear, or pinna, which is exposed to the environment, is frequently subjected to trauma. It has a minimal blood supply and does not often bleed heavily when lacerated. In glancing blows, the pinna may be partially or completely avulsed. In a folding type of injury, the cartilage may separate. Due to the poor blood supply, external ear injuries do not heal as well as other facial wounds.

The internal portions of the ear—the external auditory canal and the middle and inner ear—are well protected from trauma by the structure of the skull. Injury only results from objects forced into the ear or from rapid changes in pressure as in diving accidents or explosions. With an explosion—even with repeated small arms fire—the pinna focuses the rapidly changing air pressure and directs it into the external auditory canal. This enhanced pressure irritates or ruptures the tympanum and, if strong enough, fractures the small bones of hearing (the ossicles). The result can be temporary or permanent hearing loss. In a diving injury, the changing pressure is not equalized by the eustachian tube (also called the pharyngotympanic passage) and eventually builds until the eardrum ruptures. Water floods the middle ear and interferes with the function of the semicircular canals. The patient experiences vertigo, an extremely dangerous sensation when near weightless under water.

Basilar skull fracture may also disrupt the external auditory canal and tear the tympanum. If the dura mater is torn, cerebrospinal fluid may flood the middle ear and seep outward through the torn tympanum (Figure 8-20 ▪). As with the other mechanisms described earlier, hearing loss may result.

Tympanic injuries are not life threatening and, in many cases, repair themselves, even with a rupture that tears as much as half the tympanum. However, a victim with an acute hearing loss can be quite apprehensive and anxious. The patient may be frustrated when unable to hear and understand questions or instructions. Such a patient may also be unable to hear sounds of approaching danger such as traffic noise.

Eye Injury

Although the orbit is a very effective protective housing for the eye, penetrating and some blunt trauma may cause serious injury. The anterior eye structures are extremely specialized and, like most specialized tissues, do not regenerate effectively. If significant penetrating injury occurs, especially if accompanied by loss of the eye's fluids—aqueous or vitreous humor—the patient's sight is threatened, possibly with permanent loss. A penetrating object is likely to disturb the integrity of the anterior and possibly

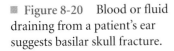 Figure 8-20 Blood or fluid draining from a patient's ear suggests basilar skull fracture.

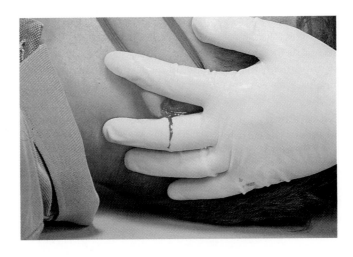

the posterior chamber. In addition, removal of the object may allow fluids to leak from the chambers and further threaten the patient's vision. Penetrating injuries may be caused by foreign bodies so small that they are difficult to see with the naked eye. Suspect the presence of such bodies if the patient reports a history of sudden eye pain and the sensation of an impaled foreign body after using a power saw or grinder, especially when working with metal.

Similarly, small foreign particles that land on the eye's surface can also cause ocular injury. The object may embed in the surface of the eyelid and then drag across the cornea as the eye blinks. Corneal abrasions or lacerations result, often causing intense and continuing pain even after the object is cleared from the eye. These lacerations are usually superficial but can be deep (Figure 8-21 ■).

Blunt trauma may result in several ocular presentations. Hemorrhage may occur in the anterior chamber pools, displaying a collection of blood in front of the iris and pupil. This condition, called **hyphema,** is a potential threat to the patient's vision and requires evaluation by an ophthalmologist and may result in hospital admission.

A less serious, but equally dramatic, eye injury is a subconjunctival hemorrhage. This may occur after a strong sneeze, vomiting episode, or direct eye trauma, such as orbital fracture. It occurs when a small blood vessel in the subconjunctival space bursts, leaving a portion of the eye's surface blood red (Figure 8-22 ■). Subconjunctival hemorrhage often clears without intervention and rarely causes any residual scars or impairment.

Blunt trauma may fracture the orbital structures surrounding the eye and produce an injury called eye avulsion. In such a case, the eye is not really avulsed but appears to protrude from the wound as the structure of the orbit is crushed and depressed. If the eye as well as the nerves and vasculature remain intact, sight in the eye can usually be salvaged.

Two other, more serious ocular problems involve the retina. **Acute retinal artery occlusion** is not an injury but rather a vascular emergency caused when an embolus blocks the blood supply to one eye. The patient complains of sudden and painless loss of vision in the eye. In **retinal detachment,** which may be traumatic in origin, the retina separates from the eye's posterior wall. The patient complains of a dark curtain obstructing part of the field of view. Both of these conditions are true emergencies in which the patient's eyesight is at risk.

Soft-tissue lacerations can occur around the eye and involve the eyelid. If not properly identified and repaired, such an injury may disrupt the function of the lacrimal duct and interrupt lubrication and oxygenation of the cornea. Another soft-tissue problem may occur if a contact lens is left in the eye of an unconscious patient. The contact lens will then obstruct the normal lacrimal fluid flow across the eye. This loss of circulation may dry out the eye's surface and cause hypoxic injury. The result is usually severe eye pain and possible damage to the cornea.

hyphema *blood in the anterior chamber of the eye, in front of the iris.*

A hyphema is a sight-threatening injury.

Occasionally, blood will completely fill the anterior chamber resulting in what is called an "eight-ball" hyphema. This can easily be missed without close examination.

acute retinal artery occlusion *a nontraumatic occlusion of the retinal artery resulting in a sudden, painless loss of vision in one eye.*

retinal detachment *condition that may be of traumatic origin and present with patient complaint of a dark curtain obstructing a portion of the field of view.*

■ Figure 8-21   Laceration of the eyelid.

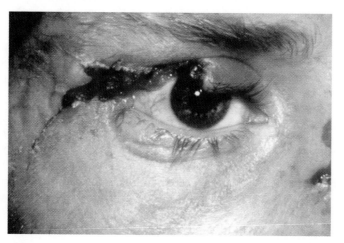

Figure 8-22 Subconjunctival hemorrhage.

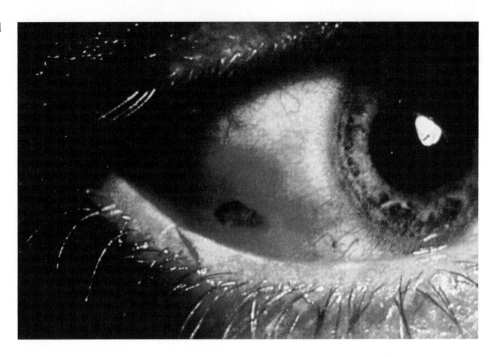

NECK INJURY

The neck is protected from impact by the more anterior head and chest and by its own skeletal and muscular structures. The neck's major skeletal component is the cervical vertebral column, which is strengthened by interconnecting ligaments. The neck muscles provide additional protection to the vital structures in the neck. They include the muscles that support and move the head through a large range of motion as well as the shoulder muscles that help move the upper extremities and act as auxiliary breathing muscles. The skeletal structures and muscles of the neck protect the airway, carotid and jugular blood vessels, and the esophagus very well from all but anterior blunt trauma and deep penetrating trauma. Such trauma may result in serious injuries to the airway, cervical spine, blood vessels, and other structures in the region.

Blood Vessel Trauma

Blunt trauma to a blood vessel may produce a serious and rapidly expanding hematoma. This hematoma may be trapped within the fascia of the region and apply restrictive pressure to the jugular veins. Laceration of the external jugular vein, or deep laceration involving the internal jugular vein or the carotid arteries, may result in severe hemorrhage due to the large size of the vessels and the volume of blood they carry (Figure 8-23 ■). Their laceration and subsequent hemorrhage can rapidly lead to hypovolemia and shock. Arterial interruption may cause subsequent brain hypoxia and infarct, mimicking the signs and symptoms of a stroke. An open neck wound affecting the external jugular vein may permit formation of an air embolism as the venous pressure drops below atmospheric pressure with deep respirations.

Airway Trauma

Trauma may also injure the trachea. Severe blunt or penetrating trauma may separate the larynx from the trachea, fracture or crush either of these two structures, or open the trachea to the environment. These injuries may result in serious hemorrhage that threatens the airway, vocal cord contusion or swelling, destruction of the integrity of the airway and collapse on inspiration, disruption of normal airway landmarks, and restrictive soft-tissue swelling.

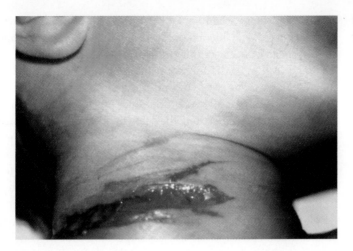

Cervical Spine Trauma

Severe blunt trauma and, in some cases, gunshot wounds to the neck may cause vertebral fracture and cervical spine instability. The wounds may cause pressure on the spinal cord, cord contusion, or severing of the cord. Such injuries will likely cause bilateral paresthesia, anesthesia, weakness (paresis), or paralysis, generally at and below the dermatome controlled by the peripheral nerve branch leaving the spinal column at the level of the injury. Neurogenic shock from these injuries may cause hypotension from vasodilation. (This is discussed in Chapter 9, "Spinal Trauma.") Blunt trauma may disrupt and injure the muscles and connective tissues of the region and result in serious pain and limited motion.

Other Neck Trauma

The neck may also demonstrate subcutaneous emphysema due to tension pneumothorax (air pushed into the skin from intrathoracic pressure that migrates to the neck) or from tracheal injury in the neck. Penetrating trauma may involve the esophagus, perforating it and permitting gastric contents or undigested material to enter the fascia. Since the fascia communicates with the mediastinum, this foreign material can physically harm mediastinal structures or provide the medium for infection, which may have devastating results. Deep penetrating trauma may disrupt the vagus nerve, causing tachycardia and gastrointestinal disturbances. More anterior and superficial injuries may damage the thyroid and parathyroid glands.

ASSESSMENT OF HEAD, FACIAL, AND NECK INJURIES

As with all trauma patients, assessment of head, facial, and neck injury patients follows the standard format, including the scene size-up, initial assessment, rapid trauma assessment/focused exam and history, and the detailed assessment as appropriate. Perform ongoing assessments frequently on these patients. With head, facial, and neck injuries, pay special attention to assuring airway patency and monitoring breathing, level of consciousness and orientation, pupillary signs, and blood pressure. With these patients, be sure to consider the need for rapid transport to a trauma center specializing in neurologic care.

SCENE SIZE-UP

Analysis of the mechanism of injury is a key part of the assessment of the patient with a possible head, face, or neck injury. During the scene size-up, consider the circumstances of injury and identify the nature and extent of forces that caused the injury. In a vehicle crash, for example, look for evidence of head impact such as the characteristic spider-web windshield. Look also for deformity of the upper steering wheel, which suggests head or neck trauma or the use of the shoulder belt without the lap belt. Identify the direction of the forces causing injury and anticipate what body structures the forces may have damaged. In motorcycle impacts, remember that helmet use reduces head injury by about 50 percent but does not spare the neck from cervical spine injury. In shootings, try to determine the caliber and type of weapon, the distance from the gun to the patient, and the approximate angle of the bullet's entry into the patient's body.

With other types of impacts, try to determine what forces were involved and how they were directed to the head, face, and neck. Use this information to anticipate injuries to the brain, airway, and sense organs. Remember that many signs of head injury may be masked by the patient's use of alcohol or other drugs, by the nature of the injury, and/or by the slow development of the wound process. Consequently, a good analysis of the MOI and the resulting indexes of suspicion are very important. Your thorough analysis must enable you to describe both the incident scene and the mechanism of injury to the attending physician at the emergency department. Remember that the mechanism of injury can often give a better indication of the seriousness of the injury than the patient's signs and symptoms.

Rule out scene hazards, and request any additional resources needed at the scene as soon as you can. Use of gloves is the minimum level of BSI protection when approaching the potential head, face, and neck injury patient. Serious head injuries pose real risks of exposure to blood or other fluids propelled by air movement or by arterial or heavy venous bleeding. Anticipate such exposures, and don splash and eye protection when contacting any patient with significant trauma to the head, face, or neck.

INITIAL ASSESSMENT

As you approach, form an initial impression of the patient's condition. Is the patient alert? Does the patient show any signs of anxiety? If there is any reason to suspect that the head or neck sustained serious impact, provide immediate manual immobilization of the head and cervical spine (Figure 8-24 ■). Quickly determine the patient's level of consciousness and then orientation to time, place, and persons early in the initial assessment. While determining the patient's level of orientation may add a few seconds to the initial assessment, assessing trends in orientation can be critical to rapid identification of a brain injury patient. Be alert to the patient's facial skin color, respiratory effort, and to pupil luster and level of responsiveness throughout the initial assessment as these factors can help you recognize internal head injury. As you gather information about the patient, continue to build and modify your general patient impression and your index of suspicion for head injury.

Apply a cervical collar at the end of the initial assessment and maintain manual head immobilization until the patient is fully immobilized to a short spine board, KED, or long spine board with a cervical immobilization device. If there are any significant injuries to the neck, do not apply the collar until you complete the assessment and provide needed care. While the cervical collar provides some neck stabilization, it does not completely immobilize the region, and its placement may be delayed so long as manual immobilization is continued.

If the patient is wearing a helmet, consider whether or not to remove it as described in Chapter 9, "Spinal Trauma." A patient's use of a helmet reduces the likelihood of soft-tissue injury and skull and facial fracture. Helmet use can also significantly reduce the incidence of brain injury, but do not be lulled into a false sense of security by the absence of outward signs of trauma. Be watchful for the early signs of internal brain injury, and be sure to inform the emergency department staff that the patient was wearing a helmet. Also alert them to any signs of impact or helmet damage suggestive of the forces of trauma that the patient experienced.

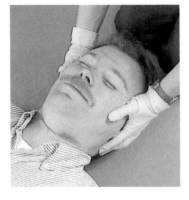

■ Figure 8-24 If spinal injury is suspected, immediately immobilize the head and neck manually.

Although determining the patient's level of orientation may add a few seconds to the initial assessment, assessing trends in orientation can be critical to rapid identification of a brain injury patient.

Always be sure to inform the emergency department staff if a patient was wearing a helmet.

Airway

Move quickly to evaluate the airway. Examine the face and neck for any deformity, swelling, hemorrhage, foreign bodies, or other signs of injury that may threaten the airway. Suction and insert an oral or nasal airway as necessary. Listen for unusual or changing voice patterns as they may be indicative of airway injury and developing edema. Swelling can quickly occlude the airway, and any hemorrhage can complicate airway maintenance as the patient loses consciousness and the gag reflex. Anticipate vomiting, possibly without warning. Assure that the airway is structurally sound and that the mandible supports the tongue well enough to keep it out of the airway. Have a large-bore suction catheter and strong suction ready to remove any fluids, and consider positioning the patient to enhance airway drainage (left lateral recumbent position) if doing so is not contraindicated by injuries. If the patient does not display a protective airway reflex or if he has an altered level of consciousness, consider early insertion of an endotracheal tube.

If there is a serious neck injury, check the structural integrity of the trachea. If the trachea is open to the environment, keep the wound clear of blood to prevent aspiration, and seal the wound unless the patient's upper airway is blocked. If an impaled object obstructs the airway, remove it, anticipating that heavy bleeding may then threaten the airway. Blunt wounds may crush the cartilage of the trachea, permitting it to close with the reduced pressure during inspiration. This type of crushing injury may require surgical opening of the trachea by needle or surgical cricothyrotomy to assure air exchange.

Breathing

Closely monitor breathing to assure that the patient is moving an adequate volume of air. Determine the rate of respirations and their rhythm. Estimate the amount of air moved with each breath, and from those numbers determine the minute volume:

$$\text{Minute Volume} = \text{Tidal Volume} \times \text{Respiratory Rate}$$

If the patient is breathing less than 12 times per minute, moving less than 500 mL of air with each breath, or has a minute volume of less than 6 liters, consider overdrive ventilation. Remember that head injury is likely to produce irregular breathing patterns and that hypoxia and carbon dioxide retention both contribute to morbidity and mortality with brain injury. Ventilations for the serious head injury patient (GCS ≤8) are guided by capnography. For the head injury patient without signs of herniation, adjust ventilation rates to maintain an end-tidal CO_2 reading of between 35 and 40 mmHg (adults at about 10 breaths per minute, children at about 20 breaths per minute, and infants at about 25 breaths per minute). For patients with suspected herniation, the end-tidal CO_2 reading should range between 30 and 35 mmHg, using ventilation rates about 10 breaths per minute faster than for patients without herniation. Also assure the oxygen saturation level is at least 95 percent for any serious head injury patient.

For a patient who is breathing adequately on his own, apply oxygen via nonrebreather mask with a flow of 15 liters per minute, to assure inspiration of high concentrations. It is advisable to apply pulse oximetry to monitor oxygenation. Attempt to keep oxygen saturation above 95 percent.

Ventilations for the serious head injury patient (GCS ≤8) are guided by capnography.

Circulation

Begin to monitor the patient's pulse rate and its rhythm early in your care and continue to do so frequently thereafter. A slow and strong (bounding) pulse may be an early sign of building intracranial pressure. Apply an ECG monitor and watch for rhythm disturbances. Quickly look for any hemorrhage from the head, face, and neck and control any moderate to severe bleeding with direct pressure and bandaging. Be cautious of open neck wounds because they may present a risk for air embolism. Cover any such wounds quickly with occlusive dressings and secure them in place.

A slow and strong (bounding) pulse may be an early sign of building intracranial pressure.

At the end of the initial assessment, you must determine whether to perform a rapid trauma assessment followed by gathering of vital signs and the patient history or to perform a focused history and physical exam followed by gathering of vital signs. With most head, face, and neck injury patients, you will perform a rapid trauma assessment because of the high likelihood of airway, vascular, special sense organ, or central nervous system injuries in these regions. If there is no significant mechanism of injury and injuries appear minor and superficial, perform an exam focused on the specific area(s) of injury.

RAPID TRAUMA ASSESSMENT

The rapid trauma assessment calls for performance of a quick and directed head-to-toe examination of a patient with a significant mechanism of injury. When head, facial, or neck injury is suggested in such a patient, pay particular attention to the procedures described in the following sections as you carry out the assessment. Manage any life-threatening injuries and conditions as you find them during the rapid trauma assessment. If the patient shows any signs of pathology within the cranium, consider rapid transport. Brain injury patients can deteriorate quickly, but rapid neurosurgical intervention can frequently alleviate life-threatening problems.

Head

Look at, then sweep, each region of the skull, feeling for deformity and bleeding with the more sensitive tips of your fingers. Interlock your fingers to sweep the posterior head, and look at your gloves to check for any blood that indicates hemorrhage there. If you find any moderate or serious hemorrhage, apply direct pressure unless you suspect skull fracture. Control the hemorrhage with gentle pressure around the wound and place a loose dressing over it. Palpate gently for any deformities, being careful, however, not to palpate the interior of open wounds (Figure 8-25 ■).

Shine a penlight into the external auditory canal and look for signs of escaping cerebrospinal fluid. This fluid loss may be difficult to notice early during assessment, so observe carefully. If blood or fluid drains from the auditory canal, cover the ear with a gauze dressing to permit fluid to move outward while providing a barrier to keep contaminants from entering. If the fluid drains on a gauze dressing or other fabric, look for the halo sign. However, you should presume (regardless of the presence or absence of halo sign) that any fluid draining from the ear contains cerebrospinal fluid. Examine the pinnae for injury and, after you complete the rapid trauma assessment, bandage and dress as needed.

■ Figure 8-25 Carefully inspect and palpate the head for bleeding and other signs of injury.

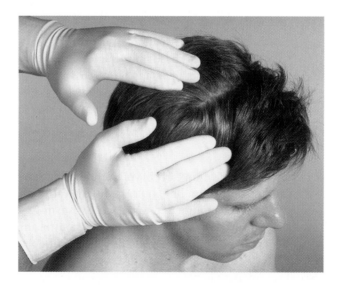

If you observe a skull deformity, palpate such a closed wound very gently. Try to determine the probability of skull fracture before swelling makes this determination more difficult. Cover any open wounds with dressings to restrict blood flow and prevent further contamination. The signs of basilar skull fracture—bilateral periorbital ecchymosis and retroauricular ecchymosis (raccoon eyes and Battle's sign)—are very late indications of this injury and are not likely to be recognizable during field assessment and care.

Head injury may cause patient seizures. Seizures are serious complications because they may compromise the airway and respirations, increase the intracranial pressure, and exacerbate any existing brain injury. If you observe a seizure or the patient or bystanders describe one as you gather the history, find out as much about the episode as you can and be prepared to describe the seizure in detail, including its origin and progression, to the attending physician. Protect the seizing patient from further injury and be especially watchful of the airway. Consider the administration of diazepam, which reduces electrical impulse transmission across the cerebrum and may limit seizure activity.

Raccoon eyes and Battle's sign are very late signs of basilar skull fracture and are not likely to be recognizable during field assessment and care.

Face

Study the patient's facial features carefully, looking for asymmetry, swelling, discoloration, or deformity. Palpate the facial region including the brow ridge, nasal region, cheek, maxilla, and mandible searching for any deformity, instability, or crepitus that suggest fracture and for any signs of soft-tissue swelling (Figure 8-26 ■). Palpate the maxilla and attempt, gently, to move it from left to right. It should be firmly attached to the facial bones and should display no crepitus. Do likewise with the mandible. It should be solid yet very mobile from left to right and up and down. Note and investigate any patient report of pain during your palpation and movement. Open the mouth and examine for any signs of trauma, excessive secretions and bleeding, or swelling. All teeth should be firmly in place (loose teeth may suggest mandibular fracture). Find any displaced teeth and prepare them for transport with the patient or suspect that missing teeth may have been aspirated. Assure that the mandible is intact and supports the airway.

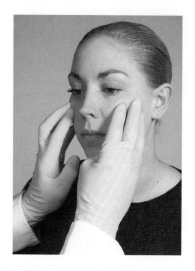

■ Figure 8-26   Carefully palpate the facial bones.

Carefully examine the eyes. In general, eye reactivity and luster reflect the oxygenation status of the brain. Watch for bright and sparkling eyes and briskly reactive pupils. Shine a bright light into the eyes—or in bright sunlight, shade them—and watch for sluggishness, nonreactivity, and constriction (or dilation). Assure that reactivity is bilateral. Note that both eyes should respond to changes in light intensity affecting only one eye (**consensual reactivity**). Both eyes should gaze together and, at rest, directly forward. Watch for a down and out gaze. Usually, an affected pupil is on the same side (ipsilateral) as a head injury. If the patient is conscious and alert, have him follow your finger up and down, left and right, with each eye. Watch for and note any limited eye movement. Restricted eye movement suggests eye muscle entrapment and nerve compression or injury and paralysis.

consensual reactivity *the response of both eyes to changes in light intensity that affect only one eye.*

Carefully examine the pupil, iris, and conjunctiva. The pupil and iris should be round, the anterior chamber clear, and the sclera free of accumulating blood. Check for contact lenses, especially in the unconscious patient. If they are noted, remove them carefully.

Restricted eye movement suggests eye muscle entrapment, nerve compression, or injury and paralysis.

Neck

Examine the anterior, lateral, and posterior neck for signs of injury including swelling, discoloration, wounds, blood loss, or frothy blood. Frothy blood is likely caused by bleeding in association with a tracheal injury and suggests serious airway compromise. Palpate the region, feeling for any changes in skin tension, deformities, or unusual masses underneath. Crepitus beneath the skin may be associated with subcutaneous emphysema from a tracheal or chest injury or a tracheal or laryngeal fracture. Identify the thyroid cartilage, beneath and posterior to the mandible. Palpate it, the cricoid cartilage, then the trachea. Assure they are not deformed by trauma and remain midline in the neck. Visually examine the depth of neck wounds to anticipate those that may involve jugular or carotid blood vessels, and cover any open wounds with occlusive dressings.

While carrying out the rapid trauma assessment, question the responsive patient about headaches and increased light sensitivity (photophobia), which are common symptoms of head injury. Also question the patient about his memory of the events preceding and following the injury to identify retrograde and anterograde amnesia. Note any repetitive questioning by the patient (inability to establish short-term memory) and any unusual behavior or confusion. Ask if the patient has any unusual fullness in the throat and any difficulty swallowing. Ask about any visual disturbances such as double vision (diplopia) and blurred vision that may indicate eye muscle entrapment. Inquire about visual acuity (the ability to distinguish objects) both near and far, and note reports of any restriction to vision, which the patient might describe as a curtain drawn across the field of view. Patient complaints of eye pain are also important and may suggest conjunctival or corneal injury. You may also note patient complaints about focal deficits. Examine any area of facial paresthesia, anesthesia, weakness, or paralysis, noting the borders of the area and whether it is unilateral or bilateral. Question the patient frequently to identify any increase or decrease in awareness and any changes in injury symptoms.

Complete the rapid trauma assessment by examining the rest of the body, paying particular attention to any region where the mechanism of injury suggests serious injury and in which the patient complains of serious symptoms. While examining the extremities, look for any signs of decreased muscle tone, flaccid muscles, diminished sensation or muscle strength, and determine if any unusual findings are bilateral or unilateral and where the deficit begins. Then gather the balance of the patient history, determine the patient's Glasgow Coma Scale score, and take a set of the patient's vital signs.

Glasgow Coma Scale Score

Determine the patient's best eye opening, motor, and verbal responses using the Glasgow Coma Scale. The Glasgow Coma Scale awards the patient points for different responses, with a total score that will range between 3 and 15 points (see the adult GCS in Table 8–2, the pediatric GCS in Table 8–3). The scale is a moderately good predictor of head injury severity. A patient with a score of between 13 and 15 is considered to have a mild head injury. A score between 9 and 12 indicates moderate injury, while a score of ≤8 represents severe head injury. Most patients with a GCS of ≤8 are in a coma.

When assessing eye-opening response, award 1 point for no response, 2 points for eye opening in response to pain, 3 points for response to verbal command, and 4 points for spontaneous eye opening. With verbal response, award 1 point for no sound or response; 2 points for incomprehensible, garbled sounds; 3 points for inappropriate words and speech that make no sense; 4 points for confused or disoriented speech; and 5 points for clear and oriented speech. With motor response, award 1 point for no movement or response, 2 points for decerebrate posturing, 3 points for decorticate posturing, 4 points for purposeful motion (withdrawal of a body part from pain), 5 points for purposeful movement (of the hand) to localize pain, and 6 points for following simple verbal commands. The lowest GCS value is 3, which represents a completely unresponsive patient. The maximum GCS value is 15, which represents the fully conscious and alert patient.

Record the best response for each of the GCS criteria (for example, as E_3, V_4, M_5) and note any differences, either from side-to-side or in the upper versus lower extremities. Also note the eye signs along with the Glasgow Coma Scale score results because they help identify the existence and nature of the patient's brain injury. Determine the

Table 8-2 | Glasgow Coma Scale

Eye Opening	
Spontaneous	4
To verbal command	3
To pain	2
No response	1
Verbal Response	
Oriented and converses	5
Disoriented and converses	4
Inappropriate words	3
Incomprehensible sounds	2
No response	1
Motor Response	
Obeys verbal commands	6
Localizes pain	5
Withdraws from pain (flexion)	4
Abnormal flexion in response to pain (decorticate rigidity)	3
Extension in response to pain (decerebrate rigidity)	2
No response	1

GCS score every 5 minutes (with the ongoing assessment) in the patient with any GCS less than 15. The pediatric patient is a special challenge to Glasgow Coma Score assessment. To arrive at an accurate value, you must modify your evaluation of the child's best verbal response as appropriate for the developmental age. See the criteria identified in the pediatric Glasgow Coma Scale (review Table 8–3).

Vital Signs

Carefully monitor the vital signs for evidence of increasing intracranial pressure. Identify and record the pulse rate and strength. Note the blood pressure and especially the pulse pressure. Lastly, note the respiratory pattern. The vital signs change with increasing ICP or injury to the brainstem. Be watchful for a slowing pulse rate, increasing systolic blood pressure, and the development of irregular respirations (Cheyne-Stokes, central neurologic hyperventilation, or ataxic respirations), which together are known as Cushing's triad.

At the conclusion of the rapid trauma assessment, determine the need for rapid transport. A history of head trauma coupled with any history of unconsciousness, a degradation in the level of orientation or consciousness, or any vital sign suggestive of brain injury requires rapid transport to the closest appropriate facility. If such signs and symptoms of brain injury exist, begin rapid transport and contact medical direction for approval to transport to the nearest neurocenter. Significant airway threats and uncontrolled hemorrhage are also indicators for rapid transport. Carefully monitor other head, face, and neck injury patients during further assessment and care for any signs of increasing intracranial pressure or expanding lesions. Identify the wounds and other injuries you have found or suspect and prioritize them for care.

At the conclusion of the rapid trauma assessment, determine the need for rapid transport.

FOCUSED HISTORY AND PHYSICAL EXAM

If your head, face, or neck injury patient has no significant mechanism of injury and no other indications of serious injury, perform a focused history and physical exam,

		Table 8–3	**Pediatric Glasgow Coma Scale**		

			> 1 Year	< 1 Year	
Eye Opening		4	Spontaneous	Spontaneous	
		3	To verbal command	To shout	
		2	To pain	To pain	
		1	No response	No response)	
			> 1 Year	**< 1 Year**	
Best Motor Response		6	Obeys		
		5	Localizes pain	Localizes pain	
		4	Flexion-withdrawal	Flexion-withdrawal	
		3	Flexion-abnormal (decorticate rigidity)	Flexion-abnormal (decorticate rigidity)	
		2	Extension (decerebrate rigidity)	Extension (decerebrate rigidity)	
		1	No response	No response	
			>5 Years	**2–5 Years**	**0–23 Months**
Best Verbal Response		5	Oriented and converses	Appropriate words and phrases	Smiles, coos, cries appropriately
		4	Disoriented and converses	Inappropriate words	Cries
		3	Inappropriate words	Cries and/or screams	Inappropriate crying and/or screaming
		2	Incomprehensible sounds	Grunts	Grunts
		1	No response	No response	No response

concentrating on the area of injury. During your assessment, however, carefully observe for any signs of a diminished level of consciousness or orientation or any evidence of previous unconsciousness or airway or vascular restriction or compromise. If you discover any of these things, complete a rapid trauma assessment and consider the patient for rapid transport to the appropriate facility. Remember, the signs of significant brain injury may not develop for some time or may be masked by drug or alcohol use or by the patient's anxiety. It is always better to err on the side of more intensive patient care.

Direct the focused history and physical exam to the areas of specific patient complaint and to areas where the mechanism of injury suggests injury. Use the assessment techniques—inspection, palpation, and so forth—suggested for the rapid trauma assessment.

When you have completed the focused assessment, obtain a set of baseline vital signs and gather a patient history. Then provide emergency care for the injuries you have found and prepare the patient for transport.

With superficial wounds to the head, face, and neck, apply dressings and bandages as for minor soft-tissue injuries but be alert for hemorrhage into the airway and vomiting that may follow it and for any signs of progressive swelling that may restrict the airway. Watch also for open neck wounds that may permit air to enter the jugular vein. Cover such wounds with occlusive dressings held firmly in place.

Inspect any soft-tissue head, facial, or neck injury very carefully before bandaging it and be prepared to describe the injury to the attending emergency department physician or nurse so they do not have to remove and replace dressings and bandages unnecessarily.

Of special concern for the head injury patient is the blood glucose level. Research has found that depressed glucose levels (hypoglycemia) increase the morbidity and mortality in these patients. It may be prudent to perform a quick blood glucose check to assure the glucose level is above 60 mg/dL. If not, administer IV glucose ($D_{50}W$).

Of special concern for the head injury patient is the blood glucose level.

DETAILED ASSESSMENT

You will normally perform a detailed assessment for the head, face, and neck injury patient during transport and only if and when you have cared for all other serious injuries. The detailed assessment is an in-depth, head-to-toe assessment searching for any other signs or symptoms suggestive of injury. Use your skills of questioning, inspection, palpation, and—as appropriate—auscultation to search out these additional injuries. Look for signs of neurologic deficit in the extremities, including flaccidity, paresthesia, anesthesia, weakness, and paralysis. Remember that early in the course of trauma, serious injuries may be masked by other more painful ones, by patient anxiety, and by drug and alcohol use. Careful evaluation is required to identify injuries at this stage of patient care.

ONGOING ASSESSMENT

Perform ongoing assessments every 5 minutes for patients with potentially serious injuries. Be especially alert for slowing of the pulse, increasing systolic blood pressure (an increasing pulse pressure), and development of deeper, more rapid, or erratic respirations. Carefully observe the patient for changes in the level of consciousness and orientation as well. Finally, watch the eyes for signs of cerebral hypoxia—they become dull and lackluster—or of increasing intracranial pressure—one pupil becomes sluggish, nonreactive, then dilated. Note any changes in any element of patient presentation, and track any trends to identify whether the patient's condition is deteriorating, improving, or remaining the same.

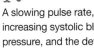

A slowing pulse rate, increasing systolic blood pressure, and the development of erratic respirations are signs of increasing intracranial pressure.

Watch pulse oximetry and blood pressure readings to assure that the patient becomes neither hypoxic nor hypovolemic. Both of these conditions are associated with increased mortality and morbidity when associated with brain injury. If you notice any sign of deterioration, provide rapid transport. Monitor the $PaCO_2$ reading on your capnography device to assure the carbon dioxide level remains between 35 and 40 mmHg.

If the patient's eyes become dull and lackluster, it is a sign of cerebral hypoxia; if one pupil becomes sluggish, nonreactive, then dilated, that indicates intracranial injury.

HEAD, FACIAL, AND NECK INJURY MANAGEMENT

The management priorities for the patient sustaining head, face, or neck trauma include care directed at maintaining the patient's airway and breathing, assuring circulation through hemorrhage control, addressing or taking steps to avoid hypoxia and/or hypovolemia, and providing appropriate medications. Once these priorities have been attended to, you may dress and care for minor head, facial, and neck wounds.

AIRWAY

The airway is one of the most important care priorities with head, face, and neck injury patients. Head, face, and neck injury can leave patients unable to control the airway due either to an altered level of consciousness or to damaged airway structures. In addition, soft-tissue trauma to the airway may cause edema that can quickly progress from restriction of the airway to its complete obstruction. Vigilant attention to the airway and aggressive airway care are the only means of assuring that the airway of these patients remains protected and patent. Airway management techniques appropriate for such patients include suctioning, patient positioning, oral and nasal airway insertion,

Vigilant attention to the airway and aggressive airway care are vital with head, facial, and neck injury patients.

endotracheal intubation, and cricothyrotomy. (You can review these techniques in Volume 1, Chapter 13, "Airway Management and Ventilation.")

Suctioning

Airway tissues are extremely vascular, bleed profusely, and swell quickly. Soft-tissue injury may cause significant hemorrhage that can compromise the airway in two ways. First, the sheer volume of blood may block the airway. Note that aspiration of blood is more often responsible for hypoxia than physical obstruction of the airway, so be certain to suction as necessary in order to remove blood from the airway.

Secondly, blood is a gastric irritant that frequently induces emesis. If a large volume of blood is swallowed, the patient may vomit, thus endangering the airway. In addition, vomiting is common with head injury patients because emesis is a frequent result of brain injury or increasing intracranial pressure. Vomiting often occurs without warning (without nausea) and can be projectile in nature. Vomiting is especially dangerous with head injury patients because they commonly have a depressed or absent gag reflex. Gastric contents are very acidic and will quickly damage the tissues of the lower airway if aspirated. Aspiration of gastric contents is associated with a high patient mortality. Be ready to suction aggressively as needed in any patients with nasal, oral, or head trauma. Use a large-bore catheter or a suction hose without a tip to clear the airway of any blood or emesis.

Patient Positioning

Consider placing the patient in a position that protects the airway early in your care (during the initial assessment). The best position for the patient with suspected head injury is on the left side with the head turned slightly and facing downward, the left lateral recumbent position. Remember, of course, that head injury patients require spinal precautions. Maintain manual immobilization until the patient is secured to a long spine board, and then be prepared to turn the patient and board as a unit to facilitate airway drainage.

It is unlikely that suction alone will evacuate all emesis from the oral cavity before the unconscious or semiconscious patient attempts an inspiration. If the patient experiencing serious oral, nasal (epistaxis), or facial bleeding is conscious and alert and no serious spinal injury is suspected, have the patient sit leaning forward to promote drainage and keep fluids from flowing into the posterior airway. If the patient has sustained an open neck injury with the danger of air embolism, place the patient on a spine board in the Trendelenburg position, with the lower part of the patient's body elevated about 12 inches. Otherwise, position the patient with potential brain injury by elevating the head of the spine board to about 30 degrees to reduce both external hemorrhage and intracranial pressure.

Oropharyngeal and Nasopharyngeal Airways

Oro- and nasopharyngeal airways each have advantages and disadvantages when used with head, face, and neck injury patients. The nasal airway does not trigger the gag reflex as easily as the oral airway and is better tolerated by the semiconscious patient. Because there is less stimulation of the gag reflex, there is also a reduction in transient increases in intracranial pressure and in the chances of increasing the severity of head injury. One hazard of nasal airway use is the possible insertion of the tube directly into the cranium through a fracture of the posterior nasal border. Always insert the nasal airway straight back, through the largest of the nares (nostrils), and use only gentle force in its introduction. If you suspect basilar skull fracture, use an oral airway or endotracheal intubation to establish and maintain the airway.

While the oral and nasal airways help to keep the respective pharynxes open, they can represent threats to the airway. The ends of the tubes sit just superior to the opening of the larynx. If a patient vomits, which frequently happens with brain injury, the vomitus is blocked from exiting the patient's mouth through the airway and remains just at the laryngeal opening. With the next breath, the patient can aspirate the gastric contents, which

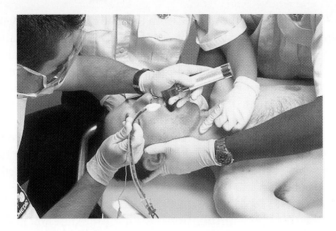

■ Figure 8-27 Oral intubation is difficult in the patient with facial trauma because landmarks may be distorted, blood may flow into the airway, and the head must remain in the neutral position.

may have serious consequences. Whenever an oral or nasal airway is in place, monitor the patient's airway carefully and be prepared to remove the airway and evacuate any emesis.

Endotracheal Intubation

Endotracheal intubation is the most definitive method of assuring a clear and patent airway in the head injury patient. Intubate early in the care of the unresponsive patient, and consider intubation for any patient with a reduced level of consciousness. Techniques useful in caring for head injury patients include orotracheal, digital, nasotracheal, retrograde, directed, and rapid sequence intubation.

Orotracheal Intubation   Orotracheal, or oral, intubation is the most common and usually the most successful technique for placing an endotracheal tube (Figure 8-27 ■). It does, however, pose some hazards for head, face, and neck injury patients. All patients who sustain serious injuries in these regions require spinal immobilization. Immobilization, however, limits the movement of the patient's head during intubation attempts, restricting you from manually bringing the oral opening, pharynx, and trachea in line. The result is often an inability to visualize the vocal folds and watch the endotracheal tube pass into the trachea, seriously reducing the chances of a successful oral intubation.

To improve visualization during oral intubation with spinal immobilization, employ a technique called the Sellick maneuver. Apply pressure directed posteriorly to the cricoid ring with the thumb and index finger, moving it downward toward the vertebral column. This brings the trachea more in line with the oral cavity and pharynx and compresses the esophagus, thus reducing the likelihood of vomitus entering the upper airway during intubation. Exercise caution to prevent the pressure from flexing the cervical spine. Be aware that the Sellick maneuver may not align the airway enough to permit visualized oral intubation.

Attempts at endotracheal intubation can increase the parasympathetic (vagal) tone. This, in turn, may increase intracranial pressure and lower the heart rate or increase the severity of other cardiac dysrhythmias already induced by the brain injury. Therefore, carry out the intubation rapidly. If possible, have the most experienced care provider attempt the procedure to reduce both intubation time and vagal stimulation. Also consider use of a pharmacologic agent, such as a topical anesthetic spray, to reduce both vagal stimulation and the retching associated with stimulation of the gag reflex.

Digital Intubation   Another technique that may be effective when intubating an unconscious patient undergoing spinal precautions is digital intubation. In this procedure, the endotracheal tube is positioned without visualization; instead, the tube

 Intubate early in the care of the unresponsive patient, and consider intubation for any patient with a reduced level of consciousness.

If possible, have the most experienced care provider attempt intubation to reduce both the length of the procedure and vagal stimulation.

is directed into the trachea from the base of the tongue by the intubator's fingers. This is a procedure best attempted by a paramedic with long thin fingers.

A slightly smaller-diameter-than-usual endotracheal tube is shaped by a stylet into a "J" configuration. The patient's mouth is held open with a bite block while you insert the first two fingers of one hand and "walk" them back along the tongue to its base. Use these fingers to locate and lift the epiglottis. Advance the tube with your other hand along the back of the tongue and direct it with your fingers past the epiglottis and toward the tracheal opening. Continue to advance the endotracheal tube with slight anterior pressure along the posterior surface of the epiglottis for about 1½ to 2½ inches. Remove the stylet and carefully confirm tube placement in the trachea, not the esophagus.

Nasotracheal Intubation   A third procedure for intubation of the patient with possible spinal injury is nasotracheal, or nasal, intubation. Insert the endotracheal tube into the largest of the nares. Then direct it posteriorly, curving it toward the floor of the nasal cavity. Advance the tube the length of an oral airway (the distance between the earlobe and the corner of the mouth). At this point, slowly continue insertion while you, with your ear at the endotracheal tube opening, listen for the sounds of respirations. Gently manipulate the tube until the respiratory sounds are loudest and then advance it during inspiration. The tube should pass directly into the trachea. The technique can be made somewhat easier using an endotracheal tube with a directable tip (such as an Endotrol). With this device, a small cord connected to the tube's end permits the user to increase or decrease the tube's curve.

The disadvantages to nasal intubation include the necessity of having a breathing patient and a quiet environment, and the danger of inserting the tube through a fractured cribiform plate and into the skull. The procedure has a lower rate of success than either oral or digital intubation. Nasal intubation also tends to raise intracranial pressure more than oral intubation because it generally takes longer and more aggressively stimulates the posterior nasal and oral pharynxes.

Retrograde Intubation   Retrograde intubation is a process in which a wire is introduced through the cricothyroid membrane into the larynx, then the pharynx, and then out through the mouth. The process begins with the placement of a catheter through the cricothyroid membrane, directed superiorly. A flexible wire is advanced through the catheter toward the oral opening. A laryngoscope may be inserted to visualize the oral cavity and identify the advancing wire. When you see the wire, use the McGill forceps to retrieve it. Then advance an endotracheal tube over the wire down to the thyroid cartilage. When the tube reaches the larynx, withdraw the wire and advance the tube into the trachea.

Retrograde intubation may be the only effective technique for intubation when the normal landmarks are disrupted by severe facial and airway trauma.

Directed Intubation   In some cases of serious facial or upper neck trauma, as in a shotgun blast, the landmarks of the upper airway are disrupted or destroyed. In such cases, obtaining and maintaining an airway may be extremely difficult. Use strong suction over the area, and use the laryngoscope to attempt to visualize the elements of the oro- and laryngopharynx. If you cannot see airway landmarks themselves, look for bubbling air escaping from the trachea with expirations. If you believe you are close to the tracheal opening and can visualize the area, have an assistant compress the chest to induce bubbling. Attempt to pass the endotracheal tube along the route of bubbles and into the trachea. With this technique, it is critically important to confirm proper placement of the endotracheal tube.

Another form of directed intubation uses a device called the bougie. The bougie is a long, malleable, gum rubber stylet you insert into the trachea while visualizing it with the laryngoscope. You then insert the endotracheal tube over the bougie and into the trachea. The bougie is withdrawn and the patient is ventilated through the endotracheal tube.

Rapid Sequence Intubation (RSI)   Occasionally, a patient who is responsive or whose teeth are clenched (trismus) needs intubation. Such cases might involve brain injury patients or patients with serious oral trauma with the risk of swelling and progressive airway obstruction. RSI is a medication-facilitated procedure that paralyzes the conscious or semiconscious patient to permit intubation. A sedative/amnestic is administered to sedate the patient and reduce anxiety. Then a quick-acting paralytic agent is given to induce muscle relaxation, including the muscles of the oral and pharyngeal cavities. The patient must then be intubated and positive pressure ventilations provided quickly because the paralytic agent paralyzes all skeletal muscles, including those associated with breathing. The paralytic also eliminates the gag reflex and the patient's ability to maintain the airway.

The drugs most commonly used for this procedure are the paralytics succinylcholine, atracurium, and vecuronium and the sedatives etomidate, diazepam, midazolam, fentanyl, and morphine. Sedative antagonists are used to reverse the effects of these drugs when given and include flumazenil (for diazepam or midazolam) and naloxone (for morphine or fentanyl). (See Volume 1, Chapter 13, "Airway Management and Ventilation" and the discussion later in this chapter.)

The process for RSI begins with reconfirmation of the indications: a patient experiencing muscle spasm (trismus) or who has an intact gag reflex (semiconscious or conscious patient) and who needs a protected airway. Apply the Sellick maneuver and ventilate or be ready to ventilate the patient as needed. Premedicate the patient with the sedative and then administer the paralytic quickly. When the muscles relax and/or the gag reflex ceases, have the most experienced care provider attempt oral or digital intubation.

The role of RSI in the prehospital management of head injury patient remains controversial. Some studies have shown that prehospital RSI actually causes a worse outcome when compared to routine airway management. Other studies seem to support its use. RSI may be best suited for services that encounter a great deal of head trauma or who have a limited number of paramedics who perform the procedure to assure that the provider remains competent in the skill. Above all, the decision to use prehospital RSI rests with the system medical director, and local protocols should be followed.

Confirmation of Tube Placement   Once the endotracheal tube is inserted using one of the techniques previously described, confirm its proper placement in the trachea. This is especially important when the tube has been placed blindly. Auscultate, at a minimum, the axillae and over the epigastrium. (Good breath sounds at the axillae reflect good ventilation to the distal alveoli.) Watch carefully for good, symmetrical chest wall excursion with each ventilation. If you hear good breath sounds bilaterally, detect no epigastric sounds, and see the chest wall move equally with each breath, the tube is most likely in the trachea. Inflate the cuff of the tube and hyperventilate the patient for a short period of time. Use an end-tidal CO_2 monitor, pulse oximetry, and observation of the patient's skin color to help confirm and monitor proper and continuing endotracheal tube placement. Remember that the endotracheal tube may dislodge from the trachea during any movement of the patient, as from the ground to the stretcher or as the stretcher is loaded into the ambulance. Reconfirm proper tube placement frequently.

The use of continuous waveform capnography provides a graphic and almost irrefutable record of endotracheal tube placement. It also provides information about tube

Confirmation of tube placement is especially important when the tube has been placed blindly.

If you hear good breath sounds bilaterally, detect no epigastric sounds, and see the chest wall move equally with each breath, the tube is most likely in the trachea.

Use of waveform capnography is highly recommended.

placement and ventilation on a breath-to-breath basis. Use of waveform capnography is highly recommended both from a medical/legal and from a patient care standpoint.

Cricothyrotomy

In some cases of face and neck trauma, the region may be so distorted or blocked that oral and nasal intubation are impossible. Here the only potential for providing a life-saving airway may be opening a surgical pathway for the air. There are two forms of this procedure: the needle cricothyrostomy and the surgical cricothyrotomy. Consult your protocols and medical direction to identify whether these advanced airway procedures or the other procedures already described may be used in your system.

With needle cricothyrostomy, one or more large-bore catheters are inserted into the cricothyroid membrane to provide a temporary airway. This technique permits only limited air exchange and does not sustain the patient. Inspirations can be enhanced by oxygen-powered ventilation (termed transtracheal jet insufflation); however, exhalations are not adequate and the patient cannot be sustained by the technique for more than several minutes.

With surgical cricothyrotomy, an incision and opening is made in the cricothyroid membrane to provide an emergency airway. The soft tissue covering the membrane that separates the thyroid and cricoid cartilages is then held open by a small oral airway or a shortened #6 endotracheal tube. The chief dangers associated with surgical cricothyrotomy are serious bleeding from the soft tissue surrounding the site (and that bleeding's threat to the airway) and damage to the thyroid and parathyroid glands just below the incision site.

To begin either the needle or surgical cricothyrotomy, don gloves, goggles, and gown. Then briskly cleanse the upper anterior neck with an alcohol swab in concentric circles outward from the base of the thyroid cartilage. Set out the needed equipment including a large-bore (14-gauge or larger) over-the-needle catheter and a syringe for the needle procedure or a sharp scalpel and a small oral airway or shortened endotracheal tube for the surgical cricothyrotomy. Palpate upward along the trachea from the sternal notch. The first, slightly larger, and firm ring you feel is the cricoid cartilage. Immediately above it, and before the next firm and even larger cartilage (the thyroid cartilage), is the cricothyroid membrane. It is found in the depression between the two cartilages (Figure 8-28 ■).

For the needle cricothyrostomy, attach the catheter to the syringe and perforate the cricothyroid membrane by inserting the needle into the skin and membrane until you

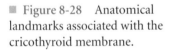

■ Figure 8-28 Anatomical landmarks associated with the cricothyroid membrane.

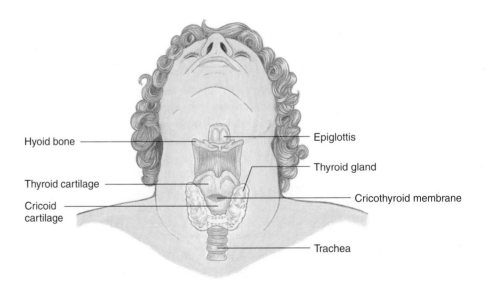

Hyoid bone

Epiglottis

Thyroid gland

Thyroid cartilage

Cricothyroid membrane

Cricoid cartilage

Trachea

feel a "pop." Advance the catheter a few centimeters over the needle and then withdraw the needle. When using a single large-bore catheter, remove the tube from a 6.0 pediatric endotracheal tube and connect it to the catheter hub. Attach the bag and valve and ventilate or use a high-flow transtracheal jet insufflation device. Use of a demand valve is not acceptable since the pressure of its oxygen flow is insufficient to adequately ventilate the patient through the needle. Give the patient a very long time to exhale as the airway is now extremely restricted. Normally, expiration through the catheter takes about four times longer than inspiration. Watch carefully for chest rise and good breath sounds.

For the surgical cricothyrotomy, insert the blade of a sterile scalpel into the skin and the cricothyroid membrane until you feel a "pop." Enlarge the opening, as needed, to accept the shortened endotracheal tube. Introduce an endotracheal tube, cut to about 4 inches in length and bent to a sharp curve, through the surgical opening. Ventilate the patient with a bag-valve-mask device using a child-sized mask or connect the bag and valve to the endotracheal tube and seal the area with sterile dressings. You may have to close the patient's mouth and nose or otherwise seal the upper airway opening to assure that the air reaches the lungs. If the airway obstruction is partial, open the mouth and nose during expiration to enhance the flow of air outward, especially when using needle cricothyrotomy.

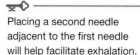

Give the patient who has received a needle crichothyrostomy a very long time to exhale because the airway is now extremely restricted.

Placing a second needle adjacent to the first needle will help facilitate exhalation.

BREATHING

Assurance of breathing is an important priority with any patient, but it becomes extremely critical with the head injury patient. Not only is reduced air exchange a problem, but excessive air exchange and the excessive depletion of carbon dioxide can also endanger the patient. Providing supplemental oxygenation and appropriate ventilation are essential with such patients.

Oxygen

Any patient who has sustained a significant head injury or who displays any indication of lowered level of consciousness, orientation, or arousal is a candidate for high-flow, high-concentration oxygen. Administer oxygen at a rate of 15 liters per minute via a nonrebreather mask with a patient who is moving an adequate respiratory volume. If the patient is not breathing adequately, supplement any positive pressure ventilations with oxygen via reservoir, again flowing at 15 liters per minute.

Any patient who has sustained a significant head injury or who displays any indication of lowered level of consciousness, orientation, or arousal is a candidate for high-flow, high-concentration oxygen.

Ventilations

Provision of a good supply of oxygen is critical to the head injury patient, but so too is the removal of carbon dioxide. Assess the patient's respiratory status and, if the patient is not moving a normal volume of air, employ overdrive respiration. Ventilations for the serious head injury patient (GCS ≤8) are guided by capnography. For the head injury patient without signs of herniation, adjust ventilation rates to maintain an end-tidal CO_2 reading of between 35 and 40 mmHg (adults at about 10 breaths per minute, children at about 20 breaths per minute, and infants at about 25 breaths per minute). For patients with suspected herniation, the end-tidal CO_2 reading should range between 30 and 35 mmHg, using ventilation rates about 10 breaths per minute faster than for patients without herniation. Also assure the oxygen saturation level is at least 95 percent for any serious head injury patient.

CIRCULATION

Your care of the patient with head, facial, and neck injury includes both control of any serious hemorrhage and support of the body's attempts to maintain blood pressure and cerebral circulation.

Hemorrhage Control

Head and facial hemorrhage is usually easy to control because most of these injuries are to the tissues that lie over facial and cranial bones. Direct pressure is commonly an effective means of controlling such bleeding, though you should take care not to put pressure directly on suspected skull or facial fractures. Wrap bandaging circumferentially, but be careful to keep the airway clear and give the patient the freedom to rid himself of vomitus should emesis occur. Watch the airway and be prepared to suction aggressively to limit danger from aspiration. Suctioning can also assure that the patient does not swallow large volumes of blood, stimulating emesis. Permit the conscious and alert patient with no suspected spinal injury who is suffering epistaxis to sit leaning forward, allowing the blood to drain. This positioning keeps blood from flowing down the pharynx and entering the esophagus.

An open neck injury carries the risk of air entering the external jugular during strong inspiration, leading to cerebral embolism with strokelike symptoms. Seal any open neck wound with an occlusive dressing held firmly in place by bandaging and tilt the patient's body head down on a backboard or stretcher, if possible. Carefully evaluate any other open wounds for frothy blood suggestive of tracheal involvement, seal those wounds on three sides with occlusive dressings, and monitor respirations.

Blunt trauma to the neck may produce the equivalent of compartment syndrome. Fasciae in the region compartmentalize muscle and anatomical structures and permit pressures to rise with rapid edema or blood accumulation. Any sign of neck edema or hematoma is an indication for rapid transport. Monitor the patient's skin tension and level of consciousness while en route to the hospital.

Severe hemorrhage associated with open neck wounds can lead quickly to hypovolemia and shock. Control the blood loss by using a dressing and gloved fingers to apply direct pressure to the source of bleeding. You may have to maintain digital pressure throughout prehospital care because application of circumferential bandaging may restrict the airway and circulation.

Blood Pressure Maintenance

Another component of circulation care for the head, face, and neck injury patient is guarding against hypotension. The brain is very dependent upon receiving a continuous supply of oxygenated blood. Any interruption of the supply, such as might be caused by hypotension in response to increasing intracranial pressure, will rapidly prove fatal. Care for the patient in whom you suspect increased intracranial pressure with fluid resuscitation, even though the patient's other injuries might not suggest that step. For example, the patient with penetrating chest trauma might not receive aggressive fluid resuscitation until the systolic blood pressure drops to below 80 mmHg. If that patient also has a head injury with increasing intracranial pressure, waiting for the blood pressure to drop to that level would be life threatening. Hence, provide rapid fluid (electrolyte) administration and other shock care measures to maintain a systolic blood pressure of 90 mmHg.

HYPOXIA

It is very important to monitor the patient with a head injury at all times in order to quickly identify and correct any hypoventilation. Hypoxia can further damage central nervous system tissue already affected by direct injury. If someone else is delivering ventilations, frequently monitor both that person's performance as well as the patient's oxygen saturation levels. Care providers often find it difficult to determine accurate ventilation rates while using a bag-valve-mask unit during the emergency. Assure that the patient is well oxygenated before any intubation attempt and hyperventilated (at 20 times per minute) for a short time after intubation. Also be watchful for interruptions in ventilations that might occur during patient movement or when changing ventilation providers.

HYPOVOLEMIA

Like hypoxia, hypovolemia and the associated hypotension reduce oxygen transport to the brain. This condition also reduces both circulation through the brain and the blood's ability to remove the products of metabolism. Since brain tissue is especially sensitive to oxygen deprivation, with head injury patients who have already suffered some damage to brain tissue, any further circulatory loss might prove devastating. The problems of hypovolemia and hypotension are compounded if there is any increase in intracranial pressure. Such an increase further restricts cerebral blood flow, and the body's autoregulatory mechanisms cannot compensate in a preexisting state of hypotension.

Provide fluid resuscitation for any patient with significant head injury in whom you suspect brain injury and who shows signs of shock compensation—rapid, thready pulse, slowed capillary refill, lowered level of consciousness, anxiety, or restlessness. Insert two large-bore catheters and administer lactated Ringer's solution or normal saline at a wide-open rate through nonrestrictive trauma IV tubing. Administer 1,000 mL of an isotonic solution, followed by additional fluids as needed to maintain a systolic blood pressure of 90 mmHg. In the child (6–12 years), young child (2–5 years), and infant (0–1 year), maintain a systolic blood pressure of at least 80, 75, or 65, respectively. Periods of hypotension, as well as hypoxia, are associated with a poor outcome from serious head injury.

In serious head injury, the blood pressure may rise. This elevation in blood pressure is a reflex response to increasing intracranial pressure and represents an attempt by the body to maintain perfusion of the brain. In the patient with probable brain injury, do not treat hypertension.

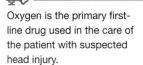
Provide aggressive fluid resuscitation for any patient with significant head injury in whom you suspect brain injury and who shows signs of shock compensation.

MEDICATIONS

Several medications may be useful in the care of the head injury patient. These medications include oxygen, diuretics (furosemide), paralytics (succinylcholine, atracurium, vecuronium), sedatives (diazepam, etomidate, midazolam, morphine, fentanyl), atropine, dextrose, thiamine, and topical anesthetic sprays.

Oxygen

Oxygen is the primary first-line drug used in the care of the patient with suspected head injury. Administration of high-flow, high-concentration oxygen provides a high inspired oxygen level and facilitates both diffusion through the alveolar and capillary walls and the highest oxygen uptake by the hemoglobin of the red blood cells. Oxygen saturation is important for the head injury patient because the brain is acutely dependent upon a good supply of oxygen. There are no contraindications nor side effects of concern for use of oxygen during prehospital emergency care. (Note, however, that hyperventilation is contraindicated in head injury patients because it reduces circulating CO_2 levels.)

Administer oxygen via a nonrebreather mask at a flow rate of 15 liters per minute for the patient who is breathing adequately. If the patient is receiving positive-pressure ventilations, supplement the ventilations with 15 liters per minute of oxygen flowing into the reservoir. Monitor oxygen administration using the pulse oximeter, and keep the saturation level above 95 percent. Also monitor skin color, respiratory excursion, orientation, and anxiety to assure the patient is well oxygenated.

Oxygen is the primary first-line drug used in the care of the patient with suspected head injury.

Diuretics

Furosemide   Furosemide (Lasix) is a loop diuretic that inhibits the reabsorption of sodium in the kidneys. It results in the increased secretion of water and electrolytes, including sodium, chloride, magnesium, and calcium. Furosemide also causes venous dilation and a reduced cardiac preload. Furosemide is generally contraindicated in pregnant patients because it may cause fetal abnormalities. Since furosemide causes diuresis, use with caution, if at all, in patients with hypotension secondary to hypovolemia.

Furosemide often comes in a preloaded syringe or a single-use vial and is given as a slow IV bolus or IM injection. It is administered at a dose of about 0.5 to 1.0 mg/kg, frequently in doses of either 40 or 80 mg. Administer the medication very slowly, over 1 to 2 minutes.

Paralytics

Paralytics are drugs that paralyze the skeletal muscles, permitting intubation in patients with whom the procedure would otherwise be impossible. Administration is a part of the rapid sequence intubation (RSI) procedure, in which you must quickly sedate, paralyze, then intubate the patient while assuring the patient is well oxygenated and the airway remains clear. RSI uses etomidate, diazepam, midazolam, fentanyl, or morphine sulfate to sedate the patient; in some cases, atropine sulfate to limit muscle fasciculations; and succinylcholine chloride, atracurium, or vercuronium to paralyze the patient.

Succinylcholine　Succinylcholine (Anectine) is an ultra-short-acting depolarizing skeletal muscle relaxant. It acts upon cholinergic receptors to cause the muscles to contract (depolarize). This action produces **fasciculations,** individual muscle contractions seen beneath the skin. Succinylcholine induces complete paralysis in 30 to 60 seconds and persists for about 2 to 3 minutes with IV administration. Onset of paralysis occurs in 75 seconds to 3 minutes with IM administration. Succinylchloline is frequently administered to achieve temporary paralysis for the intubation of patients with muscle tone, spasms, or seizures that may otherwise prevent the procedure. Succinylcholine paralyzes the muscles of respiration, so care providers must be immediately ready to intubate and ventilate the patient when the drug takes effect. Succinylcholine does not affect the patient's level of consciousness, cerebration, anxiety, or pain perception, so its use should follow the administration of a sedative/amnestic agent. Succinylcholine increases ICP, may induce vomiting, and should be used with caution, if at all, in cases of head injury. Because it slightly increases intraoccular pressure, it is contraindicated for patients with penetrating eye injuries and should be used with caution in patients who are taking digitalis because of the risk of hypokalemia.

Succinylcholine is administered rapidly in a dosage of 1 to 1.5 mg/kg IV. It may be given IM if necessary. In that case, it is usually supplied in a single-use vial with 10 mL of a 20 mg/mL solution. Storage of succinylcholine requires refrigeration. If the patient is conscious, succinlycholine is given after a sedative/amnestic to sedate the patient during the procedure. Frequently 0.5 mg of atropine is administered prior to succinylcholine to halt the fasciculations and reduce secretions.

Atracurium and Vecuronium　Atracurium (Tracrium) and vecuronium (Norcuron) are nondepolarizing skeletal muscle relaxants. They induce paralysis without causing muscle contractions and fasciculations. Both are effective agents with a more rapid onset (less than 1 minute) and shorter duration (25 to 40 minutes) than other nondepolarizing blockers. They also have fewer cardiovascular side effects than succinylcholine. Like succinylcholine, atracurium and vecuronium are used to paralyze patients with muscle tone, spasms, or seizures in order to permit endotracheal intubation. They also do not have any effect on the level of consciousness, cerebration, anxiety, or pain perception, so their use should follow administration of a sedative/amnestic agent.

fasciculations *involuntary contractions or twitchings of muscle fibers.*

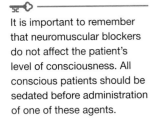

It is important to remember that neuromuscular blockers do not affect the patient's level of consciousness. All conscious patients should be sedated before administration of one of these agents.

Atracurium comes in single-use vials containing 10 mg/mL. It is administered by rapid IV bolus of 3 to 6 mg/kg. Atracurium must be refrigerated. Vecuronium is administered rapidly in a dose of 0.08 to 0.1 mg/kg IV. Vecuronium comes as 10-mg vials of powder that must be reconstituted with saline (either 5 or 10 mL) prior to administration.

Sedatives

Diazepam   Diazepam (Valium) is a benzodiazepine with both antianxiety and muscle relaxant qualities. In prehospital care, it is often used to premedicate patients to facilitate intubation. Diazepam is also a potent anticonvulsant. It is administered in a slow IV bolus of 5 to 10 mg, not to exceed 5 mg/minute, into a large vein. Diazepam is rather fast acting, with IV effects occurring almost immediately and reaching peak effectiveness in 15 minutes. Its duration is from 15 to 60 minutes. Do not mix diazepam with any other drugs, and flush the IV line before and after administration. Administer it as close to the IV catheter as possible. Do not inject it into a plastic IV bag because diazepam is readily absorbed by plastic, which quickly reduces its concentration.

Diazepam is usually supplied in single-use vials or preloaded syringes containing 2 mL of a 5 mg/mL solution (10 mg). Administer 5 to 10 mg IV every 10 to 15 minutes to a maximum of 30 mg. When an IV line is not immediately available, diazepam may be administered rectally for seizures with effects occurring quickly.

The effects of diazepam (and midazolam) may be reversed by the administration of flumazenil. Usually, 2 mL of a 0.1 mg/mL solution is given IV (over 30 seconds) with a second dose repeated at 60 seconds. Be careful in its administration as flumazenil may precipitate seizures in the head injury patient.

Etomidate   Etomidate (Amidate) is a very rapid-acting, short-duration, nonbarbiturate hypnotic with no analgesic properties. Etomidate lowers cerebral blood flow and oxygen consumption and has minimal cardiovascular and respiratory effects. Etomidate is of special interest for head injury patients as it somewhat lowers intracranial pressure. IV administration of etomidate induces hypnosis within 1 minute that lasts for 3 to 5 minutes.

Etomidate is supplied in a preloaded syringe at a concentration of 2 mg/mL and administered in a dose of 0.1 to 0.3 mg/kg over 15 to 30 seconds. It is not recommended for use in children under 10 years of age. Use with caution in hypotensive patients or those with severe asthma. Flumazenil is not effective in reversing the actions of etomidate.

Midazolam   Midazolam (Versed) is a benzodiazepine similar to diazepam though it is three to four times more potent. Onset of its effects occurs within 3 to 5 minutes. Administration of midazolam may cause cardiorespiratory arrest and hypotension, and the drug does not protect against increasing intracranial pressure that follows succinylcholine and pancuronium administration. Midazolam is frequently paired with vecuronium to achieve rapid sedated paralysis. It may cause vomiting and nausea and many of the signs and symptoms of head injury.

Administer midazolam very slowly in small increments (at no more than 1 mg/min) titrated to the desired effect or the maximum administration of 2.5 mg. Midazolam is supplied in 2-, 5-, and 10-mL vials of a 1 mg/mL concentration and may be mixed in the same syringe with morphine, meperidine, or atropine or diluted with normal saline.

Morphine   Morphine (Duramorph, Astramorph) is an opium alkaloid used to relieve pain (narcotic analgesic), to sedate, and to reduce anxiety. It may mask the signs and symptoms of head injury and mildly increase intracranial pressure. It also reduces cardiac preload by increasing venous capacitance and thus may decrease blood pressure in the hypovolemic patient. Its major side effects are respiratory depression and possible nausea and vomiting.

Morphine is available in 10-mL single-use vials or Tubex units of a 1 mg/mL solution or as 1 mL of a 10 mg/mL solution vial for dilution with 9 mL normal saline. Administer a 5- to 10-mg bolus, slowly IV, and repeat as necessary every few minutes until effective.

Fentanyl Fentanyl is an opiate narcotic, chemically unrelated to morphine, that provides immediate and effective pain control. Fentanyl's onset of action is more rapid than morphine's and it is considerably more potent, thus requiring lower doses. Fentanyl does not cause hypotension to the same degree as does morphine, which makes it an ideal agent for trauma.

Fentanyl is supplied in various doses. The typical starting dose is 25 to 50 mcg IV. Repeat doses of 25 mcg IV can be provided as needed. As with all opiates, continuously monitor the patient's vital signs.

Naloxone (Narcan) is a narcotic antagonist that can quickly reverse the effects of narcotics and should be available anytime you use morphine sulfate or fentanyl. Naloxone is administered IV bolus of 0.4 to 2 mg, repeated every 2 to 3 minutes until effective (up to 10 mg). Naloxone is a shorter acting drug than morphine, so repeat doses may be necessary.

Atropine

Atropine is an anticholinergic (parasympatholytic) agent sometimes administered as part of a rapid sequence intubation routine. It has the ability to reduce parasympathetic (vagal) stimulation associated with intubation attempts and the resultant decrease in heart rate. Atropine may reduce oral and airway secretions and limit the fasciculations associated with administration of succinylcholine. Atropine may cause pupillary dilation and other CNS signs frequently associated with head injury—headache, nausea, vomiting, and blurred vision.

Atropine is available in many concentrations from 0.05 and 0.1 mg/mL preloaded syringes to 10 mL vials of 1 mg/mL solution. For emergency administration, its usual form is 10-mL preloaded syringes of 0.1 mg/mL concentration. Atropine is usually administered as a 0.5-mg bolus for rapid sequence intubation.

Dextrose

In general, both hypoglycemia and hyperglycemia are detrimental to the patient with head injury. In the past, dextrose was given routinely to patients who were unresponsive with an undetermined cause. However, current practice calls for identifying the blood glucose level on all unresponsive patients, especially those with a possible history of chronic alcoholism or diabetes. If significant hypoglycemia is found, administer 25 mg of glucose and 100 mg of thiamine.

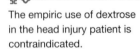
The empiric use of dextrose in the head injury patient is contraindicated.

Dextrose is supplied in preloaded syringes containing 50 mL of a 0.5 mg/mL (50 percent) solution ($D_{50}W$). It is to be administered slowly through a large vein because it is a very hypertonic solution. In severe cases of hypoglycemia, a second dose may be administered.

Thiamine

Thiamine, more commonly known as vitamin B_1, is a substance obtained from diet and needed for body metabolism. Thiamine is essential for the processing of glucose through Krebs cycle, from which the body gains its life-sustaining energy. In malnourished patients (like the chronic alcoholic), thiamine is depleted and the body tissue cannot obtain energy from glucose. The brain is especially affected since it does not store energy sources.

Thiamine is supplied in 1-mL single-use ampules, vials, and preloaded syringes containing a 100 mg/mL solution. Most commonly 100 mg are administered IV bolus or IM. It should be administered before or with glucose.

Topical Anesthetic Spray

Topical sprays use an anesthetic agent, such as xylocaine or benzocaine, to anesthetize the oral and pharyngeal mucosa. This reduces the gag reflex, making endotracheal intubation easier and reducing the impact retching has on intracranial pressure. The agent is sprayed into the oral pharynx where it is rapidly absorbed by mucosal tissue. It inhibits nerve sensation, thereby reducing the gag reflex. The effects of the agent are immediate (within 15 seconds), remain local, and last for about 15 minutes. These agents are usually supplied in 2-ounce aerosol spray cannisters with long, hollow extension tubes to direct the spray down the throat. The agent is applied by directing a spray of the material into the posterior oral cavity and pharynx. While topical anesthetic sprays permit easier intubation and reduce the associated vagal effects, they also reduce the patient's ability to remove fluids from the airway and increase the danger of aspiration.

TRANSPORT CONSIDERATIONS

There are special considerations to observe when transporting the patient with serious head injury to the hospital. Some suggest that the use of red lights, siren, rough ride (high speed), and other patient stimulation may agitate the patient, increase intracranial pressure, and induce seizures. While there is little evidence to support this claim, it is probably prudent to reduce speed and use red lights and siren sparingly.

When transporting head injury patients, limit external stimulation, such as the use of red lights and sirens, and try to provide a smooth ride.

Be cautious in considering the head injury patient as a candidate for air medical service transport. While the time saved by helicopter transport may be very important, the head injury patient is prone to seizures, especially with the physical stimulation (noise and vibration) associated with this mode of transport. Seizures aboard any type of aircraft are very dangerous. If you elect to transport by air, assure that the patient is firmly secured to a long spine board (including feet and hands) and that his airway is protected by endotracheal intubation.

EMOTIONAL SUPPORT

Identify someone to remain with the patient with the specific role of calming and reassuring him during care and transport. Have that person continuously reorient the patient to his environment. Remember, head injury patients may have trouble remembering events preceding and immediately following the incident as well as have difficulty laying down short-term memory. The person assigned the role should describe what happened to the patient and help the patient remain oriented to the current location and what is happening. This simple step aids greatly in reducing the patient's anxiety and in helping to return to a normal level of orientation.

Head injury patients may be very confused, distressed, abusive, or even combative. Do not take their behavior personally. Maintain a professional demeanor and provide emotional support during assessment, care, and transport.

SPECIAL INJURY CARE

There are certain types of head, face, and neck trauma that deserve special care. They include scalp avulsion, injury to the pinna of the ear, eye injury, dislodged teeth, and impaled objects.

Scalp Avulsion

Avulsion occurs when a glancing blow tears the scalp's border and releases a flap of scalp. The flap may remain in anatomical position, fold back exposing the cranium, or may be torn completely free. If the avulsion uncovers the cranium, cover both the open wound and the undersurface of the exposed scalp flap with a large bulky dressing. Also place padding under the fold of the scalp to prevent a sharp kinking along its border. If the region is seriously contaminated, remove gross contamination and rinse the area with normal saline before applying the dressings. Scalp avulsions tend to heal very well unless grossly contaminated or the circulation to the flap is severely disrupted.

Pinna Injury

Serious injury to the pinna, or exposed portion of the ear, often results from glancing blows and trauma, like a tearing or avulsion injury, that disrupts its structure. Such an injury is best treated by placing the pinna in as close to its anatomical position as possible. Then place a dressing between the head and medial surface of the injured ear and cover the exposed ear with a sterile dressing. Finally, bandage the dressed injury firmly to the head.

Eye Injury

Care for eye injuries involves careful assessment and protective care. Most eye wounds or injuries are best cared for by applying soft dressings to cover the closed, injured eye. The other eye, even if uninjured, is also dressed and the dressings on both eyes are held in place with gentle bandaging. This technique prevents sympathetic motion (one eye moving with the other) which may cause additional damage to the injured eye. If the eye injury is an open wound or torn eyelid, consider using a sterile dressing soaked in normal saline to reduce the pain and discomfort and prevent evaporative loss of lacrimal fluid. Place the patient in the supine position if other injuries do not prevent it.

If the patient complains of eye pain without apparent injury, suspect corneal abrasion or laceration, possibly caused by an object embedded in the conjunctiva or sclera. Gently invert the eyelid and examine for any small embedded object (Figure 8-29 ■). If

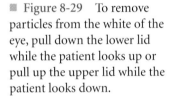 Figure 8-29   To remove particles from the white of the eye, pull down the lower lid while the patient looks up or pull up the upper lid while the patient looks down.

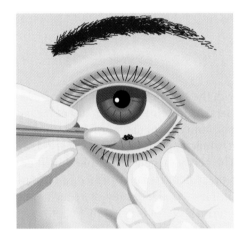

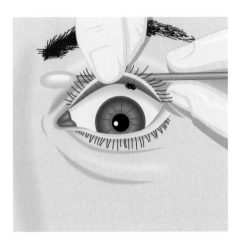

you observe one, you may attempt to remove it with a saline-moistened cotton swab. Even if you successfully remove the object, the patient is likely to continue reporting pain and the sensation of the foreign body. As with apparent wounds, cover both eyes with soft dressings and loose bandaging.

If the eye is avulsed or has an impaled object in it, cover the eye and the object with a cup or other protective material and again dress and bandage both eyes. If the patient is combative or has a significantly reduced level of consciousness, secure his hands together and then to his waist or belt. This prevents accidental dislodging of the protective dressing and possible aggravation of the eye injury.

Eye injuries and the loss of eyesight in one or both eyes can create anxiety in most patients. Be sure to calm and reassure the patient and explain in advance your actions as you move the patient from the scene to the ambulance and to the hospital.

If, during the assessment, you observe that the patient is wearing contact lenses and there is any risk that he may become unresponsive, have the patient remove the lenses. If the patient is already unresponsive, try removing the lenses yourself with a contact removal suction cup (Figure 8-30 ■). This miniature suction cup seals against the contact lens and allows easy removal. Alternatively, lift the eyelid, which may cause the lens to dislodge, or, with the eye closed, gently push the lens into the corner of the eye. Keep the lens you remove in a contact lens case where it should be soaked in a contact lens or sterile saline solution.

Dislodged Teeth

Locate any teeth that may have been dislodged by trauma and transport them to the hospital with the patient. Rinse the teeth in normal saline and wrap them in saline-soaked gauze for transport to the emergency department. If a tooth is largely intact, it may be successfully replanted.

Impaled Objects

Any object impaled in the head, face, or neck should be left in place and dressed and bandaged to assure that it does not move about during care and transport. Use bulky dressings to stabilize the object. Secure the patient's hands if there is a danger that he may dislodge the object. Only if the object obstructs or seriously threatens the airway should you consider its removal. In such cases, removal will likely increase the associated hemorrhage and possibly damage adjoining structures, but the patency of the airway is absolutely essential.

Removal of objects that pass through the patient's cheek pose the least danger for removal. With such a wound, you have ready access to both of its sides, and the wound involves no critical structures or organs. Nevertheless, expect increased hemorrhage from the wound, have dressings ready, and be prepared to apply direct pressure as soon as the object is removed.

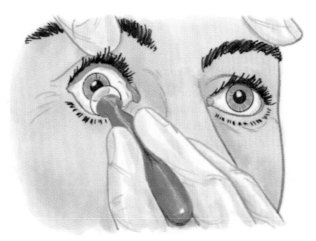

■ Figure 8-30   You can use a moistened suction cup to remove hard lenses.

Summary

The head, face, and neck contain very special and important structures—key elements of the central nervous system, the airway, the alimentary canal, and major organs of sensation. Serious trauma to the region endangers these structures and demands special assessment and care. During the scene size-up, identify possible mechanisms of injury and the injuries they suggest. Confirm the injuries during the initial and rapid trauma assessments. Identify your patient's level of consciousness and orientation early, and watch the eyes carefully for signs of cerebral hypoxia and increasing intracranial pressure. Assure that the spine is immobilized and the airway is clear and protected from aspiration and physical obstruction. Administer high-flow, high-concentration oxygen and ventilate, as necessary, being careful not to under- or overventilate the patient. Secure rapid transport for the patient with possible intracranial hemorrhage or serious lesion. Once the central nervous system, the airway, and breathing are protected, address skeletal structure fractures, minor bleeding, and open wounds. During all your care for the patient with injury to the head, face, or neck, provide emotional support and help orient the patient to what happened, to where he is, and to what will be happening during prehospital care.

You Make the Call

You are called to a scene where a young woman, in an attempt to end her life, has deeply lacerated her anterior and lateral neck. The wound is deep and produces severe flowing hemorrhage with bubbling on expiration. She also has blood gurgling and spattering from her mouth with expiration.

1. What structures are most likely injured?
2. What care would you employ?
3. What are serious life threats associated with this injury?

See Suggested Responses at the back of this book.

Review Questions

1. Retroauricular ecchymosis over the mastoid bone, indicating a basilar skull fracture, is called:
   a. Battle's sign.
   b. raccoon eye.
   c. Goblet's sign.
   d. periorbital ecchymosis.

2. Battle's sign and raccoon eyes indicate:
   a. tension pneumothorax.
   b. basilar skull fracture.
   c. abdominal injury.
   d. impending shock.

3. A sight-threatening injury, involving hemorrhage into the anterior chamber pools, is known as:
   a. ecchymosis.
   b. blepharospasm.
   c. erythema.
   d. hyphema.

4. Patients with a Glasgow Coma Scale score of _____ or less should be immediately intubated.
   a. 8
   b. 10
   c. 12
   d. 14

5. Your patient has been involved in an accident and has received open trauma to the neck and blood vessels therein. Your concern should be directed toward the danger of exsanguination and:
   a. pulmonary edema.
   b. tension pneumothorax.
   c. air embolism.
   d. subcutaneous emphysema.

6. Sudden painless loss of sight in one eye is most generally associated with:
   a. ocular trauma.
   b. acute retinal artery occlusion.
   c. retinal detachment.
   d. increasing intracranial pressure.

7. A classic sign of increasing intracranial pressure, which includes increasing blood pressure, slowing pulse, and irregular respirations, is referred to as:
   a. Cheyne-Stokes.
   b. Cushing's triad.
   c. Kernig's sign.
   d. medullary syndrome.

8. The inability to remember events that occurred after a traumatic event is known as:
   a. anterograde amnesia.
   b. retrograde amnesia.
   c. transient amnesia.
   d. morbid amnesia.

9. The connective tissue sheet covering the superior aspect of the cranium is called the galea:
   a. pericranium.
   b. periosteum.
   c. aponeurotica.
   d. subaponeurotica.

10. The meninges serve as a protective mechanism for the brain and spinal cord. The three layers of the meninges are the pia mater, the dura mater, and the:
    a. tentorium.
    b. falx cerebri.
    c. zygomatica.
    d. arachnoid.

11. Which of the following drugs may cause fasciulations and raises ICP?
    a. succinylcholine
    b. Solu-Medrol
    c. mannitol
    d. furosemide

12. The largest portion of the brain, which controls consciousness and higher mental functions, is the:
    a. brainstem.
    b. cerebellum.
    c. cerebrum.
    d. hypothalamus.

13. For the head injury patient without signs of herniation, you should adjust ventilation rates to maintain an end-tidal CO_2 reading of between:
    a. 20 and 25
    b. 25 and 30
    c. 30 and 35
    d. 35 and 40

14. Rate, depth, and rhythm of respirations are controlled by the:
    a. pons.
    b. apneustic center.
    c. aponeurotica center.
    d. medulla oblongata.

15. Your patient has presented with a facial injury secondary to blunt trauma. You note left facial abrasions and lacerations, depression over the prominence of the left cheek, diminished movement of the left ocular muscles, and diplopia. This injury pattern is consistent with:
    a. Le Fort I fracture.
    b. mandibular dislocation.
    c. basilar skull fracture.
    d. orbital fracture.

See Answers to Review Questions at the back of this book.

Further Reading

American College of Surgeons, Committee on Trauma. *Advanced Trauma Life Support Course: Student Manual.* Chicago: American College of Surgeons, 2003.

Bates, Barbara, Lynn S. Bickley, and Robert A. Hoekelman. *A Guide to Physical Examination and History Taking.* 8th ed. Philadelphia: J. B. Lippincott, 2003.

Bledsoe, Bryan E., and Dwayne E. Clayden. *Pocket-Reference for EMTs and Paramedics.* 2nd ed. Upper Saddle River, N.J.: Pearson/Prentice Hall, 1998.

Bledsoe, B. E. and D. Clayden. *Prehospital Emergency Pharmacology.* 6th ed. Upper Saddle River, N.J.: Pearson/Prentice Hall, 2005.

Butman, A., S. Martin, R. Vomacka, and N. McSwain. *Comprehensive Guide to Pre-Hospital Skills: A Skills Manual for EMT-Basic, EMT-Intermediate, and EMT-Paramedic.* St. Louis: Mosby, 1996.

Campbell, John E. *Basic Trauma Life Support for Paramedics and Other Advanced Providers.* 5th ed. Upper Saddle River, N.J.: Pearson/Prentice Hall, 2004.

Ivatury R. R., and G. C. Cayten, eds. *Textbook of Penetrating Trauma.* Media, Pa.: Williams & Wilkins, 1996.

Martini, Frederic. *Fundamentals of Anatomy and Physiology.* 6th ed. San Francisco: Benjamin Cummings, 2004.

McSwain, N. E. and S. B. Frame, eds. *Prehospital Trauma Life Support.* 5th ed. St. Louis: Mosby, 2003.

Rosen, P., and R. Barkin, eds. *Emergency Medicine: Concepts and Clinical Practice.* 5th ed. St. Louis: Mosby, 2002.

On the Web

Visit Brady's Paramedic Website at **www.bradybooks.com/paramedic**.

Spinal Trauma

Objectives

After reading this chapter, you should be able to:

7. Describe the assessment findings associated with and management for traumatic spinal injuries. (pp. 351–374)
8. Describe the various types of helmets and their purposes. (p. 365)
9. Relate the priorities of care to factors determining the need for helmet removal in various field situations including sports-related incidents. (pp. 365–366)
10. Given several preprogrammed and moulaged spinal trauma patients, provide the appropriate scene size-up, initial assessment, rapid trauma assessment or focused physical exam and history, detailed exam, and ongoing assessment and provide appropriate patient care and transportation. (pp. 334–374)

Key Terms

anterior cord syndrome, p. 349
anterior medial fissure, p. 340
ascending tracts, p. 340
autonomic hyperreflexia syndrome, p. 350
axon, p. 340
Brown-Séquard syndrome, p. 350

central cord syndrome, p. 350
dermatome, p. 343
descending tracts, p. 340
gray matter, p. 340
intervertebral disk, p. 336
laminae, p. 336
myotome, p. 343
pedicles, p. 335
posterior medial sulcus, p. 340

spinal canal, p. 335
spinal cord, p. 340
spinal nerves, p. 341
spinous process, p. 336
transection, p. 349
transverse process, p. 336
vertebra, p. 335
vertebral body, p. 335
white matter, p. 340

Case Study

Paramedics Fred and Lisa are providing stand-by service at a local high school football game. Just before the end of the third quarter, they are called onto the field when a player is thrown to the ground and "can't get up."

Upon arrival at the player's side, they find a well-developed teenager who is oriented to person but not to time and place. He states that he was hit hard from the side and now has a "tingling" in his legs and feet. Upon further questioning, the player, Bill, complains of some localized pain just above the shoulders. Bill's medical history reveals that he's had no significant previous medical problems, has no allergies, and that his tetanus vaccination is up to date.

The paramedics' physical exam reveals a patient clothed in protective football gear and helmet who has no external signs of physical injury. The patient's airway is clear, and the rate, strength, and quality of his breathing and pulse are within normal limits. Physical examination of the head is limited by the helmet, but palpation of the posterior neck reveals some localized tenderness at or slightly above the first thoracic vertebra. Respiratory excursion and diaphragm movement seem unaffected by the injury. Paresthesia appears to affect the entire chest, abdomen, and lower extremities, as well as the posterior surface of the upper extremities. The patient's upper extremity grip is strong, while the strength of foot dorsiflexion and plantar flexion appears diminished. Bill maintains both bowel and bladder control.

Fred feels it will be very difficult to immobilize Bill with the helmet and shoulder pads in place. He has the athletic trainer hold the helmet while he and Lisa release the air pressure in the bladder and begin its removal. Lisa stabilizes Bill's head, while Fred gently and carefully negotiates the helmet around Bill's facial features. Once the helmet is removed, Fred assumes manual stabilization of Bill's head, which is well above the surface of the playing field because the shoulder pads raise his shoulders more than an inch off the ground. Lisa proceeds to cut Bill's shirt and the webbing that holds the pads in place and gently removes the pads. Then, using a rope sling, Fred, Lisa, and the athletic trainer gently slide Bill with axial control onto the spine board. After the torso is immobilized to the board, they use padding and a cervical immobilization device to immobilize Bill's head about 1 inch above the board to maintain neutral alignment.

Bill's blood pressure, pulse rate and strength, and respiratory rate and volume have all remained relatively normal during these procedures. Fred notes no differences in skin temperature or capillary refill in any extremity, which reduces the likelihood of neurogenic shock from spinal cord injury. The pulse oximeter reads 98 percent, and the ECG displays a normal sinus rhythm at 68 as the paramedics load Bill into the ambulance and begin transport to the regional neurocenter.

Fred and Lisa learn from the local paper that Bill suffered a compression fracture of the seventh cervical vertebrae and will miss the rest of the season. The injury may limit Bill's athletic career but is not expected to otherwise affect his life. What the paper did not report is that, if it had been mishandled, this injury could easily have resulted in Bill spending his life in a wheelchair.

INTRODUCTION TO SPINAL INJURIES

A spinal cord injury can both threaten life and induce serious, lifelong disability. Each year more than 11,000 permanent spinal cord injuries occur, most commonly in men aged from 16 to 30. Auto and other vehicle crashes account for almost half these spinal cord injuries (48 percent), with falls (21 percent), intentional injuries (15 percent), and sports-related injuries (14 percent) also contributing significantly to the total. Further, of all patients who suffer neurologic deficit from trauma, some 40 percent have experienced cord injury. The remaining patients with neurologic deficits have suffered injuries that disrupt the spinal or peripheral nerve roots along their course.

Spinal cord injury is an especially devastating type of trauma. The spinal cord consists of highly specialized central nervous system tissue and does not repair itself when seriously injured. Permanent injury to it affects the body's major communications pathways and control over the lower extremities (paraplegia) or both upper and lower extremities (quadriplegia). Spinal cord injuries also affect the body's control over internal organs and the body's internal environment (homeostasis). A patient with a serious spinal injury is left less able to care for himself, will have a significantly altered lifestyle, and will face increased expenses associated with care and support. In fact, lifelong care costs for the victim of a permanent spinal cord injury may well exceed $1 million. This figure does not include the patient's lost earning power due to the disability.

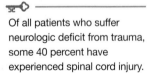

Of all patients who suffer neurologic deficit from trauma, some 40 percent have experienced spinal cord injury.

As with most trauma, the best form of care is prevention. Recent advances in motor vehicle and highway design have helped reduce the incidence of spine injury in its most common category, motor vehicle trauma. Proper use of lap and shoulder belts further reduces the incidence of spinal cord injury, as do programs to reduce drinking and driving. Education programs aimed at teaching safe practices also reduce the potential for spinal cord injury. These programs can foster such behaviors as not diving into unknown waters, developing good physical conditioning, and wearing protective equipment in sports. Following good safety practices in the workplace and in the home can also reduce both temporary and permanent spinal column and cord injury.

The danger of incurring spinal injury exists even after a traumatic event has occurred. According to the U.S. Department of Transportation, as many as 25 percent of all spinal cord injuries result from improper handling of the spinal column (and the patient) after an injury (often by bystanders). Clearly, one way to reduce this figure is to assure that patients with mechanisms of injury or any signs or symptoms that suggest potential spinal cord or column injuries receive immediate and continuing manual spinal immobilization followed rapidly by mechanical immobilization (called spinal precautions) during prehospital assessment, care, and transport.

As many as 25 percent of all spinal cord injuries result from improper handling of the spinal column (and the patient) after an injury.

SPINAL ANATOMY AND PHYSIOLOGY

The spine consists of a supporting skeletal structure, the vertebral column, and a central nervous system pathway, the spinal cord. These are important functional elements both for body posture and movement and for communication among the body's many systems. The vertebral column provides skeletal support for and permits movement of the head, assists in maintaining the shape of the thoracic cage, supports the upper body, and forms the posterior aspect of the pelvis. The spinal cord, contained and protected within the vertebral column, is the main communication conduit of the central nervous system. It is responsible for transmitting messages from the brain to the body organs and tissues and from the sensory nerves in the organs, skin, and other tissues back to the brain.

THE VERTEBRAL COLUMN

The vertebral column is a hollow skeletal tube made up of 33 irregular bones, called **vertebrae.** This column attaches to the head, to the bones of the rib cage, and to the pelvis. It provides the central skeletal support structure and a major portion of the axial skeleton. At the same time, the vertebrae provide a protective container for the spinal cord. Several components with differing functions may make up the structure of each individual vertebra.

vertebra   *one of 33 bones making up the vertebral column.*

The major weight-bearing component of a vertebra is the **vertebral body.** It is a cylinder of skeletal tissue made up of cancellous bone surrounded by a layer of hard, compact bone. It lies anterior to the other components of the vertebra.

vertebral body   *short column of bone that forms the weight-bearing portion of a vertebra.*

The size of the vertebral body varies with its location along the spinal column (Figure 9-1 ■). The first two cervical vertebrae (C-1 and C-2) do not have vertebral bodies because of their specialized functions. Below C-1 and C-2, the size of the vertebral bodies increases progressively as you move down the spine because the vertebral column is supporting an increasing portion of the upper body's weight. The lumbar spine has the strongest and largest vertebral bodies due to the weight they bear. Because of the fused nature of the sacrum and coccyx, these regions have no discernable bodies.

A component of the vertebra posterior to the vertebral body is the **spinal canal,** which is the opening, or foramen, that accommodates the spinal cord. This opening is formed by small fused bony structures that are joined together to create a ring. The lateral structures of the ring are called **pedicles,** while the two posterior structures are

spinal canal   *opening in the vertebrae that accommodates the spinal cord.*

pedicles   *thick, bony struts that connect the vertebral bodies with the transverse processes and help make up the opening for the spinal canal.*

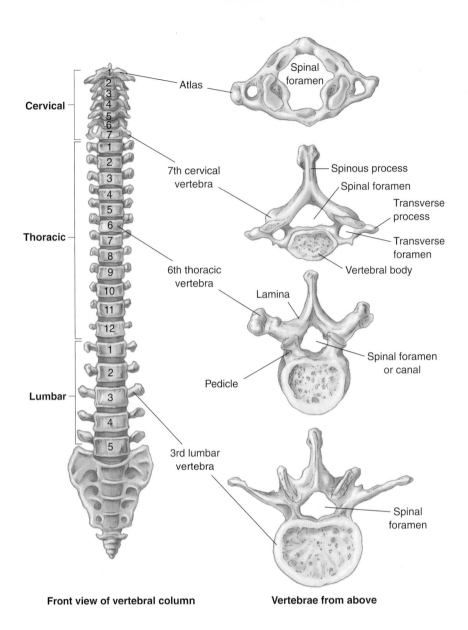

■ Figure 9-1 Changing anatomical dimensions of the vertebral column.

Cervical
Atlas
Spinal foramen

1
2
3
4
5
6
7

Thoracic

1
2
3
4
5
6
7
8
9
10
11
12

7th cervical vertebra

Spinous process
Spinal foramen
Transverse process
Transverse foramen
Vertebral body

6th thoracic vertebra

Lamina

Spinal foramen or canal

Pedicle

Lumbar

1
2
3
4
5

3rd lumbar vertebra

Spinal foramen

Front view of vertebral column   **Vertebrae from above**

laminae *posterior bones of a vertebra that help make up the foramen, or opening, of the spinal canal.*

transverse process *bony outgrowth of the vertebral pedicle that serves as a site for muscle attachment and articulation with the ribs.*

spinous process *prominence at the posterior part of a vertebra.*

intervertebral disk *cartilaginous pad between vertebrae that serves as a shock absorber.*

called **laminae.** The inferior surface of the pedicle contains a notch, called the intervertebral foramen. This notch permits the exit of a peripheral nerve root and spinal vein and the entrance of a spinal artery on each side of the spinal canal and at each vertebral junction.

At the juncture of the pedicle and lamina on each side of a vertebra, there is a bony outgrowth called the **transverse process.** There is also a bony outgrowth where the laminae join, which is called the **spinous process.** The spinous process is the posteriorly and inferiorly oriented bony protrusion that you can feel along the spine.

The spinous and transverse processes are points of attachment for ligaments and tendons. Ligaments hold the vertebrae firmly together and in place while they permit limited motion. The tendons attach muscles to the vertebral column and permit these muscles to move the spine, other bones, and the body. This attachment of muscles and capsule of ligaments protects and strengthens the vertebral column against the forces of trauma.

Between the vertebral bodies are cartilaginous **intervertebral disks.** These disks are formed of a strong yet somewhat flexible outer cover called the annulus fibrosus and a soft and gelatinous inner region called the nucleus pulposus. The intervertebral disks accommodate some motion of the adjacent vertebrae, limit bone wear, and absorb shock along the length of the spinal column. The intervertebral disks make up about 25 percent of the total length of the spinal column, and their degeneration accounts for much of the height loss associated with advancing age.

The elements of the spinal column also have numerous articular surfaces. These surfaces are found on the vertebral bodies, the pedicles, and on the transverse and spinous processes. The articular surfaces enable the spinal column to move around the spinal cord without compressing it, permit articulation with the skull and ribs, and make possible the formation of the rigid, immobile joint of the pelvis.

The vertebral bodies are held firmly together by strong ligaments to assure that the spinal foramen safely accommodates the spinal cord and that the body has a reasonable range of motion. The anterior longitudinal ligament travels along the anterior surfaces of the vertebral bodies. It provides the major stability of the spinal column and resists hyperextension. The posterior longitudinal ligament travels along the posterior surfaces of the vertebral bodies, within the spinal canal. This ligament helps to prevent hyperflexion; when it is disrupted, the result is, frequently, a spinal cord injury. Other ligaments encapsulate the spinous processes (interspinous ligaments) and the transverse processes. These ligaments strengthen and stabilize the column against excessive lateral bending, rotation, and flexion.

DIVISIONS OF THE VERTEBRAL COLUMN

The vertebral column is divided into five regions: the cervical, the thoracic, the lumbar, the sacral, and the coccygeal (Figure 9-2 ■). Each region is unique in its design and function and has a curve that reverses the curve of the spinal section(s) adjacent to it. The individual vertebrae of the column are identified by the first letter of their region and numbered from superior to inferior. For example, the most inferior of the seven cervical vertebrae is identified as C-7.

Cervical Spine

The cervical spine consists of seven cervical vertebrae located between the base of the skull and the shoulders. The cervical spine is the sole skeletal support for the head, which weighs about 16 to 22 pounds.

The first two cervical vertebrae have a unique relationship with the head and each other that permits rotation to left and right and nodding of the head. The first cervical vertebra, C-1, is called the atlas (after the Greek god who held up the world) and supports the head. It is securely affixed to the occiput and permits nodding but does not accommodate any twisting or turning motion. It and the next vertebra, C-2, differ from most vertebrae in not having discernable vertebral bodies. Vertebra C-2, called the axis, has a small bony tooth, called the odontoid process or dens, that projects upward. This projection provides a pivotal point around which the atlas and head can rotate from side to side.

The remaining cervical vertebrae permit some rotation as well as flexion, extension, and lateral bending. The range of motion provided by the cervical spine is greater than allowed by any other portion of the spinal column, while the portion of the spinal cord traveling through the region is most critical to life functions. The last cervical vertebra (C-7) is quite noticeable as its spinous process is pronounced and can be felt as the first bony prominence along the spine and just above the shoulders.

Thoracic Spine

The thoracic spine consists of 12 thoracic vertebrae. The first rib articulates individually with the first thoracic vertebra at two locations, with the transverse process and with the vertebral body. The next nine ribs articulate with the transverse process and

Review

Divisions of the Vertebral Column

Cervical spine
Thoracic spine
Lumbar spine
Sacral spine
Coccygeal spine

The range of motion provided by the cervical spine is the greatest allowed by any portion of the spinal column, yet the cord in this region is critical to life functions.

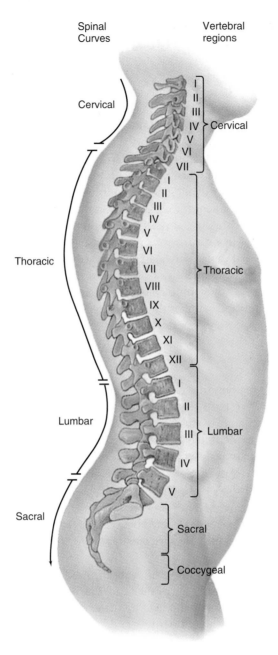

Spinal Curves

Vertebral regions

Cervical

Cervical
I
II
III
IV
V
VI
VII

Thoracic

Thoracic
I
II
III
IV
V
VI
VII
VIII
IX
X
XI
XII

Lumbar

Lumbar
I
II
III
IV
V

Sacral

Sacral

Coccygeal

the superior portion of the vertebral body as well as with the inferior portion of the vertebral body that is adjacent (superior) to it. This system of fixation limits rib movement and increases the strength and rigidity of the thoracic spine. The last two ribs articulate only with the vertebral bodies, which permits greater movement and flexibility.

Because the thoracic spine supports more of the human body than the cervical spine, the thoracic vertebral bodies are larger and stronger. The spinous and transverse processes are also larger and more prominent because they are associated with the musculature holding the upper body erect and with the movement of the thoracic cage during respiration.

Lumbar Spine

The five bones of the lumbar spine each carry the weight of the head, neck, and thorax above them. They also bear the forces of bending and lifting above the pelvis. The vertebral bodies are largest in this region of the spinal column, and the intervertebral disks are also the thickest and bear the greatest stress. The lumbar pedicles and lamina are also thick, while the transverse and spinous processes are shorter and stouter than those in the thoracic spine. The spinal foramen is largest in the lumbar region.

Sacral Spine

The sacral spine consists of five sacral vertebrae that fuse into the posterior plate of the pelvis. This plate, in conjunction with the two innominate bones of the pelvis, protects the urinary and reproductive organs and attaches the pelvis and lower extremities to the axial skeleton. The articulation with the pelvis occurs at the sacroiliac joint on the lateral surface of the sacrum. This joint is very strong and permits no movement. The upper body balances on the sacrum.

Coccygeal Spine

The coccygeal spine is made up of three to five fused vertebrae that represent the residual elements of a tail. They comprise the short skeletal end of the vertebral column.

The vertebral column curves through each region of the spine. The cervical and lumbar regions of the spine demonstrate concave curves, while the thoracic and sacral regions represent convex curves. These curves both strengthen the spine and permit a greater range of supported motion.

THE SPINAL MENINGES

The spinal meninges are similar to those covering and protecting the structures within the cranium. They consist of the dura mater, the arachnoid, and the pia mater. The meninges cover the entire spinal cord and the peripheral nerve roots as they leave the spinal column. However, the spinal meninges are not as strongly secured to the spinal column as the meninges are to the cranium. The dura mater is firmly attached to the base of the skull and to a collagen fiber called the coccygeal ligament at the top of the sacrum. These attachments and the dura mater's attachments associated with each pair of peripheral nerve roots help position the cord centrally within the spinal canal yet permit the column to move around the cord (Figure 9-3 ■).

As it does in the brain, cerebrospinal fluid bathes the spinal cord by filling the subarachnoid space. The fluid provides a medium for the exchange of nutrients and waste

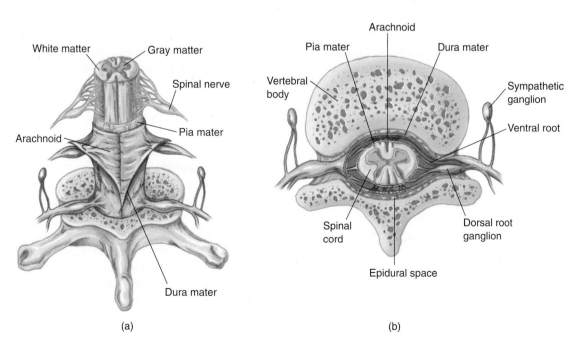

■ Figure 9-3   Structural protection of the spinal cord, including the spinal meninges.

products and absorbs the shocks of sudden movements. Cerebrospinal fluid is produced in the ventricles of the brain and then circulates through the ventricles and through the arachnoid space of the spinal meninges. The fluid is absorbed by specialized cells (the arachnoid villi) in the lower portion of the lumbar meninges, a region called the spinal cistern.

The distance between the spinal cord and the interior of the vertebral foramen varies in the different spinal regions. The region with the closest tolerance between the cord and the interior surfaces of the spinal foramen is the thoracic spine, where movement of the spinal column is most limited. Although this region is injured only infrequently, just a slight displacement into the vertebral foramen is likely to cause spinal cord injury. The greatest spacing between the cord and the interior of the vertebral column is found in upper lumbar and upper cervical (C-1 and C-2) regions.

Injuries to the mid- or lower lumbar regions do not endanger the spinal cord because the cord ends at the L-1 or L-2 level in mature adults. Injury to the lumbar spine can, however, damage the peripheral nerve roots there. The vertebral foramen below L-1 or L-2 is filled with cerebrospinal fluid and is where the fluid may be most safely removed for diagnostic testing (spinal tap).

THE SPINAL CORD

The **spinal cord** is the central nervous system (CNS) pathway responsible for transmitting sensory input from the body to the brain and for conducting motor impulses from the brain to the body muscles and organs. Through this pathway, the brain monitors and controls most body functions. Additionally, the spinal cord acts as a reflex center, intercepting sensory signals and initiating short-circuited (reflex) signaling to muscle bodies as needed. If this pathway is compromised, control of the body below the injury is lost.

In the fetus, the cord fills the entire length of the vertebral column. However, the growth of cord does not keep pace with the growth of the vertebral column. This discrepancy means that, as a person grows, the peripheral nerve roots are pulled into the spinal foramen. The sheath of the dura below L-2 is thus filled with numerous strands of peripheral nerves. The resulting structure resembles the tail of a horse and is called the cauda equina (Latin for horse's tail). In the adult, the spinal cord extends from the base of the brain (the medulla oblongata) to approximately the L-1 or L-2 level.

Like all central nervous system tissue, the spinal cord constantly needs oxygenated blood. This blood is supplied through paired spinal arteries that branch off the vertebral, cervical, thoracic, and lumbar arteries. These spinal arteries travel through intervertebral foramina, then split into anterior and posterior arteries. On the surface of the spinal cord there are numerous interconnections (anastomoses) between the arteries to provide a better chance for adequate circulation in case of vascular blockage or injury.

Anatomically, the spinal cord is a long cylinder divided into left and right halves by the **anterior medial fissure** and by the **posterior medial sulcus** (Figure 9-4 ■). In cross section, the central part of the cord has a butterfly or "H" shape and appears gray in color. This **gray matter** is made up largely of neural cell bodies and plays an important role in the reflex system.

The remaining areas, or **white matter,** then form three bundles or columns of myelinated (covered with a protein sheath) nerve fibers on each side of the cord around the gray matter: the anterior white column, the lateral white column, and the posterior white column. This white matter is composed of nerve cell pathways, called axons. It contains bundles of **axons** that transmit signals upward to the brain in what are called **ascending tracts** and bundles that transmit signals downward to the body in what are called **descending tracts.** These tracts are paired, one ascending and one descending on each side, and injury may affect either or both.

spinal cord *central nervous system pathway responsible for transmitting sensory input from the body to the brain and for conducting motor impulses from the brain to the body muscles and organs.*

anterior medial fissure *deep crease along the ventral surface of the spinal cord that divides the cord into right and left halves.*

posterior medial sulcus *shallow longitudinal groove along the dorsal surface of the spinal cord.*

gray matter *areas in the central nervous system dominated by nerve cell bodies; central portion of the spinal cord.*

white matter *material that surrounds gray matter in the spinal cord; made up largely of axons.*

axon *extension of a neuron that serves as a pathway for transmission of signals to and from the brain; major component of white matter.*

ascending tracts *bundles of axons along the spinal cord that transmit signals from the body to the brain.*

descending tracts *bundles of axons along the spinal cord that transmit signals from the brain to the body.*

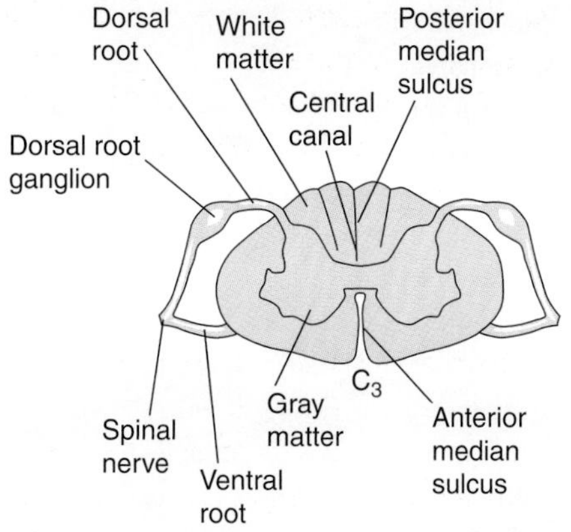

Dorsal root

White matter

Posterior median sulcus

Central canal

Dorsal root ganglion

C₃

Spinal nerve

Gray matter

Ventral root

Anterior median sulcus

■ Figure 9-4 Cross section of the spinal cord at the C₃ level.

A thorough discussion of organization and functions of the ascending and descending spinal tracts is beyond the scope of this textbook. However, knowing the functions of some motor and sensory pathways can aid you in recognizing spinal cord injury.

The important ascending (sensory) tracts or fasciculi include the fasciculus gracilis, fasciculus cutaneous, and the spinothalamic tracts. The fasciculus gracilis and fasciculus cutaneous carry sensory impulses of light touch, vibration, and positional sense from the skin, muscles, tendons, and joints to the brain. They are located on the posterior portion of the cord (posterior columns). Their injury causes disruption on the ipsilateral (same side) of the body because the left to right switching occurs at the medulla. The spinothalamic tracts include both lateral and anterior tracts. The anterior pathway conducts pain and temperature, while the lateral pathway conducts touch and pressure sensation. These pathways cross as they enter the cord; hence, injury results in contralateral (opposite side) deficits.

The important descending (motor) spinal nerve tract is the corticospinal tract. It is responsible for voluntary and fine muscle movement on the ipsilateral side of the body. This pathway lies on the posterior and lateral portions of the cord. Two other descending tracts are the reticulospinal and rubrospinal tracts. The reticulospinal tract consists of three sub-tracts, one lateral, one medial, and one anterior. It is thought to be involved with sweating and the muscular activity associated with posturing. The rubrospinal tracts are lateral pathways that affect and control fine motor function of the hands and feet. Injury affects the ipsilateral side of the body with both of these pathways.

SPINAL NERVES

Spinal nerves are the peripheral nerve roots that branch in pairs from the spinal cord (Figure 9-5 ■). They travel through the intervertebral foramina and have both sensory and motor components. They provide the largest part of the innervation of the skin, muscles, and internal organs. There are 31 pairs of spinal nerve roots. The first pair exits the spinal column between the skull and the first cervical vertebra. Each of the next seven pairs exits just below one of the cervical vertebrae and is identified as C-2 through C-8. (While there are only seven cervical vertebrae, there are eight cervical spinal nerves.) There are 12 pairs of thoracic nerves, five lumbar, five sacral, and one coccygeal. Each of these pairs originates just below the vertebra with whose name it is identified. Each spinal nerve pair has two dorsal and two ventral roots. The ventral roots carry motor impulses from the cord to the body, while the dorsal roots carry sensory impulses from the body to the cord. (C-1 and Co [coccygeal]-1 do not have dorsal [sensory] roots.)

The nerve roots often converge in a cluster of nerves called a plexus (Table 9–1). A plexus (or braiding) permits peripheral nerve roots to rejoin and function as a group. The cervical plexus, made up of the first five cervical nerve roots, innervates the neck

spinal nerves *31 pairs of nerves that originate along the spinal cord from anterior and posterior nerve roots.*

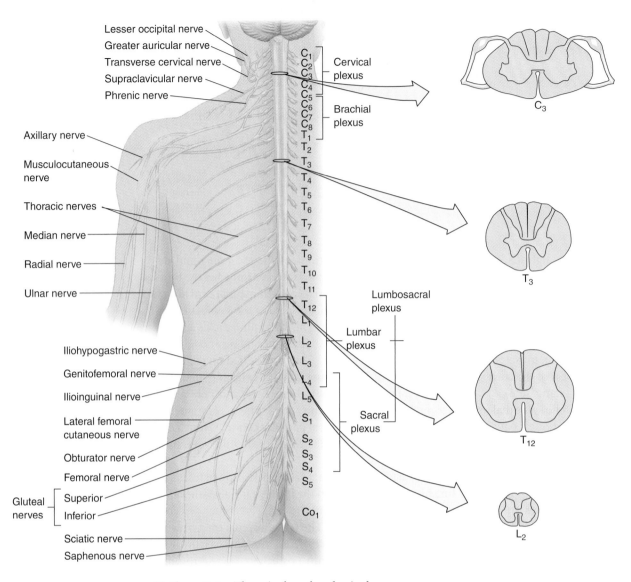

Figure 9-5   The spinal cord and spinal nerves.

Table 9–1		Spinal Nerve Plexuses		
Plexus	**Origin**	**Nerve**	**Control**	**Result of Injury**
Cervical	C-1 to C-5	phrenic	diaphragm	respiratory paralysis
Brachial	C-5 to C-8, T-1	axillary	deltoid/skin of shoulder	deltoid muscle paralysis
		radial	triceps/forearm	wrist drop
		median	flexor muscles, forearm, arm	decreased usage
		musculocutaneous	flexor muscles of arm	decreased usage
		ulnar	wrist/hand	claw hand; inability to spread fingers
Lumbar	T-12 to L-4	femoral	lower abdomen, gluteus, thighs	inability to extend leg, flex hip
		obturator	abductor muscles, medial thigh	decreased usage
Sacral	L-4 to S-3	sciatic	lower extremity	decreased usage

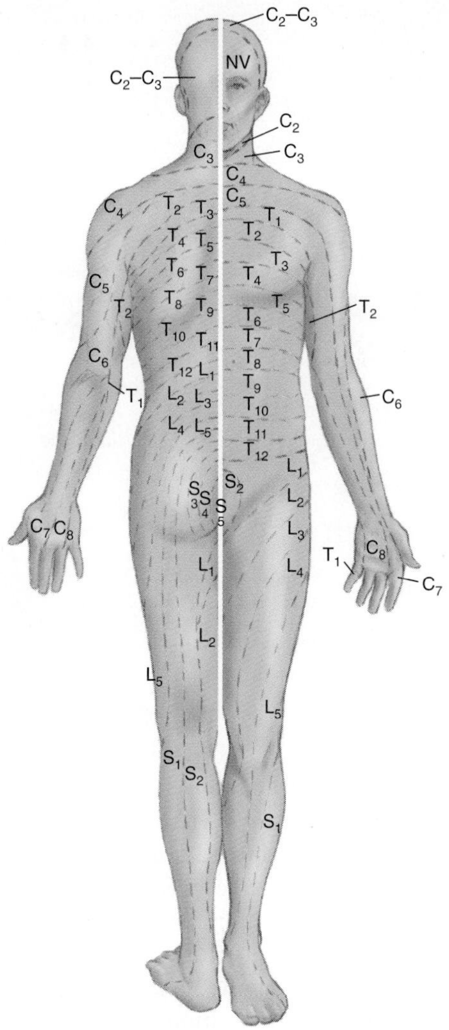

■ Figure 9-6 The dermatomes. Each dermatome corresponds to a spinal nerve.

and produces the phrenic nerve. The phrenic nerve (consisting of peripheral nerve roots C-3 through C-5) is responsible for diaphragm control. The brachial plexus joins the nerves controlling the upper extremity (C-5 through T-1). The lumbar and sacral plexuses control the innervation of the lower extremity.

The sensory components of the spinal nerves innervate specific and discrete areas of the body surface. These areas are called **dermatomes** and are distributed from the occiput of the head to the heel of the foot and buttocks (Figure 9-6 ■). Key locations to recognize for assessment include the collar region (C-3), the little finger (C-7), the nipple line (T-4), the umbilicus (T-10), and the small toe (S-1).

The motor components of the spinal nerve roots also innervate discrete tissues and muscles of the body in regions called **myotomes.** However, as the body grows and matures, some muscles merge and their control is not as specific as it is with the dermatomes. Key myotomes for neurologic evaluation include arm extension (C-5), elbow extension (C-7), small finger abduction (T-1), knee extension (L-3), and ankle flexion (S-1). Evaluation of areas controlled by both dermatomes and myotomes can help you identify the spinal cord region associated with an injury.

The spinal cord also performs some primary processing functions, speeding body responses and helping the brain maintain balance and muscle tone. These responses, called reflexes, occur as special neurons in the cord, called interneurons, intercept sensory signals (Figure 9-7 ■). For example, if you touch a hot stove, the severe pain sends

dermatome *topographical region of the body surface innervated by one nerve root.*

myotome *muscle and tissue of the body innervated by spinal nerve roots.*

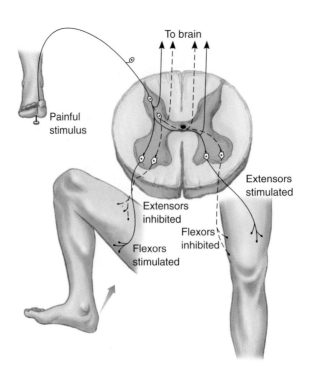

■ **Figure 9-7** The reflex response.

To brain

Painful stimulus

Extensors stimulated

Extensors inhibited

Flexors inhibited

Flexors stimulated

an intense signal to the brain. This strong signal simultaneously triggers an interneuron in the spinal cord to direct a signal to the flexor muscles telling them to contract. The limb withdraws without waiting for the signal sent to the brain to reach it, be processed, and trigger a command to be sent back to the limb. The speed of this reflex action reduces the seriousness of injury. Other reflexes help stabilize the body if it stands in one position for a length of time. As the stretch receptors report the body is moving, the interneurons signal muscles to counteract the movement to help maintain position. This again reduces the body's reaction time and allows the body to stand or maintain a steady position.

The spinal nerves can be further subdivided according to the division of the autonomic nervous system they serve and to their spinal origin. The parasympathetic nervous system controls rest and regenerative functions and consists of the peripheral nerve roots branching from the sacral region and the cranial nerves (predominantly the vagus nerve). The parasympathetic nervous system's major tasks are to slow the heart and increase digestive system activity; the system also plays a role in sexual stimulation. The sympathetic nervous system adjusts the body's metabolic rate to waking activity, provides "fight-or-flight" functions, and branches from nerves originating in the thoracic and lumbar regions. This system decreases organ and digestive activity through vasoconstriction, constricts the venous blood vessels, and affects the body's metabolic rate through the release of the adrenal hormones norepinephrine and epinephrine. In shock, the sympathetic nervous system causes systemic vasoconstriction to reduce the venous blood volume and increase peripheral vascular resistance. It also increases the heart rate to increase cardiac output in response to dropping preload and blood pressure.

PATHOPHYSIOLOGY OF SPINAL INJURY

If you understand how the events of trauma impact the spinal cord and body systems, you will be better prepared to anticipate and recognize spinal column and cord injuries. Traumatic events may cause immediate and devastating injury to the cord with no chance for the patient's recovery. Such events may also cause damage to bones or ligaments, resulting in spinal column instability and providing the potential for cord injury during patient care and transport. By understanding the mechanism of injury and the spinal problems it may produce (the pathophysiology), you can more quickly recognize and better protect the patient with spinal cord trauma.

MECHANISMS OF SPINAL INJURY

The mechanisms of injury that affect the spinal column and cord include extremes of normal motion such as flexion, extension, rotation, and lateral bending (Figure 9-8 ■). Damaging mechanisms also include stresses along the axis of the spine: axial loading and distraction. Finally, spinal injury may occur as a direct result of either blunt or penetrating trauma or as an indirect effect of trauma, when an expanding mass (edema or hematoma) compresses the cord or when a disruption in the blood supply damages it.

Extremes of Motion

Hyperextension or hyperflexion bend the spine forcibly, most commonly in the cervical or lumbar regions. A classic example of an extension injury mechanism is a rear-impact auto crash. The patient's head remains stationary while the upper torso moves rapidly and abruptly forward with the auto. The heavy head moves backwards and hyperextends the neck. The hyperextension places compressing forces on the posterior vertebral structures (the spinous processes, laminae, and pedicles) and stretching forces on the anterior vertebral ligaments. Extremes of extension may cause disk disruption, compression of the interspinous ligaments, and fracture of the posterior vertebral elements. If the forces are great enough, ligaments may tear or the vertebra may fracture, resulting in instability and bone displacement.

In frontal impact crashes, the shoulder strap may restrain the body while the head continues its forward travel. The attachment of the neck restrains the head and flexes the spine with the movement. The process is frequently forceful enough to cause a patient to literally "kiss the chest" (sometimes demonstrated by the patient's lipstick print on the shirt front). Extreme flexion may lead to wedge fractures of the anterior vertebral bodies, stretching or rupture of the posterior longitudinal and interspinous ligaments, compression injury to the cord, fracture of the pedicle(s), and disruption of the intervertebral disks with dislocation of the vertebrae.

Excessive rotation may occur both in the cervical and lumbar spine. Anatomically, the head is attached to the vertebral column at the foramen magnum, located well posterior of the midline and the head's center of mass. With lateral impact, the head turns toward the impacting force as the body moves out from under it. The cervical spine attachment restrains its motion and turns the head violently. Rotation injury normally affects the upper reaches of the cervical region, but may also be transmitted to the lumbar spine as, for example, when a tackled football player's thorax twists while his feet are firmly planted. The result is a rotational injury that may include stretching or tearing of the ligaments, rotational subluxation or dislocation, and vertebral fracture.

Lateral bending may take place along the entire vertebral column, though it is most common and likely to cause injury in the cervical and lumbar regions. As one portion of the body moves sideways and the remaining portion remains fixed, the spine absorbs the energy. The movement may compress the vertebral structures inducing compression fracture on one side of the column (toward the impact) while it tears ligaments on the opposite side. The result may be compression of the vertebral pedicles with bone fragments driven into the spinal foramen, torn ligaments, and vertebral instability. An example of this mechanism is a lateral-impact auto crash in which the forces of the crash move the thorax to the side and out from under the head, placing severe lateral

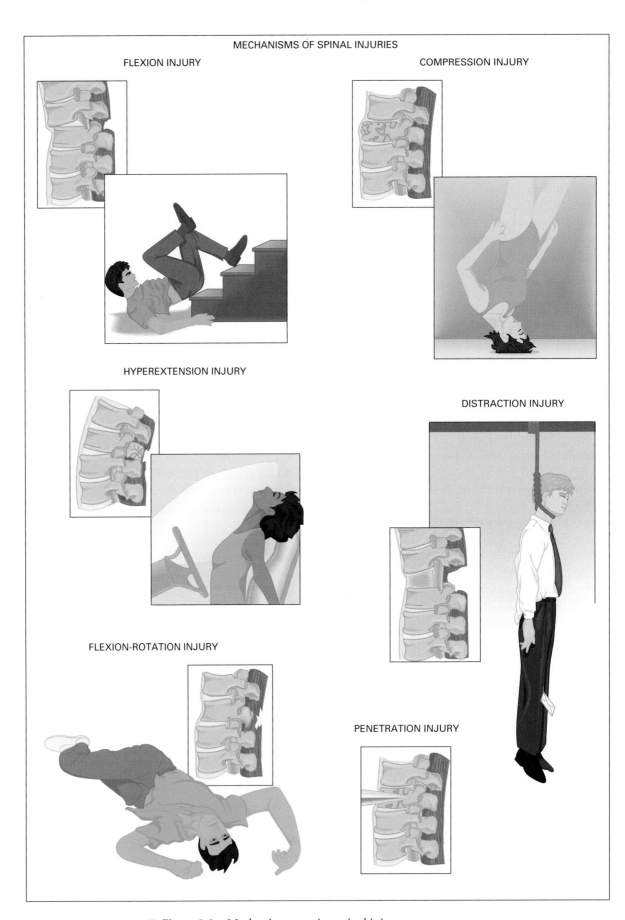

MECHANISMS OF SPINAL INJURIES

FLEXION INJURY

COMPRESSION INJURY

HYPEREXTENSION INJURY

DISTRACTION INJURY

FLEXION-ROTATION INJURY

PENETRATION INJURY

■ Figure 9-8   Mechanisms causing spinal injury.

stress on the cervical spine. Because of the structure of the spine, the forces necessary to induce injury from lateral bending are generally less than those needed to cause flexion/extension injury.

Axial Stress

Axial loading occurs as compressional stress is brought to bear along the axis of the spine. It may occur when a person lifts a weight too great for the strength of his lumbar spine or when a person falls and lands on his heels. The resulting force is transmitted up the lower extremities to the pelvis, the sacrum, and the lumbar spine. Another frequent mechanism of axial loading injury is the shallow water dive. In this case, the diver impacts the pool bottom with the head while the weight of the lower portion of the body drives the thorax into the head, crushing the cervical spine. This mechanism also occurs in auto crashes, when an occupant is propelled into the windshield by the crash forces. With these mechanisms, impact is likely to compress, fracture, and crush the vertebrae and herniate (rupture) disks, releasing their semiliquid centers into the vertebral foramina and compressing the spinal cord. The most common sites of axial loading injuries are between T-12 and L-2 (for lifting injuries and heel-first falls) and the cervical region (for head impacts).

Distraction is the opposite of axial loading. A force, such as gravity applied during hanging or at the end of a bungee jumper's travel, stretches the spinal column and tears ligaments. The process may also stretch and damage the spinal cord without causing physical damage to the spinal column. The upper cervical region is most commonly affected by this mechanism of injury.

Often the actual spinal injury process involves complicated combinations of the various injury mechanisms previously mentioned. Hanging may suspend the victim from the side of the head, causing injury from distraction and severe lateral bending directed at the C-1/C-2 region (causing a hangman's fracture). The lateral-impact auto crash may produce both lateral bending and rotational injury mechanisms affecting the cervical spine. The shallow water dive may result in both axial loading and hyperflexion as the body pushes against and bends the neck. (Note that the cervical spine is posterior to the midline of both the head and chest. In-line impacts frequently cause the head and neck to flex as the body pushes forward.)

Be aware of the distinctions among connective tissue, skeletal, and spinal cord injuries. Connective tissue and skeletal injuries do not necessarily result in spinal cord injuries. They do, however, represent potential instability of the spinal column and the danger that any subsequent motion, even normal motion, may result in spinal cord injury. Spinal cord injury can also occur without noticeable injury to the ligaments, disks, and vertebra of the spinal column. This is why, whenever a patient shows any sign of spine injury or has experienced a mechanism that suggests the possibility of spine injury, you must provide immediate manual immobilization and full mechanical immobilization as soon as possible. Maintain immobilization during all of your assessment, care, and transport.

Other Mechanisms of Injury

Other mechanisms of spine injury can involve both direct blunt and penetrating trauma. Kinetic forces may be directed at the spine when objects strike the spine posteriorly (or laterally in the neck) or when a person falls on or is thrown against an object (as in a blast). Penetrating injuries caused by objects like knives and ice picks or by missiles like blast fragments and bullets may also apply the forces of trauma directly to the spinal column. The penetrating object may harm vertebral ligaments, fracture vertebral structures, drive bone fragments directly into the spinal cord, or directly damage the cord itself. However, unlike blunt trauma, penetrating injury rarely results in ligamentous instability of the vertebral column.

Because of the structure of the spine, the forces necessary to induce injury from lateral bending are generally less than those needed to cause flexion/extension injury.

Often the spinal injury process involves a combination of mechanisms.

Connective tissue and skeletal injuries represent potential instability of the spinal column and the danger that any subsequent motion may result in spinal cord injury.

As a result of trauma, tissues adjacent to the spinal cord may swell or otherwise encroach upon the vertebral foramen. With the close tolerance between the interior surfaces of the vertebral foramen and the cord, this swelling may place pressure on the cord, producing direct compression injury and halting blood flow through the compressed tissues. Such injury may also involve the spinal nerve roots that exit the vertebral column close to the injury.

Electrocution, on rare occasions, can cause spinal injury. The extreme and uncontrolled muscular contractions associated with it can tear tendons and ligaments and fracture vertebrae, resulting in column instability and possible spinal cord injury.

A direct injury to the spinal or vertebral blood vessels or any soft-tissue or skeletal injury and the swelling associated with them may decrease the circulation to portions of the cord. This will likely result in tissue ischemia and compromise of cord function.

The coccygeal region of the spinal column can also be injured. Although it contains neither the spinal cord nor many peripheral nerve roots, injury to the region can be painful. Such injuries are usually related to direct blunt trauma, for example, "falling on one's tailbone."

RESULTS OF TRAUMA TO THE SPINAL COLUMN

Spinal injuries may damage the musculoskeletal components of the spinal column, injure the spinal cord, or both. Spinal column injury alone may damage the ligaments and skeletal elements of the column, damaging its integrity and endangering the spinal cord. Injury to the cord may endanger or destroy the ability of the central nervous system to communicate with the body distal to the injury.

Column Injury

The spine is subject to numerous types of injury. The forces of trauma or the stresses of heavy lifting may tear tendons, muscles, and ligaments, resulting in pain and a reduction in the stability of the vertebral column. Those forces may cause movement of the vertebrae from their normal position, a subluxation (partial or incomplete dislocation), or dislocation. The injury process may fracture the spinous or transverse processes, the pedicles, the laminae, or the vertebral bodies. Trauma, especially axial loading, may damage the intervertebral disks. These injuries are to the connective or skeletal tissues of the vertebral column. They may or may not be associated with injury to the spinal cord itself.

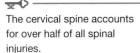

The cervical spine accounts for over half of all spinal injuries.

Several sites along the spinal column are especially subject to injury. The cervical region accounts for over half of all spinal injuries, with the atlas/axis (C-1/C-2) joint being most frequently involved. This is due to the very delicate nature of the two vertebrae, the mobility of the joint, and the great weight of the head it supports. C-7 is also injured frequently because it is located at the transition between the flexible cervical spine and the more rigid thoracic spine.

Similar injuries occur at the transition point between the thoracic and lumbar vertebrae (T-12/L-1), again due to the differences between the rigid thoracic spine and the flexible lumbar spine. The lumbosacral area (L-5/S-1) likewise is injured because the pelvis immobilizes the sacral spine. Spinal injuries not associated with the cervical spine are about equally divided between the thoracolumbar and lumbosacral regions.

Remember that the spinal cord ends at the L-1/L-2 region. Below this point, the spinal nerve roots extend until they exit the spinal column. These spinal nerve roots are more mobile than the cord and less likely to be injured within the spinal foramen during spinal column injury.

Cord Injury

The spinal cord can be injured through the mechanisms discussed earlier. Those injuries can be further described as either primary or secondary. A primary injury is one directly associated with the insult and its effects occur immediately. For example, a primary injury may be caused by cord compression, stretching, or a direct injury. A secondary injury results, as the initial injury causes swelling or ischemia, further injuring the cord tissue. It may also occur as an unstable spinal column is moved about and causes physical injury to the spinal cord. Primary and secondary injuries to the spinal cord can include concussion, contusion, compression, laceration, hemorrhage, and transection.

Concussion   Concussion of the cord, like a cerebral concussion (see Chapter 8, "Head, Facial, and Neck Trauma"), causes a temporary and transient disruption of cord function. Without associated injuries, cord concussion generally does not produce any residual deficit.

Contusion   Spinal cord contusion is simply a bruising of the cord. It is associated with some tissue damage, vascular leakage, and swelling. If blood crosses the blood–brain barrier, more significant edema may occur. But, in general, this injury is likely to repair itself with limited residual effects or none at all. The resolution of a cord contusion and its associated signs and symptoms is likely to take longer than is the case with a concussion.

Compression   Spinal cord compression may occur secondary to the displacement of a vertebra, through herniation of an intervetebral disk, from displacement of a vertebral bone fragment, or from swelling of adjacent tissue. The pressure caused by these mechanisms results in restricted circulation, ischemic damage, and possibly physical damage to the cord.

Laceration   Cord laceration can occur as bony fragments are driven into the vertebral foramen or the cord is stretched to the point of tearing. Laceration is likely to result in hemorrhage into the cord tissue, swelling due to the injury, and disruption of some portions of the cord and their associated communication pathways. In very minor lacerations, some recovery may be expected. Severe lacerations usually result in permanent neurologic deficit.

Hemorrhage   Spinal cord hemorrhage, often associated with a contusion, laceration, or stretching injury, produces injury by disruption of the blood flow, application of pressure from accumulating blood, and irritation by blood passing across the blood–brain barrier. Some of the arteries supplying the cord may affect circulation distant from the injury and result in ischemic injury above the level of physical injury.

Transection   A cord **transection** is an injury that partially or completely severs the spinal cord. In a complete transection, the cord is totally cut and the potential to send and receive nerve impulses below the site of injury is lost. With transection injuries below the beginning of the thoracic spine, the results include incontinence and paraplegia, while injuries to the cervical spine cause quadriplegia, incontinence, and partial or complete respiratory paralysis.

Incomplete cord transection involves only a portion of the cord, and some spinal tracts remain intact. There is potential for some recovery of function. There are three particular types of incomplete spinal cord transection: anterior cord syndrome, central cord syndrome, and Brown-Séquard syndrome.

Anterior cord syndrome is caused by bony fragments or pressure compressing the arteries that perfuse the anterior cord. The cord is damaged by vascular disruption and its potential for recovery is poor. The injury generally involves loss of motor function and of sensation to pain, light touch, and temperature below the injury site. The patient is likely to retain motion, positional, and vibration sensation.

 Review

Types of Primary and Secondary Spinal Cord Injuries

Concussion
Contusion
Compression
Laceration
Hemorrhage
Transection

 Review

Signs and Symptoms of Spinal Injury

Paralysis of the extremities
Pain with and without movement
Tenderness along the spine
Impaired breathing
Spinal deformity
Priapism
Posturing
Loss of bowel or bladder control
Nerve impairment to extremities

transection   *a cutting across a long axis; a cross-sectional cut.*

anterior cord syndrome   *condition that is caused by bony fragments or pressure compressing the arteries of the anterior spinal cord and resulting in loss of motor function and sensation to pain, light touch, and temperature below the injury site.*

central cord syndrome
condition usually related to hyperflexion of the cervical spine that results in motor weakness, usually in the upper extremities and possible bladder dysfunction.

Brown-Séquard syndrome
condition caused by partial cutting of one side of the spinal cord resulting in sensory and motor loss to that side of the body.

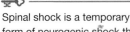

Spinal shock is a temporary form of neurogenic shock that presents with hypotension, bradycardia, and the signs and symptoms of cord injury.

autonomic hyperreflexia syndrome *condition associated with the body's adjustment to the effects of neurogenic shock; presentations include sudden hypertension, bradycardia, pounding headache, blurred vision, and sweating and flushing of the skin above the point of injury.*

Central cord syndrome is usually related to hyperextension of the cervical spine, as might occur with a forward fall and facial impact. It is often associated with a preexisting degenerative disease, such as arthritis, that has narrowed the vertebral canal. This syndrome results in motor weakness, more likely affecting the upper rather than the lower extremities, and possible bladder dysfunction. Of the three syndromes, central cord syndrome has the best prognosis for recovery.

Brown-Séquard syndrome is usually caused by a penetrating injury that affects one side of the cord (hemitransection). The damage to one side results in sensory and motor loss to that side (ipsilateral) of the body. Pain and temperature perception are lost on the opposite (contralateral) side of the body because of the switching of the associated nerves that occurs as they enter the spinal cord. This injury is rare and is usually associated with some recovery, except in cases of direct penetrating trauma.

Spinal Shock

Spinal shock is a temporary insult to the cord that affects the body below the level of injury. The affected area becomes flaccid and without feeling, and the patient is unable to move the extremities or other musculature (flaccid paralysis). There is frequently a loss of bowel and bladder control and, in the male, priapism (a prolonged, nonsexual penile erection). Body temperature control is affected, and hypotension is often present due to vasodilation. Spinal shock is often a transient problem if the cord is not seriously damaged.

Neurogenic Shock

Neurogenic (or spinal-vascular) shock results when injury to the spinal cord disrupts the brain's ability to exercise control over the body. The interruption of signals limits vasoconstriction, most noticeably in the skin below the level of injury. Lack of sympathetic tone permits the arteries and veins to dilate, expanding the vascular space, resulting in a relative hypovolemia. With the reduced cardiac preload, the atria fail to fill adequately, and their contraction does not stretch the walls of the ventricles. This reduces the strength of contraction (Frank-Starling reflex) and cardiac output. The problem is further compounded as the autonomic nervous system loses its sympathetic control over the adrenal medulla. It can then no longer control the release of epinephrine and norepinephrine. These hormones are responsible for increasing the heart rate against direct parasympathetic stimulation. Their absence restricts the increase in heart rate that normally follows reduced cardiac preload and falling blood pressure. The result of all these factors is a patient in relative hypovolemia. In addition, it is difficult for the patient to maintain blood pressure with a reduced cardiac output when the body is unable to increase peripheral vascular resistance through vasoconstriction. The patient in neurogenic shock is thus likely to present with a slow heart rate, low blood pressure, and shocklike symptoms (cool, moist, and pale skin) above the cord injury, and warm, dry, and flushed skin below the injury, as well as with priapism in the male.

Autonomic Hyperreflexia Syndrome

Autonomic hyperreflexia syndrome is associated with the body's resolution of the effects of neurogenic shock. It occurs in patients well after the initial spinal injury as the body begins to adapt to the problems associated with loss of neurologic control below the injury. After a time, the vascular system adjusts to the lack of sympathetic stimulation and the blood pressure moves toward normal. However, the body now does not respond to increases in blood pressure with vasodilation below the cord injury so only bradycardia results. Autonomic hyperreflexia syndrome is most commonly associated with injuries at or above T-6. The syndrome presents with sudden hypertension, as high as 300 mmHg, bradycardia, pounding headache, blurred vision, and sweating and flushing of the skin above the point of injury. Nasal congestion, nausea, and bladder and rectum distention are also frequently present in autonomic hyperreflexia syndrome.

Other Causes of Neurologic Dysfunction

Not all injuries that result in neurologic dysfunction affecting a dermatome or myotome are related to spinal cord injuries. An injury may occur anywhere along a nerve impulse's path of travel. For example, the C-7 nerve root travels from just below the seventh cervical vertebra through the shoulder, arm, and forearm before innervating the little finger. It may be injured by a vertebral fracture; soft-tissue injury and swelling; a shoulder, arm, or forearm fracture; penetrating trauma; or compartment syndrome.

Any of the injuries previously described will interrupt sensory impulses to the brain from the little finger region and motor signals to the region from the brain (to initiate movement and maintain muscle tone). The most obvious difference between nerve root injury and spinal cord injury is the size of the region affected. Remember, however, that an injury that is currently affecting only a single dermatome may have created a vertebral column instability that threatens the entire cord.

There are also several nontraumatic processes that affect the spinal cord. Refer to Volume 3, Chapter 3, of this series for further information on them.

The obvious difference between nerve root and spinal cord injury is that in the former a single dermatome is affected while in the latter multiple dermatomes are affected.

ASSESSMENT OF THE SPINAL INJURY PATIENT

Assessment and care for the patient with a potential spinal injury begins with special emphasis on the analysis of the mechanism of injury. During this analysis, consciously try to identify or rule out the likelihood of spinal injury. This is important because the patient who has suffered serious trauma may have other injuries that are much more painful and more obvious and that may distract you and the patient from the less obvious signs and symptoms of spinal injury. Also, a seriously injured trauma patient may have a reduced level of consciousness due to intoxication or to other processes such as shock or head injury and thus be an unreliable reporter of the symptoms of spinal injury. *For these reasons, you should consider the mechanism of injury to be the most critical indicator of spinal injury.*

Put special emphasis on your analysis of the mechanism of injury with a potential spinal injury patient.

SCENE SIZE-UP

Analyze the mechanism of injury very carefully to identify what forces were transmitted to the patient and from which direction they came (Figure 9-9 ■). Identify the likely movements of the spine during the crash or impact and determine if severe flexion, extension, lateral bending, rotation, axial loading, or distraction was likely. Also, assure that direct forces of blunt or penetrating trauma did not involve the spine. Be especially concerned about high-speed motor vehicle crashes (including motorcycles, ejections, and pedestrian collisions), any fall (especially in the elderly), any diving or shallow water injury, any serious blunt injuries above the shoulders, and any penetrating wounds close to or directed toward the spine. Also maintain a high level of suspicion regarding athletic injuries, in which blunt and twisting forces are often transmitted to the spine. If there is any reason to suspect spinal injury, be prepared to employ immediate cervical immobilization as you begin the initial assessment.

Examine the scene to determine whether the patient used a helmet or other protective gear. Remember that helmets reduce the likelihood of head injury but neither increase nor decrease the likelihood of neck injury. Whenever a patient wearing a helmet sustains moderate or severe head impact, suspect spine injury and employ spinal

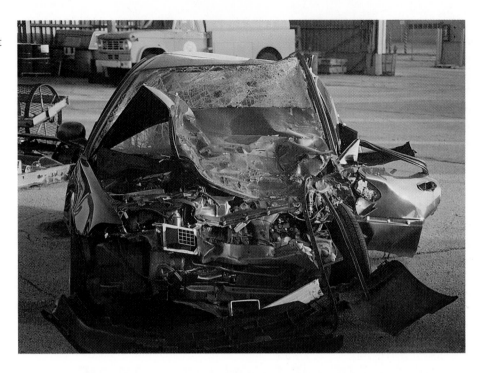

■ Figure 9-9   Often the mechanism of injury will suggest the potential for spinal column injury.

If you are unclear about the mechanism of injury or the potential for spinal involvement, always err on the side of overprotecting the patient.

If you are unclear about the mechanism of injury or the potential for spinal involvement, always err on the side of overprotecting the patient.

Provide any patient sustaining a serious injury with immediate manual spinal immobilization, followed by full mechanical immobilization from your first moments at his side until arrival at the emergency department.

precautions. Bring the helmet to the emergency department with the patient or relate the damages it displayed to the emergency department physician. Also keep in mind that while seat belt use prevents some injuries, it does not preclude spinal injury.

Even if the incident does not appear to involve a significant mechanism of injury or forces directed at the spine, look for and assure that there are no signs or symptoms of spinal injury during your early assessment. If you are unclear about the mechanism of injury or the potential for spinal involvement, always err on the side of protecting the patient. Full spinal precautions cause some patient discomfort and extend your time at the scene, but failure to provide needed immobilization may result in an unnecessary, devastating, and lifelong patient disability or even in death. Generally, a patient sustaining any serious injury receives immediate manual spinal immobilization, thereafter maintained by mechanical immobilization, from your first moments at his side until arrival at the emergency department.

Recent research is demonstrating that we can reliably identify patients who are likely to have spinal injury. The decision to continue spinal precautions is predicated on an evaluation of the injury mechanism and of patient signs or symptoms of injury. If the patient has a mechanism of injury suggestive of spinal injury you will employ spinal precautions until you can determine that the patient is a reliable reporter of injury symptoms, that there are no distracting injuries, and that there are no signs and symptoms of spinal injury. If you cannot rule out spinal injury, you will provide the patient with full spinal precautions: in-line manual immobilization of the head and spine until the patient is fully immobilized to the long spine board or full-body vacuum mattress.

INITIAL ASSESSMENT

As you approach the patient and begin your initial assessment, first manually immobilize the head and neck of the patient who has a mechanism of injury likely to cause spinal injury and then determine the patient's mental status. Initial spinal precautions are required to assure any spinal injury is not compounded during assessment and care. If the likelihood of spinal injury can be excluded (after the rapid trauma assessment), you may release immobilization of the head—as permitted by your local protocols.

The mental status evaluation is essential in determining the patient's reliability to report symptoms of spinal injury and your ability to rule out the need for spinal precautions. Assure that the patient is fully conscious, alert, and oriented. If the potential spinal injury patient is found to be intoxicated by drugs or alcohol, to have an altered level of consciousness (Glascow Coma Scale of less than 15), or seems to be significantly affected by the "fight-or-flight" response, employ full and continuing spinal precautions. You will also employ full and continuing spinal precautions whenever the patient is distracted by a serious injury, such as an open wound, or a symptom, such as dyspnea.

When evaluating a patient for possible spinal injury and the need for spinal precautions, also take into account the patient's age. The elderly often have a reduced sensitivity to pain and may not report an injury or claim it as significant. The elderly are also more likely to have sustained injury with a less significant mechanism of injury. Young children may not be able to localize or accurately report their symptoms. Therefore, whenever presented with an elderly or a very young patient with a mechanism of injury suggestive of spinal injury, be suspicious of injury and provide spinal precautions unless you can confidently rule out spinal injury.

Firmly apply manual immobilization to hold the patient's head in the neutral, in-line position before proceeding with the remaining assessment and care. (Prehospital medicine currently uses terms such as *immobilization*, *stabilization*, and *spinal motion restriction [SMR])* to describe the objective of care techniques used for the spinal injury patient. To limit confusion, we use the term *immobilization* throughout this text. With

Legal Notes

Spinal Motion Restriction (SMR): What's in a Phrase? What does a phrase really mean? As we continue developing the Emergency Medical Services System into the twenty-first century we are destined to discover new and better terminology to describe what we do. In this quest we must be careful to accept only those phrases that are specific and that accurately describe the objectives of our care. In trauma, we use phrases that describe the care objectives for the patient with a suspected spinal injury. Currently these phrases include *spinal stabilization*, *spinal immobilization*, and now *spinal motion restriction (SMR)*.

Stabilize is a word commonly used to describe protecting the spinal cord from possible injury (or further injury) when vertebral column integrity is disrupted. (Webster: *stabilize*—to make stable or firm, keep from changing or fluctuating.) Some suggest we cannot truly achieve stabilization of the spinal column.

Immobilize refers to the "splinting" of the head, neck, and torso to limit any transmission of motion to the spine. (Webster: *immobilize*—to make immobile, keep in place, or keep from moving.) Immobilizing the spine, too, may be difficult to fully achieve.

Spinal motion restriction (SMR) is now suggested as a more accurate description of modern spinal injury care. However, this phrase could be misunderstood to indicate a more limited (Webster: *restriction*—being limited or confined) "immobilization" of the spine than is currently practiced. *The application of a cervical collar alone, for example, does restrict the motion of the cervical spine*—so collar application alone could be considered to fulfill the objective of "spinal motion restriction."

If we use this new phrase, therefore, it must be with the understanding that spinal motion restriction (SMR) calls for a *complete* motion restriction of the spine—to include manual stabilization of the head and neck, application of a cervical collar, intermediate immobilization to a vest-type device (if necessary), and full mechanical immobilization to a long spine board or full-body vacuum splint or vacuum mattress.

time, however, *spinal motion restriction*, or a similar term or phrase, may become the standard used to describe the optimal handling of the spinal injury patient. When that becomes evident, we will adopt that term or phrase in subsequent editions. Manual immobilization should continue from the moment you arrive at the patient's side and suspect spinal injury until the patient receives full mechanical immobilization to a long spine board with a cervical immobilization device or vest-type immobilization device, or is immobilized in a full-body vacuum mattress, or until you can determine that spinal precautions are no longer indicated. It is best if the caregiver responsible for the overall assessment and care of the patient does not hold the manual immobilization. A well-trained EMT-Basic or First Responder may best provide this manual immobilization.

Neutral, in-line positioning is very important in the care of a spinal injury patient because it maintains the best orientation of the spinal column and the greatest clearance between the cord and the interior of the spinal foramen. This positioning permits the best circulation and thus lessens the impact of local injury and edema. As your assessment progresses, gently and smoothly move any body segment that is out of alignment toward alignment as you examine it. If the patient feels any increase in pain or if you feel resistance to movement, immobilize the head and neck or other portion of the body in the position achieved. Do not continue movement, as doing so may compromise the spinal cord. Maintain the patient's head and body position using manual immobilization until you can secure the position with full mechanical immobilization using the spine board, firm padding, and a cervical immobilization device or full-body vacuum mattress.

Once you assess the neck, consider applying a cervical collar. While the collar does not prevent flexion/extension, rotation, or lateral bending, it does limit cervical motion. However, manual immobilization of the head and neck is adequate until time and patient priorities permit you to apply the collar. Manual immobilization must continue even after a cervical collar has been applied until full mechanical immobilization is achieved.

As you move on to assess the airway, be sure that the patient's head remains in the neutral, in-line position. The airway is more difficult to control when you are required to observe spinal precautions. Be ready to carefully log roll the patient if he vomits or if necessary to drain the upper airway of fluids. Have adequate suction ready and anticipate the possible need to clear the airway during transport, should vomiting occur. To prepare for this, secure the patient firmly to a spine board and immobilize him well enough to permit 90-degree rotation of the board.

If advanced airway procedures are indicated, consider either orotracheal intubation with spinal precautions or digital intubation. Have the patient's head held firmly in the neutral, in-line position as you attempt to identify airway features and insert the endotracheal tube. Anticipate that landmarks will be hard to visualize because the head cannot be brought into the sniffing position and the upper airway aligned. During the procedure, be careful not to displace the jaw anteriorly beyond the point at which it begins to lift the neck (extension) or to permit any rotation of the head. Digital intubation has the benefit of not requiring any displacement of the head and neck, although it requires a completely unconscious patient and takes a provider skilled in the procedure and who has long fingers to direct the tube properly.

After using any modified or blind intubation technique like those just described, be very careful to assure proper tube placement by assessing for the presence of good chest excursion and bilaterally equal breath sounds and the absence of epigastric sounds with ventilation. Check the depth of tube placement by noting the number on the side of the tube and secure the tube firmly. Monitor both the tube's depth and the breath sounds frequently during your care and transport. Using the pulse oximeter or capnography are essential to assure proper tube placement and effective oxygenation.

Quickly evaluate your patient's respiratory effort. In the potential spinal injury patient, watch the motion of the chest and abdomen carefully. They should rise and fall together. Exaggerated movement of the abdomen and limited chest excursion with mo-

Manual immobilization must continue even after a cervical collar has been applied and until it is maintained with mechanical immobilization.

tion opposite to that of the abdomen suggest diaphragmatic breathing. For such a patient, immediately provide positive-pressure ventilation coordinated with the patient's respiratory effort (overdrive ventilation) while maintaining spinal precautions. Your assistance will make breathing more effective and less energy consuming. Use pulse oximetry to continuously evaluate the effectiveness of respirations.

During your check of the patient's circulation status, monitor the pulse carefully. Be very watchful of patients with bradycardia, especially when it is likely that they may be experiencing hypovolemia and shock. This bradycardia may be relative—for example, if a patient has a normal heart rate in the presence of low blood pressure and hypovolemia when a tachycardia might be expected. As you scan the body for other signs of vascular injury or shock, watch for warm and dry skin in the lower extremities while the upper portions of the body show the cool, clammy skin associated with hypovolemic compensation. This is an indication of neurogenic injury and possible shock secondary to spinal cord damage. Spinal cord injury may also induce paralysis and anesthesia below the lesion, reducing the pain or other symptoms of blood loss into an abdominal or extremity injury.

> Be very watchful for patients with bradycardia, especially when it is likely that they may be experiencing hypovolemia and shock.

RAPID TRAUMA ASSESSMENT

Once the initial assessment is complete, determine the need for the rapid trauma assessment or the focused physical exam and history. For patients with suspected or likely spinal column or cord injury, move directly to the rapid trauma assessment (Figure 9-10 ■). Even if such patients are otherwise stable, consider rapid trauma assessment, expeditious

SIGNS OF SYMPTOMS OF POSSIBLE SPINAL INJURY

- PAIN   Unprovoked pain in area of injury, along spine, in lower legs.

- TENDERNESS   Gentle touch of area may increase pain.

- DEFORMITY (rare)   There may be abnormal bend or bony prominence.

- SOFT TISSUE INJURY   Injury to the head, neck, or face may indicate cervical spine injury. Injury to shoulders, back, and abdomen may indicate thoracic or lumbar spine injury. Injury to extremities may indicate lumbar or sacral spine injury.

- PARALYSIS   Inability to move or inability to feel sensation in some part of body may indicate spinal fracture with cord injury.

- PAINFUL MOVEMENT   Movement may cause or increase pain. Never try to move the injured area.

- ALSO: Loss of bowel or bladder control, priapism, impaired breathing.

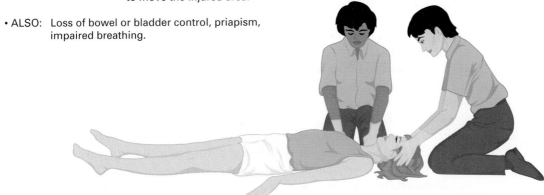

■ Figure 9-10   Provide immediate and continuing manual immobilization of the patient with possible spine injury while assessing for additional signs and symptoms.

employment of spinal precautions, and immediate transport to the trauma center. These patients are likely to deteriorate and to need neurologic intervention.

During the rapid trauma assessment, palpate the entire posterior spine. Feel for any deformity, pain, crepitus, unusual warmth, or tenderness from C-1 through L-5. It may be beneficial to repeat palpation of the spine from L-5 to C-1 as pain or tenderness may be difficult to identify in the presence of other painful injuries when minor tenderness may be the only symptom of significant vertebral column instability.

Continue your exam, inspecting each distal extremity and evaluating both motor and sensory function. If there is any limb injury, perform what spinal assessment you can while working around the injuries and assuring that you do not cause further harm to the limb.

For each upper extremity, test finger abduction/adduction (T-1) by having the patient spread the fingers of the hand while you squeeze the second, third, and fourth fingers together. You should meet with bilaterally equal and moderate resistance to your effort. Test finger or hand extension (C-7) by having the patient hold the fingers and/or wrists fully extended. Place pressure against the back of the fingers while you hold the forearm immobile. Again, you should meet bilaterally equal and moderate resistance. Finally, have the patient squeeze your first two fingers in his hand and assure that the grip is firm and bilaterally equal (Figure 9-11 ■).

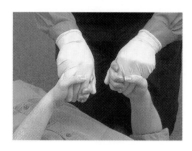

■ Figure 9-11 Compare grip strength bilaterally.

To assess for limb sensation, first ask about any abnormal feelings in the limb—inability to move (paralysis), weakness, numbness (anesthesia), tingling (paresthesia), or pain. Have the patient close both eyes and check the ability to distinguish between sensations of pain and light touch. To check pain reception (the spinothalamic tract), use the retracted tip of a ballpoint pen or another pointed object not likely to cause injury to induce slight point pain. To check for light touch (involving several tracts), use a cotton swab or a gentle touch with the pad of a finger. Responses to both pain and touch stimulation should be bilateral and equal.

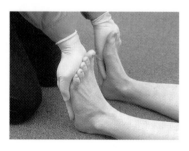

■ Figure 9-12 Compare lower limb strength bilaterally.

Also test motor and sensory function for the lower extremities (Figure 9-12 ■). Place your hand against the ball of the patient's foot and have him push firmly against it (plantar flexion, S-1 and S-2). Then place your hand on top of the toes and have the patient pull the toes and foot upwards (dorsiflexion, L-5). To evaluate pain sensation, use the same techniques you used in testing the upper extremities. Lower limb strength and sensations should be present and bilaterally equal.

During the full body exam, look for any line of demarcation between normal sensation and paresthesia or anesthesia and any differences in muscle tone. Begin the exam with the feet, and work up the body toward the head. Try not to alarm the patient because if he recognizes that your touch is not felt, his anxiety may increase. Use a sharp object not likely to cause injury and move upward. Note the level at which the patient first identifies sensation or pain and relate it to the dermatomes. You might mark the level at which sensation is first noticed on the patient with a felt-tipped pen so that you can compare the results of later tests with your initial results.

Also evaluate the myotomes to determine the level of muscular control. Suspect muscle flaccidity if a body area has muscle masses with a more relaxed tone than the rest of the body. These neurologic signs give you a good indication of the level of spinal cord disruption. Examine both sides of the body as there may be differences from side to side both in sensation and in levels of voluntary and involuntary (muscle tone) motor activity.

You may also perform a test for Babinski's sign (Figure 9-13 ■). Stroke the lateral aspect of the bottom of the foot and watch for the movement of the toes and great toe. Fanning of the toes and dorsiflexion (lifting) of the great toe is a positive sign and suggests injury along the pyramidal (descending spinal) tracts.

If discrete areas of nervous deficit exist, relate them to an injury along the nerve pathway or suspect injury to the spinal nerve root as it emerges from the spinal column. A nerve root injury suggests the possibility of a vertebral column injury and the need for spinal immobilization. Also consider that the source of a deficit may be peripheral

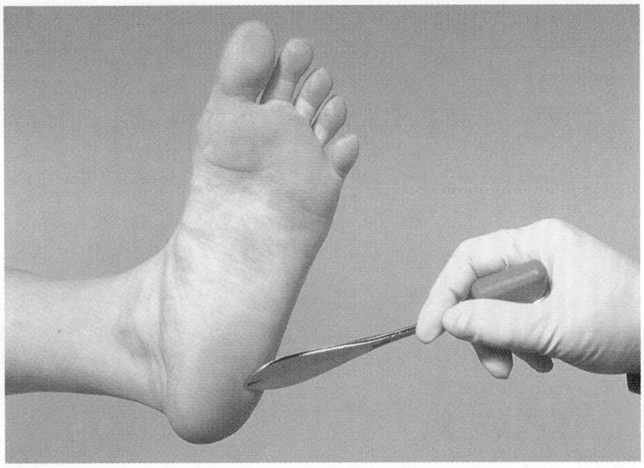

Figure 9-13 Test for Babinski's sign.

nerve damage related to soft-tissue or skeletal damage along its pathway to the affected area. Again, try to identify the associated dermatome and myotome and, thus, the likely location of the lesion along the spinal column, spinal root, or peripheral nerve.

Another sign of spinal injury is priapism. This prolonged, possibly painful erection of the male genitalia is due to unopposed parasympathetic stimulation. Disruption of the sympathetic (thoracolumbar) pathways during a cervical spinal injury can produce this sign. In many cases, the pain sensation is lost due to disruption of the sensory pathways to the brain.

Occasionally, the patient with midcervical spine injury presents with the "hold-up" position. Left on his own, the patient's arms rise to a position above the shoulders and head. This occurs because the injury paralyzes the adductor and extensor muscles while the patient maintains control over the abductors and flexors. Without the opposition of the adductors and extensors, normal muscle tone impulses or any attempt by the patient to move the limb cause it to move toward the flexed position. With such cases, simply secure the patient's wrists to his belt to hold the limbs down for transport.

If the patient is a reliable reporter of injury and does not show any signs or symptoms of spinal injury or the mechanism of injury does not suggest spinal injury, ask the patient to gently move his neck. If the patient experiences any pain or discomfort or shows any neurologic deficit, employ spinal precautions and consider transport to a neurocenter for further evaluation. Also continue to examine the extremities for signs of neurologic impairment. If any are found, immediately employ spinal precautions.

As permitted by your local protocols (Figure 9-14 ■), you may discontinue spinal precautions if all of the following three criteria are met:

★ The patient is alert and fully oriented; is not intoxicated or under the influence of drugs, including alcohol; has a Glasgow Coma Scale of 15; and is not significantly affected by the "fight-or-flight" response.

★ The patient is free of significant distracting injuries or symptoms such as a fracture, joint injury, abdominal pain, or dyspnea.

★ The patient is free of any signs or symptoms of spinal injury.

If you have any doubt about the patient's potential for spinal injury or his ability to accurately report the symptoms of such an injury, continue spinal precautions including full immobilization to the long spine board or full-body vacuum mattress.

Vital Signs

Evaluate the vital signs carefully in the patient with suspected spinal injury. Any signs of abnormally low blood pressure, slow heart rate, or absent, diaphragmatic, or shallow respirations indicate possible spinal cord injury.

Any signs of abnormally low blood pressure, slow heart rate, or absent, diaphragmatic, or shallow respirations suggest possible spinal cord injury.

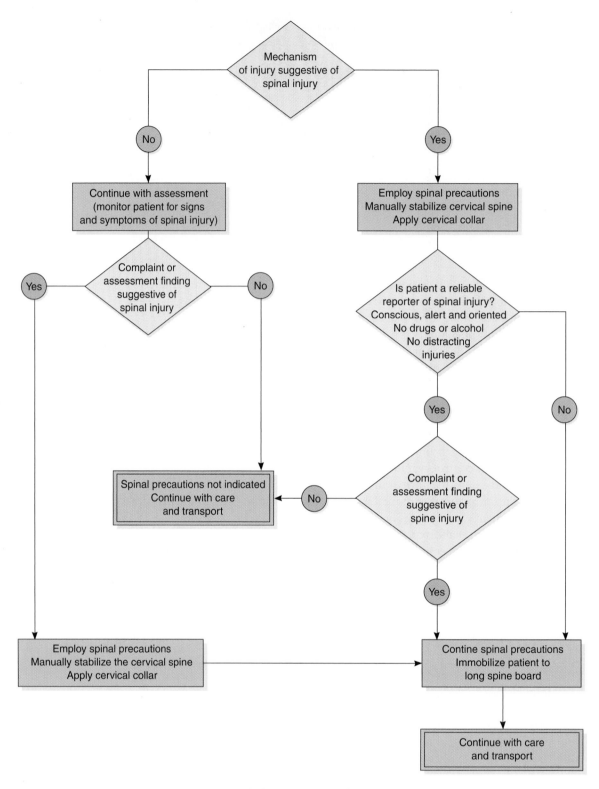

Figure 9-14   A spinal clearance protocol.

Body temperature is an important consideration when evaluating the potential spinal injury patient. Spinal injury patients are subject to fluctuations in body temperature related to ambient temperature changes. This is because those patients lose the ability to control the skin's heat conservation/dissipation function below the lesion. While this does not result in an obvious sign in the patient, that patient is highly susceptible to body temperature fluctuations. Cover the patient with blankets in all but the warmest environments and monitor the patient's temperature carefully.

At the conclusion of the rapid trauma assessment, consider the patient with any sign, symptom, or mechanism of injury suggestive of vertebral column or spinal cord injury, not otherwise excluded, for rapid transport to a nearby neurocenter or trauma center. Employ full spinal precautions, monitor for neurogenic shock, and perform frequent ongoing patient assessments.

ONGOING ASSESSMENT

During the ongoing assessment, repeat the elements of the initial assessment, take vital signs, and reevaluate any signs or symptoms of spinal cord injury every 5 minutes (Figure 9-15 ▪). Monitor carefully for any changes in neurologic signs, including the levels of orientation, responsiveness, sensation, and motor function. Observe also for any changes in the dermatomes and myotomes affected by the injury. Look for any improvement or deterioration. Watch for a slowing pulse rate or a constant pulse rate in the presence of falling blood pressure. Watch for a dropping blood pressure without

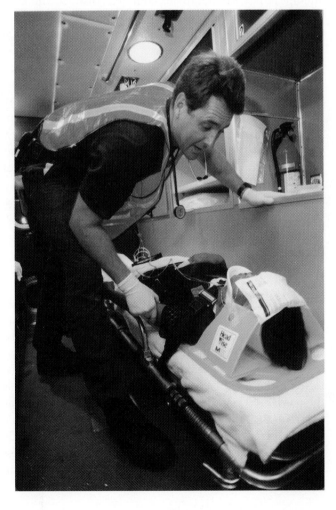

▪ Figure 9-15   Repeat the ongoing assessment every 5 minutes with seriously injured patients. (© *Craig Jackson/In the Dark Photography*)

signs of shock compensation. Remember that spinal column injury may not produce any overt associated neurologic signs or symptoms yet may still threaten the spinal cord if the patient is moved without proper precautions.

For the patient with a possible spinal injury mechanism but who has not received continuing spinal precautions, periodically question the patient about pain along the spinal column and other symptoms of spinal injury. Also perform frequent sensory and motor evaluations of the distal extremities to assure the evidence of spinal injury does not develop. If it does, employ full spinal precautions.

MANAGEMENT OF THE SPINAL INJURY PATIENT

Spinal injury care steps (spinal precautions) performed during the initial assessment include moving the patient to the neutral, in-line position, maintaining that position with manual immobilization until the patient is fully immobilized by mechanical means, and applying the cervical collar once the neck assessment is complete. The remaining steps in management of the spinal injury patient are related to maintaining the neutral, in-line position while moving the patient to the long spine board and then firmly securing him to the board for transport to the hospital.

These skills have but one major objective: maintaining the neutral, in-line position. Although this might seem a simple objective, it is not. Remember that the spine is a chain of 33 small, rather delicate bones, which is attached to other skeletal members only at the head, thorax, and pelvis. These skeletal attachments may transmit forces that attempt to flex, extend, rotate, compress, distract, and laterally bend the spine during any patient movement. The procedures and devices discussed in the following text are intended to assure that the patient remains in the neutral, in-line position throughout care, movement, and transport.

Constantly calm and reassure the patient with suspected spinal injury. Spinal injury can produce extreme anxiety in patients because of the severity of its effects and their potentially lifelong implications. The application of spinal precautions can compound this anxiety. The patient must endure complete immobilization on a rigid and relatively uncomfortable device, the long spine board. He will be unable to move and protect himself during the processes of immobilization, assessment, care, and transport to the hospital. To alleviate some of the anxiety, be sure to communicate frequently with the patient. Tell the patient why you are employing spinal precautions and explain, in advance, what you will be doing in each step of the process. Do what you can to make the patient comfortable and to provide assurance that you and your team are caring for his needs.

SPINAL ALIGNMENT

The first step of the spinal precautions process is to bring the patient from the position in which he is found into a neutral, in-line position adequate for assessment, airway maintenance, and spinal immobilization. This process involves moving the patient to the supine position with the head facing directly forward and elevated 1 to 2 inches above the ground. Remember that the spine curves in an "S" shape through its length. This leaves the head displaced forward when the posterior thorax and buttocks (supporting the pelvis) rest on a firm, flat surface. Also remember that the neutral position (also known as the position of function) is generally with the joints halfway between the extremes of their motion. In spinal positioning, this means the hips and knees should be somewhat flexed for maximum comfort and minimum stress on the muscles, joints, and spine. For complete spinal immobilization, consider placement of a rolled blanket under the knees.

Spinal precautions have one major objective: maintaining the patient in a neutral, in-line position.

It is also important to assure there are no distracting or compressing forces on the spine. If the patient is seated or standing, support the head to leave only a portion of the head's weight on the spine. Be careful not to lift the entire head as this places a distracting force on the spine. Lastly, bring the spine into line by aligning the nose, navel, and toes to assure that there is no rotation along the spine's length. The head must face directly forward and the shoulders and pelvis must be in a single plane with the body. This neutral, in-line positioning allows for the greatest spacing between the cord and inner lumen of the spinal foramen. Neutral, in-line positioning both reduces pressure on the cord and increases circulation to and through it, an especially important consideration in the presence of injury. There are many techniques for moving and immobilizing the potential spine injury patient; whichever you employ, always focus on obtaining and then maintaining neutral, in-line positioning. Doing this assures you the best opportunity to protect the vertebral column and the spinal cord of the patient during your time at his side.

The only contraindications to moving the potential spine injury patient from the position in which he is found to the neutral, in-line position are as follows: when movement causes a noticeable increase in pain; when you meet with noticeable resistance during the procedure; when you identify an increase in neurologic signs as you move the head; or when the patient's spine is grossly deformed. Pain and resistance both suggest that the alignment process may be moving the injury site and thus may be causing further injury. When you meet with resistance or increased pain during any positioning of the head or spine, immobilize the patient as he lies. The same rule applies when you note an increase in the signs of neurologic injury in the patient with movement of the spine. Finally, in cases of severe deformity of the spine, do not move the patient because any movement will further compromise the column and cord. Use whatever padding and immobilization devices are necessary to accommodate the patient's positioning and assure that no further movement occurs.

Assure that any movement of the patient during assessment or care is toward alignment. If, for example, the patient is lying twisted on the ground when you find him, assess the exposed areas, then move the patient toward alignment. If the patient is found prone, assess the patient's posterior surfaces before you log roll him (to a long spine board) for further assessment and care. Never move a patient twice before you complete your mechanical immobilization, if possible.

MANUAL CERVICAL IMMOBILIZATION

The typical trauma patient is found either seated (as in an auto) or lying on the ground. For the seated patient, initially approach from the front and carefully direct the patient not to move or turn his head. It is an almost reflexive act to turn to listen when we hear someone speak to us from behind. Such movement is dangerous in the potential spine injury patient. Ask your patient to keep his head immobile and explain to the patient that a caregiver is going to position himself behind the patient to immobilize the spine.

The assigned caregiver should then move behind the patient and bring his hands up along the patient's ears, using the little fingers to catch the mandible and the medial aspect of the heels of the hand to engage the mastoid region of the skull (Figure 9-16 ■). Gentle pressure inward engages the head and prevents it from moving. A gentle lifting force of a few pounds helps take some of the weight of the head off the cervical spine, but care should be taken not to lift the head or apply any traction to this critical region. The patient's head should then be moved slowly and easily to a position in which the eyes face directly forward and along a line central to and perpendicular to the shoulder plane.

If there is no access to the seated patient from behind, employ the same techniques of movement and immobilization from in front with the little fingers engaging the mastoid region while the heels of the hand support the mandible. When approaching from

Move any body segment that is out of alignment toward alignment as you examine it, but if the patient feels any increase in pain or if you feel resistance to movement, immobilize the head and neck or other portion of the body in the position achieved.

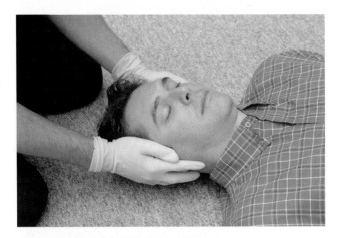

■ **Figure 9-16** Bring the head to the neutral in-line position and maintain manual immobilization until the head, neck, and spine are mechanically immobilized.

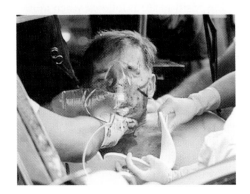

■ **Figure 9-17** When you cannot access the patient from behind to apply manual immobilization, use alternative hand placement.

the patient's side, place one hand under the mandible while using the other to support the occiput (Figure 9-17 ■).

If the patient is supine, support the head by placing your hands along the lateral and inferior surfaces of the head. Position the little fingers and heels of the hands just lateral to the occipital region of the skull to support the head. With gentle inward pressure, hold the patient's head immobile and prevent flexion/extension, rotation, and lateral bending motion. Lift the head gently off the ground to approximate the neutral position, usually 1 to 2 inches for the adult. (If the surface on which the patient is found is not flat, adjust the height accordingly.) Position a small adult's or a large child's head at about ground level. Elevate the shoulders of infants or very small children because of their proportionally larger heads (Figure 9-18 ■). Apply no axial pressure; neither push nor pull the head toward or away from the body.

If a patient is found prone or on the side, position your hands according to the patient's position. If it will be some time until the patient can be moved to the supine position, place your hands so that they are comfortable during cervical immobilization. You should then reposition your hands just before the patient is moved to the final position. If the time until moving the patient to the supine position is expected to be short, place your hands so they will be properly positioned at the conclusion of the move. This may involve initially twisting your hands into a relatively uncomfortable position.

Assessment, care, and patient movement may require the caregiver holding immobilization to reposition his hands. To accomplish this, another caregiver supports and immobilizes the patient's head and neck by bringing his hands in from an alternate position. This caregiver places one hand under the patient's occiput while the other hand holds the jaw. Once the head is stable, have the original caregiver reposition his hands, reassume immobilization, and then have the second caregiver remove his hands.

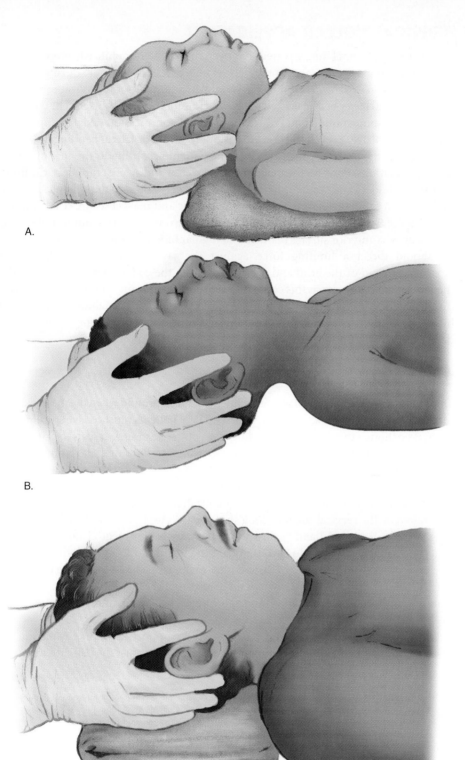

■ Figure 9-18   Neutral spinal positioning for infant, child, and adult patients. A. Due to the large heads of infants and small children you may need to raise the shoulder with padding. B. In older children or small adults, obtain neutral positioning with the shoulders and head on a flat firm surface. C. With adults, elevate the head 1 to 2 inches with firm padding.

A.

B.

C.

CERVICAL COLLAR APPLICATION

After a potential spinal injury patient has been manually immobilized, apply a cervical collar. Apply the collar as soon as the neck is fully assessed, generally during the rapid trauma assessment. The cervical collar is only an adjunct to full cervical immobilization and should never be considered to provide immobilization by itself. The collar does limit cervical spine motion and reduce the forces of compression (axial loading), but it does not completely prevent flexion/extension, rotation, or lateral bending.

To apply the cervical collar, size it to the patient according to the manufacturer's recommendations. Position the device under the chin and against the chest. Contour it over the shoulders and secure it firmly behind the neck. Be sure the Velcro closures remain clear of sand, dirt, fabric, or the patient's hair and make a secure seal behind the neck (Figure 9-19 ■). The collar should fit snugly around the neck but not place pressure against its anterior surface (carotid and jugular blood vessels and trachea). The collar should direct a limiting force against the jaw and occiput to restrict any flexion/extension of the head and neck. Assure that the collar does not seriously limit the movement of the jaw, as this could prevent the patient from ridding himself of vomitus. Once the cervical collar is in place, do not release or relax manual cervical immobilization until the patient is fully immobilized either with a vest-type immobilization device or to a long spine board with a cervical immobilization device.

STANDING TAKEDOWN

Often at vehicle crash sites, you will find patients walking around when the mechanisms of injury suggest the potential for spinal injuries. These patients must receive spinal precautions, even though they are found standing. Your objective in such cases is to bring the patient to a fully supine position for further assessment, care, immobilization, and transport.

To accomplish this, employ a standing takedown procedure that maintains the spine in axial alignment. Have the patient remain immobile while a caregiver approaches from the rear and assumes manual cervical immobilization. Quickly assess any areas that will be covered by the cervical collar or long spine board. Apply a cervical collar and place a long spine board behind and against the patient, with the caregiver holding immobilization spreading his arms to accommodate the board. Position two other caregivers, one on each side of the spine board, and have each place a hand under the patient's axilla and with it grasp the closest (preferably next higher) handhold on the board. The team should then move the patient and spine board backward, tilting the patient on his heels until the patient and board are supine (Figure 9-20 ■).

During the move, the hands in the handholds support the thorax while the caregiver holding cervical immobilization rotates his hands against the patient's head with-

A cervical collar by itself does not immobilize the cervical spine.

Always assure that the cervical collar is correctly sized for the patient or choose another one.

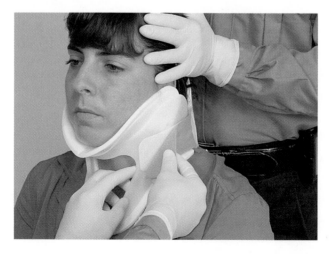

■ Figure 9-19 Properly place and secure the cervical collar on suspected spinal injury patients.

out either flexing or extending the head and neck as the patient moves from standing to supine. During this maneuver, the hands holding the patient's head must move from grasping the mastoid and mandible (standing) to grasping the lateral occiput (supine). This is not easy, because the head must rotate while the caregiver's hands remain in the same relative position. As with all movement procedures, the caregiver at the patient's head should be in control and direct the process.

Once the patient and board are on the ground, continue to maintain manual immobilization while assessing and caring for the patient. Then provide mechanical immobilization to the long spine board before moving the patient to the ambulance.

HELMET REMOVAL

Helmet use in contact sports, bicycling, skateboarding, in-line skating, and motorcycling has increased over the past decade. While these devices offer significant protection for the head during impact, they have not been proven to reduce spine injuries. Their use also complicates spinal injury care for prehospital care providers. Many helmets are of the partial variety (such as those worn while bicycling and skateboarding) and are easy to remove at the trauma scene. Some motorcycle and sports helmets, however, fully enclose the head and are very difficult to remove in the field. These helmets are also very difficult to secure to the spine board because of their spherical shapes. Further, most full helmets do not hold the head firmly within, so even fixing the helmet securely to the spine board does not result in effective cervical immobilization. Some newer contact sport helmets contain air bladders that expand and firmly hold the head in position within the helmet. These helmets immobilize the head well, but they are still difficult to firmly secure to a spine board. Consequently, most full-enclosure helmets must be removed to assure adequate spinal immobilization.

The helmet must be removed if you find any of the following conditions:

★ The helmet does not immobilize the patient's head within.

★ You cannot securely immobilize the helmet to the long spine board.

★ The helmet prevents airway care.

★ The helmet prevents assessment of anticipated injuries.

★ There are, or you anticipate, airway or breathing problems.

★ Helmet removal will not cause further injury.

Helmet removal may be a tricky endeavor. You should familiarize yourself with the types of helmets used by sporting teams in your area (e.g., high-school football).

Management of the Spinal Injury Patient   **365**

During helmet removal, have a caregiver initially stabilize the cervical spine by manually immobilizing the helmet. Remove the face mask, if present, either by unscrewing it or by cutting it off, if possible. Remove or retract any eye protection or visor and unfasten or cut away any chin strap as well. Be careful not to manipulate the helmet or otherwise transmit movement to the patient through the helmet. Then have another caregiver immobilize the head by sliding his hands under the helmet and placing them along the sides of the head, supporting the occiput, or by placing one hand on the jaw and the other on the occiput. This caregiver should choose the hand placement that works best for him and can be accommodated by the helmet. The caregiver holding the helmet should then grasp the helmet and spread it slightly to clear the ears by pulling laterally just below and anterior to the ear enclosure. That caregiver then rotates the helmet to clear the chin, counterrotates it to clear the occiput, and then rotates it to clear the nose and brow ridge (Figure 9-21 ■). The clearance is usually very tight with a well-fitted helmet.

Execute the previous procedure slowly and carefully to prevent head and neck motion and to minimize patient discomfort. For helmets with air bladders, use the same procedure, but empty the bladder after someone stabilizes the head and before you begin the removal. Helmet removal is a complicated skill that you must practice frequently before you can employ it successfully in the field.

MOVING THE SPINAL INJURY PATIENT

Once you assess and provide the essential care for a patient with a potential spinal injury, plan the movement to the long spine board carefully. If any step of assessment or patient care requires patient movement consider moving the patient onto the long spine board. Movement techniques suitable for moving the spinal injury patient to the long spine board include the log roll, straddle slide, rope-sling slide, orthopedic stretcher lift, application of a vest-type device (or short spine board), and rapid extrication. Choose a technique that affords the least spinal movement for the conditions and equipment at hand. Also select your movement technique and adjust its steps to accommodate the patient's particular injuries.

A key factor in all movement techniques for the patient with potential spinal injury is the coordination of the move. It is essential that you move the patient as a unit with his head facing forward and in a plane with the shoulders and hips. This can best be accomplished if the caregiver at the head controls and directs the move. He is able to see the other rescuers and has a focused and limited function (holding the head), which permits that person to evaluate what the other caregivers are doing. The caregiver at the head directs the move by counting a cadence such as, "Move on four—one, two, three, four." A four-count is preferable because it gives the other caregivers a good opportunity to anticipate the actual start of movement. All moves must be slowly executed and well coordinated among caregivers.

Choose a movement technique that affords the least spinal movement.

The caregiver at the head directs and controls the movement of the patient with a suspected spinal injury.

A four-count is a preferable cadence because it gives the other caregivers a good opportunity to anticipate the start of the move.

■ Figure 9-21 Helmet removal.

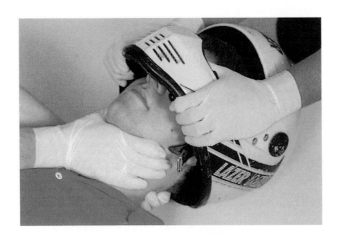

Consider what the final positioning of the patient will be when you choose a spinal movement technique. Most spinal injury patients are best served with supine positioning on a long spine board. However, a patient with a thoracic spine injury is frequently placed in a prone position on a soft stretcher. With this patient, other positioning, such as supine on a firm spine board, puts pressure on the injury site from the body's weight and any movement is more likely to cause motion of the injury site and compound any damage.

Log Roll

The log roll can be used to rotate the patient 90 degrees, insert the long spine board, and then roll the patient back. It can also be used to roll the patient 180 degrees from prone to supine or vice versa.

As you begin the 90-degree roll, assure manual spinal immobilization and apply a cervical collar. Notice that anatomically the shoulders are wider than the hips and legs. To provide a uniform roll, extend the patient's arm above his head. Then place a rolled bulky blanket between the legs (with its bulkiest portion between the feet) and tie the legs together. This reduces pelvic movement and lateral bending of the lumbar spine.

It takes four caregivers to properly perform the log roll for a spinal injury patient (Figure 9-22 ■). One caregiver holds the head, while one kneels at the patient's shoulder with the knees tight against the patient's chest. The third caregiver kneels at the patient's hip with the knees tight against the patient's hip. The last caregiver kneels at the patient's knees with the knees tight against the patient's knees.

The caregivers reach across the patient and around the opposite shoulder, hip, and knee, respectively, and grasp the patient firmly. On a count initiated by the caregiver at the head, the team, in unison, rolls the patient against their knees and up to a 90-degree angle. With a free hand, the caregiver at the knees (or an additional caregiver) slides a long spine board under the patient from the patient's side or the foot end. The board should be positioned tightly against the patient so that the head, torso, and pelvis will eventually rest solidly on the board. Then, at the count of the caregiver at the head, the team rolls the patient back 90 degrees onto the board.

The 180-degree log roll begins with placement of the long spine board between the caregivers and the patient, with the board resting at an angle on the caregivers' thighs. The caregivers reach across the board and grasp the patient as for the 90-degree log roll. The caregiver at the head must be careful to anticipate the turning motion and position his hands so they will be comfortably positioned at the end of the roll. On the count of the caregiver at the head, the team rolls the patient past 90 degrees until he is positioned against the tilted long spine board. Then they reposition their hands against the other (lower) side of the patient and slowly back their thighs out from under the patient until the board rests on the ground.

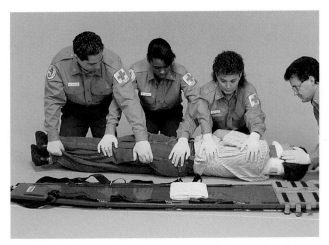

■ Figure 9-22 The four-person log roll.

Straddle Slide

Another technique effective for moving the patient with potential spinal injury is the straddle slide. In this procedure, three caregivers are positioned at the patient's head, shoulders, and pelvis, while a fourth prepares to insert the long spine board from either the patient's head or feet. The caregiver at the head holds cervical immobilization and guides the lift with a cadence. The second caregiver straddles the patient (facing the patient's head) and grasps the shoulders. The third caregiver straddles the patient (facing the head) and grasps the pelvis. All the caregivers keep their feet planted widely enough apart to permit the insertion of the long spine board. At the direction of the caregiver at the head, the three caregivers lift the patient just enough to permit the fourth caregiver to negotiate the long spine board underneath the patient. (*Note:* If the board is to be inserted from the patient's feet, the caregiver inserting the board lifts the patient's feet with one hand and slides the board into place with the other.) On a signal from the caregiver at the head, the team gently lowers the patient to the long spine board.

Rope-Sling Slide

A continuous ring or length of thick rope or other material can be used to help slide a supine patient, using axial traction, onto a long spine board. One caregiver holds cervical immobilization, while another places the rope across the patient's chest and under his arms. The rope is tied together (with a cravat) behind the patient's neck and brought out between the legs of the first caregiver. A long spine board is placed between the legs of the caregiver holding cervical stabilization. The second caregiver positions him- or herself at the head end of the spine board with the board resting on his thighs (this provides a small angle to more easily drag the patient onto the board). The second caregiver then pulls on the two strands of rope, guiding the patient onto the spine board as directed by the caregiver at the head. The caregiver holding cervical immobilization moves backwards as the patient is moved onto the spine board. (The caregiver at the head may crouch or kneel to the patient's side to hold immobilization.) The caregiver at the head must be careful to move smoothly with the caregiver pulling axial traction. That person must assure that the head moves with the body and does not pull against it.

Orthopedic Stretcher

The orthopedic stretcher, also known as the scoop stretcher, is a valuable device for positioning the patient on the spine board or helping to secure the patient to the long spine board. To apply the device, lengthen it to accommodate the patient's height and then separate it into its two halves. Maintain cervical immobilization while you gently negotiate each half of the stretcher under the patient from the sides and connect them at the top, then bottom. Be careful not to entrap the patient's skin or body parts while positioning the stretcher, especially on uneven ground. Once the device is connected, you may use the stretcher to lift the patient to the waiting spine board. Orthopedic stretchers are usually not rigid enough to use by themselves as transport devices for spinal injury patients. Rather, they are most effective in moving patients to the long spine board, where they may remain as an adjunct to full immobilization, or you may disconnect the halves, remove them, and immobilize the patient to the long spine board in the normal way.

Vest-Type Immobilization Device (and Short Spine Board)

A specialized piece of EMS equipment that may be used with some spinal injury patients is the vest-type immobilization device (Figure 9-23 ■). This device immobilizes the patient's head, shoulders, and pelvis to a rigid board so that you can move the patient from a seated position, as in an automobile, to a fully supine position. The vest-type device comes as a commercially made device that usually has the needed strapping already attached. The device is usually constructed of thin, rigid wood or plastic strips embedded in a vinyl or fabric vest. It is then wrapped and secured around the patient to provide immobilization. An alternative to the vest-type device is the short spine board, a cut-out piece of rigid plywood to which you attach strapping and padding. The basic principles of application are the same with both short-board and vest-type devices.

To apply the vest-type device, manually immobilize the patient's cervical spine and apply a cervical collar while the device is being readied for application. If the patient is positioned against a soft seat (as in an automobile), gently move the patient's shoulders and head a few inches forward to permit insertion of the vest. The caregiver holding cervical immobilization directs and coordinates the move, while a second caregiver guides and controls shoulder motion. Negotiate the device behind the patient by either inserting the head portion under and through the arms of the caregiver providing cervical immobilization, or angling it, base first, then moving it behind the patient's back. Position the device vertically so the chest appendages fit just under the arms. This positioning permits you to fasten the straps and secure the shoulders without any upward or downward movement of the device. First, secure the device to the chest and pelvis with strapping and assure that the vest is immobile. Tighten the straps firmly, but be sure that they do not inhibit respiration. Secure the thigh straps as they hold the hips and thighs in the flexed position, limiting lumbar motion. Then fill the space between the occiput and the device with noncompressible padding to assure neutral positioning. Secure both the brow ridge and chin to the device with straps, but be very careful to allow for vomiting by the patient and subsequent clearing of the airway or be prepared to release the chin strap immediately if vomiting occurs. Tie the patient's wrists together.

The vest-type immobilization device is not meant to lift the patient but rather to facilitate rotating him on the buttocks and then to tilt the patient to the supine position for further spinal immobilization (Figure 9-24 ■). Once the patient is positioned on the long spine board, gently and carefully release the thigh straps and slowly and gently extend the hips and knees. If after transfer to the spine board the patient's head remains firmly affixed to the vest-type device, leave the vest on the patient and secure the vest to the long spine board since doing this effectively secures both head and torso. If the head becomes loose during the transfer, reapply manual cervical immobilization, secure the torso with strapping, and secure the head with a cervical immobilization device.

The vest-type device is not meant to lift the patient but rather to facilitate rotating and tilting the patient to the supine position.

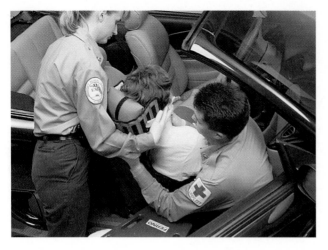

■ Figure 9-24 The vest-type immobilization device is not intended for lifting the patient, but for pivoting him.

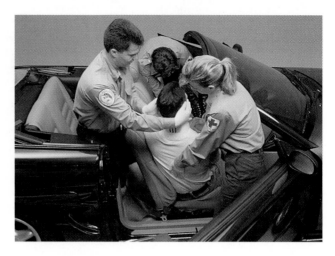

■ Figure 9-25 Rapid extrication of a patient with a spinal injury.

Rapid Extrication

Applying a vest-type immobilization device is a time-consuming process. Often the circumstances of the emergency, either issues of scene safety or the need for rapid transport to the trauma center, preclude spending the time required for standard spinal immobilization. In such cases, use a rapid extrication procedure.

With whatever personnel are available, stabilize the patient's spine, shoulders, pelvis, and legs with the patient's nose, navel, and toes kept in line. Assure that caregivers are coordinated and understand what movement is to take place. One caregiver, usually at the patient's head, should direct the move, counting a cadence to permit the crew to work together (Figure 9-25 ■). Assure that personnel involved in the extrication move the patient maintaining the alignment of the patient's nose, navel, and toes. Then, on the leader's count, they should move the patient from a seated or other position to a waiting spine board.

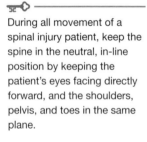

During all movement of a spinal injury patient, keep the spine in the neutral, in-line position by keeping the patient's eyes facing directly forward, and the shoulders, pelvis, and toes in the same plane.

Remember the objectives of spinal movement and stabilization: Keep the spine in the neutral, in-line position by keeping the patient's eyes facing directly forward and keeping the shoulders and pelvis in a plane perpendicular to that of the gaze. Be sure to prevent any flexion/extension, rotation, or lateral bending.

While the technique of rapid extrication does not provide maximum protection for the spine, it does permit rapid movement of the patient with a spinal injury when other considerations demand it. Use the procedure only when your patient cannot afford the time it would take for normal spinal movement techniques. Rapid extrication from the confined space of a wrecked automobile is difficult at best. Plan your move carefully and execute the rapid extrication by carefully explaining the process and individual responsibilities to your team members.

Final Patient Positioning

Once the patient is on the long spine board, consider positioning for proper mechanical immobilization. Centering the patient on the board is essential to assuring that the patient's spine remains in-line and he is effectively immobilized. Accomplish this by placing team members at the patient's head, shoulders, pelvis, and feet. The caregivers then place one hand on each side of the patient and prepare to move the patient toward the center of the board. On a cadence signaled by the caregiver at the head, they slide the portion of the patient that is out of alignment to an in-line position, centered on the long spine board.

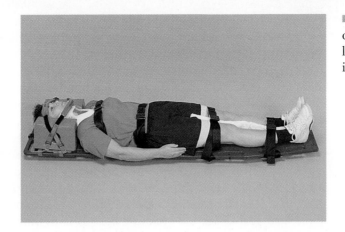

Long Spine Board

The long spine board is simply a reinforced flat, firm surface designed to facilitate immobilization of a patient in a supine or prone position (Figure 9-26 ■). While the board may immobilize patients with multisystem trauma, pelvic and lower limb fractures, and many other types of trauma, it is primarily designed for patients with spine injuries. The board has several hand and strap holes along its lateral borders for lifting and to assure effective strapping and patient immobilization. Using nylon web strapping, you can immobilize a patient with almost any combination of injuries to the board firmly enough to permit rotating the patient and board 90 degrees to clear the airway in case of vomiting.

Secure the patient to the board with the strapping, immobilizing and holding the shoulders and pelvis firmly to the board. Such strapping may cross the body and capture the shoulder and pelvic girdles. Assure that you firmly immobilize the patient to prevent lateral motion as well as cephalad (head-ward) and caudad (tail-ward) motion. Be sure that the pressure created by strapping does not come to bear on the central abdomen. That would cause forced extension of the lumbar spine. Immobilize the lower legs and feet with strapping or cravats. Tie the legs together, and place a rolled blanket under the patient's knees to immobilize them in a slightly flexed position. Once you have firmly immobilized the patient's body to the board, you can move on to immobilizing the head.

Long spine board immobilization is made more effective by use of the cervical immobilization device (CID). This device is made up of two soft, padded lateral pieces that bracket the patient's head, maintaining its position, and a base plate that permits you to easily secure the device to the board. The base plate is affixed to the long spine board before the patient is moved to it. Once you position the patient on the board, fill the void between the occiput and the CID base plate with firm, noncompressible padding. Use no padding for the small adult or older child, and pad the shoulders in the young child or infant to assure proper spinal positioning. While a caregiver maintains manual immobilization of the head, bring the lateral components of the CID against the sides of the patient's head. Use medial pressure to hold them against the head and keep the head in position. Then affix the lateral CID components to the Velcro of the CID base plate. Secure the head in position and to the long spine board using forehead and chin straps or tape. Make sure the strapping catches the brow ridge and the mandible or the upper portion of the collar. The properly secured CID must hold the patient's head in the neutral position without movement while not placing undue pressure on the neck or restricting jaw movement (in case of vomiting). Be careful that the straps do not flex, extend, or rotate the head. This procedure results in quick and effective immobilization of the head. Bulky blanket rolls, placed on each side of the head and secured both to the head and the board, will also effectively immobilize the head to the long spine board.

While the long spine board is almost universally accepted for spinal immobilization, it does have drawbacks. Because of its firm surface, the long board places extreme pressure on the skin and tissues covering the ischial tuberosities (the pelvic protuberances we sit on) and the shoulder blades. If a patient remains immobilized to the board for more than a couple of hours, ulceration injuries are likely to result.

The board also tends to encourage caregivers to immobilize the patient directly to it in a nonneutral position. In a proper neutral position, the head should be elevated about 1 to 2 inches above the board's surface and the knees should be bent at 15 to 30 degrees. This positioning relieves pressure on the cervical spine, lumbar spine, hips, and knees and increases patient comfort. You can obtain proper knee positioning by placing folded blankets under the patient's knees. You can also increase patient comfort by placing some padding under the curves of the back. Do not overpad; just fill the voids at the small of the back and neck with bulky soft dressing material.

A device that is now showing merit for spinal immobilization is the full-body vacuum mattress (Figure 9-27 ■), also known as a full-body vacuum splint. Like the vacuum splints for the limbs discussed in Chapter 7, "Musculoskeletal Trauma," the full-body vacuum mattress uses small plastic beads that maintain their position in the reduced pressure after air is evacuated from the splint. To apply the vacuum mattress, place the patient on the device and shape it around him. Evacuating the air causes the device to form to the contours of the patient's body and maintain immobilization. It is more difficult to position the patient in the vacuum mattress than on a long spine board, but use of the device can adequately immobilize the spine injury patient.

Diving Injury Immobilization

Patients injured in shallow water dives are often paralyzed from the impact. They must rely on others to protect their airways and remove them from the water. When carried out by untrained bystanders, however, these activities may compound any spinal injury. If you are present when such an incident occurs, be sure to carefully control any patient motion while he is still in the water. If necessary, turn him to a supine position, assuring that the nose, navel, and toes remain in a single plane and that the eyes face directly forward. You may accomplish this by sandwiching the patient's chest between your forearms while your arms and shoulders cradle the head. Once the patient is in the supine position, water provides an almost neutral buoyancy and, if the water is calm, helps to immobilize the patient. Move the patient by pulling on the shoulders while you cradle

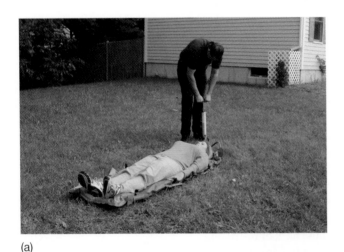

(a)

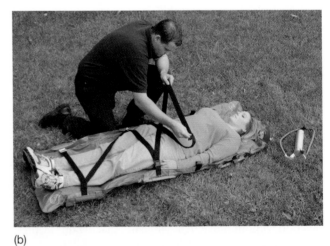

(b)

■ Figure 9-27   A full-body vacuum mattress can adequately immobilize the spine injury patient. (a) The device is shaped around the patient and air is withdrawn. (b) The patient is then secured to the rigid, confirming vacuum mattress.

Immobilize the adult patient to the long spine board with the head elevated 1 to 2 inches, the knees slightly flexed, and with limited padding at the small of the back and the space behind the neck.

the head, in the neutral position, with the forearms. Float a long spine board under the patient, strap him firmly to the board, and then lift and carry him from the water.

MEDICATIONS

There are several conditions that merit the use of medications for the patient with spine injury. These conditions include neurogenic shock and the combative patient. As noted in the following sections, recent research has changed the view of administering steroids for spinal cord injury.

Medications and Spinal Cord Injury

In the past, steroids have been used to combat the inflammation frequently associated with spinal cord injury. Recent research and other information now suggest that this treatment is not as effective as once thought, and high-dose steroid treatment is not without significant side effects. Hence the routine use of steroids for the treatment of spinal injury is no longer recommended. Please consult with your medical director and protocols for any system-specific recommendations regarding the treatment of spinal injury and the use of medications.

Routine use of steroids for spinal injury is no longer recommended.

Medications and Neurogenic Shock

The loss of sympathetic control leads to both a relaxation of the blood vessels (vasodilation) below the level of the lesion and the inability of the body to increase the heart rate. This expanded vascular system leads to a relative hypovolemia and lower blood pressure. The problem is further compounded as the heart, without sympathetic stimulation and in the presence of this relative hypovolemia, displays a normal or bradycardic heart rate. Frequently, the hypovolemia is treated with a fluid challenge, followed by careful use of a vasopressor such as dopamine. The slow heart rate is treated with atropine to reduce any parasympathetic stimulation.

The use of the PASG to combat the relative hypovolemia of neurogenic shock is somewhat controversial. The compression of the lower extremities and abdomen may counteract the vasodilation associated with the shock state, but research has not yet proven the garment's use contributes to a better outcome. Follow local protocols and consult with medical direction before using the device.

The initial treatment for hypovolemia from suspected neurogenic shock is by fluid challenge (Figure 9-28 ■). Establish an IV with a 1,000-mL bag of lactated Ringer's solution or normal saline, a nonrestrictive administration set, and a large-bore IV catheter. Administer 250 mL of solution quickly, monitor the blood pressure and heart rate, and auscultate the lungs for signs of developing pulmonary edema (crackles). If the patient responds with an increasing blood pressure, a slowing heart rate, and signs of improved perfusion, consider a second bolus, or monitor the patient and administer a second bolus if the patient's signs and symptoms begin to deteriorate. If the patient does not improve with the fluid challenge, consider vasopressor therapy, as allowed by your protocols.

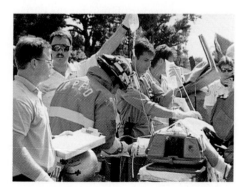

■ Figure 9-28 Aggressive fluid resuscitation may be necessary for the patient in neurogenic shock.

Dopamine (Intropin) is a naturally occurring catecholamine that, in addition to its own actions, causes the release of norepinephrine. Dopamine increases cardiac contractility and hence cardiac output and, at higher doses, increases peripheral vascular resistance, venous constriction, cardiac preload, and blood pressure. While there are no contraindications for dopamine use in the emergency setting, its common side effects include tachydysrhythmias, hypertension, headache, nausea, and vomiting.

Dopamine is frequently packaged as either a premixed solution containing 800 or 1,600 mcg/mL or as a 5-mL vial containing 200 or 400 mg of drug. Vial contents are added to 250 mL of D_5W to yield a concentration of either 800 or 1,600 mcg/mL. Dopamine is very light sensitive and once mixed should be discarded after 24 hours. If the solution is either pink or brown, discard it. Dopamine's onset of action is about 5 minutes and its half life is around 2 minutes; hence, it is administered via a continuous infusion. It should be run piggyback through an already well-established IV line as infiltration can cause tissue necrosis. It is administered initially at 2.5 mcg/kg/min, then titrated to an increase in blood pressure or a maximum of 20 mcg/kg/min. (Vasoconstriction usually begins at doses above 10 mcg/kg/min.)

Interruption of the sympathetic pathways by spinal cord injury causes unopposed parasympathetic stimulation and bradycardia (or at least prevents the compensatory tachycardia that occurs with decreased cardiac preload). The net result is a decrease in cardiac output in the neurogenic shock patient. Atropine is administered to block the parasympathetic impulse that might contribute to slow the heart rate.

Atropine is an anticholinergic agent most frequently used for symptomatic bradycardia and heart blocks in the myocardial infarction patient. It is sometimes helpful in increasing the heart rate of patients with upper spinal cord injury due to unopposed vagal stimulation. It acts by inhibiting the actions of acetylcholine, the major parasympathetic neurotransmitter. Atropine has a quick onset of action and a half life of just over 2 hours. It is available for emergency use in 5- and 10-mL preloaded syringes containing a concentration of 0.5 mg/mL. Atropine is administered rapidly in 0.5 mg (1 mL) intravenous doses every 3 to 5 minutes, up to a maximum of 2 mg. The only expected side effects in the emergency setting are dry mouth, blurred vision, and, possibly, tachycardia.

Medications and the Combative Patient

When giving a neuromuscular blocker to a conscious patient with spinal injury, always use a sedative/hypnotic first.

Frequently the patient who has sustained potentially serious spinal injury has also sustained head injury, is intoxicated, or is otherwise very uncooperative or combative. In some of these cases, sedatives may be indicated to reduce anxiety and because the patient actively resists spinal precautions and is actively moving about. Such patient motion may compromise efforts to immobilize the spine and increase the potential for further damage. Consider using meperidine (Demerol) or diazepam (Valium) to calm the patient. In extreme circumstances, consider use of the paralytics mentioned in Chapter 8, "Head, Facial, and Neck Trauma," in the discussion of facilitated intubation to paralyze the patient. Whenever you use these agents, you must carefully monitor the patient's level of consciousness and respirations. With use of paralytics, you must provide continuing ventilation for the patient during the action of the drug. Sedatives and paralytics should only be administered as permitted by your system's protocols and under the close and direct supervision of an on-line medical direction physician.

Summary

Spinal injury is a frequent consequence of serious trauma and is likely to induce serious disability or death. Injury to the spinal column may occur with only minimal signs and patient symptoms. Yet further manipulation of the injured column, either through movement by the patient or movement initiated by caregivers, may cause injury to the spinal cord. Because of this danger, prehospital care for any patient with a significant mechanism of injury—a serious auto crash, a fall from more than three times the patient's height, any significant trauma above the shoulders—or any trauma patient with a reduced level of consciousness must receive spinal precautions.

Spinal precautions include carefully bringing the patient's head to the neutral, in-line position with the eyes facing directly forward and the shoulders and pelvis in one body plane. Manually stabilize the patient's head in this position during assessment and care until you can fully immobilize the patient after movement to the long spine board. Place a cervical collar on the patient to provide additional stabilization of the cervical spine, but remember that the collar by itself is not a definitive immobilization device. Accomplish movement to the long spine board from the standing position by use of the standing takedown, from the seated position by use of the vest-type immobilization device or the rapid extrication technique, and from either the supine or prone positions by use of the log roll, straddle slide, orthopedic stretcher, or rope-sling slide. Once the patient is properly positioned on the spine board, firmly secure first the patient's torso and then head for movement to the ambulance and transport to the neurocenter. Throughout patient care, provide emotional support and calming reassurance to help alleviate your patient's anxiety.

You Make the Call

A young swimmer is found floating, face down and unconscious, at a local municipal pool. When you arrive, he is supine on a long spine board with a lifeguard holding cervical immobilization. The swimmer is now conscious and alert and is complaining of minor neck pain and some tingling in his fingers and toes.

1. What additional spinal precautions does this patient require?
2. What mechanism of injury do you suspect?
3. What other assessment and care steps does this patient require?

See Suggested Responses at the back of this book.

Review Questions

1. The most common sites of axial loading for lifting injuries and heel-first falls are located between:
   a. T-12 and L-2.
   b. C-1 and C-7.
   c. C-5 and T-4.
   d. L-3 and L-5.

2. During a trauma assessment you notice that a patient has no sensation below the lower border of the rib cage. This would suggest spinal pathology between which vertebral areas?
   a. C-1 and C-3
   b. C-3 and T-4
   c. T-4 and T-10
   d. T-10 and S-1

3. Which of the following vital signs would most likely indicate a potential spinal cord injury?
   a. hypotension, bradycardia, and shallow respirations
   b. hypertension, bradycardia, and shallow respirations

c. hypotension, tachycardia, and deep respirations

d. hypertension, tachycardia, and deep respirations

4. For which of the following patients would the anticholinergic agent atropine be best suited? A patient:

a. in early spinal shock.

b. with an injury to the upper spinal cord.

c. with an injury to the lower spinal cord.

d. with autonomic hyperreflexia syndrome.

5. The primary management objective in a patient with a suspected spinal cord injury is to:

a. administer medications to prevent further paralysis.

b. apply a cervical collar independent of spinal stabilization.

c. initiate mechanical stabilization followed by manual immobilization.

d. maintain the patient in a neutral, in-line position.

6. All of the following are primary functions of the intervertebral disks except:

a. limiting bone wear.

b. absorbing shock.

c. accommodating motion of adjacent vertebrae.

d. elevating the diaphragm during inspiratory efforts.

7. The major weight-bearing component of a vertebra is the:

a. pedicle.

b. laminae.

c. vertebral body.

d. spinal canal.

8. Priapism is defined as:

a. a sustained erection of the penis.

b. clear discharge from the nose.

c. an occasional variant of angina.

d. always associated with paralysis.

9. The most accurate definition of dermatomes is:

a. spinal nerves that innervate specific and discrete areas of the body surface.

b. spinal nerves that innervate specific organs and organ systems.

c. spinal nerves that pinpoint the exact location of the injury site.

d. spinal nerves that innervate discrete tissues and muscles in the body.

10. Which of the following statements regarding cervical collars is true?

a. They serve as an adjunct to full cervical immobilization.

b. They serve to accentuate axial loading and prevent flexion/extension.

c. They serve to immobilize the cervical, thoracic, and lumbar spine.

d. They serve to prevent axial loading when utilized before manual stabilization.

11. All of the following are signs or symptoms of spinal shock except:

a. priapism.

b. hypertension.

c. loss of bladder control.

d. flaccid paralysis.

12. Which of the following best defines spinal shock?

a. a permanent insult to the cord that affects the body above the level of the injury

b. a permanent insult to the cord that affects the body through extravasation of blood volume

c. a permanent insult to the cord that affects the body above and below the level of the injury

d. a temporary insult to the cord that affects the body below the level of the injury

13. The central nervous system is made up of the:
    a. brain and cervical spine.
    b. brain and spinal cord.
    c. spinal cord only.
    d. brain and meninges.

14. Which of the following articulates with the ribs and serves as the site for muscle attachment?
    a. spinous process
    b. vertebral pedicle
    c. intervertebral disk
    d. transverse process

15. The most accurate description of the function of cerebrospinal fluid is that it provides:
    a. a medium for exchange of all cells that are specific to immunity.
    b. stabilization and nutrients to the cervical spine and lumbar spine.
    c. a medium for exchange of micro and macro proteins as well as electrolytes.
    d. a medium for exchange of nutrients and waste products, while absorbing the shock of sudden movements.

See Answers to Review Questions at the back of this book.

Further Reading

American College of Surgeons, Committee on Trauma. *Advanced Trauma Life Support Course: Student Manual.* Chicago: American College of Surgeons, 2003.

Bates, Barbara, Lynn S. Bickley, and Robert A. Hoekelman. *A Guide to Physical Examination and History Taking.* 8th ed. Philadelphia: J. B. Lippincott, 2003.

Bledsoe, B. E. and D. Clayden. *Prehospital Emergency Pharamacology.* 6th ed. Upper Saddle River, N.J.: Pearson/Prentice Hall, 2005.

Butman, A., S. Martin, R. Vomacka, and N. E. McSwain. *Comprehensive Guide to Pre-Hospital Skills: A Skills Manual for EMT-Basic, EMT-Intermediate, and EMT-Paramedic.* St. Louis: Mosby, 1996.

Campbell, John E. *Basic Trauma Life Support for Paramedics and Other Advanced Providers.* 5th ed. update. Upper Saddle River, N.J.: Pearson/Prentice Hall, 2004.

Martini, Frederic. *Fundamentals of Anatomy and Physiology.* 6th ed. San Francisco: Benjamin Cummings, 2004.

McSwain, N. E. and S. B. Frame, eds. *Prehospital Trauma Life Support.* 5th ed. St. Louis: Mosby, 2003.

Rosen, P. and R. Barkin, eds. *Emergency Medicine: Concepts and Clinical Practice.* 5th ed. St. Louis: Mosby, 2002.

On the Web

Visit Brady's Paramedic Website at **www.bradybooks.com/paramedic**.

Thoracic Trauma

Objectives

After reading this chapter, you should be able to:

1. Describe the incidence, morbidity, and mortality of thoracic injuries in the trauma patient. (pp. 380–381)

2. Discuss the anatomy and physiology of the organs and structures related to thoracic injuries. (pp. 381–392)

3. Predict thoracic injuries based on the mechanism of injury. (pp. 393–395)

4. Discuss the pathophysiology of, assessment findings with, and the management and need for rapid intervention and transport of the patient with chest wall injuries, including:
   a. Rib fracture (pp. 396–397, 417)
   b. Flail segment (pp. 398–399, 418)
   c. Sternal fracture (pp. 397–398)

5. Discuss the pathophysiology of, assessment findings with, and management and need for rapid intervention and transport of the patient with injury to the lung, including:
   a. Simple pneumothorax (pp. 399–400)
   b. Open pneumothorax (pp. 400–401, 418–419)
   c. Tension pneumothorax (pp. 401–403, 419–421)
   d. Hemothorax (pp. 403, 420–421)
   e. Hemopneumothorax (p. 403)
   f. Pulmonary contusion (pp. 403–405)

6. Discuss the pathophysiology of, findings of assessment with, and management and need for rapid intervention and transport of the patient with myocardial injuries, including:
   a. Myocardial contusion (pp. 405–406, 421)
   b. Pericardial tamponade (pp. 406–407, 421)
   c. Myocardial rupture (pp. 407–408)

7. Discuss the pathophysiology, assessment, and management for the patient with vascular injuries, including injuries to:
   a. Aorta (pp. 408–409, 421)
   b. Vena cava (p. 409)
   c. Pulmonary arteries/veins (p. 409)
8. Discuss the pathophysiology of, findings of assessment with, and management and need for rapid intervention and transport of patients with diaphragmatic, esophageal, and tracheobronchial injuries. (pp. 409–410, 421)
9. Discuss the pathophysiology of, findings of assessment with, and management and need for rapid intervention and transport of the patient with traumatic asphyxia. (pp. 410–411, 421–422)
10. Differentiate between thoracic injuries based on the assessment and history. (pp. 411–415)
11. Given several preprogrammed and moulaged thoracic trauma patients, provide the appropriate scene size-up, initial assessment, rapid trauma assessment or focused physical exam and history, detailed exam, and ongoing assessment and provide appropriate patient care and transportation. (pp. 411–422)

Key Terms

aneurysm, p. 407
atelectasis, p. 389
co-morbidity, p. 380
electrical alternans, p. 407
epicardium, p. 391
flail chest, p. 398
great vessels, p. 389
hemopneumothorax,
  p. 403

hemoptysis, p. 405
hemothorax, p. 403
hypoxic drive, p. 387
ligamentum arteriosum,
  p. 392
myocardium, p. 391
pericardial tamponade,
  p. 406
pericardium, p. 391

pneumothorax, p. 399
precordium, p. 406
pulmonary hilum, p. 384
pulsus paradoxus, p. 407
tension pneumothorax,
  p. 401
tracheobronchial tree,
  p. 380
xiphisternal joint, p. 382

Case Study

Medic 101 responds to a shooting call at a Southside tavern where a man was reportedly shot during a robbery attempt. Victoria and Christian are the responding paramedics. They quickly size up the scene and determine it to be safe. Police are on the scene, have the assailant in custody, and have controlled the gathering crowd.

On their arrival, they find the patient supine, just inside the tavern door. The tavern owner reports the man had tried to take cash from the register when he shot him with a .38 caliber hand gun at close range. The initial assessment reveals a pale, ashen, weakly combative patient, who is confused. He gives his name as Conrad and his age as 34. His trachea is midline, the jugular veins are full, and there is no apparent use of accessory muscles of respiration. The paramedics note minimal bleeding without air leak from wounds found just below the left clavicle, just left of the upper sternum, just to the right of the lower sternum, and close to the right nipple. Conrad is tachypneic with symmetrical chest rise and has slightly diminished breath sounds on the right. Radial pulses are not palpable, but weak, thready carotid pulses are present. No exit wounds are noted when the patient is log rolled and placed on a long backboard to stabilize the potential thoracolumbar spinal injury. The carotid pulse suggests a blood pressure between 60 and 80 mm Hg.

Conrad is immediately placed on high-flow, high-concentration oxygen via nonrebreather mask and his color improves somewhat. He is rapidly loaded into the ambulance, where bilateral antecubital large-bore IV lines are initiated and run wide open to administer 500 mL en route to Southside Hospital. Christian alerts medical direction and asks to have a trauma team standing by. As Victoria treats initial life threats identified during the initial assessment, she quickly reassesses the chest and notes that respirations are more labored and chest rise is no longer symmetrical. The right chest is somewhat hyperexpanded and demonstrates decreased breath sounds in comparison to the left. Conrad appears more ashen, with carotid pulses now absent. His trachea appears somewhat deviated to the left with jugular venous distention also developing. Christian, suspecting tension pneumothorax, quickly recontacts medical direction and receives an order to decompress the right chest. Victoria inserts a 14-gauge IV catheter in the second intercostal space, along the right midclavicular line and notes a significant rush of air. She observes improvement in the patient's color and better chest rise with less labored breathing. A subsequent ongoing assessment now finds that the weak, thready carotid pulses have returned as the ambulance arrives at the hospital.

The emergency department physician and trauma team take over Conrad's care, initiate an O-negative blood transfusion, intubate him, and place bilateral chest tubes for pneumothoraces. A trauma x-ray series reveals one bullet in the area of the left scapula, another right of the thoracic spine, one in the right upper abdominal quadrant, and one in the midline upper abdomen. Continuing assessment now reveals the abdomen to be distended and that hypotension is continuing despite aggressive resuscitation with blood. The patient is rapidly transferred to the operative suite and an abdominal exploration is performed, revealing a liver laceration and partial abdominal aorta laceration. These injuries are repaired, and Conrad survives.

INTRODUCTION TO THORACIC INJURY

tracheobronchial tree the structures of the trachea and the bronchi.

Twenty-five percent of all motor vehicle deaths are due to thoracic trauma (about 12,000 per year in the United States).

co-morbidity associated disease process.

The thoracic cavity contains many vital structures including the heart, great vessels, esophagus, **tracheobronchial tree,** and lungs. Trauma to any one of these structures could lead to a life-threatening event. Twenty-five percent of all motor vehicle deaths are due to thoracic trauma (about 12,000 per year in the United States). The majority of these deaths are secondary to injury to the heart and great vessels. In addition to life threats from intrathoracic injuries, abdominal injuries are also common in patients with traumatic chest injury and can cause significant **co-morbidity.**

The incidence of blunt thoracic trauma has increased with the development of the modern automobile (Figure 10-1 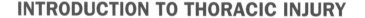). Together with the development of a national highway system, more people are traveling greater distances, at greater speeds, and roadways are becoming more congested. This allows for an increased incidence of motor vehicle collisions (MVCs) and thus an increase in the incidence of thoracic injuries and subsequent deaths, as most blunt thoracic trauma deaths are MVC related. An increase in

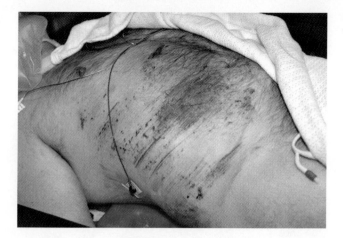

■ Figure 10-1 An example of blunt trauma to the chest. *(Edward T. Dickinson, MD)*

penetrating trauma has also been observed in urban areas associated with violent crime. The weapons used in violent crime in years past were likely to be of the "Saturday night special" variety: cheap, small-caliber revolvers often producing just single wounds. The weapons of choice now are more likely to be large-caliber semiautomatic or automatic weapons that increase the likelihood of multiple missile injuries. With multiple wounds, there is a higher likelihood of injury to vital structures and therefore a higher mortality. Many advances in the treatment of penetrating thoracoabdominal trauma have been made during military conflicts, and the incidence of mortality from these wounds has decreased from 8 to 40 percent during World War II to 3 to 18 percent today.

Prevention efforts have the potential to reduce the occurrence of these injuries. Such efforts include gun control legislation, firearm safety courses, seat belt laws, and better design of automobiles including the development of passive restraint systems such as air bags. Statistics indicate that these efforts have already decreased the incidence of these injuries and the related morbidity and mortality.

In this chapter, we will discuss thoracic trauma in relation to penetrating and blunt injury. These mechanisms have more clinical significance than simple injury categories. Certain injuries are almost exclusively associated with one type of chest trauma but unlikely with the other. For example, pericardial tamponade is almost exclusively associated with penetrating thoracic trauma while cardiac rupture is almost exclusively caused by blunt thoracic trauma. By considering the mechanism of injury, understanding the pathology of the various injuries, and by being aware of the patient's physical signs of injury and symptoms, you will be better able to predict, identify, and treat potential life threats.

Penetrating trauma is increasing in urban areas.

ANATOMY AND PHYSIOLOGY OF THE THORAX

The thoracic cage is the chamber that moves air in and out and where oxygen and carbon dioxide are exchanged to support the body's metabolism. It consists of the thoracic skeleton, diaphragm, and associated musculature. It is also the location of the heart, major blood vessels, and other important structures essential for body function. It contains the trachea, bronchi, lungs, and the mediastinum. Finally, the dynamics of the chest (ventilation) are controlled by a series of centers in the brain and blood vessels.

THORACIC SKELETON

The thoracic skeleton is defined by 12 pairs of C-shaped ribs, which articulate posteriorly with the thoracic spine and then extend in an anterior and inferior direction (Figure 10-2 ■). The upper seven pairs join the sternum at their cartilaginous endpoints. The 8th through 10th ribs have cartilage at their distal anterior ends that join

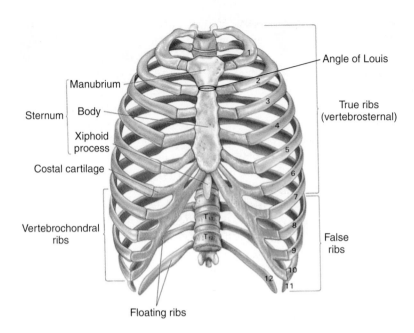

the cartilage of the 7th rib at the inferior margin of the sternum. The 11th and 12th ribs are often termed the floating ribs and have no anterior attachment. The sternum completes the anterior bony structure of the thorax and is made up of three sections: the manubrium, the body of the sternum, and the xiphoid process. The manubrium is the superior portion of the sternum and is the medial endpoint of the clavicle and first rib. The sternal angle (also known as the angle of Louis) is the junction of the manubrium and the body of the sternum and is palpable through the skin as an elevation or prominence. This structure has clinical significance as it is the site of attachment of the second rib and quickly allows the paramedic to identify the second intercostal space. This location is important because it is where you may be required to perform a needle decompression of the chest in the event of a tension pneumothorax. The xiphoid process is the most inferior portion of the sternum and meets the body at the junction of the costal cartilages of the lower ribs.

The thorax is divided by imaginary vertical lines used to describe positions lateral to the sternum. These lines include the midclavicular line, the anterior axillary line, the midaxillary line, and the posterior axillary line. When combined with a rib level, these lines serve as good landmarks for describing wounds, locating underlying structures, and for identifying locations to perform procedures. The space just inferior to each rib is called an intercostal space and is given the number of the rib above it. For example, the anterior axillary line extends from the anterior margin of the axilla (armpit) inferiorly along the thoracic wall. Its intersection with the fifth intercostal space is generally used in the emergency department to place a thoracostomy tube in patients with pneumothorax or hemothorax. It is not frequently used for prehospital needle decompression because this site is often obscured by the patient's arms or by immobilization devices, strapping, and blankets.

The thoracic inlet is the superior opening in the thorax. It is narrow in comparison to the thoracic outlet, and is defined by the curvature of the first rib, with its posterior attachment at the first thoracic vertebra and ending anteriorly, at the manubrium. The thoracic outlet is formed posteriorly by the 12th vertebra, laterally by the curvature of the 12th rib, and extends anteriorly and superiorly along the costal margin to the **xiphisternal joint.**

xiphisternal joint *union between xiphoid process and body of the sternum.*

DIAPHRAGM

The diaphragm is a muscular, domelike structure that separates the abdominal cavity from the thoracic cavity. It is affixed to the lower border of the rib cage, while its central and superior margin may extend to the level of the fourth intercostal space anteriorly and the sixth intercostal space posteriorly during maximal expiration. This superior positioning may allow penetrating wounds of the lower half of the thorax to penetrate the diaphragm and enter the abdominal cavity. The aorta, esophagus, and inferior vena cava exit the thoracic cavity through separate openings in this structure. The diaphragm is a major muscle of respiration, contracting to displace the floor of the thoracic cavity downward during inspiration and relaxing and moving upward with expiration.

ASSOCIATED MUSCULATURE

The chest wall musculature along with the shoulder musculature, clavicles, scapula, and humerus provide additional protection to the vital structures within the upper thorax (Figure 10-3 ■). The clavicles articulate laterally with the acromion process of the scapula. The scapula covers the posterior and lateral aspects of the first six ribs and articulates with the humerus to complete the shoulder girdle. Chest wall muscles found between the ribs, called the intercostal muscles, along with the diaphragm and the sternocleidomastoid muscles are the major muscles of respiration. The sternocleidomastoid muscles raise the upper rib and sternum and, with the sternum, the anterior attachments of the next nine ribs. The intercostal muscles contract to further elevate the ribs and increase the anterior-posterior dimension of the thorax. Simultaneously, the diaphragm, which forms the floor of the thorax, contracts and flattens to further increase the volume of the thoracic cavity. As the thoracic volume increases, the pressure within it becomes less than atmospheric. Air rushes in through the tracheobronchial tree and into the alveoli to equalize this pressure gradient, filling the lungs.

As the musculature relaxes, the diaphragm again intrudes upward into the thoracic cavity, the ribs and sternum move inferiorly, and the ribs move closer together in an inferior and posterior direction. This decreases the thoracic volume and increases the intrathoracic pressure. When the pressure within the thorax exceeds that of the surrounding atmosphere, air rushes out. Therefore exhalation in the resting state is

Normal inspiration is an active process, while normal expiration is a passive process.

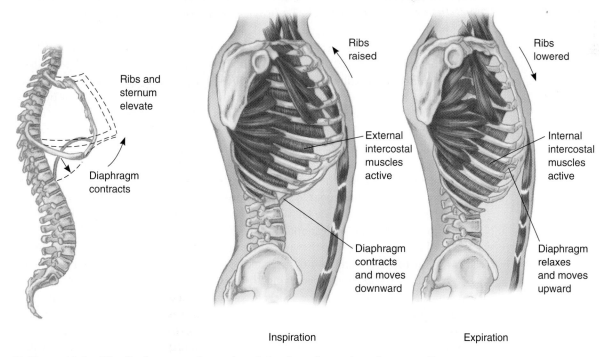

Ribs and sternum elevate

Diaphragm contracts

Ribs raised

External intercostal muscles active

Diaphragm contracts and moves downward

Ribs lowered

Internal intercostal muscles active

Diaphragm relaxes and moves upward

Inspiration

Expiration

■ Figure 10-3 The diaphragm and muscles of the chest change its volume to effect respirations.

largely a passive activity aided by the elastic recoil of the lungs. Gravity helps facilitate this action with downward displacement of the ribs in either the upright or supine position. This changing of volume to move air in and out is called the bellows effect.

The changing volume and pressure within the thoracic cage also assist with the pumping of blood to and venous return from the systemic circulation. The decreased intrathoracic pressure of inspiration helps move venous blood toward the thorax and heart, while the increased pressure of expiration helps move arterial blood away from the heart and thorax. The changing intrathoracic pressure affects the blood pressure and pulse strength. Normally, the systolic blood pressure and pulse strength fall during inspiration and rise during expiration.

The diaphragm is the primary muscle of respiration. The intercostal muscles are recruited to increase the depth of respiration. As the rate, depth, and work of respiration increase due to exercise or stress from trauma or infection, more accessory muscles of ventilation are recruited. These include the sternocleidomastoid and scalene muscles of the neck for inspiration and the anterior abdominal muscles to aid in forceful exhalation. The rhomboid muscles lift, abduct, and rotate the scapulae to help lift the upper chest with inspiration. The cough reflex, important to keeping the airways clear and alveoli expanded, depends on the addition of the latissimus dorsi muscles located along the posterior and lateral thoracic wall and the erector spinae muscles along the spine to allow for forceful contraction of the thorax.

TRACHEA, BRONCHI, AND LUNGS

Contained within the thoracic cavity are the tracheobronchial tree and the lungs (Figure 10-4 ■). The trachea is the hollow and cartilage-supported respiratory pathway through which air moves in and out of the thorax and lungs. It enters through the thoracic inlet and divides into the right and left mainstem bronchi at the carina, located in the upper central thorax. The right and left mainstem bronchi extend for about 3 centimeters and enter their respective lungs at the **pulmonary hilum.** The pulmonary hilum is also where the pulmonary arteries enter and the pulmonary veins exit the lungs and is the sole point of fixation of the lung in the thoracic cage. The bronchi then further divide into bronchioles, which ultimately terminate in the alveoli. The lungs contain millions of these tiny "grape"-shaped alveoli, which are the basic unit of structure and function in the lungs. As air fills the alveoli during ventilation, the oxygen diffuses across the single cell membrane of the alveolus into the capillary (the alveolar-capillary interface) and carbon dioxide diffuses out, and the air is then exhaled (Figure 10-5 ■). This process is external respiration, also referred to as ventilation. Internal respiration occurs at the cellular level, where oxygen diffuses into and carbon dioxide diffuses out of the interstitial and cellular tissues. The alveoli must remain expanded to function in gas exchange.

Each lung occupies one side of the thoracic cavity and is divided into lobes. The right lung has three lobes: the upper, middle, and lower. The left lung has two lobes, the upper and lower. The left upper lobe contains the cardiac notch against which the heart rests. The lower section of the left upper lobe (the lingula) projects around the lateral border of the heart and corresponds to the middle lobe of the right lung.

The lungs are covered by the visceral pleura, a smooth membrane that lines the exterior of the lungs. It folds over on itself at the pulmonary hilum and then lines the inside of the thoracic cavity, becoming the parietal pleura. This dual layer forms a potential space called the pleural space. It contains a small amount of serous (pleural) fluid for lubrication and permits the lungs to expand and contract easily. This dual layer also creates the seal that causes the lungs to expand and contract with the changing volume of the thoracic cavity. If air is allowed to freely enter this potential space, the lung will collapse, producing a pneumothorax.

pulmonary hilum *central medial region of the lung where the bronchi and pulmonary vasculature enter the lung.*

The layers of the pleura and the small volume of fluid between them permit the lungs to move freely with the thoracic cage.

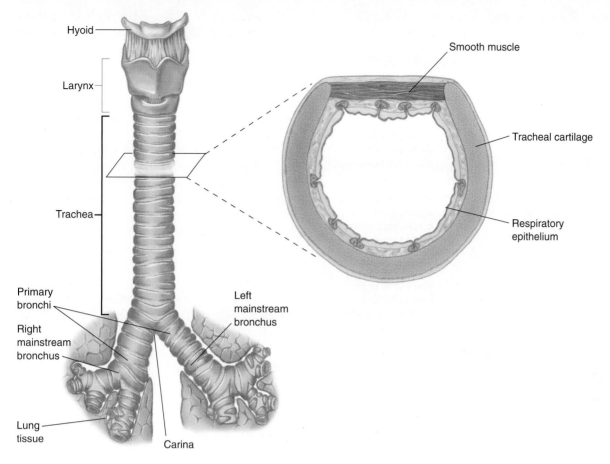

Hyoid

Larynx

Trachea

Primary
bronchi

Right
mainstream
bronchus

Lung
tissue

Carina

Left
mainstream
bronchus

Smooth muscle

Tracheal cartilage

Respiratory
epithelium

■ Figure 10-4   Anatomy of the lower airway.

Lung Volumes

The volume of gas in the lungs at any one time depends on the mechanics of the chest wall musculature, the use of accessory respiratory muscles, and the lung's ability to expand and contract (elasticity). There are four standard lung volumes and four standard lung capacities (Figure 10-6 ■).

Lung Volumes

★ *Tidal volume* is the volume of air entering or leaving the lungs with each breath (approx. 500 mL in a 70-kg adult during resting, quiet respiration).

★ *Residual volume* is the volume of gas left in the lungs after forced maximal expiration (about 1,200 mL in a 70-kg adult).

★ *Expiratory reserve volume* is the volume of gas expelled during forced maximal exhalation starting at the end of normal tidal expiration (about 1,200 mL in a 70-kg adult).

★ *Inspiratory reserve volume* is the volume of gas inhaled into the lungs during a forced maximal inhalation starting at the end of a normal tidal inspiration (about 3,600 mL in a 70-kg adult).

Standard Lung Capacities

★ *Functional residual capacity* is the volume of air left in the lung after a normal tidal exhalation and is equal to the residual volume plus the expiratory reserve volume.

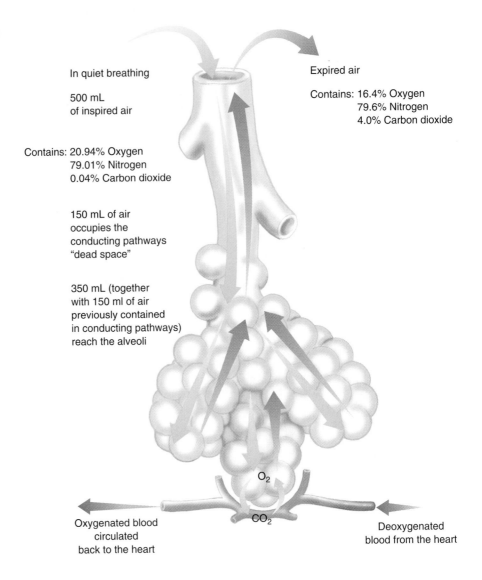

■ **Figure 10-5** Air movement and gas exchange during respiration.

In quiet breathing

500 mL
of inspired air

Contains: 20.94% Oxygen
79.01% Nitrogen
0.04% Carbon dioxide

150 mL of air
occupies the
conducting pathways
"dead space"

350 mL (together
with 150 ml of air
previously contained
in conducting pathways)
reach the alveoli

Expired air

Contains: 16.4% Oxygen
79.6% Nitrogen
4.0% Carbon dioxide

O_2

CO_2

Oxygenated blood
circulated
back to the heart

Deoxygenated
blood from the heart

★ *Inspiratory capacity* is the maximum volume of air inhaled into the lungs after a normal expiration and is equal to the tidal volume plus the inspiratory reserve volume.

★ *Total lung capacity* is the volume of air in the lungs after a maximal inspiratory effort and is the sum of all four of the lung volumes (about 6,500 mL in a normal 70-kg adult).

★ *Vital capacity* is the volume of air forcefully exhaled after a maximal forced inspiration and equals the total lung capacity minus the residual volume.

Other Lung Volumes and Spaces

★ *Minute volume* describes the volume of air exhaled in 1 minute and equals the tidal volume times respiratory rate.

★ *Dead space volume* is divided into two main categories, anatomical and alveolar.

★ *Anatomical dead space* is the volume of air that remains in the tracheobronchial tree and does not reach the alveoli for gas exchange.

★ *Alveolar dead space* is the volume of air in the alveoli that is not perfused and in which no gas exchange with the alveolar capillary bed occurs.

★ *Physiological dead space* is the sum of alveolar and anatomical dead space.

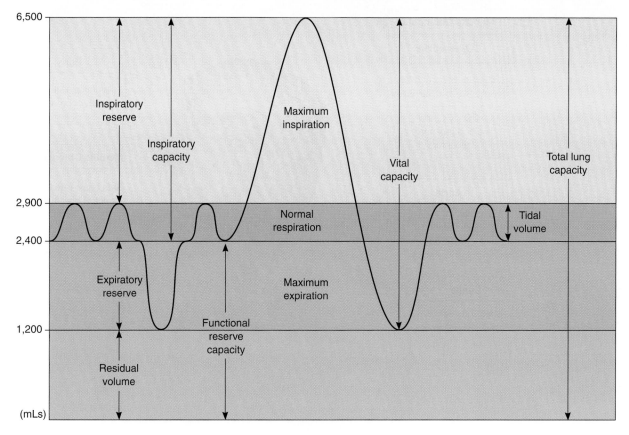

■ Figure 10-6   Respiration volumes.

Respiratory Control

Respiratory centers within the brainstem control respiration (Figure 10-7 ■). Inspiration and expiration occur automatically and are triggered by impulses generated in the respiratory center of the medulla oblongata during normal respiration (eupnea). The medullary respiratory center contains central chemoreceptors that respond to changes in the CO_2 and pH levels in the cerebrospinal fluid. CO_2 rapidly diffuses across the blood–brain barrier into the cerebrospinal fluid (CSF) while hydrogen ions and bicarbonate ions (HCO_3^-) do not. Hypoventilation and increasing CO_2 levels in the blood stimulate the respiratory rate and increase respiratory volume while hyperventilation and decreasing CO_2 levels decrease the blood and CSF pH and inhibit the respiratory rate and decrease the respiratory volume. This mechanism also permits the respiratory system to play an active role in controlling the blood's pH by increasing respiration (hyperventilation and respiratory alkalosis) in the presence of acidosis or decreasing ventilation (hypoventilating and respiratory acidosis) when the pH rises. These processes provide rapid compensatory mechanisms when the body is exposed to metabolic pH disturbances like metabolic acidosis or alkalosis. Because bicarbonate does not diffuse across the barrier, it is possible to have a metabolic acidosis with a CSF alkalosis that will lead to hypoventilation and subsequent worsening of the peripheral acidosis. The central chemoreceptors do not respond to blood oxygen levels, and specifically, hypoxia.

Peripheral chemoreceptors in the carotid and aortic bodies also help regulate respiration. Hypoxemia ($PaO_2 < 60$ mmHg) stimulates the peripheral chemoreceptors to increase the respiratory rate but to a lesser degree than the effect CO_2 has on the medullary respiratory center. In chronic obstructive pulmonary disease (COPD), where there is chronic CO_2 retention, the chemoreceptors become desensitized to high CO_2 levels and do not respond by increasing the respiratory rate. The **hypoxic drive** is then

hypoxic drive   *mechanism that increases respiratory stimulation when PaO_2 falls and inhibits respiratory stimulation when PaO_2 climbs.*

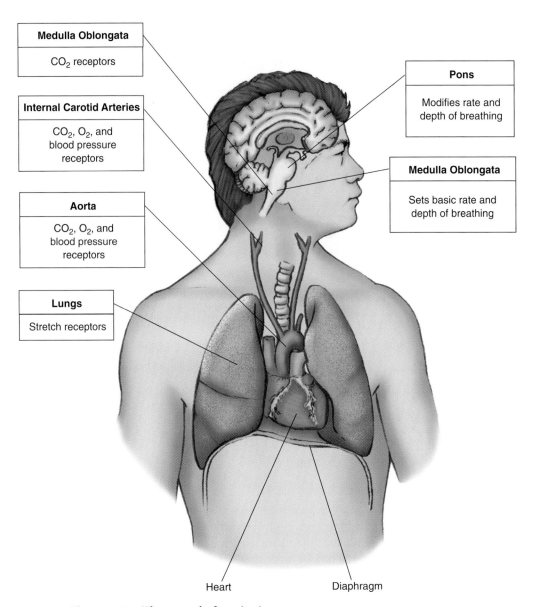

Medulla Oblongata	Pons
CO_2 receptors	Modifies rate and depth of breathing

Internal Carotid Arteries	Medulla Oblongata
CO_2, O_2, and blood pressure receptors	Sets basic rate and depth of breathing

Aorta

CO_2, O_2, and blood pressure receptors

Lungs

Stretch receptors

Heart   Diaphragm

■ Figure 10-7   The control of respiration.

the main stimulus to ventilation. That is why it becomes important not to raise the arterial PO_2 much above 60 torr in the COPD patient who uses the hypoxic drive to control respiration. There is also some input to the respiratory center by peripheral baroreceptors in the carotids and aorta that respond to blood vessel stretch or increases in blood pressure by decreasing respiratory rate and producing bronchodilation.

Two respiratory centers in the pons also contribute to the control of respiration. The apneustic center located in the lower pons acts as the shut-off switch to inspiration. If it becomes nonfunctional, the respiratory pattern exhibits prolonged inspiration interrupted by occasional expirations. The pneumotaxic center is located in the upper pons, above the apneustic center, and acts to moderate the activity of the apneustic center and provide further fine tuning of the respiratory pattern.

Two respiratory reflexes are protective of the air passages. The sigh reflex is a deeper than normal inspiration followed by a slower than normal exhalation that irregularly and occasionally occurs in the normal physiologic state. This reflex recruits and expands the alveoli that may become atelectatic (collapsed) with normal quiet respira-

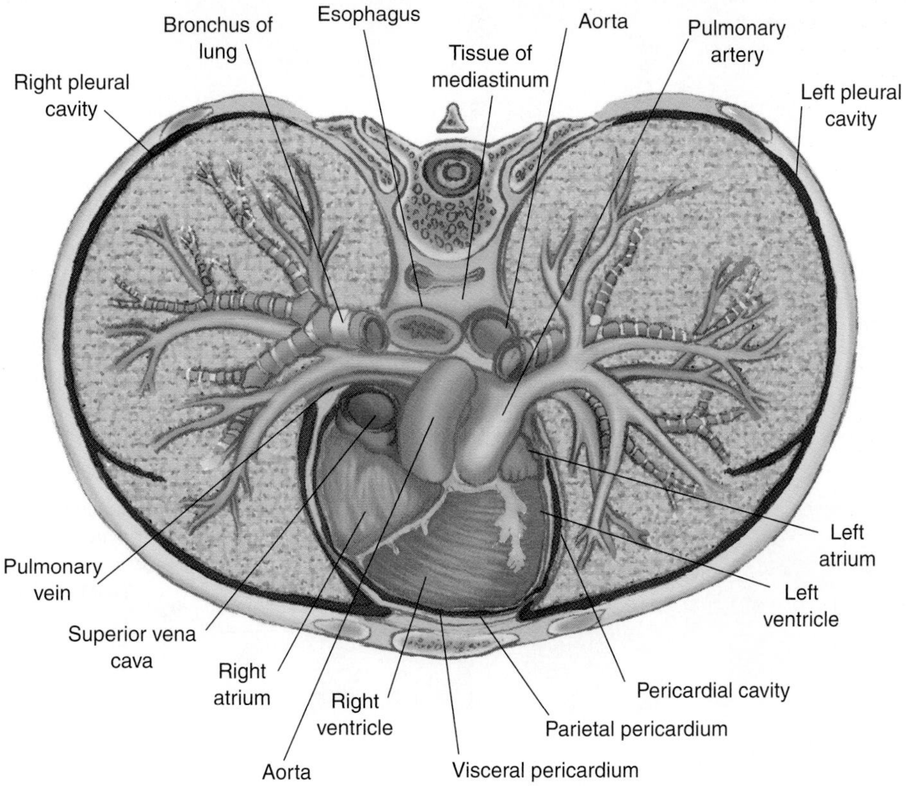

Right pleural cavity

Bronchus of lung

Esophagus

Tissue of mediastinum

Aorta

Pulmonary artery

Left pleural cavity

Pulmonary vein

Superior vena cava

Right atrium

Right ventricle

Aorta

Visceral pericardium

Parietal pericardium

Pericardial cavity

Left ventricle

Left atrium

■ Figure 10-8   Structures of the mediastinum and thorax.

tion. If mechanical ventilation is required after traumatic chest injury, a sigh is often programmed into the ventilator settings to prevent **atelectasis.** The cough reflex is a spasmodic contraction of the diaphragm to expel foreign material from the bronchi, trachea, and larynx.

atelectasis   *collapse of a lung or part of a lung.*

MEDIASTINUM

The mediastinum is the central space within the thoracic cavity bounded laterally by the lungs, inferiorly by the diaphragm, and superiorly by the thoracic inlet (Figure 10-8 ■). The heart is located within and fills most of the mediastinum. Through this structure the **great vessels** traverse to and from the heart, and the trachea and esophagus enter the thorax. The esophagus then courses anterior to the aorta before exiting through the diaphragm at the thoracic outlet (esophageal hiatus or foramen). The vagus nerve, which provides parasympathetic innervation of thoracic and abdominal viscera, enters the thorax bilaterally through the thoracic inlet and traverses the mediastinum giving branches to the larynx, esophagus, trachea, bronchi, and heart. The vagus nerve then exits the thorax through the esophageal opening in the diaphragm to innervate the abdominal viscera. The phrenic nerve (originating from the third, fourth, and fifth cervical nerve roots) also enters the thorax through the thoracic inlet and traverses the thorax to innervate the diaphragm.

great vessels   *large arteries and veins located in the mediastinum that enter and exit the heart.*

The thoracic duct (part of the lymphatic system) also traverses the thorax from the thoracic outlet where it enters through the aortic opening in the diaphragm. It typically crosses the midline from the right side of the aorta in the posterior mediastinum at the level of the fifth thoracic vertebra and then ascends above the level of the left clavicle before arching back downward to empty into the left internal jugular vein. The thoracic duct carries most of the body's lymphatic drainage (all but the right side of the head, neck, thorax, and right upper extremity).

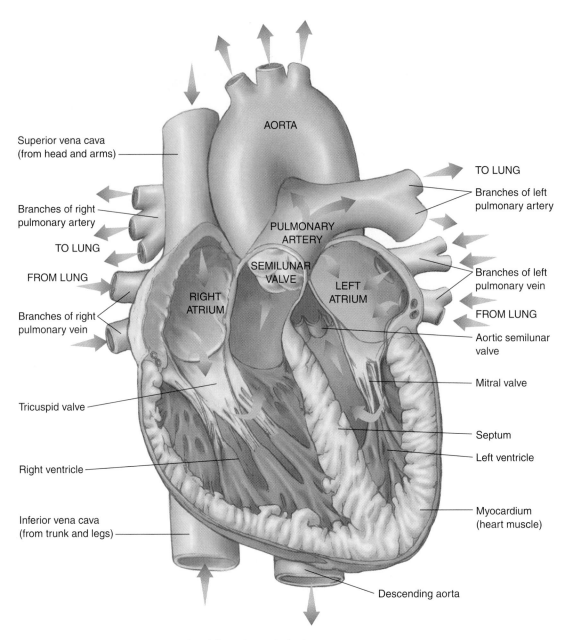

Superior vena cava
(from head and arms)

AORTA

Branches of right
pulmonary artery

TO LUNG

FROM LUNG

Branches of right
pulmonary vein

Tricuspid valve

Right ventricle

Inferior vena cava
(from trunk and legs)

PULMONARY
ARTERY

SEMILUNAR
VALVE

RIGHT
ATRIUM

LEFT
ATRIUM

TO LUNG

Branches of left
pulmonary artery

Branches of left
pulmonary vein

FROM LUNG

Aortic semilunar
valve

Mitral valve

Septum

Left ventricle

Myocardium
(heart muscle)

Descending aorta

▧ Figure 10-9   Blood flow through the heart.

HEART

The heart is a four-chambered pump, divided into right and left sides (Figure 10-9 ▧).
Each side has an upper chamber termed an atrium, and a lower chamber termed a ventricle. The right heart circulates blood to the lungs and the left heart circulates blood to
the rest of the body. The blood enters the heart at the right atrium, and traverses the tricuspid valve to enter the right ventricle. Blood then leaves the right heart through the
pulmonary semilunar valve and travels through the pulmonary arteries (right and left)
to the lungs where it is oxygenated and carbon dioxide is eliminated in the alveolar capillary bed. Blood then returns to the heart via the pulmonary veins (4) and enters the
left atrium before passing through the mitral valve to the left ventricle. From the left
ventricle, it exits the heart through the aortic semilunar valve into the aorta and on to
the systemic circulation.

The heart muscle receives its blood supply via the coronary arteries, which leave the
aorta just above the aortic semilunar valve leaflets. The coronary arteries primarily fill in

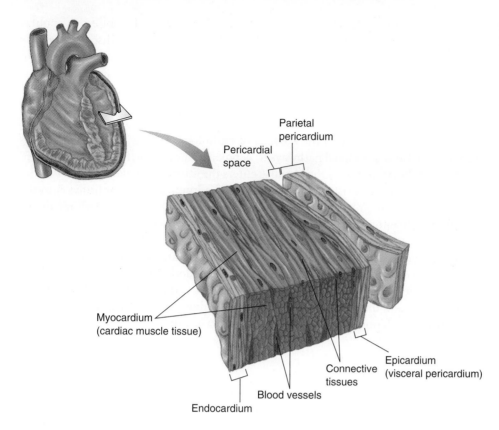

Parietal
pericardium

Pericardial
space

Myocardium
(cardiac muscle tissue)

Connective
tissues

Epicardium
(visceral pericardium)

Blood vessels

Endocardium

diastole. Tachycardia can therefore limit coronary artery blood flow. The endocardial (within the heart muscle) vessels are also constricted somewhat by the systolic contraction of the myocardium, further limiting coronary blood flow and increasing the risk for ischemia. Atherosclerosis accentuates this limitation in coronary blood flow. The epicardial blood flow is not affected by systolic muscular contraction because the epicardial vessels lie on the surface of the heart muscle and do not suffer external compression by the muscle. The more internal cardiac muscle tissue is, therefore, more susceptible to ischemia.

A membranous lining, the **pericardium,** surrounds the heart and the space containing it and is similar to the pleura of the lungs (Figure 10-10 ■). The portion of this lining that covers the outer surface of the heart is the **epicardium,** or visceral pericardium. It then extends to the root of the great vessels before folding back on itself to form the parietal pericardium, which forms the outer lining of the pericardial sac that surrounds the heart. These two layers make up the serous pericardium and, like the pleura, also form a potential space, the pericardial space. The pericardial space may be filled with a straw-colored pericardial fluid secreted by the visceral pericardium. The space usually contains a small amount of fluid and no more than 35 to 50 mL in the normal physiological state. The fluid functions mainly as a lubricant between the visceral and parietal layers. It also may provide some protection against local infection from adjacent structures such as the lungs or pleural space. External to the serous pericardium is a tough fibrous sac called the fibrous pericardium that, unlike the serous pericardium, resists distention. The fibrous pericardium originates at the base of the great vessels and surrounds the heart and serous pericardium before fusing with the central tendon of the diaphragm. This pericardial structure somewhat fixes the heart in the mediastinum and prevents the kinking of the great vessels. If the pericardial space rapidly fills with blood, the fibrous pericardium resists the passive filling of the heart and thereby reduces cardiac output (pericardial tamponade).

The **myocardium** is the muscular layer of the heart. It consists of very specialized muscle cells that require a constant supply of oxygenated circulation to provide their

pericardium *fibrous sac that surrounds the heart.*

epicardium *serous membrane covering the outer surface of the heart; the visceral pericardium.*

myocardium *the cardiac muscle tissue of the heart.*

continuous pumping function. These specialized cells have the ability to spontaneously depolarize and have specialized structures (intercalated discs) to rapidly conduct impulses throughout the myocardium, allowing the atria and ventricles to contract separately as units. The heart also contains specialized conduction tissue that functions as the heart's pacemaker. The sinoatrial (SA) node, located in the right atrium, is the most rapidly depolarizing area of the conduction system and by overdrive suppression (the most rapidly depolarizing tissue takes over as the pacemaker) sets the heart rate in the absence of pathology. The impulse then traverses the interatrial and intraatrial pathways to depolarize the atria before entering the AV junction. In the AV junction the impulse enters the atrioventricular node (AV node) that delays the impulse as the atria contract. The impulse then continues into the bundle of His before traversing the bundle branches (right and left), Purkinje fibers, and ultimately entering the ventricular musculature to facilitate ventricular contraction.

The innermost lining of the heart is called the endocardium. This layer also covers the heart valves and becomes continuous with the endothelial lining of the great vessels. It provides a smooth inner surface to the heart and prevents clotting along the chamber walls and the exchange of oxygen, carbon dioxide, nutrients, and waste products between the blood in the chambers and the myocardium.

GREAT VESSELS

ligamentum arteriosum
cordlike remnant of a fetal vessel connecting the pulmonary artery to the aorta at the aortic isthmus.

The great vessels are those large arteries and veins that enter and leave the heart and are found in the mediastinum. They are the aorta, the superior and inferior vena cava, the pulmonary arteries, and the pulmonary veins. Injury to these large vascular structures can lead to significant blood loss and death if the condition is not quickly recognized and repaired. The aorta, which is fixed at three positions within the thorax, is not only susceptible to penetrating injury, but also to blunt injury by rapid deceleration or shear forces. It is fixed at the annulus where it attaches to the heart, at the **ligamentum arteriosum** near the bifurcation of the pulmonary artery, and at the aortic hiatus where it passes through the diaphragm and enters the abdomen.

Other major vessels that branch from the great vessels in the upper thorax include the subclavian arteries and veins, the common carotid arteries, and the brachiocephalic artery (which is the first large branch off the aortic arch dividing into the right common carotid and right subclavian). The internal mammary vessels are inferior branches of the subclavians running along the anterior surface of the pleura, posterior to the costochondral (rib-cartilage) junction. They are often harvested for coronary artery bypass grafts. The intercostal arteries are branches of the thoracic aorta (except for the first two, which arise from branches of the subclavian) that run along the lower margins of the ribs along with the intercostal nerves. Finally, the bronchial arteries (one right and two left) are usually branches of the thoracic aorta that nourish the nonrespiratory tissues of the lung.

ESOPHAGUS

The esophagus enters the thorax through the thoracic inlet with and just posterior to the trachea. It continues the length of the mediastinum and exits through the esophageal hiatus of the diaphragm. It is a muscular tube that is contiguous with the posterior wall of the trachea and conducts food and drink from the oral pharynx to the stomach. It moves food and liquid toward the stomach through a rhythmic muscular contraction called peristalsis. During vomiting, peristalsis reverses and propels the emesis up the esophagus.

PATHOPHYSIOLOGY OF THORACIC TRAUMA

Thoracic trauma is classified into two major categories by mechanism: blunt and penetrating. It is important to examine these injury mechanisms and their effects on the organs of the thorax.

BLUNT TRAUMA

Blunt thoracic trauma is injury resulting from kinetic energy forces transmitted through the tissues. These injuries may be further subdivided by mechanism into blast, crush (compression), and deceleration injuries.

Blast injuries result from an explosive chemical reaction that creates a pressure wave travelling outward from the epicenter. This pressure wave causes tissue disruption by dramatic compression and then decompression as the wave passes. In the thorax, this action may tear blood vessels and disrupt the alveolar tissue. These injuries may lead to hemorrhage, pneumothoraces, and air embolism (air entering the disrupted pulmonary vasculature and subsequently returning to the central circulation). Other injuries associated with a blast mechanism can include disruption of the tracheobronchial tree and traumatic rupture of the diaphragm. When the blast occurs in a confined space, the pressure wave may be contained and accentuated. The result is an increase in the incidence and severity of the associated injuries.

Crush injuries occur when the body is compressed between an object and a hard surface. This leads to direct injury or disruption of the chest wall, diaphragm, heart, or tracheobronchial tree. If the victim remains pinned between two objects, significant restriction in ventilation and venous return may occur, also known as traumatic asphyxia.

Deceleration injuries occur when the body is in motion and impacts a fixed object, such as when the chest impacts against the steering column in a front-end collision (Figure 10-11 ■). This impact causes a direct blunt injury to the chest wall while the internal organs of the thoracic cavity continue in motion. The organs and structures then impact with the internal surface of the thoracic cavity and may be compressed as more posterior structures collide with them. If the organ or structure has points of fixation, as with the aorta at the ligamentum arteriosum, the force of the organ moving against this point of fixation (shear force) can lead to a traumatic disruption. These sudden deceleration and shear forces can cause disruption of the myocardium, great vessel, lung,

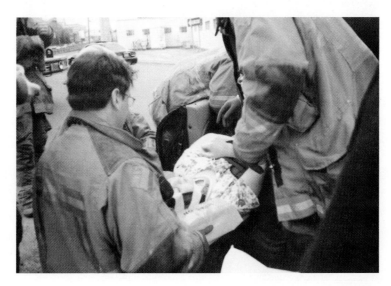

■ Figure 10-11   Frontal impact auto crashes frequently result in chest trauma.

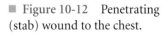

The age of the blunt trauma victim may affect the seriousness of the trauma received.

trachea, and bronchi. The rapid compression of the chest, especially against a closed glottis, may also cause alveolar and tracheobronchial rupture and pneumothorax.

The age of the blunt trauma victim may affect the trauma received and its seriousness. The cartilaginous nature of the pediatric thorax spares the infant or child from rib fractures but more easily transmits the energy of trauma to the vital organs below. The result is less significant signs of injury, few rib fractures, and a greater incidence of serious internal injury. The geriatric patient responds very differently to blunt chest trauma. That patient will suffer more frequent rib fracture than the younger adult due to calcification of the skeletal system. Though the greater incidence of rib fracture may somewhat protect the underlying organs, preexisting disease and the progressive reduction of respiratory and cardiac reserves result in a greater morbidity and mortality from serious chest trauma.

PENETRATING TRAUMA

Penetrating thoracic trauma induces injury as an object enters the chest and causes either direct trauma or secondary injury from transmitted kinetic energy forces related to the cavitational wave of high-velocity projectiles. Penetrating chest trauma can be subdivided into three categories: low energy, high energy, and shotgun wounds.

Low-energy wounds are those caused by arrows, knives, hand guns, and other relatively slow-moving objects (Figure 10-12 ■). They cause injury by direct contact or very limited creation of temporary cavities. The injury that occurs from this type of wound is related to the direct path that the missile or object takes.

High-energy wounds are caused by military and hunting rifles (and some high-powered hand guns at close range) that fire missiles at very high velocity. Their veloc-

■ Figure 10-12   Penetrating (stab) wound to the chest.

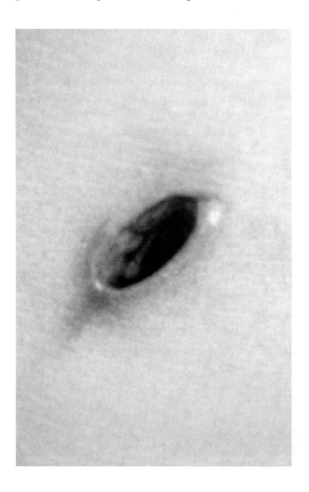

ity gives the projectile very high kinetic energy. As the projectile passes through tissue, it creates a shock wave, tissue movement (including compression and stretching), and a large temporary cavity. These wounds cause extensive tissue damage perpendicular to the track of the projectile.

Shotgun wounds are classified according to the distance between the victim and the shotgun. A smaller gauge (a larger caliber) of shotgun and a larger size of shot also increase the effective range and penetrating power of the weapon and its potential to cause tissue damage. Type I injuries are those where the target is greater than 7 meters from the gun barrel at discharge. The pellets usually penetrate the skin and subcutaneous tissue but rarely penetrate the deep fascia to cause body cavity penetration. Type II injuries occur at a distance of 3 to 7 meters and often permit the pellets to penetrate the deep fascia with internal organ injury possible. Type III injuries occur at a distance of less than 3 meters and usually involve massive tissue destruction and life-threatening injury.

Shotgun wounds within 3 meters of the discharging barrel cause serious tissue destruction and are frequently life threatening.

Penetrating thoracic trauma is often related to the structures involved. Lung tissue is very resilient when impacted by high-energy projectiles. The "spongy" nature of the air-filled alveoli absorbs the energy of cavitation and reduces the size of the temporary cavity and injury associated with the compression and stretching. The great vessels and heart (if it is distended with blood) respond much differently. The fluid transmits the kinetic energy very well and may result in cardiac or vessel rupture. With slower moving projectiles, or if the heart is struck while in diastole, the result may be a simple penetration. While a projectile tends to move in a straight line, it is easily deflected by contact with a rib, clavicle, scapula, or the spinal column. Contact with skeletal structures may also fragment the projectile (as well as the skeletal structure), increasing the rate of energy exchange and the seriousness of injury. Penetrating trauma frequently leads to pneumothorax, which may be bilateral, depending on the track of the missile or knife. Table 10–1 lists common injuries associated with penetrating thoracic trauma.

CHEST WALL INJURIES

Chest wall injuries are by far the most common injuries encountered in blunt chest trauma. As previously discussed, an intact and moving chest wall is necessary to develop

Chest wall injuries are by far the most common injuries encountered in blunt chest trauma.

Table 10–1	Injuries Associated with Penetrating Thoracic Trauma
Closed pneumothorax	
Open pneumothorax (including sucking chest wound)	
Tension pneumothorax	
Pneumomediastinum	
Hemothorax	
Hemopneumothorax	
Laceration of vascular structures, including the great vessels	
Tracheobronchial tree lacerations	
Esophageal lacerations	
Penetrating cardiac injuries	
Pericardial tamponade	
Spinal cord injuries	
Diaphragmatic penetration/laceration/rupture	
Intra-abdominal penetration with associated organ injury	

the pressures essential for air movement into and out of the lungs (the bellows effect). Chest wall injury may disrupt this motion and result in respiratory insufficiency. Closed injuries of the chest wall include contusions, rib fractures, sternal fractures/dislocations, and flail chest. Open injuries to the chest wall are almost entirely due to penetrating trauma and are often associated with deep structure injury in addition to disruption of the changing intrathoracic pressure necessary for respiration.

Chest Wall Contusion

Chest wall contusion is the most common result of blunt injury to the thorax. The injury damages the soft tissue covering the thoracic cage and causes pain with respiratory effort. Like contusions elsewhere, contusion of the chest wall may present with erythema initially, then ecchymosis. The discoloration may outline the object that caused the trauma, may outline the ribs as the soft tissue is trapped between the ribs and the offending agent, or may outline a combination of both. The most noticeable symptom of chest wall contusion is pain, made worse with deep breathing and possibly resulting in reduced chest expansion. The area will be tender at the contusion site, and you may observe decreased chest wall movement due to pain. You may auscultate limited breath sounds because of decreased air movement due to limited chest expansion.

The pain of chest wall contusion and associated limiting of deep inspiration may lead to hypoventilation. Hypoventilation may not be apparent in a young, otherwise healthy individual and may not pose a significant life threat due to the individual's significant pulmonary reserves. The aged patient, however, often has preexisting medical problems, little pulmonary reserve, and does not tolerate this injury as well. Such a patient quickly becomes hypoxemic (low oxygen levels in the blood) without proper respiratory support. In a pediatric patient, the ribs are very flexible, resist fracture, and easily transmit the forces of trauma. The result may be chest wall contusion and internal injury without rib fracture.

Rib Fracture

Rib fractures are found in more than 50 percent of cases of significant chest trauma from blunt mechanisms. Rib fractures are likely to occur at the point of impact or along the border of the object that impacts the chest (Figure 10-13 ■). Fractures may also occur at a location remote from the injury site. The thoracic cage is a hollow cylinder that has some flex to it. As the compressional force of blunt trauma deforms the thorax, the ribs flex and may fracture at their weakest point, the posterior angle (along the posterior axillary line).

Ribs 4 through 8 are the most commonly fractured as they are least protected by other structures and are firmly fixed at both ends (to the spine and sternum). It takes great force to fracture ribs 1 through 3 because the shoulder, scapula, and the heavy musculature of the upper chest protect them. Their fracture is more likely associated with severe intrathoracic injuries (tracheobronchial tree injury, aortic rupture, and other vascular injuries), especially if multiple ribs are involved. Ribs 9 through 12 are less firmly attached to the sternum, are relatively mobile, and are thus less likely to fracture. However, they better transmit the energy of trauma to internal organs and may permit intra-abdominal injury without fracture. Fractures of ribs 9 through 12 are frequently associated with serious trauma and splenic or hepatic injury.

The incidence and significance of rib fracture varies with age. The pediatric patient has very cartilaginous ribs that bend easily. The ribs resist fracture and transmit kinetic forces to the thoracic and abdominal structures underneath. The pediatric patient hence has a decreased incidence of rib fracture and an increase in the incidence of underlying injury. The geriatric patient, however, has ribs that are calcified, less flexible, and more easily fractured. The geriatric patient is also more likely to have co-morbidity like COPD, which reduces respiratory reserves and compounds the effects of rib injury. If multiple rib fractures are noted in a young adult, they are probably associated with severe trauma

Chest wall contusion is the most common result of blunt injury to the thorax.

✓ Review

Signs and Symptoms of Chest Wall Injuries

Blunt or penetrating trauma to chest
Erythema
Ecchymosis
Dyspnea
Pain on breathing
Limited breath sounds
Hypoventilation
Crepitus
Paradoxical motion of chest wall

Rib fractures are found in more than 50 percent of cases of significant chest trauma from blunt mechanisms.

Ribs 4 through 8 are the most commonly fractured.

In pediatric patients, more flexible ribs permit more serious internal injury before fracture occurs.

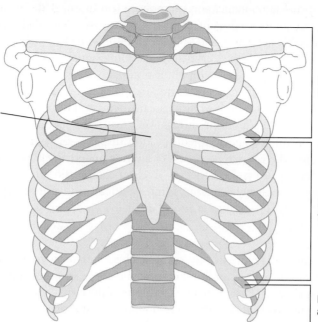

Great force is required for sternal fractures.

Ribs 1-3 are well protected by shoulder bones and muscles.

Ribs 4-8 are most frequently fractured.

Ribs 9-12 are relatively mobile and fracture less frequently.

■ Figure 10-13   Rib fractures.

and may lead to significant pain, splinting, hypoventilation, and inadequate cough. They also are likely to be associated with significant internal injuries. The mortality associated with rib fractures increases with the number of fractures, extremes of age (the very young or very old), and associated chronic respiratory or cardiac problems, especially in the elderly trauma victim.

The rib fracture is likely to be associated with an overlying chest wall contusion and presents with those signs and symptoms. The fracture site may also demonstrate a grating sensation (crepitus) as the bone ends move against each other, either during chest wall movement or during direct palpation. The pain associated with rib fracture is greater than that with chest wall contusion and will more greatly limit respiratory excursion. This reduced chest wall excursion frequently leads to hypoxia, hypoventilation, and muscle spasms at the fracture site. Hypoventilation can result in a progressive collapse of alveoli called atelectasis. This collapse reduces the lung surface available for gas exchange and contributes to hypoxia. These atelectatic segments also may become filled with blood or tissue fluid due to the injury and set the stage for secondary infection such as pneumonia. While pneumonia does not develop in the emergency setting, it is the cause of a significant mortality in blunt chest injury patients. Serious internal injuries may also result as the jagged rib ends move about and lacerate structures beneath them. Laceration of the intercostal arteries may result in hemothorax, while damage to the intercostal nerves may result in a neurologic deficit. Fracture and displacement of the lower ribs may injure the liver (right) or spleen (left).

Rib fracture mortality increases with the number of fractures, extremes of age, and associated disease.

Sternal Fracture and Dislocation

Sternal fractures and dislocations are usually associated with blunt anterior chest trauma. Sternal fracture results only from severe impact, as this region of the chest is well supported by the ribs and clavicles. The most likely mechanism is a direct blow, a fall against a fixed object, or the blunt force of the sternum against the steering wheel or dashboard in a motor vehicle crash. The overall incidence of sternal fracture in thoracic trauma patients is between 5 and 8 percent. However, the mortality associated with it is between 25 and 45 percent due to underlying myocardial contusion, cardiac rupture,

Sternal fracture is frequently associated with serious myocardial injury.

pericardial tamponade, and pulmonary contusion. If the surrounding ribs or costochondral joints are disrupted, the injury may result in a flail chest. The injury results in a noticeable deformity and possible crepitus with chest wall movement or palpation.

Dislocation at the sternoclavicular joint is uncommon and also requires significant force. It too may occur with blunt trauma to the anterior chest or with a lateral compression mechanism, as in side impact collisions or falls with the patient landing on the shoulder. The clavicle may dislocate from the sternum in one of two ways, anteriorly or posteriorly. The anterior dislocation creates a noticeable deformity anterior to the manubrium. The posterior dislocation displaces the head of the clavicle behind the sternum where it may compress or lacerate underlying great vessels or compress or injure the trachea and esophagus. Tracheal compression may result in stridor and voice change, though any deformity is more difficult to identify except that the shoulder may noticeably displace anteriorly and medially.

Flail Chest

Flail chest is a segment of the chest that becomes free to move with the pressure changes of respiration. The condition occurs when three or more adjacent ribs fracture in two or more places (Figure 10-14 ■). It is one of the most serious chest wall injuries because it is often associated with severe underlying pulmonary injury (contusion) and it reduces the volume of respiration and increases the effort associated with it. This underlying injury adds to mortality in serious thoracic trauma (between 20 and 40 percent), as does age, head injury, shock, and other associated injuries. The most common mechanisms of injury causing flail chest are blunt traumas from falls, motor vehicle crashes, industrial injuries, and assaults.

The flail segment created by this injury is no longer a controlled component of the chest wall and bellows system. Increasing intrathoracic pressure associated with expiration moves the flail segment outward while the rest of the chest moves inward, pushing air under the moving segment that would normally be exhaled. This reduces the change in chest volume caused by the breathing effort as well as the volume of air expired and draws the mediastinum toward the injury. During inspiration, the intrathoracic pressure falls as the respiratory muscles move the chest wall outward and the diaphragm drops caudally (tail-ward). The reduced pressure draws the flail segment inward. The lung beneath it moves away from the inward-moving segment, reducing the

flail chest *defect in the chest wall that allows for free movement of a segment. Breathing will cause paradoxical chest wall motion.*

■ Figure 10-14 Flail chest occurs when three or more adjacent ribs fracture in two or more places.

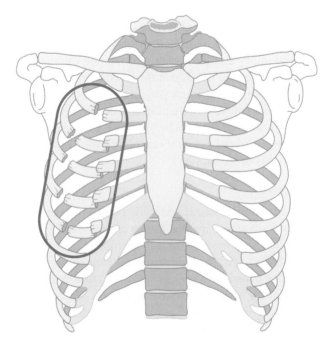

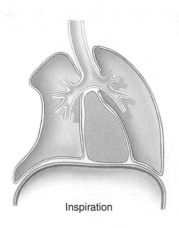
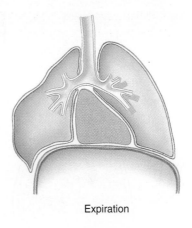

Inspiration   Expiration

■ Figure 10-15   Paradoxical movement of the chest wall seen in flail chest.

volume of air moving into the thorax and displacing the mediastinum away from the injury. In summary, the injury produces a segment of the chest wall that moves in opposition to the chest's normal respiratory effort (paradoxical movement), it reduces the volume of air moved with each breath, and it displaces the mediastinum toward and then away from the injury site with each breath (Figure 10-15 ■). In flail chest, the patient takes more energy to move less air and the respiratory volume is further reduced as the rib fracture pain produces a natural splinting of the chest.

It takes tremendous energy to create these six fracture sites (three or more ribs fractured in two or more places) and, accordingly, flail chest is often associated with serious internal injury. In addition, the movement of the flail segment, which is opposite to the rest of the chest wall, is damaging to surrounding tissue. With each breath, the bone fracture sites move against one another causing further muscle damage, soft-tissue damage, and pain. Small flail segments may go undetected as the associated intercostal muscle spasm naturally splints the segment. With time, however, these muscles suffer further injury and fatigue and the flail segment's paradoxical movement may become more and more apparent.

Positive-pressure ventilation of the patient with flail chest reverses the mechanism that causes the paradoxical chest wall movement, restores the tidal volume, and reduces the pain of chest wall movement. It accomplishes this by pushing the chest wall and the flail segment outward with positive pressure. Passive expiration then may cause both the flail segment and the rest of the chest to move inward, again, together. However, in the presence of underlying injury, positive-pressure ventilation may induce pneumothorax.

Over time, the muscles splinting the flail segment will fatigue, and paradoxical respiration will become more evident.

PULMONARY INJURIES

Pulmonary injuries are injuries to lung tissue or injuries that damage the system that holds the lung to the interior of the thoracic cavity. They include the simple pneumothorax, open pneumothorax, tension pneumothorax, hemothorax, and pulmonary contusion.

Simple Pneumothorax

Simple **pneumothorax** (also known as closed pneumothorax) occurs when lung tissue is disrupted and air leaks into the pleural space (Figure 10-16 ■). While there may be an external, and possibly penetrating, wound, there is no communication between the pleural space and the atmosphere. The pressure within the thorax does not exceed normal expiratory pressures and there is no associated mediastinal shift. As more and more air accumulates in the pleural space, the lung collapses. With lung collapse, the alveoli collapse (atelectasis) and blood flowing past the collapsed alveoli does not exchange oxygen and carbon dioxide. As more and more of the alveoli collapse, this condition, called ventilation/perfusion mismatch, becomes more pronounced and begins to lower

pneumothorax   *air in the pleural space.*

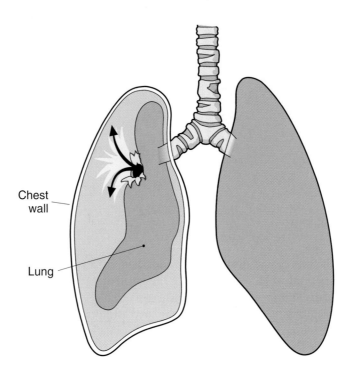

Chest
wall

Lung

the blood oxygen level (hypoxemia). This soon becomes life endangering, especially if there are other associated injuries or shock.

Simple pneumothorax can occur with penetrating and blunt mechanisms. Blunt trauma may cause a pneumothorax when a rib fracture directly punctures the lung. Another mechanism may cause alveolar rupture from a sudden increase in intrathoracic pressure as the chest impacts the steering column with fully expanded lungs and a closed glottis (much like a paper bag filled with air and compressed suddenly between two hands). The incidence of pneumothorax in serious thoracic trauma is between 10 and 30 percent and its morbidity is related to the amount of atelectasis and the degree of perfusion mismatch. Penetrating trauma to the chest is frequently associated with simple pneumothorax, or with an injury that allows air to enter the pleural space through an external wound (open pneumothorax).

A simple pneumothorax reduces the efficiency of respiration and quickly leads to hypoxia. The hypoxia and increase in blood levels of CO_2 cause the medulla to increase the respiratory rate (tachypnea) and volume. If only a very small portion of the lung is involved, there may be no apparent signs or symptoms. A larger pneumothorax may cause mild dyspnea, or complete lung collapse may result in severe dyspnea and hypoxia. The signs, symptoms, and significance of simple pneumothorax increase with preexisting disease. Pneumothorax may produce local chest pain with respiration as the pleurae become irritated (respirophasic pain). The pathology may cause the chest to hyperinflate and breath sounds to diminish on the affected side (usually in the extremes of the upper and lower lung first). A small pneumothorax involving collapse of less than 15 percent of the affected lung may be difficult to detect clinically and requires only supportive measures. Often the small pneumothorax will seal itself and the air in the pleural cavity will be absorbed. A larger pneumothorax is often clinically apparent and requires more aggressive therapy such as high-flow, high-concentration oxygen and chest tube placement (in the emergency department).

Open Pneumothorax

Open pneumothorax is most commonly noted in military conflicts when a high-velocity bullet creates a significant wound in the chest wall (usually the exit wound). Recently use of high-velocity assault weapons has become more common in civilian

 Review

**Signs and
Symptoms of
Pneumothorax**

Trauma to chest
Chest pain on inspiration
Hyperinflation of chest
Diminished breath sounds
  on affected side

Content

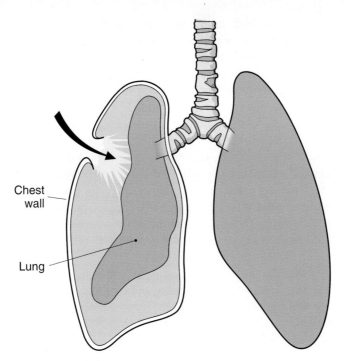

■ Figure 10-17 Open pneumothorax (sucking chest wound).

Chest wall

Lung

settings and thus the frequency of these injuries is on the increase. Another cause of open pneumothorax is a shotgun blast at close range with an associated large wound to the chest wall. This chest wall disruption leads to the free passage of air between the atmosphere and the pleural space (Figure 10-17). Air is drawn into the wound as the chest moves outward and the diaphragm moves downward during inspiration. The internal thoracic pressure drops and air rushes through the wound and into the chest cavity. This air replaces the lung tissue and permits lung collapse and results in a large functional dead space. The inspiratory effort of the intact side of the chest draws the mediastinum toward it and away from the injury. This prevents the uninjured lung from fully inflating. On exhalation, the contracting chest wall and rising diaphragm increase the internal pressure and force air outward through the wound. This movement of air into and out of the chest through the wound is the cause of the "sucking" sound that leads to the wound's common name, "sucking chest wound."

For air movement to occur through the opening in the chest wall, the opening must be at least two thirds the diameter of the trachea. Remember, the size of the trachea is about the size of the patient's little finger. This must be the size of the opening into the chest, not the size of the wound. The thickness and resiliency of the chest wall often closes the wound to air movement unless it is quite large. Then the remaining defect may permit the free movement of air and create an open pneumothorax.

The open pneumothorax can be recognized by the large open wound to the thorax and the characteristic air movement (or sound) it produces. Air passage through the wound and the wound's associated hemorrhage may produce frothy blood around the opening, another characteristic of the open pneumothorax. The patient is likely to experience severe dyspnea, and possibly hypovolemia from associated injury and hemorrhage. The patient's condition is further compromised because the reduced intrathoracic pressures developed during inspiration do not complement venous return to the heart as they do with the intact thorax and respiratory effort.

Tension Pneumothorax

Tension pneumothorax is an open or simple pneumothorax that generates and maintains a pressure greater than atmospheric pressure within the thorax. It may be caused by a traumatic mechanism and injury or possibly by positive-pressure ventilation of a

✓ **Review**

Signs and Symptoms of Open Pneumothorax

Penetrating chest trauma
Sucking chest wound
Frothy blood at wound site
Dyspnea
Hypovolemia

For air movement to occur through the opening in the chest wall, the opening must be at least two thirds the diameter of the trachea.

tension pneumothorax
buildup of air under pressure within the thorax. The resulting compression of the lung severely reduces the effectiveness of respirations.

patient with chest trauma or congenital defect affecting the respiratory tree. Tension pneumothorax may also occur as an open pneumothorax is sealed and an internal injury or defect permits the build-up of pressure.

Tension pneumothorax occurs because the mechanism of injury (either the external wound, or the internal injury) forms a one-way valve. Air flows into the pleural space through the defect during inspiration as the pressure within the pleural space is less than atmospheric. With expiration, the increasing pleural pressure closes the defect and does not permit air to escape. With each breath, the volume of air and the pressure within the pleural space increase. The increasing intrapleural pressure collapses the lung on the ipsilateral (same or injury) side, causes intercostal and suprasternal bulging, and begins to exert pressure against the mediastinum. As the pressure continues to build, it displaces the mediastinum, compressing the uninjured lung and crimping the vena cava as it enters the thorax through the diaphragm or where it attaches to the heart. This reduces venous return (which reduces cardiac output), results in an increase in venous pressure, causes the jugular veins to distend (JVD), and narrows the pulse pressure. Tracheal shift may occur as the mediastinal structures are pushed away from the increasing pressure. This is a very late and rare finding and is more commonly seen in the young trauma victim as the pediatric mediastinum is more mobile than the adult's. Atelectasis occurs in the ipsilateral side from the initial lung collapse and on the contralateral (uninjured or opposite) side from the mediastinal shift and compression of that lung. These mechanisms lead to ventilation/perfusion mismatch, further hypoxemia, and systemic hypoxia.

Tension pneumothorax begins with the presentation of a simple or open pneumothorax (Figure 10-18 ■). As the pressure in the pleural space begins to increase, dyspnea, ventilation/perfusion mismatch, and hypoxemia develop. The ipsilateral side of the chest becomes hyperinflated, hyperresonant to percussion, and respiratory sounds

✓ Review

Signs and Symptoms of Tension Pneumothorax

Chest trauma
Severe dyspnea
Ventilation/perfusion
　mismatch
Hypoxemia
Hyperinflation of affected
　side of chest
Hyperresonance of affected
　side of chest
Diminished, then absent
　breath sounds
Cyanosis
Diaphoresis
Altered mental status
Jugular venous distention
Hypotension
Hypovolemia

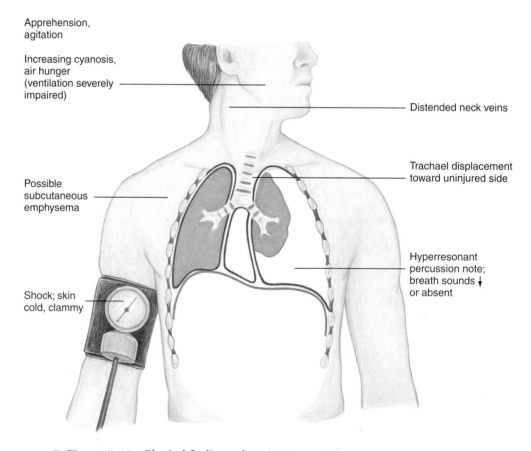

Apprehension, agitation

Increasing cyanosis, air hunger (ventilation severely impaired)

Distended neck veins

Trachael displacement toward uninjured side

Possible subcutaneous emphysema

Hyperresonant percussion note; breath sounds ↓ or absent

Shock; skin cold, clammy

■ Figure 10-18　Physical findings of tension pneumothorax.

become very faint, then absent. The pressure may cause the intracostal tissues to bulge. The opposite or contralateral side of the chest becomes somewhat dull to percussion, with progressively fainter respiratory sounds as the tension pneumothorax becomes worse. Severe hypoxia results in cyanosis, diaphoresis, and an altered mental status while the increased intrathoracic pressure reduces venous return and may cause JVD and hypotension. If the condition is not quickly recognized and promptly treated, it may lead to death.

Tension pneumothorax is a serious and immediate life threat. It is corrected by relieving the intrapleural pressure by inserting a needle through the chest wall to convert the tension pneumothorax to an open pneumothorax. If a valve is added to the decompression needle, it may permit the escape of air during expiration. If there is no continuing internal defect, this may progressively reexpand the collapsed lung and return effective respiration.

Hemothorax

Hemothorax is simply the accumulation of blood in the pleural space due to internal hemorrhage. It can be very minor and not detectable in the field or, when associated with serious or great vessel injury, may result in rapid patient deterioration. Serious hemorrhage may displace a complete lung, accumulate over 1,500 mL of blood quickly, and produce a mortality rate of 75 percent, with most (two thirds) of those dying at the scene. Hemothorax is primarily a blood loss problem as each side of the thorax may hold up to 3,000 mL of blood (or half the total blood volume). However, the blood lost into the thorax reduces the tidal volume and efficiency of respiration in a patient who has already suffered trauma and is likely to move quickly into shock.

Hemothorax is frequently associated with rib fractures and can be associated with either blunt or penetrating mechanisms. It often accompanies pneumothorax (a **hemopneumothorax**) and occurs 25 percent of the time with penetrating trauma. Hemorrhage into the pleural space may occur from a lung laceration (most common) or laceration of the intercostal arteries, pulmonary arteries, great vessels, or internal mammary arteries. The intercostal arteries can bleed at a rate of 50 mL/min. The bleeding into the chest is more rapid than would occur elsewhere because the pressure within the chest is often less than atmospheric pressure (law of Laplace). The blood lost into the hemothorax contributes to hypovolemia and displaces lung tissue. If the accumulation is significant, it may cause significant hypovolemia and shock, hypoxemia, respiratory distress, and respiratory failure.

The patient with hemothorax will have either a blunt or penetrating injury like those associated with open or simple pneumothorax. The patient may also display the signs and symptoms of shock and some respiratory distress (Figure 10-19 ■). The blood pools in the lower chest in the seated patient or posterior chest in the supine patient. The lungs present with normal percussion and breath sounds except directly over the accumulating fluid. There the lung percussion is very dull and breath sounds are very distant, if they can be heard at all.

Pulmonary Contusion

Pulmonary contusions are simply soft-tissue contusions affecting the lung. They are present in 30 to 75 percent of patients with significant blunt chest trauma and are frequently associated with rib fracture. Pulmonary contusions range in severity from very limited, minor, and unrecognizable injuries, to those that are extensive and quickly life threatening. They result in a mortality rate of between 14 and 20 percent of serious chest trauma patients.

There are two specific mechanisms of injury that allow the transfer of energy to the pulmonary tissue and result in pulmonary contusions. They are deceleration and the pressure wave associated with either passage of a high-velocity bullet or explosion. Deceleration injury occurs as the moving body strikes a fixed object. A common

Review

Signs and Symptoms of Hemothorax

Blunt or penetrating chest trauma
Signs and symptoms of shock
Dyspnea
Dull percussive sounds over site of collecting blood

Content

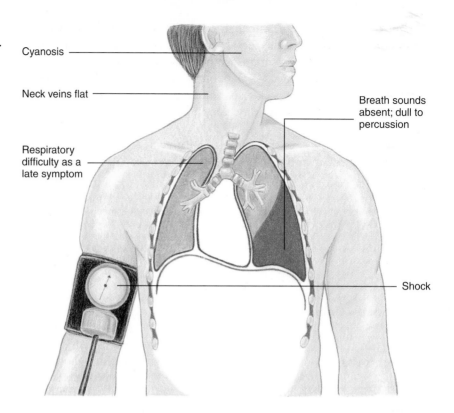

■ Figure 10-19 Physical findings of massive hemothorax.

Cyanosis

Neck veins flat

Respiratory difficulty as a late symptom

Breath sounds absent; dull to percussion

Shock

example of this mechanism is chest impact with the steering wheel during an auto crash. As the chest wall contacts the wheel and stops, the lungs continue forward, compressing and stretching the alveolar tissue or shearing it from the relatively fixed tracheobronchial tree. This causes disruption at the alveolar/capillary membrane leading to microscopic hemorrhage and edema. The second mechanism, the pressure wave of an explosion or bullet's passage, dramatically compresses and stretches the lung tissue. Due to the nature of the lung tissue (air-filled sacs surrounded by delicate and vascular membranes), the passage of this pressure is partially reflected at the gas/fluid (alveolar/capillary) interface. This leaves small, flame-shaped areas of disruption throughout the membrane leading to microhemorrhage and edema (called the Spalding effect). Pulmonary contusion is not generally associated with low-speed penetration of the chest and laceration of the lung tissues and structures.

The overall magnitude of pulmonary injury depends on the degree of deformity or stretch, and the velocity at which it occurs. Similar pulmonary contusions may result from different mechanisms. For example, an AK-47 round fired at 2,300 ft/sec striking body armor and deforming the chest wall instantaneously by 1 to 2 cm (high velocity) may cause pulmonary contusions similar to a chest impact during an MVA where the chest is deformed 50 percent as it strikes the steering wheel at 50 ft/sec (low velocity).

Microhemorrhage into the alveolar tissue associated with pulmonary contusion may be extensive and result in up to 1,000 to 1,500 mL of blood loss. This hemorrhage into the tissue of the alveoli also causes irritation, initiates the inflammation process, and causes fluid to migrate into the region. The accumulation of fluid in the alveolar/capillary membrane (pulmonary edema) progressively increases its dimension and decreases the rate at which gases, and especially oxygen, can diffuse across it. The fluid accumulation also stiffens the membrane, makes the lung less compliant, and increases the work necessary to move air in and out of the affected tissue.

The thickening wall reduces the efficiency of respiration and results in hypoxemia, while the stiffening makes respiration more energy consuming. The development of edema also increases the pressure necessary to move blood through the capillary beds.

This increases the pressure within the pulmonary vascular system (pulmonary hypertension) and the workload of the right heart. In combination, these effects lead to atelectasis, hypovolemia, ventilation/perfusion mismatch, hypoxemia, hypotension, and, possibly, respiratory failure and shock. Although isolated pulmonary contusions can occur, they are frequently associated with chest wall injury and injuries elsewhere (87 percent of the time).

The patient with pulmonary contusion presents with a mechanism of injury and evidence of blunt or penetrating chest impact. While the associated injuries may display immediate signs and symptoms (as in the pain of a rib fracture), the signs and symptoms of the pulmonary contusion take time to develop. The patient will likely complain of increasing dyspnea, demonstrate increasing respiratory effort, and show the signs of hypoxia. Oxygen saturation may gradually fall as the pathology develops. Careful auscultation of the chest may reveal increasing crackles and fainter breath sounds. Serious pulmonary contusion may cause **hemoptysis** (coughing up blood) and the signs and symptoms of shock.

CARDIOVASCULAR INJURIES

Cardiovascular injuries are the subset of thoracic trauma that leads to the most fatalities. They include myocardial contusion, pericardial tamponade, myocardial aneurysm or rupture, aortic aneurysm or rupture, and other vascular injuries.

Myocardial Contusion

Myocardial contusion is a frequent result of trauma and may occur in 76 percent of all serious chest trauma. It carries a high mortality rate and occurs most commonly with severe blunt anterior chest trauma. Here, the chest is struck by or strikes an object. The heart, which is relatively mobile within the chest, impacts the inside of the anterior chest wall and then may be compressed between the sternum and the thoracic spine as the thorax flexes with impact. The resulting contusion will most likely affect the right atrium and right ventricle (Figure 10-20). This is related to the heart's position in the chest, rotated somewhat counterclockwise and presenting the right atrium and ventricle surfaces toward the sternum.

 Review

Signs and Symptoms of Pulmonary Contusion

Blunt or penetrating chest trauma
Increasing dyspnea
Hypoxia
Increasing crackles
Diminishing breath sounds
Hemoptysis
Signs and symptoms of shock

hemoptysis *coughing of blood that originates in the respiratory tract.*

Cardiovascular injuries are the subset of thoracic trauma that leads to the most fatalities.

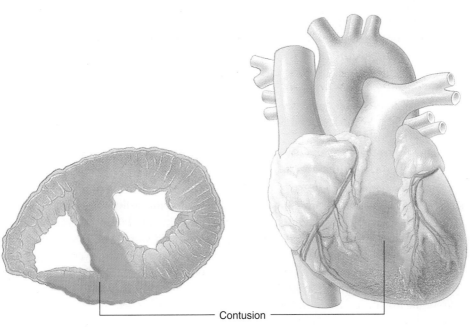

■ Figure 10-20 Myocardial contusion most frequently affects the right atrium and ventricle as they collide with the sternum.

Contusion

The cardiac contusion is similar to a contusion in any other muscle tissue. The injury disrupts the muscle cells and microcirculation, resulting in muscle fiber tearing and damage, hemorrhage, and edema. The injury may reduce the strength of cardiac contraction and reduce cardiac output. Because of the automaticity and conductivity of the cardiac muscle, contusion may also disturb the cardiac electrical system. If the injury is serious, it may lead to hematoma, hemoperitoneum (blood in the peritoneal sac), and necrosis and may result in cardiac irritability, ectopic (abnormal origin) beats, and conduction system defects such as bundle branch blocks and dysrhythmias. If the injury is very extensive, it may lead to tissue necrosis (death), decreased ventricular compliance, congestive heart failure, cardiogenic shock, myocardial aneurysm, and acute or delayed myocardial rupture. In contrast to a myocardial infarction from coronary artery disease, the cellular damage from myocardial contusions heals with less scarring and there is no progression of the injury in the absence of associated coronary artery disease.

The patient experiencing myocardial contusion will have a history of significant blunt chest trauma, most likely affecting the anterior chest. The patient will likely complain of chest or retrosternal pain, very much like that of myocardial infarction and may have associated chest injuries such as anterior rib or sternal fractures. Cardiac monitoring most frequently reveals sinus tachycardia (though it may be caused by pain, hypovolemia, or hypoxia from associated chest injury). Other dysrhythmias associated with myocardial contusions are atrial flutter or fibrillation, premature atrial or ventricular contractions, tachydysrhythmias, bradydysrhythmias, bundle branch patterns, T wave inversions, and ST segment elevations. A pericardial friction rub and murmur may be auscultated over the **precordium** but is more likely to occur weeks after the injury and is associated with the development of an inflammatory pericardial effusion.

Pericardial Tamponade

Pericardial tamponade is a restriction to cardiac filling caused by blood (or other fluid) within the pericardial sac. It occurs in less than 2 percent of all serious chest trauma patients and is almost always related to penetrating injury. Gunshot wounds are the most frequent mechanism and carry a high overall mortality, though they often result in rapid hemorrhage through the myocardial wall and then out the defect in the pericardium. The frequency of gunshot wound mortality is probably related to the depth of injury, the degree of cardiac tissue damage caused by the cavitational wave, and a more rapid progression of the pathology.

The pathology of pericardial tamponade begins with a tear in a superficial coronary artery or penetration of the myocardium. Blood seeps into the pericardial space and accumulates (Figure 10-21 ■). The fibrous pericardium does not stretch and the accumulating blood exerts pressure on the heart. The pressure limits cardiac filling, first affecting the right ventricle where the pressure of filling is the lowest. This restricts venous return to the heart, increases venous pressure, and causes jugular vein distention. The reduced right ventricular output limits outflow to the pulmonary arteries and then venous return to the left heart. The result is a decreasing cardiac output and systemic hypotension. The pressure exerted by the blood in the pericardium also restricts the flow of blood through the coronary arteries and to the myocardium. This may result in myocardial ischemia and infarct. It takes about 150 to 300 mL of blood to exert the pressure necessary to induce frank tamponade, while removing as little as 20 mL may provide significant relief. The progression of pericardial tamponade depends on the rate of blood flow into the pericardium. It may occur very rapidly and result in death before the arrival of emergency medical services or may gradually progress over hours.

The patient experiencing pericardial tamponade will likely have penetrating trauma to the anterior or posterior chest, though blunt trauma can also cause this problem. While the trajectories of missiles and knife blades are difficult to predict, consider

Review

Signs and Symptoms of Cardiac Contusion

Blunt injury to chest
Bruising of chest wall
Rapid heart rate—may be irregular
Severe nagging pain not relieved with rest but may be relieved with oxygen

precordium   *area of the chest wall overlying the heart.*

pericardial tamponade   *a restriction to cardiac filling caused by blood (or other fluid) within the pericardial sac.*

Review

Signs and Symptoms of Pericardial Tamponade

Dyspnea and possible cyanosis
Jugular venous distention
Weak, thready pulse
Decreasing blood pressure
Shock
Narrowing pulse pressure

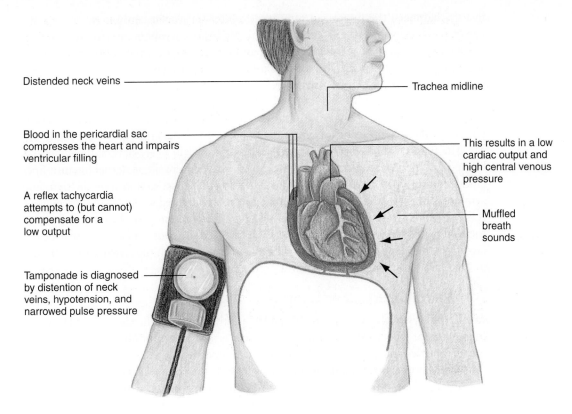

Distended neck veins

Trachea midline

Blood in the pericardial sac compresses the heart and impairs ventricular filling

This results in a low cardiac output and high central venous pressure

A reflex tachycardia attempts to (but cannot) compensate for a low output

Muffled breath sounds

Tamponade is diagnosed by distention of neck veins, hypotension, and narrowed pulse pressure

■ Figure 10-21   Physical findings of cardiac tamponade.

pericardial tamponade with any thoracic or upper abdominal penetrating wound, especially if it is over the precordium (central lower chest). Pericardial tamponade will diminish the strength of pulses, decrease the pulse pressure, and distend the jugular veins (JVD). The patient will likely be agitated, tachycardic, diaphoretic, and ashen in appearance. Cyanosis may be noted in the head, neck, and upper extremities. Heart tones may be muffled or distant sounding. Beck's triad (JVD, distant heart tones, and hypotension) is indicative of pericardial tamponade but may not be recognized early in the injury's progression. Another sign of pericardial tamponade is Kussmaul's sign, the decrease or absence of JVD during inspiration. As the patient inspires, the reduced intrathoracic pressure increases venous return and decreases the pressure the accumulating pericardial fluid exerts on the heart. This then translates to a better venous return and cardiac output during inspiration and the effect then seen in the jugular veins.

Other findings during pericardial tamponade may include pulsus paradoxus and electrical alternans. **Pulsus paradoxus** is a drop in systolic blood pressure of greater than 10 mmHg as the patient inspires during the normal respiratory cycle. (Normally the systolic blood pressure drops just slightly with each inspiration.) Pulsus paradoxus results because cardiac output increases with the minimal relief of the tamponade associated with the reduced intrathoracic pressure of inspiration. **Electrical alternans,** which is only rarely seen in acute pericardial tamponade, is noted on the cardiac rhythm strip as the P, QRS, and T amplitude decreasing with every other cardiac cycle. In profound pericardial tamponade, the heart displays a rhythm without producing a pulse (PEA).

Myocardial Aneurysm or Rupture

Myocardial **aneurysm** or rupture occurs almost exclusively in extreme blunt thoracic trauma, such as automobile collisions. It also has been reported in cases where the blunt forces are not extreme, such as a result of CPR. The condition can affect any of the

pulsus paradoxus *drop of greater than 10 mmHg in the systolic blood pressure during the inspiratory phase of respiration that occurs in patients with pericardial tamponade.*

electrical alternans *alternating amplitude of the P, QRS, and T waves on the ECG rhythm strip as the heart swings in a pendulum-like fashion within the pericardial sac during tamponade.*

aneurysm *a weakening or ballooning in the wall of a blood vessel.*

heart's chambers, the interatrial septum, the interventricular septum, or involve the valves and their supporting structures. Multiple heart chambers or structures are involved 30 percent of the time. Aneurysm and delayed myocardial rupture also occur secondary to necrosis from a myocardial infarction, repaired penetrating injury, or myocardial contusion. Necrosis usually develops around 2 weeks after the injury as inflammatory cells degrade the injured cells, weakening the tissue, and leading to aneurysm of the ventricular wall and/or subsequent rupture. Rupture can also occur with high-velocity projectile injury as the bullet impacts the engorged heart chamber.

The patient who experiences myocardial rupture will likely have suffered serious blunt or penetrating trauma to the chest and may have severe rib or sternal fracture. Specific symptoms may depend on the actual pathology. The victim may have the signs and symptoms of pericardial tamponade if the rupture is contained within the pericardial sac. If the pathology only affects the valves, the patient may present with the signs and symptoms of right or left heart failure. If there is a myocardial aneurysm, rupture may be delayed. When it happens, the patient will suddenly present with the absence of vital signs or the signs and symptoms of pericardial tamponade.

Traumatic Aneurysm or Rupture of the Aorta

Aortic aneurysm and rupture are extremely life-threatening injuries resulting from either blunt or penetrating trauma. The aorta is most commonly injured by blunt trauma, carries an overall mortality of 85 to 95 percent, and is responsible for 15 percent of all thoracic trauma deaths. Aneurysm and rupture are usually associated with high-speed automobile crashes (most commonly lateral impact) and in some cases with high falls. Unlike myocardial rupture, a significant number, possibly as high as 20 percent, of these victims will survive the initial insult and aneurysm. Some 30 percent of these initial survivors will die in 6 hours if not treated, increasing to about 50 percent at 24 hours, and just under 70 percent by the end of the first week. It is this subset of patients that survive the initial impact and are alive at the scene that you can benefit the most by recognizing the potential injury and then by rapidly extricating, packaging, and transporting the patients to the trauma center.

The aorta is a large high-pressure vessel that provides outflow from the left ventricle for distribution to the body. It is relatively fixed at three points as it passes through the thoracic cavity and, because of this, experiences shear forces secondary to severe deceleration of the chest. The areas of fixation are the aortic annulus where the aorta joins the heart, the aortic isthmus where it is joined by the ligamentum arteriosum, and the diaphragm where it exits the chest (Table 10–2). Traumatic dissecting aneurysm occurs infrequently to the ascending aorta and, most commonly, to the descending aorta. With severe deceleration, shear forces separate the layers of the artery, specifically the interior surface (the tunica intima) from the muscle layer (the tunica media). This allows blood to enter and, because it is under great pressure, it begins to dissect the aortic lining like a bulging inner tube. It is likely to rupture if it is not surgically repaired.

The patient with aortic rupture will be severely hypotensive, quickly lose all vital signs, and die unless moved into surgery immediately. Dissecting aortic aneurysm progresses more slowly, though the aneurysm may rupture at any moment. The patient will

Table 10–2	Incidence and Anatomical Location of Traumatic Aortic Rupture
Aortic annulus	9%
Aortic isthmus	85%
Diaphragm	3%
Other	3%

probably have a history of a high fall or severe auto impact and deceleration. Lateral impact is an especially high risk factor for aortic aneurysm. The patient may complain of severe tearing chest pain that may radiate to the back. The patient may have a pulse deficit between the left and right upper extremities and/or reduced pulse strength in the lower extremities. Blood pressure may be high (hypertension) due to stretching of sympathetic nerve fibers present in the aorta near the ligamentum arteriosum, or the pressure may be low due to leakage and hypovolemia. Auscultation may reveal a harsh systolic murmur due to turbulence as the blood exits the heart and passes the disrupted blood vessel wall.

OTHER VASCULAR INJURIES

The pulmonary arteries and vena cava are other thoracic vascular structures that can sustain injury during chest trauma. Their injury, and the resulting hemorrhage, may cause significant hemothorax, possibly leading to hypotension and respiratory insufficiency. The blood may also flow into the mediastinum and compress the great vessels, esophagus, and heart. Penetrating trauma is the primary cause of injury to the pulmonary arteries and vena cava.

The patient with pulmonary artery or vena cava injuries will likely have a penetrating wound to the central chest or elsewhere with a likelihood of central chest involvement. These injuries present with the signs and symptoms of hypovolemia and shock and result in hemothorax or hemomediastinum and the signs and symptoms associated with those pathologies.

OTHER THORACIC INJURIES
Traumatic Rupture or Perforation of the Diaphragm

Traumatic rupture or perforation of the diaphragm can occur in both high-speed blunt thoracoabdominal trauma as well as in penetrating trauma. Incidence is estimated from 1 to 6 percent of all patients with multiple trauma. It is more common in patients sustaining penetrating trauma to the lower chest, which has as much as a 30 to 40 percent incidence of abdominal organ and tissue involvement. Remember that during expiration the diaphragm may move superiorly to the level of the fourth intercostal space (nipple level) anteriorly and the sixth intercostal space posteriorly. Any penetrating injuries at these levels or below may penetrate the diaphragm. Diaphragmatic perforation and herniation occur most frequently on the left side because assailants are most frequently right handed and the size and solid nature of the liver protect the diaphragm on the right. The liver is also unlikely to herniate through the torn diaphragm unless the injury is sizeable.

Suspect diaphragmatic perforation with any penetrating injury to the lower thorax.

If traumatic diaphragmatic rupture occurs, the abdominal organs may herniate through the defect into the thoracic cavity causing strangulation or necrosis of the bowel, restriction of the ipsilateral lung, and displacement of the mediastinum. Mediastinal displacement occurs when the displaced abdominal contents place pressure on the lung and mediastinal structures, moving them toward the contralateral side through much the same mechanism as is seen in tension pneumothorax.

Diaphragmatic rupture presents with signs and symptoms similar to tension pneumothorax, including dyspnea, hypoxia, hypotension, and JVD. The patient will have a history of blunt abdominal trauma or penetrating trauma to the lower thorax or upper abdomen. The abdomen may appear hollow, and bowel sounds may be noted in one side of the thorax (most commonly the left). The patient may be hypotensive and hypoxic if the herniation is extensive. The patient may complain of upper abdominal pain, though this symptom is often overshadowed by other injuries. Diaphragmatic rupture may be recognized at the time of injury or may be missed if not extensive and may present with delayed herniation months to years later.

Traumatic Esophageal Rupture

Traumatic esophageal rupture is a rare complication of blunt thoracic trauma. The incidence of it related to penetrating trauma of the thorax is somewhat higher but still only about 0.4 percent. Since the esophagus is rather centrally located within the chest, its injury usually coincides with other mediastinal injuries. (Esophageal rupture may also be the result of medical problems such as violent emesis, carcinoma, anatomical distortion, or gastric reflux.) Esophageal rupture carries a 30 percent mortality, even if quickly recognized, and mortality is much greater if this injury is not diagnosed promptly. The life threat from esophageal rupture is related to material entering the mediastinum as it passes down the esophagus or as emesis comes up. This results in serious infection or chemical irritation and serious damage to the mediastinal structures. Air may also enter the mediastinum through an esophageal rupture, especially during positive pressure ventilations.

The patient with esophageal rupture will probably have deep penetrating trauma to the central chest and may complain of difficult or painful swallowing, pleuritic chest pain, and pain radiating to the midback. The patient may also display subcutaneous emphysema around the lower neck.

Tracheobronchial Injury (Disruption)

Tracheobronchial injury is a relatively infrequent finding in thoracic trauma with an incidence of less than 3 percent in patients with significant chest trauma. It may occur from either a blunt or a penetrating injury mechanism and carries a relatively high mortality similar to esophageal rupture of 30 percent. In contrast to patients with esophageal rupture, who usually die days after injury, 50 percent of patients with tracheobronchial injury die within 1 hour of injury. Disruption can occur anywhere in the tracheobronchial tree but is most likely to occur within 2.5 cm of the carina.

The patient with disruption of the trachea or mainstem bronchi is generally in respiratory distress with cyanosis, hemoptysis, and, in some cases, massive subcutaneous emphysema. The patient may also experience pneumothorax and, possibly, tension pneumothorax. Intermittent positive-pressure ventilation drives air into the pleura or mediastinum and makes the condition worse.

Traumatic Asphyxia

Traumatic asphyxia occurs when severe compressive force is applied to the thorax and leads to a reverse flow of blood from the right heart into the superior vena cava and into the venous vessels of the upper extremities. (Traumatic asphyxia is not as much a respiratory problem as it is a vascular problem.) Traumatic asphyxia engorges the veins and capillaries of the head and neck with desaturated venous blood, turning the skin in this region a deep red, purple, or blue. The back flow of blood damages the microcirculation in the head and neck, producing petechiae (small hemorrhages under the skin) and stagnating blood above the point of compression. The back flow may damage cerebral circulation, resulting in numerous small strokes in the older patient whose venous vessels are not very elastic. If flow restriction continues, toxins and acids accumulate in the blood and may have a devastating effect when they return to the central circulation with the release of pressure. If the thoracic compression continues, it restricts venous return and may prevent the victim from ventilating. This results in hypotension, hypoxemia, and shock. Death may follow rapidly. Extrication of the patient may result in rapid hemorrhage from the injury site with release of the pressure. Release of the compression may likewise result in rapid patient deterioration and death.

The traumatic asphyxia patient will have suffered a severe compression force to the chest that is likely to continue until extrication. The result of the compression, the back flow of blood and restricted blood flow, will be dramatic and cause the classical discoloration of the head and neck regions. The face appears swollen, the eyes bulge, and there

You must be ready to immediately handle the complications of traumatic asphyxia as soon as the patient is released from entrapment.

Detecting the Effects of Thoracic Trauma The thoracic cavity contains three general regions: the pericardial region, the pulmonary region, and the mediastinum. The pericardial region contains the heart and the origin of the great vessels. The pulmonary region contains the lungs, the airways, and the pulmonary vasculature. The mediastinum contains the esophagus, the vagus nerve, the thoracic duct, and other essential structures. Despite these, the thoracic cavity primarily involves respiratory and cardiac functions. Thus, with any thoracic injury, you would expect to see first a variation in respiratory function, cardiac function, or both. With a pneumothorax, you initially will see a subtle increase in respiratory rate and then, as the process progresses, increased respiratory effort and, finally, signs and symptoms of poor oxygenation. If this is allowed to progress untreated, cardiovascular impairment will follow. Cardiovascular impairment can result from incomplete ventricular filling due to increased intrathoracic pressure or from blood loss within the lung parenchyma.

Similarly, a penetrating injury to the heart can lead to cardiovascular collapse. With low-energy wounds, such as knife stab wounds, the pericardial sac may fill with blood, thus preventing adequate ventricular filling (pericardial tamponade). This will be manifest as an initial increase in heart rate, narrowing of the pulse pressure (due to restricted ventricular filling), and distended neck veins. As cardiac efficiency declines, the pulmonary vasculature can become congested, resulting in poor oxygenation. High-energy wounds, such as gunshot wounds, that penetrate the heart are usually mortal wounds—even in the best of EMS systems and trauma centers.

Any time you have a patient with a suspected thoracic injury, first look at the respiratory and circulatory systems for signs of impairment. These findings can help guide you to the nature of your patient's injury.

---

are numerous conjunctival hemorrhages. The patient may have severe dyspnea related to the compression and injuries associated with severe chest impact. Once the pressure is released, the patient may show the signs of hypovolemia, hypotension, and shock as well as signs related to any co-existing respiratory problems.

ASSESSMENT OF THE CHEST INJURY PATIENT

The proper assessment of the patient with a severe chest injury mechanism is critical to anticipating injury and providing the correct interventions. While the approach to this patient follows the standard format for assessment, special considerations regarding chest trauma occur during the scene size-up, initial assessment, and especially during the rapid trauma assessment. The ongoing assessment is also critical for monitoring the thoracic trauma patient for the progression of injuries sustained during serious chest trauma.

SCENE SIZE-UP

Chest injury care, like that for any other serious trauma, requires body substance isolation procedures with gloves as a minimum. Consider a face shield if you will be attending to the airway and a gown for splash protection with serious penetrating thoracic trauma. Assure the scene is safe, including protection from the assailant, if penetrating trauma is suspected.

Examine the mechanism of injury carefully and try to determine if the central chest (heart, great vessels, trachea, and esophagus) might be in the pathway of penetrating trauma. In gunshot injuries, determine the type of weapon, caliber, distance between the gun barrel and the victim, and the probable pathway of the projectile. Determine the direction of blunt trauma impact as it may also have a bearing on which organs sustain injury. Anterior impact may rupture lung tissue and contuse the lung and heart. Lateral impact may tear the aorta as the heart displaces laterally and stresses the aorta's ligamentous attachments.

INITIAL ASSESSMENT

During the initial assessment, determine the patient's mental status and the status of the airway, breathing, and circulation. Intervene as necessary to correct life-threatening conditions. It is during the initial assessment that you will first identify the signs and symptoms of serious chest trauma. Be especially watchful for any dyspnea; asymmetrical, paradoxical, or limited chest movement; hyperinflation of the chest; or an abdomen that appears hollow. Notice any general patient color reflective of hypoxia such as cyanosis or an ashen discoloration. Look for distended jugular veins, costal or suprasternal retractions, and the use of accessory muscles of respiration.

Assure that ventilation is adequate and administer high-flow, high-concentration oxygen by nonrebreather mask. Administer any positive-pressure ventilations with care as thoracic injury may weaken the lung tissue and make the patient prone to pneumothorax or tension pneumothorax. Aggressive (or even cautious) ventilations may induce these problems. Be suspicious of internal hemorrhage and initiate at least one large-bore intravenous catheter and line in anticipation of hypovolemia, hypotension, and shock. With anterior blunt or penetrating trauma that may involve the heart, attach the ECG electrodes, and monitor for dysrhythmias. Attach a pulse oximeter and monitor oxygen saturation to evaluate the effectiveness of respiration. If there is any mechanism suggesting serious trauma to the chest or any physical signs of either hypoventilation or hypovolemia compensation, perform the rapid trauma assessment with a special focus on the chest and prepare for rapid patient transport to the trauma center.

RAPID TRAUMA ASSESSMENT

During the rapid trauma assessment you will examine the patient's chest in detail, carefully observing, questioning about, palpating, and auscultating the region.

Observe

Observe the chest for evidence of impact. Look for the erythema that develops early in the contusion process, especially as it outlines the ribs or forms a pattern reflecting the contours of the object the chest hit. Look carefully for penetrating trauma and try to determine the angle of entry and depth of penetration. Also look for exit wounds. Lateral chest injury is likely to involve the lungs, while a pathway of energy through the central chest is likely to involve the heart, great vessels, trachea, or esophagus. Injury to the mediastinal structures is also likely to result in serious hemorrhage, hypovolemia, and shock. Look for intercostal and suprasternal retractions as well as external jugular vein distention. Remember, JVD is present in supine normotensive patients and may be exaggerated in them or may continue when the patient is moved to the seated position if venous pressure is elevated.

Watch chest movement carefully during respiration. The chest should rise and the abdomen should fall smoothly with inspiration and return to their positions during expiration. Any limited motion, either bilaterally or unilaterally, suggests a problem. Watch for the paradoxical motion of flail chest. That movement will be limited due to muscle spasm during early care, but continued motion will further damage the surrounding soft tissue and the intracostal muscles will fatigue. This will lead to a more obvious paradoxical motion and greater respiratory embarrassment with time. Look, too, for any hyperinflation of one side of the chest and any deformity that may exist from

Administer ventilations with care in the patient with chest trauma.

rib fracture, sternal fracture or dislocation, or subcutaneous emphysema. Assess the volume of air effectively moved with each breath and assure that the minute volume is greater than 6 liters. If not, consider overdrive ventilation with the bag-valve mask. Examine any open wound for air movement in or out, which is indicative of an open pneumothorax. Observe the patient's general color. If a patient's skin is dusky, ashen, or cyanotic, suspect respiratory compromise. If the head and neck are red, dark red, or blue, suspect traumatic asphyxia.

Question

Question the patient about any pain, pain on motion, pain with breathing effort (pleuritic pain), or dyspnea. Note if the pain is crushing, tearing, or is described otherwise by the patient. Have the patient describe the exact location of the pain, its severity, and any radiation of the pain. Question about other sensations and carefully monitor the patient's level of consciousness and orientation.

Palpate

Palpate the thorax carefully, feeling for any signs of injury (Figure 10-22 ■). Feel for any swelling, deformity, crepitus, or the crackling of subcutaneous emphysema. Compress the thorax between your hands with pressure directed inward. Then apply downward pressure on the midsternum. Such pressure will flex the ribs and should elicit pain from any fracture site along the thorax. (Apply pressure only if you have found no signs or symptoms of chest injury. If you suspect rib or sternal fracture, provide appropriate care but do not aggravate the injury.) Rest your hands on the lower thorax and let the chest lift your hands with inspiration and let them fall with expiration (Figure 10-23 ■). The motion should be smooth and equal. If not, determine the nature of any asymmetry.

You may have to rely on your palpation skills to assess chest injuries when scene noise is excessive.

Auscultate

Auscultate all lung lobes, both anteriorly and posteriorly (Figure 10-24 ■). Listen for both inspiratory and expiratory air movement and note any crackles, indicating edema from contusion or congestive heart failure, or any diminished breath sounds, suggesting hypoventilation. Compare one side to the other and one lobe to another. Be sensitive for distant or muffled respiratory or heart sounds.

Percuss

Percuss the chest and note the responses (Figure 10-25 ■). Determine if the area percussed is normal, hyperresonant, or dull. A dull response suggests collecting blood or

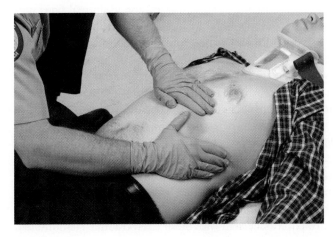

■ Figure 10-22 Carefully palpate the thorax of a patient with a suspected injury to the region. (© Maria A. H. Lyle)

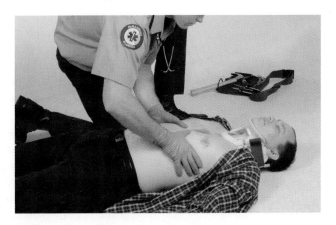

■ Figure 10-23 Place your hands on the lower thorax and let them rise and fall with respiration. (© Maria A. H. Lyle)

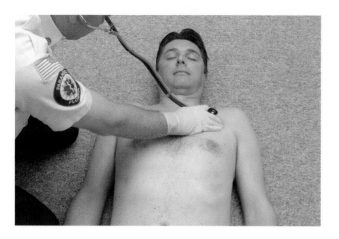

■ Figure 10-24 Auscultate all lung lobes, both anteriorly and posteriorly.

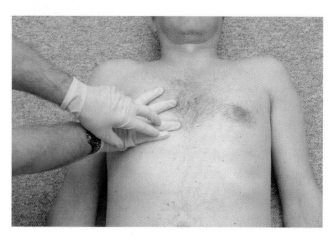

■ Figure 10-25 Percuss all lung lobes, listening for a dull response or hyperresonance.

other fluid, while hyperresonance suggests air or air under pressure as in a pneumothorax or tension pneumothorax.

Your findings from the rapid trauma assessment may suggest an injury or multiple injuries. Identify the likely cause of the signs and symptoms you find and suspect and anticipate the worst. You are likely to note clear evidence of chest wall injury and some signs of internal injuries if they exist. As mentioned earlier, blunt and penetrating trauma present with different typical injuries.

Blunt Trauma Assessment

In blunt trauma, you commonly find slight discoloration of the surface of the chest reflective of contusions. The contusions also cause the patient pain, generally in an area or region, and somewhat limit respiration. As the impact energy increases, it may cause fractures of ribs 4 through 8 and a greater possibility of underlying injury. If the upper ribs or ribs 9 through 12 fracture, suspect serious underlying injury. Sternal fracture takes great energy and is also associated with a higher incidence of internal injury. Rib fractures generate a point-specific pain (at the fracture site) and crepitus upon deep breathing or your flexing of the patient's chest during the rapid trauma assessment. That pain may further limit chest excursion during respiration. As the energy of trauma and the seriousness of chest trauma increase, more ribs may fracture, causing a flail chest. Remember that a flail chest's paradoxical motion is initially limited by muscular splinting and grows more noticeable and causes more respiratory distress as the time since the collision increases.

In blunt injury to the chest, you must anticipate and assess for additional signs suggesting internal injury. Signs specific for lung injury include increasing dyspnea, signs of hypoxemia, accessory muscle use, and intracostal and suprasternal retractions. Auscultation will help you differentiate between pulmonary contusion and pneumothorax. Contusions demonstrate progressively increasing crackles, while pneumothorax presents with diminished breath sounds on the ipsilateral side. Further, with pneumothorax the affected side may be hyperinflated and resonant to percussion. If the pneumothorax progresses to tension pneumothorax, you will likely note progressing dyspnea and hypoxia, use of accessory muscles, distended jugular veins, tracheal shift toward the contralateral side (a late finding), and hyperresonance of the ipsilateral chest on percussion. Subcutaneous emphysema may develop, especially if the lung defect was caused by or is associated with a rib fracture that disturbs the integrity of the parietal pleura. Hemothorax is noticeable due to the vascular loss, more so than for the respiratory component of the pathology. Suspect it if you find the signs of hypovolemia associated with blunt chest trauma. Hemothorax, when sizeable, may cause dyspnea and a lung field that is dull to percussion.

Blunt mediastinal injury will probably affect the heart, great vessels, and trachea. Heart injury may present with chest pain similar to that of the myocardial infarction and, if serious enough, with the signs of heart failure or cardiogenic shock. The ECG may reveal tachycardia, bradycardia, cardiac irritability, and, in cases of severe cardiac contusion, may demonstrate ST elevation. Cardiac rupture presents with the signs of sudden death, while pericardial tamponade is unlikely in blunt chest trauma. Injury to the great vessels (aneurysm) is most frequently associated with lateral impacts or feet-first high falls and may produce a tearing chest pain and pulse deficits in the extremities. If the aneurysm ruptures, rapidly progressing hypovolemia, hypotension, shock, and death ensue. Tracheobronchial injury results in rapidly developing pneumomediastinum or pneumothorax and possible subcutaneous emphysema, hemoptysis, dyspnea, and hypoxia. Positive-pressure ventilations may increase the development and severity of signs. Traumatic asphyxia presents with jugular vein distention, discoloration of the head and neck, severe dyspnea, and possibly the signs of hypovolemia and shock.

Penetrating Trauma Assessment

Penetrating injury displays a different set of signs associated with different injuries. Inspect a chest wound for frothy blood or sounds of air exchange with respirations (open pneumothorax). Remember that a wound needs to be rather large (high-velocity bullet exit wound or close-range shotgun blast) for these signs to occur. A penetrating wound, however, commonly induces a simple pneumothorax with its associated signs and symptoms. A hyperinflated chest, distended jugular veins, tracheal shift away from the injury, distant or absent breath sounds, hyperresonance to percussion, and severe dyspnea and hypotension suggest tension pneumothorax. The pressure of tension pneumothorax may push air outward through a penetrating wound or cause subcutaneous emphysema around the wound. Some degree of hemothorax is likely to be associated with penetrating chest trauma and, if extensive, may reveal diminished or absent breath sounds and a chest region that is dull to percussion. Hemothorax also causes or significantly contributes to hypovolemia and shock.

Penetrating trauma to the heart is likely to cause pericardial tamponade and present with jugular vein distention, distant heart sounds, and hypotension (Beck's triad). Pulsus paradoxus may be present and jugular filling may occur with inspiration (due to a paradoxical rise in venous pressure during inspiration, known as Kussmaul's sign, that is associated with pericardial tamponade). Both pulsus paradoxus and jugular filling are indicative of pericardial tamponade. Additionally, with pericardial tamponade, heart sounds are distant, pulses are weak, and the patient experiences increasing hypotension and shock (Figure 10-26 ■). Penetrating trauma to the heart may also cause myocardial rupture and immediate death (Figure 10-27 ■). The patient demonstrates vital signs that fall precipitously as the vascular volume is pumped into the mediastinum.

ONGOING ASSESSMENT

While the ongoing assessment simply repeats elements of the initial assessment, the taking of vital signs, and examination of any injury signs discovered during earlier assessment, it takes on great importance for the patient with chest trauma. With any serious chest impact or any penetrating injury to the chest, observe the respiratory depth, rate, and symmetry of effort. Auscultate the lung fields for equality and crackles and monitor the distal pulses, oxygen saturation, skin color, and blood pressure for signs of progressing hypovolemia (Figure 10-28 ■). If any signs change between assessments, search out the cause and rule out progressing chest injury. Be especially suspicious of developing tension pnuemothorax, pericardial tamponade, extensive and evolving pulmonary contusion, and hypovolemia associated with hemothorax. If any of these is found, institute the appropriate management steps.

Remember, the severity of internal injury associated with penetrating trauma may be great despite seemingly minor entrance and/or exit wounds.

Continuous reassessment of the patient with chest injury is essential because deterioration may occur within a matter of seconds.

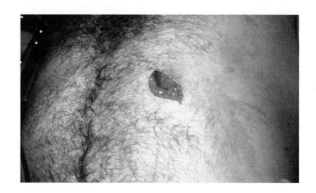

■ Figure 10-26 Penetrating stab wound to the chest involving the heart.

MANAGEMENT OF THE CHEST INJURY PATIENT

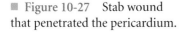

General management of the patient with serious chest trauma requires assurance of good oxygenation and adequate respiratory volume and rate.

The general management of the patient with significant chest injury focuses on assuring good oxygenation and adequate respiratory volume and rate. Administer high-flow, high-concentration oxygen using the nonrebreather mask. Assure the airway is patent and consider endotracheal intubation if there is any significant loss in the level of consciousness or orientation. Consider intubation early in your care, as patients with thoracic trauma are likely to get worse with time. Rapid sequence intubation may be needed for the combative patient. Endotracheal intubation also makes ventilation of the flail chest or pulmonary contusion patient easier.

Carefully evaluate the minute volume of the patient (breaths per minute times volume) and if it is less than 6,000 mL consider overdrive ventilation. Bag-valve mask the conscious patient with severe dyspnea at a rate of 12 to 16 full breaths per minute, trying to match the patient's respiratory rate. Closely monitor pulse oximetry, level of consciousness, and skin color. Bag-valve masking may also be beneficial for the patient with serious rib fractures and flail chest. The positive pressure displaces the chest outward, reducing the movement of the fracture site and moving the flail segment with the chest. It may also be beneficial to the patient who is exhausted from the increased breathing effort associated with pulmonary contusion. In this case, the positive pressure of assisted ventilations helps push any fluids back into the vascular system to relieve edema.

■ Figure 10-27 Stab wound that penetrated the pericardium.

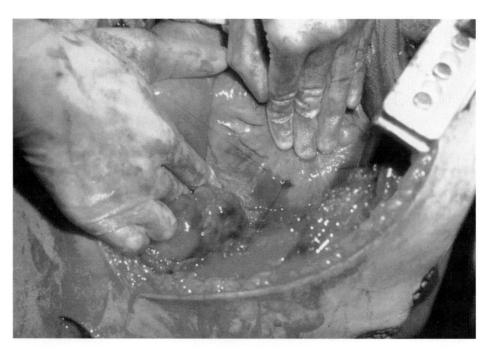

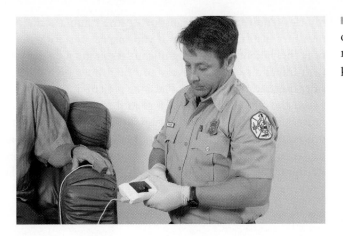

■ Figure 10-28 With pulse oximetry, you can continuously monitor the percentage of the patient's oxygen saturation.

Remember, however, that positive-pressure ventilations change the dynamics of respiration from a less than atmospheric to a greater than atmospheric process and may exacerbate respiratory problems like tracheobronchial injury, pneumothorax, and tension pneumothorax.

Anticipate heart and great vessel compromise with thoracic injury and be ready to support the patient's cardiovascular system. Initiate at least one large-bore IV site if the patient has a serious mechanism of chest trauma and place two lines if there are any signs of hypovolemia or compensation. Be prepared to administer fluids quickly (in 250 to 500 mL boluses) if the patient's systolic blood pressure is below 80 mmHg. Use of the PASG is contraindicated for penetrating chest trauma as it may increase the rate and volume of blood loss and disrupt the clotting process.

IV fluid infusion for the patient with chest trauma should be conservative. Rapid fluid administration may increase the rate of hemorrhage and dilute the clotting factors, further adding to the problem. Additional fluid also increases the edema associated with pulmonary contusion, increasing the rate and extent of its development. Anytime you administer fluids to the chest trauma patient, auscultate all lung fields carefully and reduce the fluid resuscitation rate whenever you hear respiratory crackles or the patient's dyspnea increases.

Care is specific for thoracic injuries including rib fractures, sternoclavicular dislocation, flail chest, open pneumothorax, tension pneumothorax, hemothorax, cardiac contusion, pericardial tamponade, aortic aneurysm, tracheobronchial injury, and traumatic asphyxia.

Remember, aggressive fluid resuscitation in the patient with chest trauma can result in hemodilution and loss of clotting factors.

RIB FRACTURES

Rib fractures, either isolated or associated with other respiratory injuries, may produce pain that significantly limits respiratory effort and leads to hypoventilation. In these patients you may consider administering analgesics to grant greater patient comfort and improve chest excursion. Assure that the patient is hemodynamically stable, that there is no associated abdominal or head injury, and that the patient is fully conscious and oriented. Consider administration of diazepam, morphine sulfate, or meperidine as described in Chapter 7, "Musculoskeletal Trauma." Note that use of nitrous oxide is contraindicated in chest trauma as the nitrous oxide may migrate into a pneumothorax or tension pneumothorax.

STERNOCLAVICULAR DISLOCATION

Supportive therapy with oxygen is usually all that is required for an isolated sternoclavicular dislocation. However, hemodynamic instability indicates associated injuries requiring rapid transport to the trauma center with aggressive resuscitation measures instituted en route. If you suspect posterior sternoclavicular dislocation and note the patient to be in significant respiratory distress that is not effectively treated with initial airway maneuvers and high-flow, high-concentration oxygen, then consider dislocation reduction. Place the patient in the supine position with a sandbag between the shoulder blades. The sandbag helps to pull the shoulders backward and moves the head of the clavicle laterally and away from the trachea. Do not perform this procedure for the multiple-trauma patient due to the probability of spine injury. An alternative reduction method is to place the patient supine and grasp the clavicle near the sternum. Pull it upward and laterally, directly perpendicular to the sternum. This distracts the clavicle forward, alleviating its impingement of the airway.

FLAIL CHEST

Place the patient on the side of injury if spinal immobilization is not required, or secure a large and bulky dressing with bandaging against the flail segment to stabilize it (Figure 10-29 ■). Employ high-flow, high-concentration oxygen therapy; monitor oxygen saturation with pulse oximetry; and monitor cardiac activity with the ECG. If there is significant dyspnea, evidence of underlying pulmonary injury, or signs of respiratory compromise, these measures will not suffice. Then consider endotracheal intubation, positive pressure ventilations, and high-flow, high-concentration oxygen. Positive-pressure ventilations internally splint the flail segment, expand atelectatic areas of the lung, and also treat underlying pulmonary contusion. Use of sandbags to support the flail segment is not indicated because it may diminish chest movement, adding to hypoventilation, atelectasis, and subsequent hypoxemia. Rapid transport to the trauma center is indicated as this injury, its complications, and associated injuries are often life threatening.

Consider early intubation of the patient with flail chest, especially when oxygenation remains impaired despite the provision of high-flow, high-concentration oxygen.

OPEN PNEUMOTHORAX

Support the patient with open pneumothorax by administering high-flow, high-concentration oxygen and monitoring oxygen saturation and respiratory effort. If you find a penetrating injury, cover it with a sterile occlusive dressing (sterile plastic wrap) taped on three sides (Figure 10-30 ■). This process converts the open pneumothorax into a closed pneumothorax, prevents further aspiration of air, and relieves any building pressure (tension pneumothorax) through the valvelike dressing. If the dyspnea diminishes somewhat but still continues, provide positive pressure ventilations and intubate as indicated. Carefully monitor the patient when you employ intermittent positive-pressure ventilation because its use may lead to a tension pneumothorax. If, after the dressing has been applied, the patient has progressive breathing difficulty, appears to be hypoventilating and hypoxemic, has decreasing breath sounds on the injured side, and has increasing jugular distention, remove the occlusive dressing. If you hear air rush out and the patient's respirations improve, reseal the wound, monitor breathing carefully,

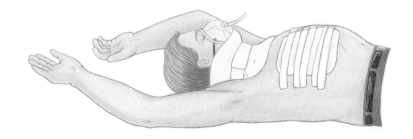

■ Figure 10-29 Flail chest should be treated with administration of oxygen and gentle splinting of the flail segment with a pillow or pad.

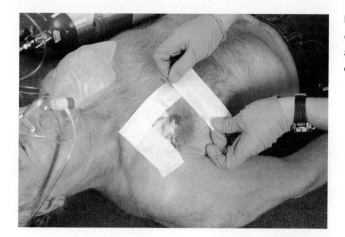

and again remove the dressing if any respiratory signs or symptoms redevelop. If removing the dressing does not relieve the increasing signs and symptoms, suspect and treat for tension pneumothorax.

TENSION PNEUMOTHORAX

Confirm possible tension pneumothorax by auscultating the lung fields for diminished breath sounds, percussing for hyperresonance, and observing for severe dyspnea, hyperinflation of the chest, and jugular vein distention. Successful treatment depends on rapid recognition of this condition and then pleural decompression. As you prepare to decompress the affected (ipsilateral) side, apply high-flow, high-concentration oxygen if the airway is intact and the patient is able to demonstrate adequate ventilatory effort. Pleural decompression should only be employed if the patient demonstrates significant dyspnea and distinct signs and symptoms of tension pneumothorax.

Provide ventilations with the bag-valve mask and supplemental oxygen and intubate if the patient is unable to maintain an airway or continues to show signs/symptoms of hypoxemia on high-flow, high-concentration oxygen. Perform needle thoracentesis by inserting a long 14-gauge intravascular catheter into the second intercostal space, midclavicular line on the side of the thorax with decreased breath sounds and hyperinflation (Figure 10-31 ■). Attach a syringe filled with sterile water or saline to the needle hub of the catheter. Then advance the catheter through the chest wall while maintaining gentle traction on the syringe plunger. Assure you enter the thoracic cavity by passing the needle just over the rib. The intercostal artery, vein, and nerve pass just under each rib and may be injured if the needle's track is too high. As you enter the pleural space, you will feel a pop and note bubbling air through the fluid in the syringe. Advance the catheter into the chest and then withdraw the needle and syringe.

If the patient remains symptomatic, place a second or third catheter to more rapidly facilitate decompression. Secure the catheter in place with tape, being careful not to block the port or kink the catheter. Leaving the catheter open to air converts the tension pneumothorax into a simple pneumothorax and stabilizes the patient. You may create a flutter valve by cutting the finger off a latex glove, making a small perforation in its tip, and securing it to the catheter hub, or use a commercially available Heimlich valve. Monitor the patient's respirations and breath sounds for a recurring tension pneumothorax. If signs and symptoms again appear, decompress the chest again. Frequently, the initial catheter will clog or kink and necessitate replacement by another.

Rapidly transport the patient to the trauma center for definitive treatment (usually with a chest tube). Be cautious in using IV crystalloid infusion if the patient is

⚷━◇ ─────────────
Tension pneumothorax is an occasional complication of multiple trauma. Always assess for it and decompress the chest when indicated.

⚷━◇ ─────────────
Pleural decompression should only be employed if the patient demonstrates significant dyspnea and distinct signs and symptoms of tension pneumothorax.

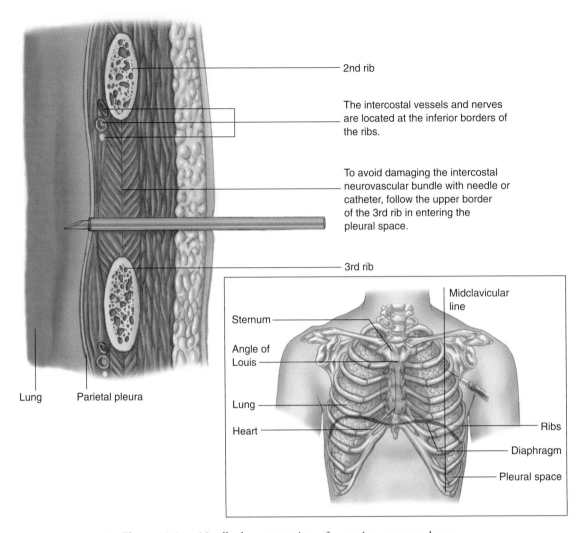

2nd rib

The intercostal vessels and nerves are located at the inferior borders of the ribs.

To avoid damaging the intercostal neurovascular bundle with needle or catheter, follow the upper border of the 3rd rib in entering the pleural space.

3rd rib

Midclavicular line

Sternum

Angle of Louis

Lung

Heart

Ribs

Diaphragm

Pleural space

Lung   Parietal pleura

■ Figure 10-31   Needle decompression of a tension pneumothorax.

hemodynamically stable. An underlying pulmonary contusion may lead to edema, which is made worse with overaggressive fluid therapy. If your patient remains hypotensive after chest decompression and respirations do not become adequate, consider the possibility of internal hemorrhage and the need for (conservative) fluid resuscitation. If respirations do not dramatically improve, assess for a contralateral tension pneumothorax or pericardial tamponade as the cause.

HEMOTHORAX

Treat the patient with suspected hemothorax with oxygen administration and ventilatory support, as needed. Initiate two large-bore intravenous catheters, readied to infuse large volumes of fluid. Be conservative in fluid administration. Maintain a blood pressure of 80 mmHg but do not attempt to return it to preinjury levels. Carefully listen to breath sounds during any infusion because the increasing vascular volume may increase the edema and congestion of pulmonary contusion. It may also increase the pressure, rate, and volume of internal hemorrhage. If the pulmonary contusion is extensive and the patient cannot be adequately oxygenated by high-flow, high-concentration oxygen, positive pressure ventilations are indicated and may limit further edema that contributes to the injury.

MYOCARDIAL CONTUSION

In serious frontal impact collisions, suspect myocardial contusion and administer high-flow, high-concentration oxygen. Monitor cardiac electrical activity and watch for tachycardias, bradycardias, ectopic beats, and conduction defects. Establish an IV line in the event that antidysrhythmics (such as amiodarone) are needed, and monitor the patient for great vessel injury. Employ the pharmacological care measures recommended for advanced cardiac life support (Volume 3, Chapter 2, "Cardiology"). Rapidly transport the patient to the trauma center for further evaluation and continued monitoring.

PERICARDIAL TAMPONADE

Maintain a high index of suspicion for pericardial tamponade in the patient with central thoracic penetrating trauma. While there is little prehospital care other than the administration of oxygen and IV fluids to maximize venous return, definitive care is to remove some of the fluid accumulating in the pericardial sac. This action is rarely permitted in the field; hence, the patient needs to be transported as rapidly as possible to the emergency department. Note that a relatively simple procedure can relieve this problem and can be adequately administered by an emergency physician. If a physician-staffed emergency department is significantly closer to you than the trauma center, it may be the best choice for the patient with pericardial tamponade. After the pericardiocentesis is performed, the patient may then be directed to the closest trauma center.

If pericardial tamponade is suspected, consider diverting to the closest hospital with a physician-staffed emergency department where emergency pericardiocentesis can be performed.

AORTIC ANEURYSM

Care for the patient with dissecting aortic aneurysm is performed through gentle but rapid transport to the trauma center. Any jarring during extrication, assessment, care, packaging, or transport increases the risk of rupture and rapidly fatal exsanguination. Initiate IV therapy en route, but be very conservative in fluid administration. Mild hypotension may be protective of the injury site. If the aneurysm ruptures, as indicated by an immediate deterioration in vital signs, provide rapid administration of fluids. Anxiety and its effect on cardiac output and blood pressure may increase the likelihood of aneurysm rupture. Place a special emphasis on calming and reassuring the patient during very gentle care and transport.

TRACHEOBRONCHIAL INJURY

Support the tracheobronchial injury patient with high-flow, high-concentration oxygen and clear the airway of blood and secretions. If you are unable to maintain a patent airway or adequately oxygenate the patient, then intubate the trachea and provide positive pressure ventilations. Observe the patient carefully for the development of a tension pneumothorax, which may result as a complication of positive pressure ventilations, and treat as previously prescribed. Provide rapid transport as soon as the patient can be extricated and stabilized. This is important because these patients can rapidly destabilize and then require emergency surgical intervention.

TRAUMATIC ASPHYXIA

Administer oxygen and support the airway and respiration of the traumatic asphyxia patient. This may require using positive-pressure ventilations with the bag-valve mask to assure adequate ventilation during the entrapment and possibly thereafter. Establish two large-bore IV lines for rapid infusion of crystalloid in anticipation of rapidly developing hypovolemia with chest decompression. Once the compressing force is removed, the direct effects of traumatic asphyxia spontaneously resolve; however, serious internal hemorrhage may begin. Prepare to transport immediately after release from entrapment because the patient will likely have severe coexisting injuries.

If the patient remains entrapped for a prolonged time, consider the administration of sodium bicarbonate. Prolonged stagnant blood flow and a hypoxic cellular environment may cause accumulation of metabolic acids. As the compression is released, this blood returns to the central circulation, much as it does with entrapped limbs during crush injury. Consider the administration of 1 mEq/kg of sodium bicarbonate just before or during decompression of the chest if entrapment has lasted more than 20 minutes. Employ this therapy as discussed in Chapter 5, "Soft-Tissue Trauma."

Summary

Thoracic trauma by either blunt or penetrating mechanisms has a great potential for posing a threat to a patient's life. In fact, 25 percent of all traumatic deaths are secondary to injuries in this region. In assessing these patients, the mechanism of injury, when considered along with the clinical findings, may help in differentiating among the many possible injuries. The assessment, in turn, helps guide your interventions and determines the need for rapid extrication and transport. Aggressive airway management, oxygenation, ventilation, and fluid resuscitation, when indicated, can make the difference between the patient's survival or death. Specific interventions, such as pleural decompression or stabilization of a flail segment, can also affect mortality and morbidity from chest trauma. Understanding the pathological processes affecting the chest during trauma and employing proper assessment and care measures will assure the best possible outcome for your patients.

You Make the Call

Medic 101 responds to the interstate where they are called to a crash scene. An older pick-up truck has struck a bridge abutment, apparently after the driver fell asleep while driving home from the night shift. The scene survey reveals that the State Patrol has deployed appropriate warning flares and controlled traffic to allow safe access to the scene. The paramedics approach the truck and find a 20-year-old male patient unconscious behind the wheel. The paramedics note that no seat belt has been worn and no air bag has deployed. The steering wheel is displaced somewhat upward and bent inward against the dash. The windshield is starred.

The initial assessment reveals an unconscious male patient with central cyanosis, poor air exchange, and no peripheral (radial) pulses palpable. With in-line stabilization, the patient is rapidly extricated to a long board, the airway is opened by a jaw thrust (with cervical precautions), and an oral airway is then placed with respiratory assistance provided via BVM with reservoir attached to oxygen at 15 L/min. Little improvement is noted in the patient's color, air exchange, level of consciousness, and peripheral pulses. The trachea appears midline, but jugular vein distention is present. As the patient's clothes are cut away, subcutaneous emphysema is palpable along the left anterior and lateral chest wall. There is a pronounced inward movement of a section of anterior chest wall with the patient's inspiratory efforts.

1. Considering the mechanism of injury and what is known about the patient, what thoracic pathophysiology may explain the patient's presentation?

2. As the treating paramedic, what is your next step in stabilizing this patient?

3. What further emergency treatment is likely indicated by the absence of breath sounds on the left side and a relatively normal abdominal exam?

See Suggested Responses at the back of this book.

Review Questions

1. The union between the xiphoid process and the body of the sternum is called the:
   a. manubrium.
   b. thoracic duct.
   c. costal margin.
   d. xiphisternal joint.

2. During a football game, a 17-year-old male is tackled and knocked to the ground. Although he reports hearing a "bone crack," he initially appears to be stable. The team manager summons the paramedics. By the time they arrive, the patient states that he is "feeling funny" and having difficulty breathing. Upon initial assessment, a rapid, weak pulse and a low B/P are noted. The patient's appearance suggests that he may be developing shock. You suspect a fractured rib and possibly:
   a. traumatic asphyxia.
   b. pericardial tamponade.
   c. tension pneumothorax.
   d. traumatic aortic rupture.

3. Secondary to a severe chest wall contusion, which of the following signs/symptoms is most commonly seen?
   a. retractions
   b. hypoventilation
   c. deep, gasping respirations
   d. use of accessory muscles

4. You have elected to apply an occlusive dressing to your patient who has sustained a stab wound to the chest. You realize that you should secure the dressing:
   a. on two sides.
   b. on four sides.
   c. on three sides.
   d. loosely over the wound.

5. Your patient has received significant deceleration trauma to his chest. He presents with absent radial and brachial pulses in the left upper extremity and severe hypotension. He reported that he felt a tearing sensation in his chest before quickly losing consciousness. He most likely has experienced a:
   a. severe rib fracture.
   b. pericardial tamponade.
   c. pulmonary contusion.
   d. traumatic aortic aneurysm.

6. The type of crash impact most commonly associated with aortic rupture when the patient has been involved in a motor vehicle collision is:
   a. lateral.
   b. frontal.
   c. rollover.
   d. rotational.

7. The following mechanism of injury most likely to cause traumatic asphyxia is:
   a. blunt trauma, low impact.
   b. penetrating trauma, low velocity.
   c. penetrating trauma, high velocity.
   d. blunt trauma, compressive force.

8. You and your partner are called to the scene of a motor vehicle collision. When you arrive, you note that a car has struck a parked vehicle. Your 30-year-old female patient complains of difficulty breathing and you note that breath sounds are diminished bilaterally. The patient states that, at the last minute, she anticipated the impending accident and held her breath. You suspect "paper-bag syndrome" in which the sudden pressure exerted on her expanded lungs, with closed glottis preventing the escape of air, caused the rupture of:
   a. alveoli.
   b. arteries.
   c. the spleen.
   d. the diaphragm.

9. The most appropriate prehospital management for a patient with a flail segment and no other suspected underlying injury is:
   a. chest tube insertion.
   b. positive-pressure ventilation.
   c. needle decompression.
   d. sandbag placed on the injured side.

10. The most appropriate prehospital management for a patient with a traumatic rupture of the aorta is to:
    a. initiate two large-bore IVs prior to transport.
    b. delay transport to complete application of the PASG garment.
    c. begin a rapid IV drip of plasma expanders bilaterally, prior to transport.
    d. expedite transport to a trauma center; administer conservative IV fluids en route.

See Answers to Review Questions at the back of this book.

Further Reading

American College of Surgeons, Committee on Trauma. *Advanced Trauma Life Support Course: Student Manual.* Chicago: American College of Surgeons, 2003.

Bates, Barbara, Lynn S. Bickley, and Robert A. Hoekelman. *A Guide to Physical Examination and History Taking.* 8th ed. Philadelphia: J. B. Lippincott, 2003.

Bledsoe, B. E. and D. Clayden. *Prehospital Emergency Pharamacology.* 6th ed. Upper Saddle River, N.J.: Pearson/Prentice Hall, 2005.

Butman, A., S. Martin, R. Vomacka, and N. McSwain. *Comprehensive Guide to Pre-Hospital Skills: A Skills Manual for EMT-Basic, EMT-Intermediate, and EMT-Paramedic.* St. Louis: Mosby, 1996.

Campbell, John E. *Basic Trauma Life Support for Paramedics and Other Advanced Providers.* 5th ed. update. Upper Saddle River, N.J.: Pearson/Prentice Hall, 2004.

Clemente, C. D. *Anatomy: A Regional Atlas of the Human Body.* 4th ed. Baltimore: Lippincott, Williams & Wilkins, 1997.

Hall-Craggs, E. C. B. *Anatomy as a Basis for Clinical Medicine.* 3rd ed. Baltimore: Lippincott, Williams & Wilkins, 1995.

Martini, Frederic. *Fundamentals of Anatomy and Physiology.* 6th ed. San Francisco: Benjamin Cummings, 2004.

McSwain, N. E. and S. B. Frame, eds. *Prehospital Trauma Life Support.* 5th ed. St. Louis: Mosby, 2003.

Rosen, P., and R. Barkin, eds. *Emergency Medicine: Concepts and Clinical Practice.* 5th ed. St. Louis: Mosby, 2002.

Wilkins, E. W. *Emergency Medicine: Scientific Foundations and Current Practice.* 3rd ed. Baltimore, MD: Williams and Wilkins, 1989.

Zuidema, G. D., R. B. Rutherford, and W. F. Ballinger. *The Management of Trauma.* 4th ed. Philadelphia: W. B. Saunders, 1985.

On the Web

Visit Brady's Paramedic Website at **www.bradybooks.com/paramedic**.

11

Abdominal Trauma

Objectives

After reading this chapter, you should be able to:

1. Describe the epidemiology, including morbidity/mortality, for patients with abdominal trauma as well as prevention strategies to avoid the injuries. (pp. 428–429)

2. Apply the epidemiologic principles to develop prevention strategies for abdominal injuries. (pp. 428–429)

3. Describe the anatomy and physiology of organs and structures related to abdominal injuries. (pp. 429–437)

4. Predict abdominal injuries based on blunt and penetrating mechanisms of injury. (pp. 437–445)

5. Describe open and closed abdominal injuries. (pp. 437–440)

6. Identify the need for rapid intervention and transport of the patient with abdominal injuries based on assessment findings. (pp. 445–451)

7. Explain the pathophysiology of solid and hollow organ injuries, abdominal vascular injuries, pelvic fractures, and other abdominal injuries. (pp. 440–445)

8. Describe the assessment findings associated with, and the management of, solid and hollow organ injuries, abdominal vascular injuries, pelvic fractures, and other abdominal injuries. (pp. 445–454)

9. Differentiate between abdominal injuries based on the assessment and history. (pp. 445–451)

10. Given several preprogrammed and moulaged abdominal trauma patients, provide the appropriate scene size-up, initial assessment, rapid trauma or focused physical exam and history, detailed exam, and ongoing assessment and provide appropriate patient care and transportation. (pp. 428–454)

Key Terms

Case Study

Janice and her paramedic partner Doug respond to a "shots fired" call in the early hours of Saturday morning. They arrive at an apartment complex, noting that there are several police vehicles on scene. The officers tell the paramedics that the wife is in custody and are directed by an officer to a hallway where a middle-aged male sits propped against a wall. The man holds what appears to be a blood-soaked towel against his abdomen.

Janice introduces herself as a paramedic and begins the patient's initial assessment. The victim, Marty, is a 43-year-old who was shot by his wife during a domestic dispute. He reports "she shot me once with my 9-mm handgun" at close range. Janice coaxes Marty to lift the towel and observes a small entrance wound to the left upper quadrant, oozing just a small amount of blood. Inspection of Marty's back and flank reveals no exit wound. Doug assesses vital signs and obtains a blood pressure of 110/86, a strong and regular pulse at a rate of 80, and respirations of 22. Marty's ECG traces a normal sinus rhythm, and his oxygen saturation is 99 percent. He is alert and oriented to time, place, and person. He describes his abdominal pain as sharp in the region of the wound, although the area surrounding the wound feels "burning" in nature.

Janice applies oxygen using a nonrebreather mask at 15 liters per minute and covers the wound with a small dressing, taping it firmly in place. She and Doug prepare to move Marty quickly to the waiting stretcher and then to the ambulance.

As Janice prepares Marty for the ride to the hospital, Doug informs her that the nearest trauma center has just received several seriously injured patients from an auto crash, and Janice and Doug are directed to a more distant Level II trauma center.

En route, Janice initiates an IV line with a large-bore catheter, trauma tubing, and a 1,000-mL bag of lactated Ringer's solution, running at a to-keep-open rate. During transport Janice questions Marty about his symptoms and now notes that he complains of shoulder pain and some thirst. Janice's ongoing assessment reveals a blood pressure of 112/94, a strong pulse at 86, and respirations that are now somewhat shallow at 24. Oxygen saturation remains at 99 percent and the ECG still displays a normal sinus rhythm. Blood is no longer draining from the entrance wound, and further examination does not reveal an exit wound. Janice auscultates the chest and abdomen and, though road sounds limit the clarity of auscultation, she hears only clear breath sounds in the chest and no bowel sounds.

Janice completes a final set of vital signs as they arrive at the emergency department. Marty's pulse is 88, blood pressure is 112/96, and respirations are 22 and somewhat shallow. Janice quickly reports her assessment findings and care to the trauma team as they prepare Marty for possible surgery. She helps them quickly load Marty to the hospital gurney and watches them whisk him away.

During her next trip to the trauma center the staff informs Janice that Marty's surgery was successful. They found the stomach to be perforated, the spleen to be torn, and over 1,000 mL of blood was in the abdomen. Marty did well during surgery and is on his way to a quick recovery.

INTRODUCTION TO ABDOMINAL TRAUMA

Injury to the abdomen does not present as dramatically as it does elsewhere in the body and often occurs without overt signs.

The abdominal cavity is one of the body's largest cavities and contains many organs essential to life. Serious direct or secondary injury may damage these vital organs. In addition, large volumes of blood can be lost in the cavity before the loss becomes evident. In the abdomen, however, injury does not always present as dramatically as it does elsewhere in the body. Injury often occurs without overt signs because few skeletal structures protect the abdomen. The signs of transmitted injury—deformity, swelling, and the discoloration of contusions—take time to develop and are not often seen in the prehospital setting. These considerations make the anticipation of possible abdominal injuries and careful abdominal assessment critical for the patient with trauma to this region.

Over the past decade, the relative mortality and morbidity for the various abdominal injuries has declined due to improved surgical and critical care techniques. Reduced injury-to-surgery times have also contributed to this decline as EMS systems have recognized the necessity of rapid surgical intervention. The severity of injuries and the number of deaths associated with blunt trauma have also decreased thanks to improvements in highway design and vehicle structure and to a greater use of seat belts and other safety practices. However, the overall mortality and morbidity from penetrating trauma is on the rise due to the increasing violence in our society, most specifically in the growing use and power of hand guns. Penetrating trauma is approaching trauma associated with auto crashes as the number one trauma killer. Nowhere is this more apparent than with injuries to the abdomen.

Prevention of abdominal injuries, as with most other types of trauma, is the best way to reduce mortality and morbidity. As noted, highway and vehicle design improvements and the following of safety practices at home and in the workplace play important roles in reducing both the incidence and seriousness of abdominal injury.

There remains room for further improvements in safety practices, however. For example, many people still do not use seat belts. Failure to use the seat belt increases the incidence of abdominal injury secondary to impact with the steering wheel, dash, or other parts of the auto's interior and of impact after ejection. (Side impact air bags have the potential to reduce the incidence of pelvic fracture and internal abdominal injuries frequently associated with this mechanism of injury.)

One area of special concern is the proper application of the auto lap belt. If the belt rides too high on the abdomen, with deceleration the belt directs forces both to the contents of the abdominal cavity and to the lumbar spine. Severe compression may result in serious associated abdominal injury. Proper placement, in which the belt rests on the iliac crests, transmits the forces of severe deceleration to the pelvis and the body's skeletal structure, thus sparing the abdominal contents and the spine from injury. Proper positioning of seat belts is especially important with children.

Mortality and morbidity associated with penetrating trauma can also be reduced by reducing violence in society and by reducing the availability of hand guns.

ABDOMINAL ANATOMY AND PHYSIOLOGY

The abdominal cavity is bound by the diaphragm, superiorly; the pelvis, inferiorly; the vertebral column, the posterior and inferior ribs, and the back muscles (psoas and paraspinal muscles), posteriorly; the muscles of the flank, laterally; and the abdominal muscles, anteriorly (Figure 11-1 ■). The cavity is divided into three spaces: the **peritoneal space** (containing those organs or portions of organs covered by the abdominal (peritoneal) lining); the **retroperitoneal space** (containing those organs posterior to the peritoneal lining); and the **pelvic space** (containing the organs within the pelvis). Anatomical landmarks of this area include the centrally located umbilicus (the navel), the xiphoid process (tip of the sternum) at the upper and central abdominal border, the bony ridges of the pelvis (the iliac crests) inferiorly and laterally, and the pubic prominence inferiorly.

The abdomen is divided into four subregions by vertical and horizontal lines intersecting at the umbilicus (navel) and forming the right and left upper and lower quadrants. The right upper quadrant contains the gallbladder, right kidney, most of the liver, some small bowel, a portion of the ascending and transverse colon, and a small portion of the pancreas. The left upper quadrant contains the stomach, spleen, left kidney, most of the pancreas, and a portion of the liver, small bowel, and transverse and descending colon. The right lower quadrant contains the appendix, and portions of the urinary bladder, small bowel, ascending colon, rectum, and female genitalia. The left lower quadrant contains the sigmoid colon and portions of the urinary bladder, small bowel, descending colon, rectum, and female genitalia.

The major structures within the abdomen include the digestive tract, the accessory organs of digestion, the structures and organs of the urinary system, the spleen, and, in the female, the genitals. The digestive tract (also called the alimentary canal) is the muscular tube that physically and chemically breaks down and absorbs the fluids and nutrients from the food we eat. The accessory organs of digestion include the liver, gallbladder, and pancreas. These organs prepare and store digestive enzymes and perform

peritoneal space *division of the abdominal cavity containing those organs or portions of organs covered by the peritoneum.*

retroperitoneal space *division of the abdominal cavity containing those organs posterior to the peritoneal lining.*

pelvic space *division of the abdominal cavity containing those organs located within the pelvis.*

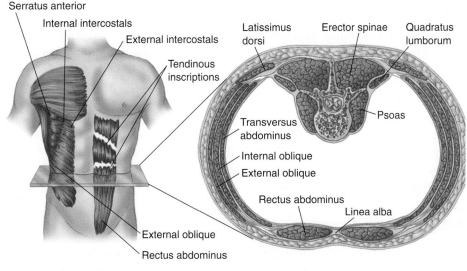

a. Anterior view of the trunk, showing superficial and deep members of the oblique and rectus groups.

b. Diagrammatic sectional view through the abdominal region.

■ Figure 11-1 Muscles protecting the organs of the abdominal cavity.

other important body functions. The spleen is a component of the immune system, while the paired kidneys and ureters, the urinary bladder, and the urethra comprise the urinary system. In the female, the ovaries, fallopian tubes, uterus, and vagina also occupy some of the abdominal cavity.

DIGESTIVE TRACT

digestive tract *internal passageway that begins at the mouth and ends at the anus.*

The **digestive tract** is a thin, 25-foot-long hollow muscular tube responsible for churning the material to be digested, for excreting digestive juices to be mixed with it, and for absorbing nutrients and then water (Figure 11-2 ■). Abdominal components of the digestive tract consist of the stomach, the small bowel (duodenum, jejunum, and ileum), the large bowel (or colon), the rectum, and the anus. These structures fill the anterior and lateral aspects of the abdominal cavity, except for the area occupied by the liver.

The esophagus enters the abdomen through the hiatus of the diaphragm (just posterior to the xiphoid process) and then deposits its contents into the stomach. The stomach is a J-shaped muscular container that mixes the ingested material with hydrochloric acid and enzymes (both produced in the gastric wall) into a thick fluid called **chyme.** The acid released by the stomach increases the gastric acidity (pH) to between 1.5 and 2.0. This is a very acidic fluid that would damage the stomach and the initial lining of the small bowel if not for the continuous production of a protective mucus. The stomach is highly variable in size, depending on the amount of material it contains. It can distend to hold as much as 1.5 liters of food after a large meal.

chyme *semifluid mixture of ingested food and digestive secretions found in the stomach and small intestine.*

Chyme is released in small boluses into the first component of the small bowel, the duodenum. The duodenum is approximately 1 foot in length and is where the digesting material is mixed with bile from the liver (stored in the gallbladder) and pancreatic digestive juices. These agents raise the pH of the chyme (returning it towards neutral) and help release the nutrients it contains.

peristalsis *wavelike muscular motion of the esophagus and bowel that moves food through the digestive system.*

The digesting food is propelled along the small and large bowel by waves of contraction called **peristalsis.** The muscles of the digestive tract constrict the bowel's lumen behind a mass of food, then progressively constrict the lumen in the direction of desired movement. The resulting rhythmic constriction moves the digesting material through the tract. As chyme enters the next two segments of the small bowel (the jejunum and the ileum), the mixing decreases and the nutrients, released by the physical and chemical digestion processes, are absorbed, directed to the liver for detoxification, and then released into the circulatory system.

As the food continues its travel through the digestive tract, it arrives at the large bowel. Here masses of bacteria assist in releasing vitamins and fluid from the digesting food while the large bowel absorbs most of the remaining fluid content. The water serves to hydrate the body while the digestive juices are reabsorbed and reprocessed to rejoin the digestive process upstream again. The large bowel ascends superiorly along the right side of the abdomen (ascending colon), traverses the abdomen just below the liver and stomach (transverse colon), then descends along the left lateral abdomen (descending colon). It aligns with the rectum through the S-shaped sigmoid colon where the end waste products of the digestive process (feces) await excretion (defecation) through the terminal valve, the anus.

ACCESSORY ORGANS

The liver is a vascular structure responsible for detoxifying the blood, removing damaged or aged erythrocytes, and storing glycogen and other important agents for body metabolism. The liver also assists in the osmotic regulation of fluids in the blood and plays a role in the clotting process. Finally, the liver detoxifies materials absorbed by the digestive system and either stores or releases nutrients to assure the body's metabolic

The Digestive System

ORGANS OF THE DIGESTIVE SYSTEM

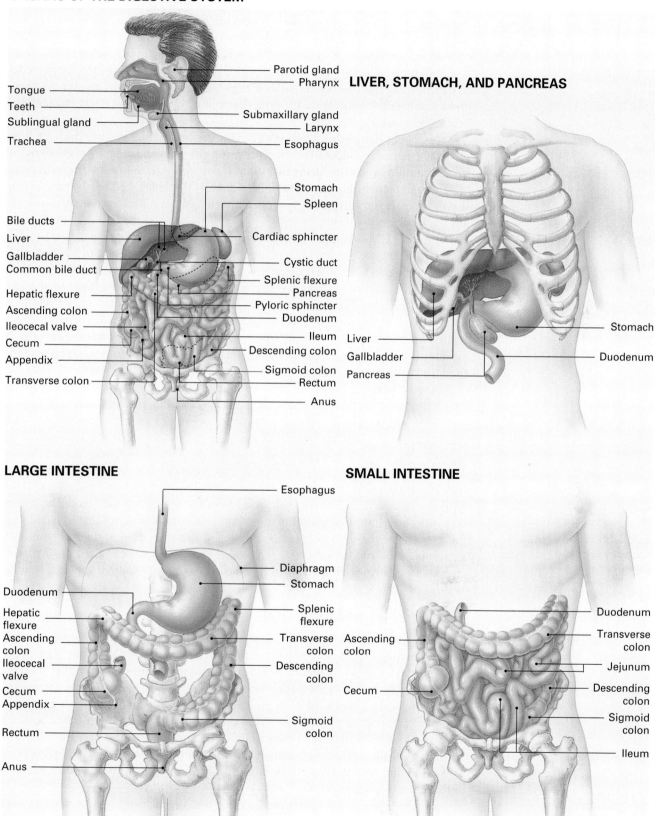

Parotid gland
Pharynx
Tongue
Teeth
Sublingual gland
Submaxillary gland
Larynx
Trachea
Esophagus

LIVER, STOMACH, AND PANCREAS

Stomach
Spleen
Bile ducts
Liver
Cardiac sphincter
Gallbladder
Common bile duct
Cystic duct
Splenic flexure
Hepatic flexure
Pancreas
Ascending colon
Pyloric sphincter
Ileocecal valve
Duodenum
Cecum
Ileum
Appendix
Descending colon
Transverse colon
Sigmoid colon
Rectum
Anus

Liver
Stomach
Gallbladder
Duodenum
Pancreas

LARGE INTESTINE

Esophagus
Duodenum
Diaphragm
Stomach
Hepatic flexure
Ascending colon
Splenic flexure
Ileocecal valve
Transverse colon
Cecum
Descending colon
Appendix
Rectum
Sigmoid colon
Anus

SMALL INTESTINE

Duodenum
Ascending colon
Transverse colon
Jejunum
Cecum
Descending colon
Sigmoid colon
Ileum

■ Figure 11-2   The digestive tract and accessory organs.

needs are met. It is located in the right upper quadrant, just below the diaphragm, and extends into the medial portion of the left upper quadrant. It is the largest abdominal organ, accounting for 2.5 percent of total body weight. It receives about 25 percent of cardiac output and holds the greatest blood reserve of any body organ. The lower portion of its mass can occasionally be palpated just below the margin of the rib cage. It is suspended in its location by several ligaments including the ligamentum teres, and connects to the omentum inferiorly. The liver is a solid organ but is rather delicate in nature. It is contained within a fibrous capsule (visceral peritoneum) that serves to retard hemorrhage and helps hold the liver together if injured by blunt trauma. When injured, the liver will regenerate to some degree but will not function as efficiently as before the injury.

The gallbladder is a small hollow organ located behind and beneath the liver. It receives bile (a waste product from the reprocessing of red blood cells) from the liver and stores it until it is needed during digestion of fatty foods. It then constricts and sends bile through the bile duct and into the duodenum. Bile helps the body by emulsifying (breaking apart and suspending) ingested fats that would otherwise remain as clumps during the digestive process.

The other accessory digestive organ is the pancreas. It is responsible for the production of glucagon and insulin, hormones responsible for the regulation of blood glucose levels and the transport of glucose across cell membranes. The pancreas also produces very powerful digestive enzymes that help return the pH of the chyme toward normal and break down proteins. These enzymes enter the duodenum through the common bile duct. Like the liver, the pancreas is a solid, though delicate, organ, encapsulated in a serous membrane. It is located in the medial and lower portion of the left upper quadrant and extends into the medial portion of the right upper quadrant. The duodenum wraps around the right pancreatic border. If the cells of the pancreas are damaged, the pancreatic enzymes may become active and begin to "self-digest" pancreatic tissue. If these enzymes are released into the retroperitoneal space, they will also damage surrounding tissue.

SPLEEN

The spleen is not an accessory organ of digestion but rather a part of the immune system. It is a very vascular organ about the size of the palm of the hand and is located behind the stomach and lateral to the kidney in the left upper quadrant. The spleen performs some immunological functions and also stores a large volume of blood. It is the most fragile abdominal organ, though well protected in its location by the rib cage, spine, and flank and back muscles. The spleen, however, can be injured during blunt trauma, especially with impacts affecting the left flank; when injured, it bleeds heavily.

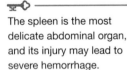

The spleen is the most delicate abdominal organ, and its injury may lead to severe hemorrhage.

URINARY SYSTEM

The urinary system consists of the kidneys (or renal glands), the ureters, urinary bladder, and urethra (Figure 11-3 ■). The kidneys are located in the posterior portions of the right and left upper quadrants and are protected by the musculature of the back, the thoracic and lumbar spine, and the muscles of the flanks. The kidneys have direct connections with the abdominal aorta and receive a more than abundant blood supply. They collect the waste products found in the bloodstream and concentrate them in a watery fluid called urine. They exert significant regulatory control over the salt/water (osmotic) balance of the body by retaining or releasing water or sodium and other body salts. The kidneys also play an important role in controlling body pH and monitoring and maintaining blood pressure.

Just above and attached to the kidneys are the adrenal glands. These structures are a part of the endocrine system and are responsible for the production and release of the

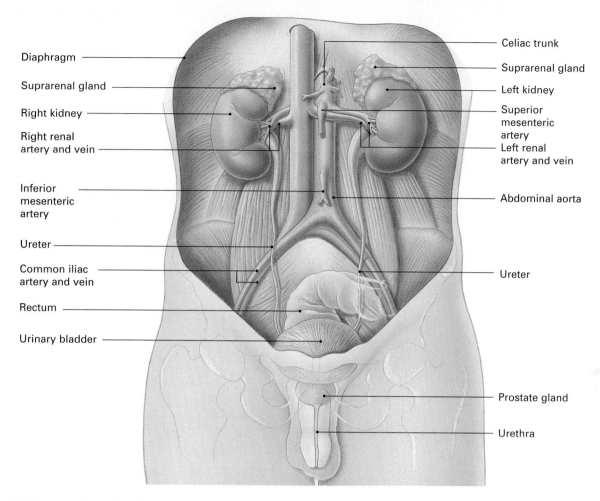

Diaphragm

Suprarenal gland

Right kidney

Right renal
artery and vein

Inferior
mesenteric
artery

Ureter

Common iliac
artery and vein

Rectum

Urinary bladder

Celiac trunk

Suprarenal gland

Left kidney

Superior
mesenteric
artery

Left renal
artery and vein

Abdominal aorta

Ureter

Prostate gland

Urethra

Figure 11-3 Major elements of the urinary system.

sympathetic hormones epinephrine and norepinephrine. Adrenal injury can have a profound effect on autonomic control of the body. However, since there are two kidneys and also two adrenal glands, it is unlikely that both would be seriously injured at the same time.

The kidneys each connect to a small tube, called a ureter, which transports urine to the urinary bladder. The bladder is a hollow muscular organ located along the floor of the pelvic space and just posterior to the pubic bone. Urine is stored here until it is convenient or necessary to void. After urination, the bladder contains about 10 mL of fluid. However, when fully distended it may contain as much as 500 mL. Urine is excreted from the body through the urethra, a small tube slightly more than 1 inch (25 to 30 mm) long in the female and 7 to 8 inches (18 to 20 cm) long in the male.

GENITALIA

The sexual organs of the female are located internally within the peritoneum and the lower abdominal cavity (Figure 11-4 ■). These organs consist of the ovaries, fallopian tubes, uterus, and vagina. The ovaries are almond-shaped solid organs that store, mature, and then release an unfertilized egg approximately every 28 days. The egg is released into the abdominal cavity and directed to the adjacent fallopian tube, through which it then travels to the uterus. The uterus is a pear-shaped muscular organ located within the central pelvis. It is about 3 inches long and 2 inches in diameter at its largest

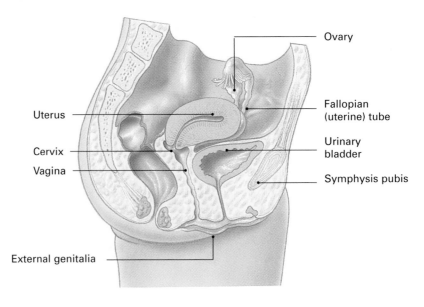

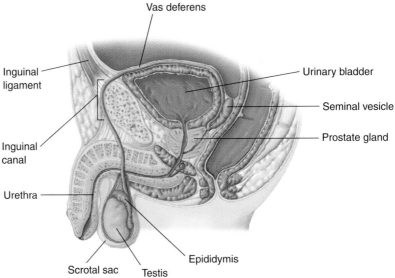

point. A fertilized egg will attach itself to the inner surface of the uterus or be sloughed off if fertilization does not occur. The inferior portion of the uterus is the cervix, a muscular valve that contains the developing fetus until time for delivery. The cervix opens to the vaginal canal, the female organ of copulation and the canal for passage of the delivering fetus. The vagina opens at the base of the pelvis, just behind the pubic bone. The vagina, uterus, and fallopian tubes represent an open passage to the interior of the abdominal cavity.

The sexual organs of the male are external to the abdomen, just anterior to the pubic bone. They include the testes, the sac that contains them (called the scrotum), and the penis. The testes generate sperm, which moves through a small, convoluted tube, the epididymis, to the prostate. At sexual climax, the sperm is mixed with seminal fluid, propelled through the prostate and the urethra, and expelled.

Pregnant Uterus

The dynamics of pregnancy greatly affect the anatomy of the female abdominal cavity (Figure 11-5 ■). The uterus and its contents grow rapidly from the time of conception until delivery and are well protected during the first trimester (3 months) of pregnancy.

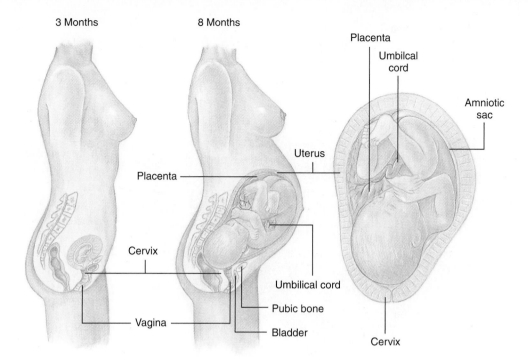

3 Months

8 Months

Placenta

Umbilcal cord

Amniotic sac

Uterus

Placenta

Cervix

Umbilical cord

Pubic bone

Vagina

Bladder

Cervix

■ Figure 11-5   The pregnant uterus.

During the second trimester (12 to 24 weeks), the progressive enlargement of the uterus displaces most of the abdominal contents upward as the growing uterus rises out of the pelvis and its upper border extends above the umbilicus. By 32 weeks and until the end of the pregnancy, the uterus fills the abdominal cavity to the level of the lower rib margin. This enlarging mass in the abdomen also increases the intra-abdominal pressure and displaces the diaphragm upward. This displacement reduces lung capacity at the same time that the physiological changes of pregnancy increase the tidal volume.

Pregnancy also affects the maternal physiology by raising the circulatory volume by about 45 percent and, by the third trimester, raising the cardiac rate by about 15 beats per minute and the cardiac output by up to 40 percent. The increase in the vascular volume is accompanied by a less significant increase in the number of erythrocytes. The result is a relative anemia that becomes an important consideration with aggressive fluid resuscitation for the mother in shock. In the last trimester of pregnancy, the uterus is significant in both size and weight and may compress the vena cava, reducing venous return to the heart and inducing a temporary hypotension in the supine patient (**supine hypotensive syndrome**). Finally, the developing fetus means there are now two lives to protect when the mother suffers any trauma, especially involving the abdomen.

supine hypotensive syndrome *inadequate return of venous blood to the heart, reduced cardiac output, and lowered blood pressure resulting from pressure on the inferior vena cava by the fetus and uterus late in pregnancy.*

VASCULATURE

The abdominal contents are supplied with blood via the abdominal aorta, which travels along and to the left of the spinal column. It sends forth many branches to discrete organs and the bowel (Figure 11-6 ■). The abdominal aorta bifurcates at the upper sacral level into two large iliac arteries. These eventually become the femoral arteries as they traverse and then exit the pelvis. The attachment of these arteries to the pelvic structure is quite firm and may result in their tearing if the pelvis is fractured and displaced. The inferior vena cava is located along the spinal column and collects venous blood from the lower extremities and the abdomen, relatively parallel to the arterial system, returning it to the heart. The abdomen also houses a special circulatory system,

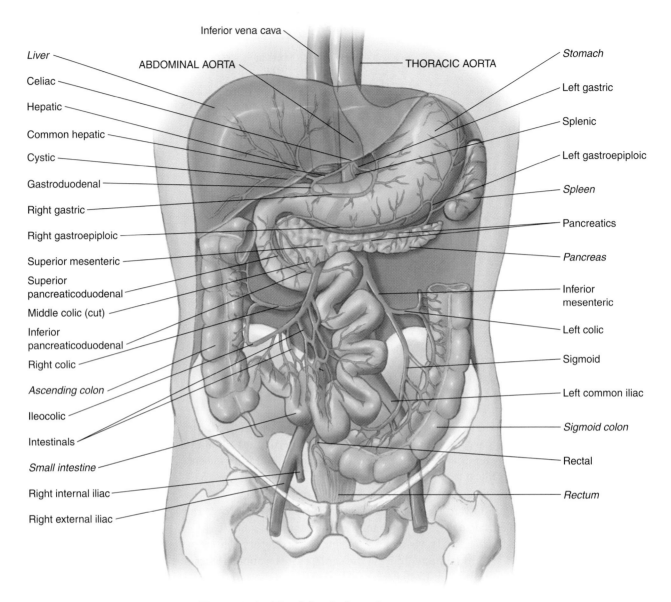

Liver
Celiac
Hepatic
Common hepatic
Cystic
Gastroduodenal
Right gastric
Right gastroepiploic
Superior mesenteric
Superior pancreaticoduodenal
Middle colic (cut)
Inferior pancreaticoduodenal
Right colic
Ascending colon
Ileocolic
Intestinals
Small intestine
Right internal iliac
Right external iliac

Inferior vena cava
ABDOMINAL AORTA
THORACIC AORTA

Stomach
Left gastric
Splenic
Left gastroepiploic
Spleen
Pancreatics
Pancreas
Inferior mesenteric
Left colic
Sigmoid
Left common iliac
Sigmoid colon
Rectal
Rectum

■ Figure 11-6   The abdominal arteries.

the portal system. This venous subsystem collects venous blood as well as the fluid and nutrients absorbed by the bowel and transports them to the liver. The liver detoxifies the fluid, stores excess nutrients, adds nutrients when they are deficient, and then sends the blood/nutrient/fluid mixture into the inferior vena cava, just below the heart. There it mixes with venous blood and is circulated through the heart and then the rest of the body.

PERITONEUM

peritoneum *fine fibrous tissue surrounding the interior of most of the abdominal cavity and covering most of the small bowel and some of the abdominal organs.*

Many of the abdominal organs are covered by a serous membrane called the **peritoneum** (Figure 11-7 ■). This tissue resembles the pleura of the lungs and functions in a similar manner. The parietal peritoneum covers most of the interior surface of the anterior and lateral abdominal cavity, while the visceral peritoneum covers the individual organs. A small amount of fluid is found between the peritoneal layers and permits free movement of the bowel during digestion. The digestive tract is restrained and pre-

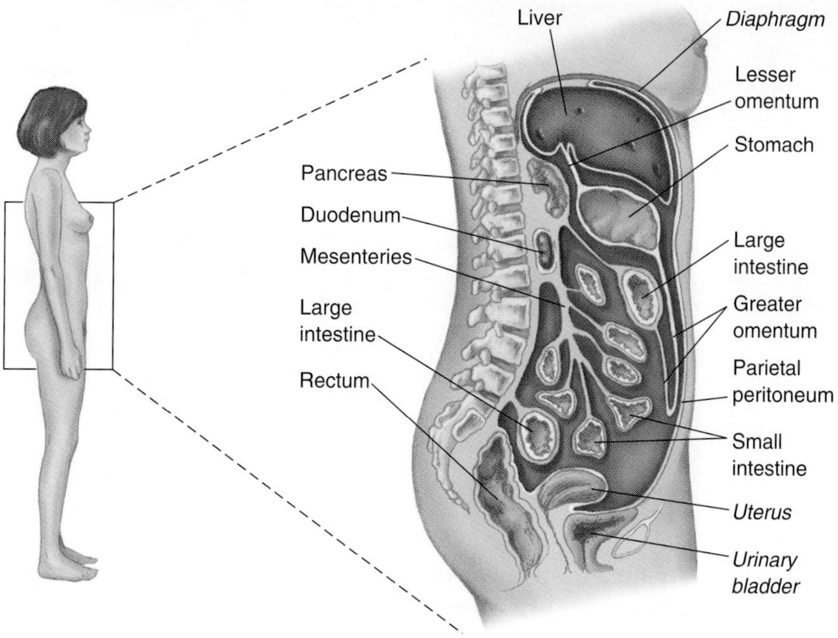

■ Figure 11-7 Reflections of the peritoneum.

Labels in figure: Liver, Diaphragm, Lesser omentum, Stomach, Pancreas, Duodenum, Mesenteries, Large intestine, Greater omentum, Parietal peritoneum, Large intestine, Rectum, Small intestine, Uterus, Urinary bladder

vented from tangling by a structure called the **mesentery.** The mesentery is a double fold of peritoneum containing blood vessels, lymphatic vessels, nerves, and fatty tissue. It suspends the bowel from the posterior abdominal wall. An additional fold of mesentery, called the omentum, also covers, insulates, and protects the anterior surface of the abdomen. The thickness of the omentum varies with the size and percentage of body fat of the patient. It may be several inches thick in the obese patient or very narrow in the thin and muscular patient. Most of the abdominal structures are covered by peritoneum, excepting the kidneys, spleen, duodenum, pancreas, urinary bladder, the posterior portions of the ascending and descending colon, and the rectum. Most of the major vascular structures within the abdomen are also retroperitoneal. An organ's relation to the peritoneum becomes important in trauma because irritation of the peritoneum (peritonitis) presents with more apparent signs and symptoms than does hemorrhage or the release of other fluids into the retroperitoneal space.

The abdominal cavity is a dynamic place. The diaphragm moves up and down, displacing the abdominal contents with each breath. With deep expiration, the central portion of the diaphragm moves as far upward as the fourth intercostal space, anteriorly (the nipple line), and the seventh intercostal space (the inferior tips of the scapulae), posteriorly. (The edge of the diaphragm attaches to the border of the rib cage.) During forced and maximal expiration, the diaphragm moves as much as 3 inches (9 cm) inferiorly. This movement displaces the abdominal contents up and down with each breath. Additionally, the volume of substance within the hollow organs varies—an empty (10 mL) versus a distended (500 mL) bladder or a full (1.5 L) versus an empty stomach. The digestive tract is also suspended from the back of the abdominal cavity and is permitted some movement as it digests food. This dynamic movement becomes an important consideration when anticipating abdominal injury due to blunt or penetrating trauma.

PATHOPHYSIOLOGY OF ABDOMINAL INJURY

MECHANISM OF INJURY

Unlike the other major body containers (skull, spine, and thorax), the abdomen is bound by muscles rather than skeletal structures. This results in a freer transmission of

mesentery *double fold of peritoneum that supports the major portion of the small bowel, suspending it from the posterior abdominal wall.*

Because the abdomen is bound by muscles rather than skeletal structures, there is a freer transmission of the energy of trauma to the internal organs and structures.

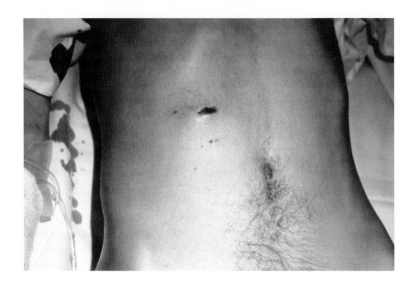

■ Figure 11-8   Stab wound to the right upper quadrant.

the energy of trauma to the internal organs and structures. Concurrently, the overt physical signs of this energy transmission are limited.

Penetrating Trauma

Penetrating trauma imparts its energy directly to the tissues touched by the offending object (Figure 11-8 ■) or, as with high-velocity projectiles (from hand guns, shotguns, and rifles), transmits energy and injury some distance from the projectile pathway. The bullet injury process causes damage as the projectile contacts tissue, sets that tissue and surrounding tissue in motion, then compresses and stretches surrounding tissue. The projectile adds to the damage as it draws debris and contaminants into the wound, causing wound infection and poor healing. The disruption of tissue from penetrating trauma may permit uncontrolled hemorrhage, organ damage, the spillage of hollow organ contents, and, eventually, irritation of the abdominal lining, the peritoneum. Gunshot wounds to the abdomen, especially those from rifles, high-powered hand guns, and shotguns at close range impart tremendous energy to the tissue and organs of the region and tend to cause a mortality and morbidity about 10 times greater than that associated with the lower velocity stab wounds. When penetrating trauma induces injury, it affects the liver 40 percent of the time, the small bowel about 25 percent of the time, and the large bowel about 10 percent of the time. Injuries to the spleen, kidneys, and pancreas follow in decreasing order of incidence.

A special type of penetrating trauma is induced by a blast from a shotgun. The shotgun delivers numerous round pellets (called shot) through the hollow gun barrel. The aerodynamics of the shot and the rapid expansion of their distribution (the pattern) cause the energy of impact to decrease rapidly the farther the projectiles move from the barrel. Generally, shotgun blasts at short range (under 3 yards) are extremely lethal. Between 3 and 7 yards, the penetration of the projectiles is great but often survivable. At distances greater than 7 yards, the depth of penetration and subsequent injury fall off quickly. These parameters change somewhat with the decreasing gauge size (gun barrel diameter) and the size of the projectiles. (See Chapter 3, "Penetrating Trauma.")

Blunt Trauma

Blunt trauma to the abdomen produces the least visible signs of injury and causes trauma through three mechanisms: deceleration, compression, and shear (Figure 11-9 ■). As the exterior of the abdomen decelerates (or accelerates) during impact, its contents slam into one another in a chain reaction. They are first injured by the force changing their veloc-

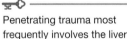

Penetrating trauma most frequently involves the liver and small bowel.

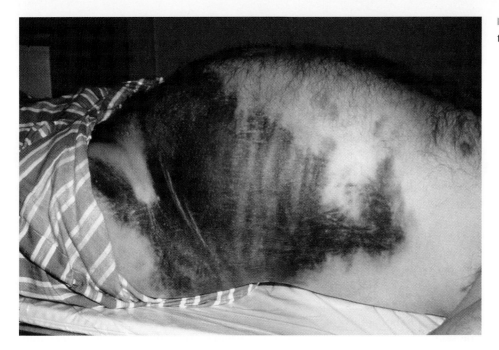

ity, then by the forces of compression, as they are trapped between the impacting energy and the more posterior organs. The entire contents of the cavity may be compressed between the force impacting the anterior abdominal cavity and the spinal column. Shear forces induce damage when one part of an organ is free to move while another part is restricted by the forces of trauma or by ligamentous or vascular attachments. Blunt trauma is responsible for about 40 percent of the incidences of splenic injury and a little more than 20 percent of hepatic (liver) injury. The bowel and kidneys are the next most frequently injured abdominal structures in blunt trauma.

Blast injuries to the abdomen involve both blunt and penetrating mechanisms. Shrapnel and debris propelled by the blast act as projectiles and create penetrating trauma. However, because of the irregular shapes of the objects and their poor aerodynamic properties, they tend to produce serious injury only in close proximity to the blast's center. The pressure wave generated by the explosion causes blunt trauma as it dramatically compresses and relaxes air-filled organs and is likely to contuse organs or rupture them. Since the stomach and bowel are only occasionally distended with air, they are neither as frequently nor as seriously injured as the lungs by the blast pressure wave. Abdominal injury is a secondary concern with blast injury patients.

Careful evaluation of the mechanism of injury, including identification of the force and direction of impact as it relates to the abdomen, is important to anticipating injuries within the region. Pay special attention to the potential for seat belt injury or direct injury as the abdomen impacts the steering wheel in a vehicle crash, impacts with objects or the ground during a fall, or is struck during an assault. Remember that the early presentation of a contusion will likely be a simple reddening (erythema) of the affected area. Hence it is critically important to carefully analyze the mechanism of injury, identify a high index of suspicion for intra-abdominal injury, and investigate the abdomen for signs and symptoms of injury. The abdominal wall, hollow organs, solid organs, vascular structures, mesentery, and peritoneum all respond differently to trauma.

INJURY TO THE ABDOMINAL WALL

Any injury to the contents of the abdomen must disrupt or be transmitted through the abdominal wall. Since the skin and muscular lining of the abdomen are more resistant

Blunt trauma most frequently involves the spleen and liver.

With trauma to the abdomen, the discoloration of ecchymosis and noticeable swelling require several hours to develop.

evisceration *a protrusion of organs from a wound.*

to injury than many of the internal organs, they are likely to be uninjured or minimally injured by blunt trauma forces that cause serious injury within. Even when injured, the skin and underlying muscle may only show erythema during the first hour or so. The more visible discoloration of ecchymosis and noticeable swelling require several hours to develop. Penetrating wounds may also be difficult to assess properly because the musculature and skin tension close the wound opening. Bullet and knife wounds look especially small and may appear much less lethal than they are.

Penetrating abdominal injury may permit abdominal contents to protrude through the opening. This type of injury, called an **evisceration,** occurs most frequently through the anterior abdominal wall and is usually associated with a large and deep laceration. The omentum and/or small bowel are most likely to protrude. The evisceration endangers the protruding bowel because of compromised circulation and the drying of this delicate intra-abdominal tissue. However, replacing the protrusion risks introducing bacteria into the peritoneal space. If the bowel is torn, there is the additional danger of its contents leaking into the peritoneal space if it is replaced.

Penetrating trauma to the thorax, buttocks, flanks, and back may also enter the abdomen and injure its contents. The abdominal organs extend well into the thorax and move up to the nipple line, anteriorly, and to the tips of the scapulae, posteriorly, during deep expiration. Injury to the lower portion of the chest may lacerate the diaphragm and injure the stomach, liver, spleen, or gallbladder. The flank, back, and buttock muscles are thick and resist penetrating trauma very well. However, deep wounds in these locations can penetrate into the abdominal cavity and cause injury to adjacent organs. High-powered projectiles, especially those from hunting or military rifles, may have enough energy to deflect when striking bone and enter the abdomen from as far away as a proximal extremity wound.

Tears in the diaphragm may also disrupt the abdominal container. These tears may occur when the patient holds his or her breath just before an impact or with penetrating injury to the lower thorax or upper abdomen. Not only may such an injury compromise the important role of the diaphragm in respiration, but it may also permit or force abdominal contents (like those of the stomach, liver, or a portion of the small bowel) to enter the thoracic cavity. This reduces the volume of the thoracic cage available during respiration and compromises the blood supply to the herniated organs. Diaphragmatic injury occurs from stab injuries most frequently on the left side because this is where right-handed assailants strike. Gunshot wounds affect both sides equally. Small tears are unlikely to permit abdominal contents to enter the thorax nor are they likely to greatly affect respiration. Large tears are more likely to do both.

INJURY TO THE HOLLOW ORGANS

Hollow organs like the stomach, small bowel, large bowel, rectum, urinary bladder, gallbladder, and pregnant uterus may rupture with compression from blunt forces, especially if the organ is full and distended. They may also tear as penetrating objects disrupt their structure. (The small bowel is the most frequently injured hollow abdominal organ during penetrating trauma because it rests anteriorly and just beneath the thin anterior abdominal muscles and omentum.) Damage to the hollow organs results in hemorrhage and in the spillage of their contents into the retroperitoneal, peritoneal, or pelvic spaces. The jejunum, ileum, colon, and rectum contain progressively higher bacterial concentrations, and their rupture and the subsequent leakage of material into the abdomen will likely induce severe but delayed infection (called sepsis). The other hollow organs are more likely to release contents that cause a chemical irritation of the abdominal lining. The urinary bladder will release urine; the gallbladder, bile; and the stomach and duodenum, chyme; which is acidic and rich in digestive enzymes. Injury to the hollow organs may result in frank blood in the stool (**hematochezia**), blood in emesis (**hematemesis**), and blood in the urine (**hematuria**).

hematochezia *blood in the stool.*

hematemesis *the vomiting of blood.*

hematuria *blood in the urine.*

INJURY TO THE SOLID ORGANS

Solid organs such as the spleen, liver, pancreas, and kidneys are also subject to blunt and penetrating trauma. These organs are especially dense and are not held together as strongly as the more muscular hollow organs of the body. They are prone to contuse, resulting in organ damage and minimal bleeding, or to rupture. If the organ's capsule remains intact, it will limit the hemorrhage. However, if the capsule is disrupted by penetrating trauma or torn by the mechanism of blunt trauma, unrestricted hemorrhage may result.

The spleen is especially well protected by the lower ribs, the back and flank muscles, and the spinal column. It is not, however, protected by a strong peritoneal capsule and is very fragile in nature. It may be injured with severe abdominal compression, blunt left flank trauma, or penetrating injury to the region (Figure 11-10 ■). The spleen then bleeds profusely, frequently resulting in shock and a life threat to the patient. The blood loss may accumulate against the diaphragm (especially in the supine patient) and result in referred pain to the left shoulder region.

The pancreas is central to the upper abdomen, somewhat less delicate than the spleen, and well protected from blunt trauma by its location deep in the central abdominal cavity. Penetrating trauma may lacerate its structure and permit blood and digestive enzymes to flow into the abdominal cavity. These digestive juices may actually begin to digest pancreatic and surrounding tissues, leading to severe internal injury. Pancreatic injury does sometimes result from severe blunt trauma to the upper abdomen that compresses the spleen between the trauma force and the vertebral column. This may occur when a patient impacts a steering wheel or the handlebars of a motorcycle during a crash. Such a patient frequently complains of upper abdominal pain that may radiate to the back.

The kidneys are equally well protected by their location deep in the abdominal cavity. They are somewhat more resistant to injury than the pancreas, have a more substantial serous capsule, and are attached by large renal arteries to the aorta. They are most frequently injured with trauma to the flanks. Renal injury may result in regional (back or flank) pain as well as hematuria.

The liver is the largest single organ within the abdomen. Being a peritoneal organ, it is surrounded by the strong visceral peritoneum, which resists injury and will hold the organ together if injured. The liver is firmer than both the spleen and pancreas and is somewhat protected by the inferior border of the thorax. When the forces of trauma are directed to this region, however, they are likely to damage the liver, especially if they induce lower rib fracture on the right side (Figure 11-11 ■). The liver is restrained from forward motion by the ligamentum teres. During severe deceleration, the weight of the liver forces it into the ligament, causing shear forces, laceration, and hemorrhage. Liver injury often presents with tenderness along the right lower border of the thoracic cage and, as blood accumulates against the diaphragm, pain in the upper right shoulder.

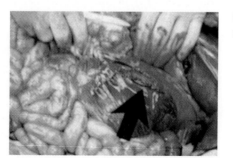

■ Figure 11-10   Penetrating trauma to the spleen.

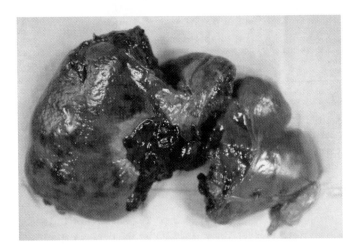

INJURY TO THE VASCULAR STRUCTURES

Arteries and veins within the abdomen are prone to injury with serious consequences. The abdominal aorta and its major tributaries can be injured by direct blunt or penetrating trauma or may be injured as abdominal organs decelerate and pull on their vascular attachments during an auto crash or similar impact. Penetrating trauma does not frequently involve the very large vessels of the abdomen, but when the aorta or other major artery is damaged, internal hemorrhage can be severe. The vena cava and its tributaries can likewise be injured. Most vascular injuries (97 percent) are associated with penetrating trauma. As blood accumulates in the abdomen of a supine patient, it will come to rest against the diaphragm. There it irritates the muscular structure and produces a referred pain in the shoulder region. However, other signs of significant hemorrhage may be limited.

Vascular injury in the peritoneal, retroperitoneal, and pelvic spaces can be serious for several reasons. These spaces are easily expandable, and hemorrhage may continue without the increase in pressure exerted by surrounding tissue that would occur if the vascular injury were within a mass of muscle elsewhere in the body. Without this pressure, both the rate and volume of blood loss do not diminish. These spaces also contain organs that require significant circulation supplied by rather large arterial and venous vessels. The dynamic nature of the abdomen and its anatomical size mean that a greater volume of blood can be accommodated there before its presence becomes noticeable. Further, due to vagal stimulation caused by the presence of blood in the peritoneal cavity, an increasing heart rate (a common sign of internal hemorrhage) may not be present.

INJURY TO THE MESENTERY AND BOWEL

The mesentery provides the bowel with circulation, innervation, and attachment. Blunt injury occurs as the mesentery stretches during impact. This type of injury occurs most frequently at points of relative immobility such as the duodenal/jejunal juncture (where the small bowel is affixed by the ligament of Trietz) or where the small bowel joins the large bowel at the ileocecal junction. Injury involving the mesentery may disrupt blood vessels supplying the bowel and eventually cause ischemia, necrosis, and possible rupture. Mesenteric injuries do not usually bleed profusely because the peritoneal layers contain the hemorrhage. Deceleration or compression may tear or rupture the full bowel. With penetrating trauma, the omentum is frequently disrupted and the bowel may be torn anywhere along its length, though tears to the small bowel (jejunum and ileum) are the most likely because of its central and anterior location. Expect a tear

Most vascular trauma is associated with penetrating injury.

to release bowel contents into the peritoneal space, but remember that signs and symptoms of such release are delayed. The duodenum is less frequently injured because of its location deep within the abdomen. Penetrating trauma to the lateral abdomen is likely to injure the large bowel (ascending colon on the right and descending colon on the left).

INJURY TO THE PERITONEUM

The peritoneum is the very delicate and sensitive lining of the anterior abdominal cavity. Its inflammation, called **peritonitis,** can be caused by two major mechanisms, bacterial and chemical irritation. Bacterial peritonitis is an irritation due to infection, which is often released into the space by a torn bowel or open wound. It takes the bacteria between 12 and 24 hours to grow in sufficient numbers to produce the inflammation and hence the condition is usually not apparent during prehospital care. Chemical peritonitis occurs more rapidly than bacterial peritonitis because the caustic nature of digestive enzymes and acids (from the stomach or duodenum), and, to a lesser degree, urine quickly irritate the peritoneum and induce the inflammatory response. Blood induces limited peritoneal inflammation, and hence serious hemorrhage into the peritoneal cavity will not, by itself, cause this condition.

Peritonitis is a progressive process that presents with characteristic signs and symptoms. It usually begins with a slight tenderness at the location of injury. Over time, the area of inflammation expands, as does the area of tenderness. Any jarring of the abdomen, as occurs with percussion or when you quickly release the pressure of deep palpation, causes a twinge of pain (**rebound tenderness**). In response to pain induced by any movement of the irritated abdominal tissue, the anterior abdominal muscles contract, even in the unconscious patient. This is called **guarding.** If the pain becomes severe, the abdominal muscles assume an extreme contraction and leave the abdominal wall with a rigid, boardlike feel. When assessing the abdomen, be aware that local muscle injury caused by trauma may result in local or regional abdominal muscle tenderness and spasm that mimics peritonitis. Tenderness or frank pain from the physical injury may coexist with the signs of peritonitis.

INJURY TO THE PELVIS

A pelvic fracture represents a serious skeletal injury, serious and often life-threatening hemorrhage, and potential injury to the organs within the pelvic space. These organs—the ureters, bladder, urethra, female genitalia, prostate, rectum, and anus—can all be injured by the severe kinetic forces, the crushing nature of the injury, or by displaced bone fragments. Pelvic fracture can also cause serious injury to the pregnant uterus. Pelvic hemorrhage and fracture have been discussed in Chapter 7, "Musculoskeletal Injuries."

Sexual assault may also injure the reproductive structures located internally in the female and externally in the male. Direct trauma to the external female genitalia or injury caused by objects inserted into the vagina may tear the soft tissues of this region. Since these tissues are both very sensitive and vascular, the injury may bleed heavily and be very painful. The same is true for the male genitalia, though they are more prone to injury because of their more external location.

INJURY DURING PREGNANCY

Trauma is the number one killer of pregnant females. Penetrating abdominal trauma alone accounts for as much as 36 percent of overall maternal mortality. Gunshot wounds to the abdomen of the pregnant female also account for fetal mortality rates of

Expect a tear of the small bowel to release bowel contents into the peritoneal space, but remember that signs and symptoms of such release are delayed.

peritonitis *inflammation of the peritoneum caused by chemical or bacterial irritation.*

rebound tenderness *pain on release of the examiner's hands, allowing the patient's abdominal wall to return to its normal position; associated with peritoneal irritation.*

guarding *protective tensing of the abdominal muscles by a patient suffering abdominal pain; may be a voluntary or involuntary response.*

When assessing the abdomen, be aware that local muscle injury caused by trauma may result in local or regional abdominal muscle tenderness and spasm that mimics peritonitis.

Trauma is the number one killer of pregnant females and penetrating abdominal trauma alone accounts for as much as 36 percent of overall maternal mortality.

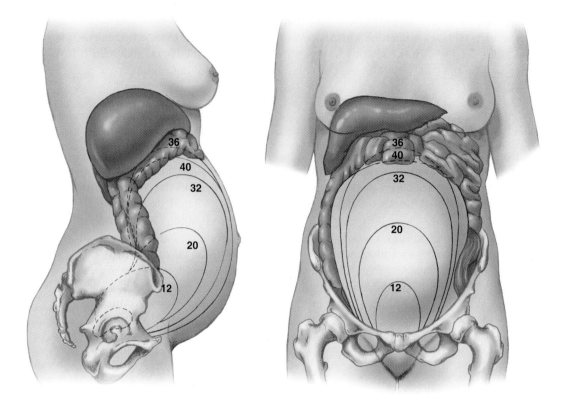

■ Figure 11-12 Changing dimensions of the pregnant uterus. Numbers represent weeks of gestation.

between 40 and 70 percent. In blunt trauma, auto collisions are the leading cause of maternal and fetal mortality and morbidity. Proper seat belt placement can significantly reduce injury to the pregnant mother and fetus, while improper placement increases the incidence of both uterine rupture and separation of the placenta from the wall of the uterus. Unrestrained mothers in serious auto collisions are four times more likely to suffer fetal mortality.

The physiological changes associated with pregnancy protect both the mother and her abdominal organs. With the increasing size of the uterus, most of the abdominal organs are displaced higher in the abdomen (Figure 11-12 ■). This generally protects them, unless blunt or penetrating trauma impacts the upper abdomen. If that happens, then the injury may involve numerous organs with increased morbidity and mortality. Direct penetrating injury to the central and lower abdomen of the late pregnancy mother often spares her from serious injury; the resulting injury, however, often damages the uterus and endangers the fetus.

The late term female is at additional risk of vomiting and possible aspiration. Increasing uterine size increases intra-abdominal pressure, while the hormones of pregnancy relax the cardiac sphincter (the valve that prevents reflux of the stomach contents). The bladder is displaced superiorly early in pregnancy and then becomes more prone to injury and, when injured, bleeds more heavily.

The increasing size and weight of the uterus and its contents have several effects on the mother, especially when trauma strikes. The uterus of a supine patient in late pregnancy may compress the inferior vena cava and reduce the venous return to the heart. This may induce hypotension in the uninjured patient and have severe consequences in the hemorrhaging trauma patient. The increased intra-abdominal pressure along with the compression of the inferior vena cava by the uterus raise venous pressure in the pelvic region and lower extremities. This pressure engorges the vessels and increases the rate of venous hemorrhage from pelvic fracture or lower extremity wounds.

The increased maternal vascular volume (up by 45 percent) helps protect the mother from hypovolemia. However, this protection does not extend to the fetus because fetal blood flow is affected well before there are changes in the maternal blood pressure or pulse rate. In fact, it may take a maternal blood loss of between 30 and 35 percent before changes in maternal blood pressure or heart rate are evident. Therefore, it becomes very important to assure early and aggressive resuscitation of the potentially hypotensive pregnant mother.

In the pregnant female, the thick and muscular uterus contains both the developing fetus and amniotic fluid. This container is strong, distributing the forces of trauma uniformly to the fetus and thereby reducing chances for injury. Significant blunt trauma may cause the uterus to rupture or penetrating trauma may perforate or tear it. The dangers of severe maternal hemorrhage and disruption of the blood supply to the fetus present life threats to both. The potential release of amniotic fluid into the abdomen is also of great concern. The risk of uterine and fetal injury increases with the length of gestation and is greatest during the third trimester of pregnancy.

If an open wound to the uterus does occur, there may be added risk to the mother (in addition to hemorrhage) if she is Rh negative and the fetus is Rh positive. (However, this situation does not impact prehospital assessment or care.) Penetrating or severe blunt trauma may permit some fetal/maternal blood mixing and lead to compatibility problems. Frank uterine rupture is a rare complication of trauma, but it does occur with severe blunt impact, pelvic fracture, and—very infrequently—with stab or shotgun wounds.

Blunt trauma to the uterus may cause the placenta to detach from the uterine wall because the placenta is rather inelastic while the uterus is very flexible. This condition, called **abruptio placentae,** presents a life-threatening risk to both mother and fetus because the separation permits both maternal and fetal hemorrhage (Figure 11-13 ▣). More frequently than not, this hemorrhage is contained within the uterus and does not extend to the vaginal outlet. Blunt trauma may also cause the premature rupture of the amniotic sac (breaking of the "membranes" or "bag of waters") and may induce an early labor.

INJURY TO PEDIATRIC PATIENTS

Another special patient with regard to abdominal injuries is the child. Children have poorly developed abdominal musculature and a reduced anterior/posterior diameter. The rib cage is more cartilaginous and flexible and more likely to transmit injury to the organs beneath. These factors increase the incidence of pediatric abdominal injury, especially to the liver, spleen, and kidney. Children also compensate very well for blood loss and may not show any signs or symptoms until they have lost over half of their blood volume. This is especially important with abdominal injuries, because a great volume of blood may be lost into the abdomen with little pain or noticeable distention.

ASSESSMENT OF THE ABDOMINAL INJURY PATIENT

Assessment of the patient who has sustained abdominal trauma is somewhat abbreviated because definitive care for such injury is often surgical intervention. Hence, it is imperative that you quickly assess the patient and, if indications of serious abdominal injury exist, you should package and transport him expeditiously. Assessment of the abdominal injury patient is like that for any trauma patient, with pertinent and significant information gained during the scene size-up, initial assessment, rapid trauma assessment (or focused exam and history), and serial ongoing assessments.

While a pregnant mother is somewhat protected from hypovolemia, the fetus is not so protected.

abruptio placentae *a condition in which the placenta separates from the uterine wall.*

ABRUPTIO PLACENTAE

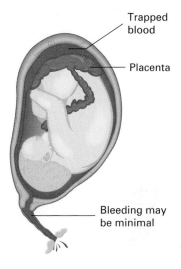

Trapped blood

Placenta

Bleeding may be minimal

▣ Figure 11-13 Abruptio placentae.

Pediatric Abdominal Trauma Serious trauma is typically a surgical disease, and the prehospital response is generally aggressive intervention and rapid transport to the nearest trauma center. However, research has shown that speed and drastic care steps are not always the most prudent response. Today, the hemodynamically stable pediatric patient with blunt abdominal trauma is often not managed with "bright lights and cold steel" but receives a more conservative approach than we might anticipate for their adult counterparts.

In the pediatric patient, the most commonly injured abdominal organs are the liver and spleen. Experience has found that injury to these organs and the associated hemorrhage is generally self-limiting. Further, splenectomy carries a significant risk of serious, even life-threatening, infection—especially from bacteria that are encapsulated.

If a pediatric blunt-trauma patient maintains a relatively normal blood pressure and pulse rate or can be stabilized through the administration of IV fluids or limited transfusion, the patient is assessed by CT scan or ultrasound and carefully observed. Those who have an altered level of consciousness, are unstable, or need other surgical intervention may be exceptions to this approach.

Clearly, medicine is looking carefully at what is done and considering modificaitons of current practice in the interest of improving patient outcome.

SCENE SIZE-UP

Assure that the scene is safe for you, fellow rescuers, bystanders, and the patient. Be ready to use appropriate body substance isolation procedures before moving to the patient's side. Also determine the number of expected patients and need for additional EMS, police, fire, and other service personnel.

For the patient who has sustained abdominal injury, the analysis of the mechanism of injury is the most important element of the scene size-up and possibly of the entire assessment.

For the patient who has sustained abdominal injury, the analysis of the mechanism of injury is the most important element of the scene size-up and possibly of the entire assessment. However, forming an index of suspicion for individual abdominal injuries is very difficult because the signs and symptoms are, for the most part, limited and nonspecific. In fact, more than 30 percent of patients with serious abdominal injury may present with no specific signs or symptoms of abdominal injury whatsoever. Additionally, other less life threatening but more painful injuries may overshadow signs and symptoms of the patient's abdominal injury. Also, those signs and symptoms that are present may become less specific in nature with time and the progressive nature of peritonitis. Lastly, the patient's reporting of his condition may be unreliable due to the effects of alcohol or drug ingestion, head injury, or shock.

If the patient has suffered blunt trauma, identify the strength and direction of the forces and where on the body they were delivered. Focus your observation and palpation on that site during the initial and rapid trauma assessments and place your highest suspicion of injury there. Begin to develop a list of possible organs injured (the index of suspicion) and the immediate and delayed effects they will have on the patient's condition. In serious blunt trauma or deep penetrating trauma, expect internal and uncontrolled hemorrhage.

If the patient was involved in an auto crash, identify if seat belts were used and if they were used properly (Figure 11-14 ■). Remember that improper placement (above the iliac crests) may increase the likelihood of abdominal compression (and lumbar spine) injury. Lack of seat belt use increases the incidence and severity of all types of injuries, including abdominal injury. Examine the vehicle interior for signs of impact like the deformity of a bent steering wheel, a deflated air bag, or a structural intrusion into

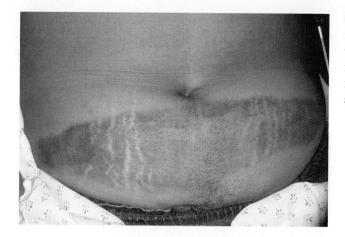

■ Figure 11-14 Use the mechanism of injury to identify where signs of injury might be found—for example, contusions resulting from compression by a seat belt. (© Mark C. Ide)

the passenger compartment. Frontal impact is most likely to compress the abdomen, injuring the liver and spleen and possibly rupturing distended hollow organs like the stomach and bladder. Right side impact frequently induces liver, ascending colon, and pelvic injury, while left side impact induces splenic, descending colon, and pelvic injuries. Pedestrians, and especially children, are likely to sustain lower abdominal injury, especially if the vehicle impacts the patient's midsection. It is important to determine the velocity of impact and the distance the patient was thrown. Motorcyclists and, to a lesser degree, bicyclists are likely to sustain abdominal injury as they are propelled forward while the handlebars restrain the pelvis and lower abdomen. In assaults and other isolated impacts, be observant for left flank impact and splenic or renal damage and right-side impact causing renal or hepatic (liver) injury. If the impact involves the superior abdomen, suspect liver, stomach, spleen, and pancreatic injury, while impact to the middle or lower abdomen will likely damage the small bowel, kidneys, and bladder.

With a patient who has experienced penetrating trauma, determine the nature of the offending agent. If it is a knife, arrow, or impaled object, determine the probable angle and depth of insertion (Figure 11-15 ■). Do not move or remove the impaled object.

With gunshot wounds, determine whether the weapon was a hand gun, shotgun, or rifle; the distance from the gun to the victim; and the gun's caliber. Also determine the number of shots fired, if possible, and the angle from which the gun was fired. Be prepared to examine the flanks, the buttocks, and the back for any sign of additional or exit wounds. Attempt to estimate the amount of blood lost at the scene and communicate this, with the other information previously listed, to the emergency department physician.

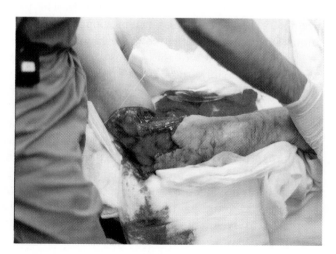

■ Figure 11-15 Analyze the mechanism of a penetrating trauma in an attempt to determine the probable angle and depth of the wound. (© Mark C. Ide)

Assessment of the Abdominal Injury Patient **447**

Gunshot wounds provide a challenge to assessment. The damage done does not correlate well to the appearance of the entrance or exit wound. It is more related to the bullet's kinetic energy (velocity and mass) as it enters the body and to its energy exchange characteristics as it travels into and through tissue. Low-velocity bullets cause little damage beyond the bullet's actual path. However, these projectiles are easily deflected from their paths by contact with clothing, bone, or, in some cases, soft tissue. They also carry pieces of clothing and other debris into the body and do not tend to pass through the body.

High-velocity weapons and the wounds they cause were once seen only in the military setting, but now more powerful hand guns are causing similar wounds and internal injuries in the civilian world. Their projectiles cause injury well beyond the bullet's path and injure tissue as the projectile creates a cavity and compresses and stretches neighboring tissue (cavitation). The wounding process also draws debris into the wound, where the damaged and devitalized (without circulation) tissue forms a good medium for bacterial growth. The wounding process may create secondary projectiles as the bullet hits bone, breaks it apart, and then drives the fragments into adjacent tissue. The high-velocity bullet may also fragment and transmit its injuring potential to several pathways.

With either significant blunt or any penetrating trauma to the abdomen, suspect serious and continuing internal hemorrhage. Be especially watchful of the patient during your assessment and initiate shock care at the first signs and symptoms of hypoperfusion. These signs and symptoms include diminishing level of consciousness or orientation, increasing anxiety or restlessness, thirst, increasing pulse rate, decreasing pulse pressure, and increasing capillary refill time.

Information you gather at the scene is invaluable to the attending emergency department physician. That information, however, will be unavailable unless you document it carefully and report it upon your arrival at the hospital. Doing this is essential to assuring that the patient receives the best care in both the prehospital and in-hospital settings.

INITIAL ASSESSMENT

As you begin the initial assessment, carefully note your patient's level of consciousness and orientation as well as any indication that he may be affected by alcohol, drugs, head injury, or shock. These agents and conditions reduce the reliability of your patient's reporting of the signs and symptoms of abdominal injury. Any decrease in the level of orientation or consciousness should alert you to the need to maintain a higher index of suspicion for abdominal injury and to perform more careful initial and rapid trauma assessments. The patient may also complain of dizziness or light-headedness when moving from a supine to a seated or standing position. (Do not ask the patient to move; however, he may have moved on his own before your arrival.) Any of these signs and symptoms should lead you to suspect hypovolemia, possibly from an abdominal injury. Use your initial evaluation as a baseline against which to trend any changes in the patient's level of consciousness or orientation.

As you evaluate airway, breathing, and circulation, be observant for any associated signs and symptoms of hypovolemia, especially if they occur early in your care or are out of proportion with the obvious or expected injuries. Note any rapid shallow respirations, diminished pulse pressure, rapid pulse rate, slow capillary refill time, or thirst. Limited chest movement may be due to the pain of peritonitis or blood irritating the diaphragm. Shallow respirations may be due to abdominal contents in the thorax from a ruptured diaphragm. Be prepared to protect the airway because abdominal trauma patients are likely to vomit.

RAPID TRAUMA ASSESSMENT

Perform the usual full rapid trauma assessment, but if you have developed a high index of suspicion for abdominal injury, pay particular attention to that region. Carefully examine the abdomen for evidence of injury as suggested by the mechanism of injury or by signs or symptoms observed during the initial assessment. When you suspect that the patient has received blunt trauma, look carefully over the entire abdominal surface for the slight reddening of erythema or minor abrasions associated with superficial soft-tissue injury. Remember that any trauma must pass through the exterior of the abdomen before it can do damage within.

Quickly examine the anterior surface of the abdomen and then flanks, then carefully and gently log roll the patient to examine the back, looking for any signs of injury, erythema, ecchymosis, contusions, or open wounds, including eviscerations and impaled objects (Figure 11-16 ■). Also look at the abdomen's general shape and any signs of distention. Visualize the inguinal area for signs of injury or hemorrhage. Jeans may contain hemorrhage without any indication of the accumulation, so they should be cut away or removed to assess this region when injury is suspected. Remember that the abdominal cavity can contain a very large volume of blood (on the order of 1.5 liters) before it becomes noticeably distended. In obese patients the volume of blood loss may be even greater before distention is visible. Also be aware that the signs and symptoms of hemoperitoneum or retroperitoneal hemorrhage are minimal.

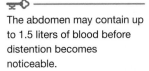

The abdomen may contain up to 1.5 liters of blood before distention becomes noticeable.

Visualize and palpate the pelvis for signs of injury or instability. Apply gentle pressure directed posteriorly, then medially, on the iliac crests, then place pressure downward on the symphysis pubis. If you note any crepitus or instability, suspect pelvic fracture and both injury to the organs of the lower abdomen and severe internal hemorrhage. If you already suspect pelvic injury, do not test or apply any pressure and be very careful during movement to the ambulance and transport to the hospital. Any manipulation of the fracture site may restart or increase hemorrhage.

Question the patient about pain or discomfort in each quadrant, then palpate the quadrants individually, leaving any quadrant with anticipated injury or patient complaint of pain to last. If you palpate an injured quadrant first, the pain may lead the patient to guard during any remaining palpation. Feel for any spasm or guarding as you palpate, then note any patient report of pain when you quickly release the pressure of your palpation (rebound tenderness). If you palpate an abdomen that is board hard, expect injury to the pancreas, duodenum, or stomach, especially if the time since the injury has been short.

Also note any unusual pulsations in the abdomen. You may visualize some pulsing in the thin, young, healthy, athletic patient, but most patients will not have any visible

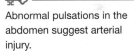

Abnormal pulsations in the abdomen suggest arterial injury.

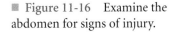

■ Figure 11-16 Examine the abdomen for signs of injury.

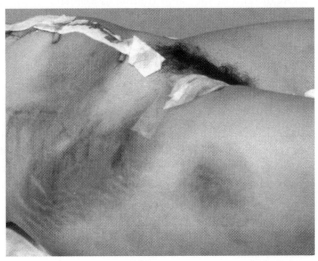

Auscultation for bowel sounds is not recommended during assessment of the abdominal trauma patient.

or palpable pulses in the abdomen. Abnormal pulsation suggests arterial injury. Injuries to the thorax or pelvis also suggest abdominal injury, especially if there are lower rib fractures or the pelvic ring is unstable. Auscultation is not recommended during assessment of the abdominal trauma patient. It takes a great deal of time to adequately listen for bowel sounds, and their presence or absence neither confirm nor rule out possible injury.

When evaluating the patient with penetrating trauma to the abdomen, look carefully at the entrance wound, and note its appearance, size, and depth. Point-blank discharge of a gun against tissue will introduce the barrel exhaust into the wound created by the bullet. You may notice powder debris and the crackling of subcutaneous emphysema. Look for contamination and any signs of serious blood loss. Then examine the patient for an exit wound. Exit wounds may look more "blown out" in nature and are generally larger and more serious in appearance than entrance wounds. Count the number of entry and exit wounds and note whether they are paired or if an inequality suggests that some projectiles did not exit. The wounds from a projectile may be very small and difficult to see, while still carrying the potential to cause lethal injury. Anticipate the injuries that occurred as the object or bullet sped into and through the body, but remember that it is not uncommon for a bullet to alter its path. Be suspicious of any projectile wound in the proximal extremities because the projectile may travel along the limb and into the body's interior. Also keep in mind that a bullet wound to the thorax may then deflect and penetrate the abdomen, or vice versa.

While performing the rapid trauma assessment, carefully question the patient about the characteristics of any pain he feels and ask specifically about any abdominal sensations or other symptoms. Serious injury may result while the patient feels limited pain or injury sensation, especially when other more painful injuries elsewhere might be distracting them. The evaluation of abdominal pain from the patient's complaint may, however, be subjective as patients often vary in their response to pain. In the male, retroperitoneal pain may be referred to the testicular region. Thirst may be one of the few symptoms of abdominal injury as significant hemorrhage draws down the body's blood volume. Be sure to record any symptoms in the patient's own words and assure these comments and your findings are documented on the prehospital care report and reported to the attending physician.

When investigating the rest of the patient history, give special consideration to the last oral intake. The bladder, bowel, and stomach are much more likely to rupture if full and distended. Ask about when the patient last ate or drank and how much he consumed. Relate the intake to the type of impact received, especially blunt trauma to the trunk.

Conclude the rapid trauma assessment by gathering a set of baseline vital signs.

At the end of the rapid trauma assessment, reevaluate the patient's priority for transport. The potential for an abdominal injury must factor into this determination. Remember that serious internal hemorrhage from blunt or penetrating trauma frequently occurs with few overt signs and symptoms. Any patient with a history of significant blunt or any penetrating trauma to the torso is a candidate for rapid transport to the trauma center. Always err on the side of providing more patient care and early transport rather than underestimating the seriousness of trauma to the abdomen.

Any patient with a history of significant blunt or any penetrating trauma to the torso is a candidate for rapid transport to the trauma center.

Special Assessment Considerations with Pregnant Patients

If the patient you are treating is pregnant, pay special attention to the abdomen and the possibility of injury. Remember that the maternal blood volume is increased by up to 45 percent in the third trimester and blood loss can exceed 30 percent before the normal signs and symptoms of hypovolemia reveal themselves. Watch for the earliest signs of shock. Assure that the uterus does not compress the vena cava by placing the noticeably pregnant mother in the left lateral recumbent position. If spinal injury is also suspected, immobilize her firmly to the spine board and, when placed on the stretcher,

Place the late pregnancy patient on her left side to prevent compression of the inferior vena cava.

rotate her onto her left side. Carefully evaluate the maternal vital signs and remember that the fetus is likely to experience distress before the mother shows any signs of hypotension or hypoperfusion.

Trauma to the abdomen in late pregnancy may cause several specific uterine injuries and requires careful assessment. The normal uterus will be firm and round to palpation. It will be palpable above the iliac crests after the first 12 weeks of pregnancy and progress upward in the abdominal cavity until it reaches the costal border at about 32 weeks. Your palpation may result in tenderness and muscular contractions of the uterus, which are normal secondary to uterine contusions. These contractions will often be self-limiting; however, any tenderness, pain, or contractions should raise your suspicions of abruptio placentae. The mother may complain of cramping, generally related to palpable uterine contractions and, in some cases, experience vaginal hemorrhage. Abruptio placentae represents a serious risk to the fetus and mother and is a true emergency requiring rapid transport.

Palpation of the uterus that reveals an asymmetrical uterus or permits you to recognize the irregular features of the fetus suggests uterine rupture. This condition may also present with uterine contractions, but the fundus of the uterus is not palpable and the mass does not harden with the contractions.

If uterine rupture or abruptio placentae are suspected or if you suspect any serious injury to the abdomen of the pregnant patient, ask for the mother's Rh status and report it to the emergency department. Alert the emergency department well before your arrival if you are transporting a pregnant mother who was injured by trauma. This allows department personnel to prepare for the special monitoring necessary for both the mother and fetus.

ONGOING ASSESSMENT

The ongoing assessment is an essential part of the continuing care process for the patient with possible abdominal injury. During it, you will look for the signs of progressing abdominal injury or continuing hemorrhage. Perform it every 5 minutes in patients with any significant suggestion of abdominal injury. Often the progressive nature of peritonitis leads to greater and greater patient complaints or may make abdominal signs and symptoms more evident as you care for and reduce the pain of other injuries. The signs of ongoing hemorrhage are equally progressive and may not clearly present until well into your patient care.

Pay close attention to the signs of hidden hemorrhage during ongoing assessments of the patient with potential abdominal injury. Watch the blood pressure, pulse rate, capillary refill time, and the patient's appearance and level of consciousness and orientation. A decrease in the difference between the systolic and diastolic blood pressures (the pulse pressure) suggests the body is compensating for shock. An increasing pulse rate (especially if the strength of the pulse is diminishing) and an increasing capillary refill time both suggest hypovolemic compensation. Also observe for the skin becoming cool, clammy, cyanotic, or ashen, and watch for pulse oximetry readings that become more erratic. A change in either the level of consciousness or, more subtly, a lowering of the patient's orientation suggests the brain is being hypoperfused. These findings all indicate the body is employing increasing levels of shock compensation. If you cannot account for a continuing blood loss elsewhere, suspect internal and continuing abdominal hemorrhage. Subtle changes may be the only apparent signs of gradually worsening shock.

Another sign of continuing blood loss from an abdominal hemorrhage is aggressive fluid resuscitation that appears ineffective. Note your patient's response to fluid resuscitation. If his or her vital signs do not improve and all external hemorrhage is controlled, suspect continuing internal hemorrhage.

Another sign of continuing blood loss from an abdominal hemorrhage is aggressive fluid resuscitation that appears ineffective.

MANAGEMENT OF THE ABDOMINAL INJURY PATIENT

Content

Management of the Abdominal Injury Patient

Position the patient properly
Assure oxygenation and ventilation
Control external bleeding
Be prepared for aggressive fluid resuscitation
Apply PASG if not contraindicated

Management of the patient with abdominal injuries is supportive, with the major emphasis on bringing the patient to surgery as quickly as possible. Prehospital care centers on rapid packaging and transport and fluid resuscitation, as needed. Specific care steps for the abdominal injury patient include proper positioning, general shock care, fluid resuscitation, PASG application, and care for specific injuries (open wounds and eviscerations).

The patient with minor or severe abdominal pain should be positioned for comfort (unless the positioning is contraindicated by suspicion of spinal injury). Flex the patient's knees to relax the abdominal muscles. If the injuries permit, place the patient in the left lateral recumbent position to maintain knee flexure and the relaxed state of the abdominal muscles, and facilitate the clearing of emesis from the airway.

Assure good ventilation and consider early administration of high-flow, high-concentration oxygen for the abdominal injury patient. The pain associated with peritonitis or diaphragmatic irritation may reduce respiratory excursion, adding to the potential for early shock development in these patients.

Control any moderate or serious external hemorrhage with direct pressure and bandaging. Minor bleeding may be controlled during transport if at all.

When a serious mechanism of injury is found and the patient does not present with the signs and symptoms of shock, act in anticipation of it.

When a serious mechanism of injury is found and the patient does not present with the signs and symptoms of shock, act in anticipation of it. Start a large-bore IV line with trauma tubing and 1,000 mL of lactated Ringer's solution or normal saline. Be prepared to administer repeated fluid boluses if any signs of shock develop. Monitor the pulse rate and blood pressure. If the pulse does not slow and the pulse pressure does not rise, consider increasing the number of fluid boluses. Institute a second line with a non-flow-restrictive saline lock using a large-bore catheter. Use this access if the patient's blood pressure begins to drop below 80 mmHg. Do not delay transport to initiate any IV access. Start the IV access en route to the hospital, if necessary. Prehospital infusion is usually limited to 3,000 mL of fluid. Titrate your administration rate to maintain a systolic blood pressure of 80 mmHg and assure that you do not exceed this volume of fluid during field care and transport.

As you should with all serious trauma patients, communicate frequently with the abdominal injury patient to reduce anxiety and provide emotional support. Also watch for any changes in the patient's description of the pain or injury's character or intensity. Be wary of patient hypothermia, especially when providing fluid resuscitation. Provide ample blankets, keep the patient compartment of the vehicle warm, take patient complaints of being cold seriously, and warm infusion fluids when possible. Hypothermia is a special consideration with pediatric patients because they have a disproportionately large body surface area to body volume and will rapidly lose heat to the environment.

Cover any exposed abdominal organs with a dressing moistened with sterile saline (Procedure 11-1). Be careful to keep the region clean and do not replace any exposed organs. Cover the wet dressing with a sterile occlusive dressing like clear plastic wrap to keep the site as clean as possible and yet retain the moisture. If the transport is lengthy, check the dressing from time to time and remoisten as necessary.

Stabilize impaled objects to prevent further injury and reduce associated hemorrhage.

Another wound that deserves special attention is the impaled object. Do all that you can to keep the object from moving and do not remove it from the victim. Any motion causes further injury, disrupts the clotting mechanisms, and continues the hemorrhage. Removal may withdraw the object from a blood vessel, thereby permitting increased internal and uncontrollable hemorrhage. Pad around the object with bulky trauma dressings and wrap around the trunk with soft, self-adherent roller bandaging to secure it firmly. Apply direct pressure around the object if hemorrhage is anything but minor. If the object is too long to accommodate during transport or it is affixed to

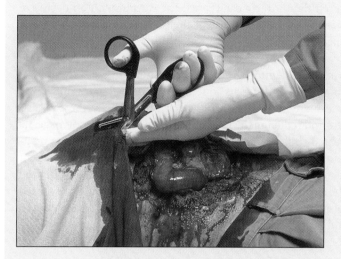

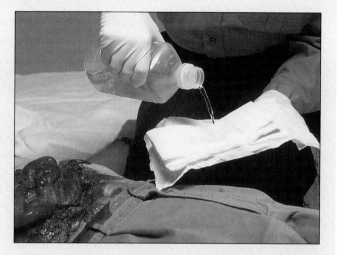

11-1a Remove clothing from around the abdominal wound.

11-1b Cover the wound with a sterile dressing soaked with sterile normal saline.

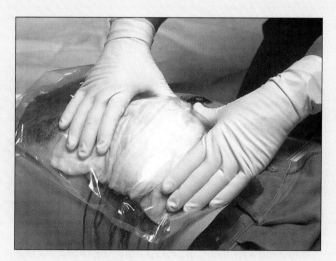

11-1c Cover the moistened dressing with a sterile occlusive dressing to prevent evaporative drying.

an immovable object, attempt to cut it. Use a saw, cutter, or torch, but be very careful to assure that vibration, jarring, and heat are not transmitted to the patient.

Carefully observe and care for penetrating wounds that may traverse both the abdominal and thoracic cavities. If the wound is large and may have penetrated the diaphragm or otherwise entered the thoracic cavity, seal the wound with an occlusive dressing taped on three sides to permit the release of the buildup of air pressure that occurs in a tension pneumothorax. Be especially watchful of respiratory excursion and effort.

The PASG is indicated for the patient with abdominal injury and the early signs of shock. However, it should not be used if there is concurrent penetrating trauma to the chest. The PASG applies circumferential pressure to the abdominal cavity, thereby raising intra-abdominal pressure and reducing the rate of intra-abdominal hemorrhage. Its use is generally contraindicated (inflate the leg sections only) in females in late pregnancy, abdominal evisceration patients, or patients with impaled objects. If the patient with an evisceration experiences a blood pressure below 50 mmHg, consider inflating the abdominal section of the garment as the risks associated with injury to the exposed bowel are less than those of profound hypotension. Incrementally inflate the PASG to maintain blood pressure and pulse rate, not to return them to preinjury levels.

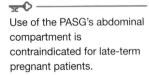

Inflate the PASG in increments to maintain blood pressure and pulse, not to return them to preinjury levels.

MANAGEMENT OF THE PREGNANT PATIENT

Special care is offered to the pregnant patient because of the anatomical and physiological changes induced by pregnancy. Place the late-term mother, when possible, in the left lateral recumbent position. This assures that the weight of the uterus does not compress the vena cava, reduce blood return to the heart, and cause hypotension. It also facilitates airway care. Administer high-flow, high-concentration oxygen early in your care because the mother's respiratory reserve volume is diminished, because the work necessary for her to move air is greater because of the increased intra-abdominal pressure, and because the fetus is especially susceptible to hypoxia. If necessary, employ intermittent positive-pressure ventilation early in your care. Also consider aggressive airway care. The pregnant mother is prone to vomiting and aspiration. If she has a significantly reduced level of consciousness, consider rapid sequence intubation.

Maintain a high index of suspicion for internal hemorrhage since the increased blood volume of the third-trimester mother may permit an increased blood loss before the signs and symptoms of hypovolemia become evident. The fetus may be at risk early in the blood loss, well before the mother displays any signs. Initiate IV therapy early, but remember that pregnancy induces a relative anemia and that aggressive fluid resuscitation may further dilute the erythrocyte concentrations and lead to ineffective circulation. Consider using the PASG, inflating the leg sections first. Use of the PASG may be beneficial for the patient in early pregnancy (first-term) as the pressure of the trouser is well distributed within the uterus by the amniotic fluid. However, for the late-term pregnant patient, use of the PASG's abdominal segment is contraindicated because the pressure of the garment may push the uterus more firmly against the inferior vena cava, reducing venous return to the heart, and increasing the effects of hypovolemia.

Use of the PASG's abdominal compartment is contraindicated for late-term pregnant patients.

Summary

Blunt or penetrating abdominal trauma can result in serious organ damage and life-threatening hemorrhage. Concurrently, the signs of injury are limited, nonspecific, and do not reflect the seriousness of abdominal pathology. It is thus very important for your assessment to carefully determine the mechanism of injury and the region of the abdomen it affects. This information must be communicated to the emergency department to assure its personnel acknowledge the significance of your first-hand knowledge of the mechanism of injury.

Care for significant abdominal injury is provided by rapid transport to the trauma center. Most significant abdominal injury results in serious internal bleeding or organ injury that can neither be cared for nor stabilized in the prehospital setting. Further, the definitive care for the patient with serious abdominal injury is provided via surgery. The patient must be transported to a facility capable of providing immediate surgical intervention when needed. This is a trauma center. Prehospital care is supportive of the airway and breathing, and preventive for shock.

The pregnant patient with abdominal injury deserves special attention because her vascular volume is increased and she will likely not show the signs of shock until the fetus is at risk. Careful observation while preparing for rapid transport to the trauma center is in order. If any of the slightest signs of hypoperfusion is noted, initiate fluid resuscitation.

You Make the Call

You arrive at the scene of a car–pedestrian collision. The victim is a young female about 12 years of age. She is lying on her side, in the fetal position, on the ground. She is conscious and alert, though confused as to where she is and what happened. The patient complains of right shoulder pain, although there is no injury visible in the region. Physical assessment reveals a tender left upper quadrant, just below the margin of the rib cage, with some guarding and no rebound tenderness.

1. Given the signs and symptoms, what is the most likely injury and why?
2. What relation does the right shoulder pain have to the suspected injury?
3. What care will you provide for this patient?

See Suggested Responses at the back of this book.

Review Questions

1. Your patient has a history of trauma to the left flank and complains of pain in that region. Which of the following organs might you suspect to be injured?
   a. liver
   b. heart
   c. spleen
   d. gallbladder

2. All of the following statements regarding bile are correct except:
   a. bile is a waste product of the reprocessing of red blood cells.
   b. bile is released into the colon in response to fatty foods.
   c. bile aids in the digestion of fats.
   d. bile is produced by the gallbladder.

3. The kidneys serve the body in all of the following ways except:
   a. pH regulation.
   b. waste product collection
   c. salt/water balance control
   d. fat emulsification.

4. Penetrating trauma most frequently involves the _____ and small bowel.
   a. liver
   b. spleen
   c. kidneys
   d. aorta

5. A protrusion of organs from a wound is called an:
   a. extravasation.
   b. evisceration.
   c. ecchymosis.
   d. exsanguination.

6. One of the functions of the pancreas is:
   a. destroying spent RBCs.
   b. producing new RBCs.
   c. secreting glucagon.
   d. manufacturing new WBCs.

7. _____ is the number one killer of pregnant females.
   a. Hypertension
   b. Toxemia
   c. Trauma
   d. Sepsis

8. The appendix and portions of the urinary bladder, small bowel, ascending colon, rectum, and female genitalia are located in the:
   a. left lower quadrant.
   b. right upper quadrant.
   c. right lower quadrant.
   d. left upper quadrant.

9. The spleen is not an accessory organ of digestion but rather a part of the _____ system.
   a. digestive
   b. respiratory
   c. nervous
   d. immune

10. It is very important to assure early fluid resuscitation of the potentially hypotensive pregnant mother. This statement is true because it may take a maternal blood loss of between _____ and _____ percent before changes in maternal blood pressure or heart rate are evident.
   a. 10 and 15
   b. 20 and 25
   c. 30 and 35
   d. 40 and 45

See Answers to Review Questions at the back of this book.

Further Reading

American College of Surgeons, Committee on Trauma. *Advanced Trauma Life Support Course: Student Manual.* Chicago: American College of Surgeons, 2003.

Bates, Barbara, Lynn S. Bickley, and Robert A. Hoekelman. *A Guide to Physical Examination and History Taking.* 8th ed. Philadelphia: J. B. Lippincott, 2003.

Bledsoe B. E. and D. Clayden. *Prehospital Emergency Pharmacology.* 6th ed. Upper Saddle River, N.J.: Pearson/Prentice Hall, 2005.

Butman, A., S. Martin, R. Vomacka, and N. McSwain. *Comprehensive Guide to Pre-Hospital Skills: A Skills Manual for EMT-Basic, EMT-Intermediate, and EMT-Paramedic.* St. Louis: Mosby, 1996.

Butman, Alexander M., and James L. Paturas. *Pre-Hospital Trauma Life Support.* Akron, Ohio: Emergency Training, 1999.

Campbell, John E. *Basic Trauma Life Support for Paramedics and Other Advanced Providers.* 5th ed. update. Upper Saddle River, N.J.: Pearson/Prentice Hall, 2004.

Ivatury R. R., and G. C. Cayten, eds. *Textbook of Penetrating Trauma.* Williams & Wilkins, Media, PA, 1996.

Martini, Frederic. *Fundamentals of Anatomy and Physiology.* 6th ed. San Francisco: Benjamin Cummings, 2004.

McSwain, N. E. and S. B. Frame, eds. *Prehospital Trauma Life Support.* 5th ed. St. Louis: Mosby, 2003.

Rosen, P., and R. Barkin, eds. *Emergency Medicine: Concepts and Clinical Practice.* 5th ed. St. Louis: Mosby, 2002.

On the Web

Visit Brady's Paramedic Website at **www.bradybooks.com/paramedic**.

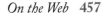

Shock Trauma Resuscitation

Objectives

After reading this chapter, you should be able to:

1. Identify the morbidity and mortality associated with blunt and penetrating trauma. (p. 460)
2. Explain the concept, value, and elements of injury prevention programs. (pp. 461–463)
3. Describe assessment of seriously and nonseriously injured trauma patients. (pp. 463–481)
4. Identify the aspects of assessment performed during the scene size-up, initial assessment, rapid trauma assessment, focused assessment and history, detailed physical exam, and ongoing assessment for the trauma patient. (pp. 464–481)
5. Identify the importance of rapid recognition and treatment of shock in trauma patients. (pp. 481–483)
6. Identify and explain the value of the components of shock trauma resuscitation. (pp. 481–485)
7. Describe the special needs and assessment considerations when treating pediatric and geriatric trauma patients. (pp. 485–493)
8. Explain the importance of good communications with other personnel within the emergency medical services system. (pp. 493–494)
9. Identify the benefits of helicopter use, and list the criteria for establishing a landing zone. (pp. 495–501)
10. Describe the preparation of a patient for air medical transport. (p. 501)
11. Identify the value of trauma care research and how it has impacted prehospital skills. (pp. 501–503)

Key Terms

Case Study

An outlying basic life support unit calls for Metro Rescue 9, an advanced life support unit. A farmer's son is trapped under a tractor, bleeding profusely. While en route, Alex, the paramedic on Rescue 9, calls dispatch to have the Life Flight helicopter placed on stand-by.

Upon arrival, Alex and the crew find a young male with his leg pinned beneath an overturned tractor and the adjoining ground soaked with blood. The patient is pale with cool, moist skin. Alex finds him conscious but anxious and somewhat combative. The patient, Peter, is unsure of what happened. He is breathing with shallow breaths, has a weak radial pulse of 120, and a 3-second capillary refill time. The initial assessment reveals no injuries, except those that are suspected on the limb trapped under the tractor. Blood pressure is 90 by palpation, respirations are 22 and shallow, oxygen saturation is 92 percent, and Peter's level of consciousness is diminishing. Extrication is expected in 6 minutes. Rescue 9 asks dispatch to send Life Flight to the scene.

Alex starts two IV lines with large-bore catheters and trauma tubing. One 1,000-mL bag of normal saline and one of lactated Ringer's solution are hung, one running to administer a 500 mL fluid bolus. High-flow, high-concentration oxygen is applied via nonrebreather mask, while the pneumatic anti-shock garment (PASG) is readied on a long spine board. Alex contacts medical direction and relays both the situation and pertinent patient information.

Removal of the tractor reveals a crush wound to Peter's right thigh. Alex locates the source of hemorrhage and applies direct digital pressure to it. Bleeding slows and pressure dressings replace digital pressure. Alex and the crew then move Peter to the long spine board, where they apply and inflate the PASG. Next, they load him into the ambulance to await the helicopter, which is only minutes from landing.

A second set of vital signs reveals respirations at 26 with very shallow breaths, a blood pressure of 70 by palpation, a carotid pulse of 136, and an oxygen saturation level of 86 percent. The patient now responds only to verbal stimuli. When Life Flight arrives, Alex gives its crew an abbreviated patient report, and Peter is quickly moved to the helicopter. They administer a second fluid bolus, and the lactated Ringer's solution is replaced with one unit of O-negative blood.

Twelve minutes later, the helicopter arrives at the trauma center. There has been some improvement in Peter's respirations, his pulse rate has slowed, and his oxygen saturation has risen to 90 percent. At the emergency department, blood is drawn, typed, and cross-matched. Meanwhile, a second unit of O-negative blood is administered. The physician's assessment and x-rays reveal no femur fracture. The ED team takes the young man to surgery, where a surgeon repairs the torn femoral artery. Three days later, Rescue 9 receives a call from Peter's parents thanking the crew. Their son is doing fine and will be coming home that weekend.

INTRODUCTION TO SHOCK TRAUMA RESUSCITATION

In the mid-1960s, trauma was identified as the neglected disease of a modern society. At that time, more than 150,000 persons died each year from trauma, while even greater numbers suffered some level of disability. Health care leaders, recognizing that no organized system existed to care for these victims, took the first steps toward forming what has grown into today's emergency medical service system. Thirty-five years later, EMS has become a highly sophisticated system, yet 150,000 lives are still lost yearly to trauma (Figure 12-1 ■). Most of these lives are taken, not at the end of a progressive disease in the later years of life, but from young and active members of society. Today, research has indicated that the skills that have been mainstays of prehospital trauma care often do not affect patient outcome and, worse, they occasionally increase patient mortality and morbidity.

As professionals in the field of prehospital emergency care, we need to look carefully and honestly at our actions and assure that they best serve our patients. We must do several things to secure a future for prehospital emergency care and to assure that our patients receive the best chances for survival. We must help strike at trauma at its source by supporting and promoting injury prevention in our society. We need to assure that our practices are current and truly benefit those who receive our care. Finally, we need to function as an integrated component of the health care system serving our patients and our communities. To help accomplish these objectives, this chapter examines injury prevention, trauma assessment, shock trauma resuscitation, care for special patients, care provider interaction, air medical service, and trauma research.

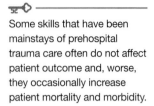

Some skills that have been mainstays of prehospital trauma care often do not affect patient outcome and, worse, they occasionally increase patient mortality and morbidity.

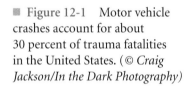

■ Figure 12-1   Motor vehicle crashes account for about 30 percent of trauma fatalities in the United States. (© *Craig Jackson/In the Dark Photography*)

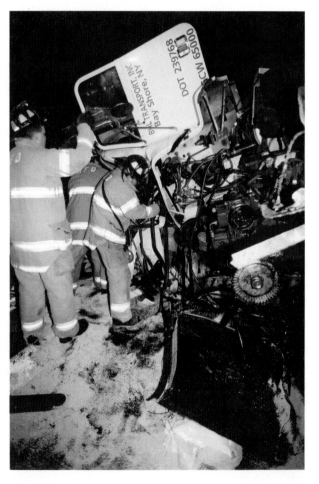

INJURY PREVENTION

Of all the care procedures and advanced interventions available to treat the trauma patient, none has more promise for reducing mortality and morbidity than prevention. Here, we in emergency medical services can learn a great deal from the fire service. The efforts of the fire service in encouraging smoke detector use, promoting more rigorous fire codes and inspections, and educating the public—especially children—about both the dangers of fire and the techniques to preserve life during fire are credited with greatly decreasing fire incidence and mortality. These fire service efforts are a valuable model for programs aimed at reducing death and disability from trauma.

If EMS is to maintain a leadership role in prehospital emergency care, we must place a new and continuing emphasis on injury prevention. The "Let's not meet by accident" campaign, developed jointly by a trauma system and prehospital care providers, is just one example of a prevention education program. It aims both to acquaint high school students with EMS and to alert them to the trauma hazards in our society. Other citizen groups have formed to help increase public awareness of social behaviors that lead to trauma. One such group, Mothers Against Drunk Driving, draws attention to the highway death toll associated with driving while alcohol or substance impaired. The EMS system must encourage or conduct programs like these with active participation from prehospital care providers to fulfill its responsibilities to the community.

A new program, sponsored by EMS and modeled after the fire service approach to prevention, is the home inspection (Figure 12-2 ■). After a significant event, such as the birth of a child, local EMS personnel perform a voluntary home inspection. The inspectors survey the home for potential hazards, notify the family of their findings, and suggest changes that would increase home safety. For example, inspectors might check the temperature of the hot water tank (and suggest lowering it when necessary) to prevent scalding injury to children; examine infant cribs to assure the slats are close enough to prevent strangulation and other injuries; and test child auto seats for proper fit and instruct parents in their proper use. They might also check for ground fault outlets in bathrooms, overloaded electrical sockets or circuits, electrical cords under rugs, and other improper electrical connections. The inspectors can recommend installation of railings or replacement of treads on stairways, porches, and other potential locations of falls. While in the home the crew also assures there are adequate smoke detectors with fresh batteries. While carrying on the inspection, the EMS crew can also promote other safe practices such as the use of helmets and other protective equipment for motorcycling, skateboarding, in-line skating, and bicycling. In addition, they can instruct the family on the best way to access police, fire, and medical services in the event of emergency. Widespread adoption of programs like these carries a tremendous potential to reduce trauma mortality and morbidity by reducing trauma in the home. These programs also introduce family members to the EMS team before an emergency strikes, thus helping to foster a good public image for the EMS system.

Currently, the Occupational Safety and Health Administration (OSHA) and other governmental agencies have developed and are enforcing workplace standards for safety. Their efforts assure that the workplace is reasonably safe and that workers are provided both with training in safe practices and with protective equipment appropriate to their work environment. The Department of Transportation is constantly improving motor vehicle safety through encouragement of better highway and vehicle design, testing, and inspection. These DOT programs assure that the highways are safer and crashes are more survivable. Other governmental and quasigovernmental agencies monitor the safety of various products like children's toys, electronic equipment, and other consumer products.

One important fact to keep in mind when considering any safety education program is the impact of serious trauma on the young male population. Males between 13 and 35 years of age account for about 27 percent of all serious trauma injuries and over

Of all the care procedures and advanced interventions available to treat the trauma patient, none has more promise for reducing mortality and morbidity than prevention.

Males between 13 and 35 years of age account for about 27 percent of all serious trauma injuries and over 30 percent of all trauma deaths.

Welcome to the World Injury Prevention Survey
Orange County Emergency Medical Services

09/20/98

EMS DATA	
Date	
Paramedic Name/Number	
Trip Number	
IRV Number/Zone	
Grid Number	
On Scene Time	
Back In Service Time	

Family's Name

Phone Number

Address   City   Zipcode

Mother's Name   Mothers Age

Father's Name   Father's Age

Individual Interviewed: ☐ Mother ☐ Father ☐ Other   Number of people living in home   Adults: Children:

Childs Name	Date of Birth	Last Non-Sick MD Visit

Home Info

Building Type: ☐ Apartment ☐ Rented Room/Floor ☐ Mobile Home   Ownership: ☐ Public Housing

☐ Duplex ☐ Condominium ☐ Single Unit House   ☐ Rented ☐ Owned

Number of Stories (levels): 1 2 3 4   Interior Stairway: Yes No   No. of Doorway Exits: ____   Pool: Yes No   Latched Gate between House and Pool: Yes No

Fire Prevention and Safety

Smoke Detector 1 Location: Ceiling Wall   Beep: Yes No

Smoke Detector 2 Location: Ceiling Wall   Beep: Yes No

Smoke Detector 3 Location: Ceiling Wall   Beep: Yes No

No. of Batteries Provided:

Smoke Detector Provided: Yes No

Education

Discuss Smoke Detector Pamphlet

Fire Extinguisher 1 Location: Charged: Yes No   Fire Extinguisher 2 Location: Charged: Yes No

Fire Exit Plan: Yes No   Have had Practice Drill: Yes No   If Yes to Drill, How often: Monthly Yearly Other _____

Space Heater 1 Location: Type: Kerosene Electrical   Space Heater 2 Location: Type: Kerosene Electrical

Are Woodstoves/Fireplaces used at this site: Yes No   If Yes, When was the Chimney last cleaned: ☐ < 1 Year ☐ > 1 Year

Discuss Fire Prevention and Emergency Exit Materials

Advise to have Chimney cleaned if not done in the past 1 year.

First Aid

First Aid Kit in home: Yes No   First Aid Kit provided: Yes No   Emergency Numbers posted in visible place near phone: Yes No

Medications out of Reach: Yes No   Medications Locked up: Yes No   Poison Control Center Number posted visibly near phone:

Cleaning Supplies out of Reach: Yes No   Cleaning Supplies Locked up: Yes No   Yes No

Discuss 911 and Poison Control Information

Firearms

Do you keep firearms locked up: Yes No   How many firearms in the home _____

Are any firearms loaded? Yes No   Are all firearms locked up: Yes No   If not locked up, are trigger locks used: Yes No

Discuss Firearm Safety

AC

Are Electrical Outlets in Child's Bedroom and Playareas covered: Yes No   AC Outlet Covers provided: Yes No

Discuss Electrical Risk

Water

Where do you bathe your child ☐ Kitchen Sink ☐ Bathroom Sink ☐ Bathroom Tub

(Test 2 Locations)   Temperature _____   Temperature _____   Temperature _____

Temperature should be < or = to 120 degrees

Crib

Crib railings spaced less than 2 3/8 inches apart: Yes No   Is Crib near any cords (ie window blinds): Yes No

Crib Mattress fits snugly (less than 2 fingers space between mattress and crib around all edges): Yes No

Discuss Crib Safety and Strangulation Risk

Car Seats

Is there an infant car seat for the newborn: Yes No   Where does the **infant** ride in the car: ☐ Front ☐ Rear

Does the Vehicle have a passenger side air bag: Yes No   ☐ Rear Facing ☐ Forward Facing

Do Children over 40 lbs wear seatbelts: Yes No   Are car seats available for all other children under 40 lbs: Yes No

Discuss Car Seat Safety Materials

W Bag/Referrals

Were the contents of the Welcome Bag reviewed with the parent: Yes No

Follow-up Visit or Referrals Requested: ☐ Smoke Detector / Batteries ☐ Health Department-Health Services

☐ Rental Without Smoke Detector ☐ Health Department-Safety Services

☐ Other _____ ☐ Health Department-Special Programs

Record Details of Each Item in the Comment Area

Comments/Concerns

Family contacted and declines visit ☐   Please Write Additional Comments or Concerns on the back of this form   Paramedic Signature:

■ Figure 12-2   A sample home safety inspection form.

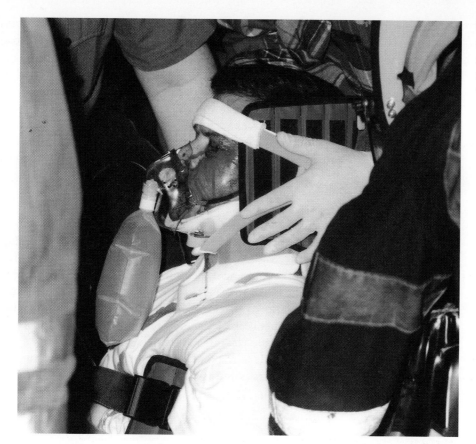

■ Figure 12-3 Young males account for a disproportionate representation of mortality and morbidity among trauma victims. (© Mark C. Ide)

30 percent of all trauma deaths (Figure 12-3 ■). At the same time, this group represents less than 20 percent of the total population. Thus, trauma among young males represents an epidemic of serious proportions. It is probable that the risk-taking nature of young males and an associated disregard for safe practices (like failure to use seat belts and motorcycle helmets and a willingness to drink and drive) contribute to this mortality. Encouraging behavioral changes in this population would likely have a marked effect on the overall incidence of trauma and the associated death and disability. Since many people entering EMS are of this gender and age group, we need to both speak to the problem and demonstrate safe practices by example to our peers.

TRAUMA ASSESSMENT

Assessment of the trauma patient is essential both to determining the priority for patient transport and identifying and prioritizing patient injuries for care. During the preceding chapters, we have discussed trauma related to body regions or systems. During these discussions, we examined how the elements of assessment were applied to each system or region. In this chapter, we will review the elements of assessment in a comprehensive way, much as you would when presented with a seriously injured trauma patient.

Trauma assessment progresses through the scene size-up, the initial assessment, either the rapid trauma assessment or the focused exam and history, and is then followed by serial ongoing assessments. However, your first opportunity to begin the assessment process is through a review of the dispatch information.

DISPATCH INFORMATION

The dispatch information provides critical information that you must evaluate while responding to the scene. The information provides the nature of the call. Often, it

Dispatch information provides the nature of the call and may suggest hazards at the scene.

specifies the mechanism of injury (like a fall, shooting, or auto crash) or the nature of the injury (like a broken leg, head injury, or deep laceration). This information permits you to begin preparation for patient care and to think about how to approach the scene. Occasionally, the dispatch information may suggest the scene is too dangerous to approach until it is secured by the police (such as cases of violence like shootings, stabbings, or domestic altercations with injuries). In such cases, you should remain at a distance from the scene until police arrive and notify you that it is secure. At other times, the dispatch information may alert you to potential hazards such as a toxic gas release or downed electrical wires for which you may need to request specialized response teams to secure the scene.

Use the dispatch information to anticipate and prepare for the care of injuries. To speed your response at the scene, locate the equipment you will be likely to use. If appropriate, lay the equipment out on the stretcher so it can be taken immediately to the patient. (It is always easier to have a first responder or bystander return a piece of equipment to the ambulance than it is to ask them to go to the ambulance, find it, and bring it to the patient's side.) Inspect the equipment, check to see that it is working properly, and review its application and use. If you expect severe injuries, set up an IV bag and administration set in the ambulance for later use on the patient. This saves time that would otherwise be taken from patient care to assemble the administration equipment. Finally, review the assessment and care you intend to provide and, as necessary, review your protocols to assure you are ready to respond to the emergency. These actions will help you move quickly through the required care steps and to offer the optimum patient care in the shortest span of time.

SCENE SIZE-UP

Trauma scene size-up involves four major elements (Figure 12-4 ■). They are determining the mechanism of injury, identifying scene hazards including the need for body substance isolation, accounting for and locating all patients, and requesting any additional resources. Initially you will don gloves because all patient contact calls for this elementary form of body substance isolation. As you progress through the analysis of the mechanism of injury and anticipate injuries, you may increase your level of personal protection as indicated in the following sections. The mechanism of injury analysis is also essential to help you identify all scene hazards.

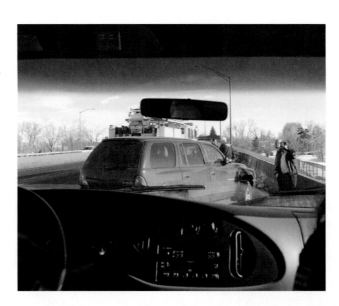

■ Figure 12-4 Assess the emergency scene quickly and carefully, looking for scene hazards, possible mechanisms of injury, the location of patients, and the possible need for additional resources.
(© Jeff Forster)

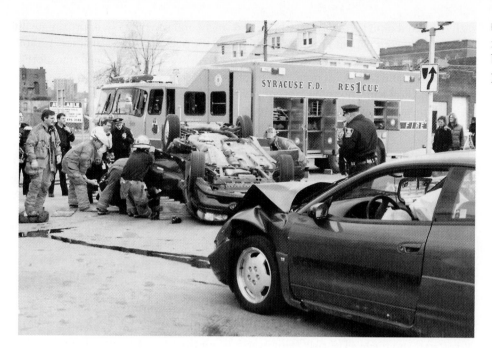

Figure 12-5 Analyze the forces of a vehicle collision, and based on that analysis, anticipate possible patient injuries.

Mechanism of Injury Analysis

Analyze the mechanism of injury by recreating the incident in your mind, and from that, anticipating the nature and severity of your patient's injuries (the index of suspicion). Take the evidence available to you as you arrive at and first view the scene, and use that evidence to determine exactly how the forces were expressed to the patient. If two autos came together, for example, determine what vehicle surfaces impacted, from which direction the vehicles were traveling, and which patient surfaces were impacted (Figure 12-5 ■). Use the amount of vehicular damage to approximate the strength of the impact, and then determine whether restraints or other protective mechanisms were used that may have reduced the potential for injury. Frontal and rear impacts afford the vehicle occupants the most protection, especially if seat belts are properly worn and air bags deploy. Lateral and rollover impacts are likely to cause the most serious injuries. In motorcycle, bicycle, and pedestrian-vs.-vehicle collisions, identify the relative speed of impact and appreciate the lack of protection afforded the victim. In other nonvehicular blunt trauma, examine the height of the fall or other indications of the energy of impact and the point of impact as well as the path of transmission of those forces through the body.

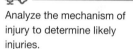

Analyze the mechanism of injury to determine likely injuries.

When assessing the mechanism of injury for a patient affected by penetrating trauma, look at the speed of the offending agent or projectile. Remember that an increase in mass directly increases the force's energy, while an increase in speed greatly increases (a squared relationship) the impact energy and the potential for serious patient injury. With gunshot wounds, identify the nature of the weapon (hand gun, shotgun, or rifle), the relative power and profile (caliber), and then the distance and angle between the gun barrel and the impact point. Visualize the pathway taken by the bullet and its destructive power as it travels through human tissue. Head, central chest, and upper abdominal injuries are most lethal. Remember, however, that the path of a bullet is frequently deflected from a straight line. In other penetrating trauma, mentally recreate the injury process and use the kinetic energy principles to analyze the nature, process, and severity of the injury. Try to determine the length of the object and the depth and angle of insertion.

From your re-creation of the injury process, identify the individual organs affected and the extent of the injury to them. Approximate what significance their injury will have on the patient's condition and how it will affect him as time progresses. Assign each suspected injury a priority for both assessment and care. Finally, approximate the seriousness of your patient's overall condition and the potential need for either (1) rapid transport with most care provided en route or (2) on-scene care and then transport or (3) treatment and release (as permitted by protocol). Remember that patients with pre-existing medical conditions, patients of advanced age, and the very young are at greatest risk when seriously injured. If there is more than one patient, identify the most seriously injured and order your patient assessment and care accordingly.

Hazard Identification

The mechanism of injury analysis helps you to identify many possible hazards at the scene. Search out all hazards and protect yourself, your patient, bystanders, and fellow rescuers from them. These hazards include the mechanism that injured your patient and may range from traffic associated with the auto crash to the assailant who is still holding the hand gun. Search for additional sources of blunt and penetrating trauma such as the broken glass and jagged metal at an auto crash scene or moving machinery at an industrial accident site. Also search out and exclude any hazards from fire, heat, explosion, electricity, toxic chemicals, radiation, or deadly gas at each and every scene. Look for hazardous material placards. Your ambulance should carry the Department of Transportation's *Emergency Response Guidebook,* which will help you identify the type of material and the level of risk. (However, it is not the job of EMS to address the risks of hazardous materials. That responsibility lies with the hazardous material team or the fire department.)

Your ambulance should carry the Department of Transportation's Emergency Response Guidebook.

Be aware of the presence and mood of family members, bystanders, and crowds at the emergency scene. These people may welcome your assistance or provide a serious threat to your well-being.

Analyze the scene carefully to identify each of these hazards and exclude them from the scene or be prepared to deal with each before you approach the patient. Your well-being and that of your patient depend on it. If you are injured at the scene you will be less able to help your patient and may, in fact, yourself become a patient rather than a caregiver.

Body Substance Isolation

Realize that the risk of infection from body substances extends to your patient and yourself, especially when dealing with trauma.

A special type of hazard existing at almost every emergency scene is the presence of body fluids and substances with the potential to spread infection (Figure 12-6 ▦). Realize that the risk of infection extends to both you and your patient, especially when dealing with trauma. While a patient's open wound releases blood that poses an infection threat to you, the open wound also creates a pathway through which infection can enter your patient's body. The use of gloves and other body substance isolation equipment and procedures protects both you and your patient. Assure that all rescuers who may

▦ **Figure 12-6** Analyze the scene carefully to determine the need for body substance isolation procedures.

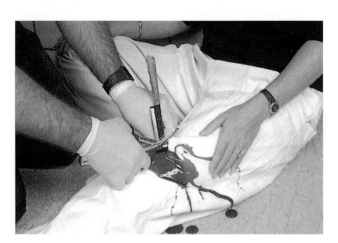

come into contact with the patient also employ appropriate body substance isolation procedures as you prepare to approach the scene.

In all patient contacts, it is essential to don gloves in anticipation of contact with blood, saliva, mucus, urine, or fecal material. If the scene size-up reveals multiple patients, put on two or three sets of gloves, one over the other. Then peel gloves off as you move from one patient to another. If you prefer not to double glove, be sure to carry additional pairs of gloves and change them with each patient contact. Remember that the body fluids from one patient are potentially as infectious to another patient as they are to you and that with open wounds the risk of infection increases.

Your analysis of the mechanism of injury may also suggest airway or chest trauma or possible external arterial hemorrhage. These injuries may result in spurting blood or in blood or other fluids being propelled or coughed into the air. In such cases, wear both eye protection and splatter protection for your clothing. A mask may also be advisable. Consider wearing a mask if you have any type of respiratory infection, again to protect your patient. Assure that all rescuers use the appropriate personal protective equipment (PPE). Once at the patient's side, your further evaluation may reveal the need for a higher level of body substance isolation than the scene size-up suggested; for that reason, always have goggles, gowns, masks, and additional gloves handy.

Accounting For and Locating All Patients

During your scene size-up, identify the number of likely patients and their locations around the emergency scene. During a collision, patients may be thrown from the auto or trapped within a twisted wreck and completely out of sight (this often occurs with infants). A patient may also leave the vehicle and mill about the scene with bystanders, leave in an attempt to find help, or simply wander from the scene in confusion. Search for evidence that suggests the number and types of patients. Consider the number of vehicles involved in a crash; the number of spider-webs on the windshields; purses or articles of clothing; and child seats, clothing, or toys. As you arrive at the scene, question the apparent patients and bystanders to better determine the number and locations of any additional patients.

Anticipate the number of patients at the trauma scene and search them out as you arrive.

Resource Needs Determination

Once you determine the likely number of patients and their injuries, approximate the type and nature of any other emergency medical resources that will be needed at the scene (Figure 12-7 ■). This may include additional ambulances, one for each seriously injured patient, and air medical service for patients who meet trauma triage criteria at a scene more than 30 minutes from the nearest trauma center.

Also determine the resources needed to control the hazards identified in your analysis of the scene. These resources may include the police for traffic control or for

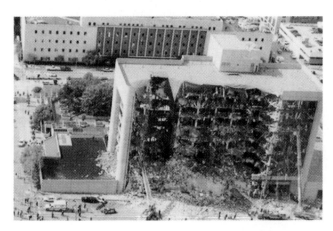

■ Figure 12-7 Assess the emergency scene to determine the need for any additional resources.

scene security with gathering crowds, the heavy rescue unit for extrication, the hazardous material team for fuel and oil spill cleanup, the power company for downed electrical lines, or the fire service for potential fire control at vehicle crashes. It is essential that you contact dispatch early so needed equipment and trained personnel are quickly en route to the scene. Waiting until later in the call delays their arrival and may hinder your ability to access and care for patients.

At the end of the scene size-up, you should have the information necessary to organize the overall response to the incident and to determine the special focus of your assessment for each patient. Take a few seconds to organize how you will address the scene and coordinate the additional resources as they arrive. Identify in your mind what you wish each respective service to accomplish and how these functions can best work together to meet your patient's needs. Then think through your initial assessment and what specific problems you might expect to find with each element of that evaluation for each patient (Figure 12-8 ■).

INITIAL ASSESSMENT

The initial assessment is intended to identify immediate patient life threats and correct them before a more detailed assessment continues. It consists of applying spinal precautions when needed, and assessing the patient's mental, airway, breathing, and circulatory status. If any serious or life-threatening problems are found, correct them immediately. As you carry out these steps, you will add to the information you gathered during the scene size-up and develop a general impression of the patient.

Spinal Precautions

Employ immediate spinal precautions in *any* of the following circumstances:

★ The mechanism of injury suggests the possibility of spinal injury.

★ You suspect any extreme of flexion/extension, lateral bending, axial loading, distraction, or rotation.

★ Any penetrating or blunt force has been directed to the neck or spinal cord.

★ The patient has any significant injury above the shoulders.

Per your local protocols, maintain initial spinal precautions until you determine *all* of the following—or, once spinal precautions have been provided and assessment has been completed, consider discontinuing spinal precautions if you find *all* of the following:

★ The patient is alert and fully oriented, has a Glasgow Coma Scale score of 15, is not significantly affected by the "fight-or-flight" response, and is not intoxicated or under the influence of drugs, including alcohol.

★ The patient has no distracting injuries (e.g., serious long-bone fracture, other painful injury, shortness of breath).

★ The patient does not complain of nor does your assessment identify any signs or symptoms of spinal injury.

However, if you have an unreliable patient, significant distracting injuries, or any signs or symptoms of spinal injury, provide and continue spinal precautions, including the application of a cervical collar and full patient mechanical immobilization to a long spine board or full-body vacuum mattress.

When in doubt, err on the side of full spinal immobilization for your patient. In children and the elderly, signs and symptoms of spinal injury may not be as specific or

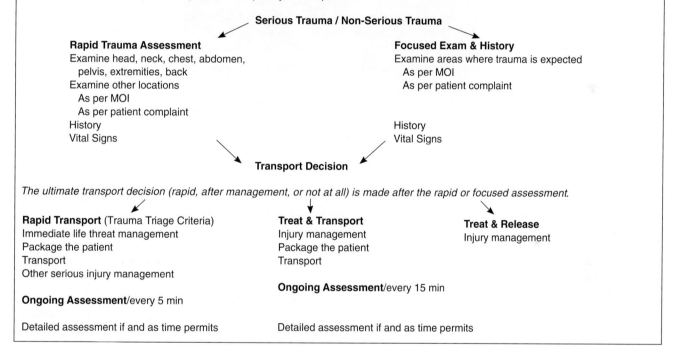

Trauma Assessment Format

Scene Size-up
Body substance isolation
Scene safety
Mechanism of injury
Locate all patients
Request additional resources

Initial Assessment
Spinal precautions
General patient impression
Mental status
Airway
Breathing
Circulation

The decision to employ rapid trauma assessment is based on an evaluation of the forces of trauma and the results of the initial assessment. Here you will also make a preliminary decision on priority of transport.

Serious Trauma / Non-Serious Trauma

Rapid Trauma Assessment
Examine head, neck, chest, abdomen,
   pelvis, extremities, back
Examine other locations
  As per MOI
  As per patient complaint
History
Vital Signs

Focused Exam & History
Examine areas where trauma is expected
  As per MOI
  As per patient complaint

History
Vital Signs

Transport Decision

The ultimate transport decision (rapid, after management, or not at all) is made after the rapid or focused assessment.

Rapid Transport (Trauma Triage Criteria)
Immediate life threat management
Package the patient
Transport
Other serious injury management

Ongoing Assessment/every 5 min

Detailed assessment if and as time permits

Treat & Transport
Injury management
Package the patient
Transport

Ongoing Assessment/every 15 min

Detailed assessment if and as time permits

Treat & Release
Injury management

■ Figure 12-8   A trauma assessment form can help you organize priorities at any emergency scene.

obvious. Hence, maintain full spinal precautions, even if the previously listed criteria are met.

General Impression

While you evaluate the patient's mental status, airway, breathing, and circulation, develop a general impression of him. Combine the information you gathered during the mechanism of injury analysis with the information gathered during the ABC check, and add to it the general appearance and mental status you observe during these first few minutes at the patient's side. The result is a general patient impression (Figure 12-9 ■). It is your determination of the seriousness of the patient injury's and the priority for

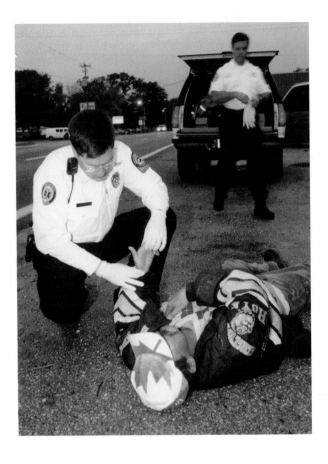

■ Figure 12-9 Form a general impression of the patient during the initial assessment and refine it during the rest of your time at the patient's side. (© *Craig Jackson/In the Dark Photography*)

If your general patient impression and the mechanism of injury suggest different levels of injury severity, base your care on the worst case scenario.

care and transport. This determination is very difficult to make early in your career; however, with experience your level of comfort in judging the severity of a patient's injuries and the need for either rapid transport or on-scene care will grow.

In some cases, your general patient impression will conflict with the seriousness of trauma suggested by the mechanism of injury or with the signs and symptoms you gather during the initial assessment. In most cases, you attend a patient very soon after an incident. In those circumstances, hemorrhage does not have the chance to accumulate and demand of the body the serious compensation that comes with time and produces the most noticeable signs and symptoms of shock. However, the mechanism of injury may not reflect the severity of the actual injuries and the patient may appear worse than expected. In all cases, base your management of the patient on the worst case scenario. As time and further assessment continues, modify your general patient impression and the care it suggests.

Mental Status

Evaluate the patient's mental status. Begin by introducing yourself, identifying your level of training, and explaining your desire to offer care to the patient. Ask the patient what happened and what is bothering him the most. This permits the patient to refuse care, assures that he knows who you are and that your intentions are helpful, and calls for a verbal response. Listen carefully to any responses as you continue your initial assessment.

At a minimum, identify the patient's level of consciousness using the AVPU mnemonic (*A*lert; responsive to *V*erbal stimuli, responsive to *P*ain, or *U*nresponsive). Even better, attempt to identify your patient's level of orientation. Does he know the day and time of day (orientation to time); recognize where he is (orientation to place); recognize friends and family (orientation to persons); and recognize who he is (orientation to own person)? (Patients will usually lose orientation in this order.) Orientation is scored from 4 to 0 with the alert and completely oriented patient being alert and oriented times 4 (A + O × 4). Some systems combine other persons and own person into a single element, resulting in a best orientation of "A+O times 3." Determining a patient's level of orientation provides a baseline reading of the patient's mental status against which improvement/deterioration can be trended in ongoing assessments.

When the patient is not responsive to verbal stimuli, check for the specific response to noxious stimuli. For example, if you apply a noxious stimulus (usually by squeezing the fleshy region between the thumb and first finger or trapezius muscle of the shoulder), does the patient move away from the stimulus (purposeful); move, but not effectively, away from the stimulus (purposeless); or does he not move at all in response to noxious stimulus? Some patients move toward a specific body position, or posture, in response to painful stimuli. With decorticate posturing, the patient's body moves toward extension with elbows flexing, while with decerebrate posturing the body and elbows extend. Determining a baseline response permits you and other care providers to track patient deterioration or improvement throughout the course of care.

Airway

It is easy to evaluate the airway in the conscious patient by listening to him speak. If he can talk clearly, you know that the patient has control over an open airway, is breathing adequately enough to speak in full sentences, and has cerebral oxygenation enough to support conscious thought. If the speech is broken or forced, there are unusual airway sounds, or the statements are confused or unintelligible, suspect and evaluate further for airway or breathing problems.

In the unconscious patient, airway assessment is more difficult. Look, listen, and feel carefully for air movement. Watch to see if the chest rises and falls. Place your ear just in front of or over your patient's mouth and listen for the sound of air moving during respirations and feel the volume of air escaping during exhalation. Remember that eupnea and apnea are the quietest and most difficult respirations to evaluate. If you do not hear air moving through the airway and/or you feel an insufficient volume of moving air, reposition the patient's head and jaw with the head-tilt/chin-lift or the jaw thrust. If repositioning improves air movement, then insert a nasal or oral airway. Be cautious in using the nasal airway if there is any serious head trauma because a basilar skull fracture may have opened the nasal cavity to the brain. Suction as needed to remove any excessive airway fluids or if necessary, turn the patient onto the side to let gravity help drain the airway. If the patient does not have protective airway reflexes, consider early intubation, either now (if the airway is at immediate risk) or at the end of the initial assessment.

If you note airway sounds like stridor, snoring, gurgling, or wheezing, presume a partial airway obstruction that will get worse during assessment and care. Trauma to the soft tissue of the airway will likely cause swelling and progressive airway restriction. Expect swelling to seriously obstruct respiration and again consider early intubation.

Breathing

Apply oxygen using a nonrebreather mask with oxygen flowing at 12 Lpm. This helps assure inspiration of high-flow, high-concentration (90 to 100 percent) oxygen for any moderately to seriously injured trauma patient. Watch for symmetrical chest and abdominal movement with each breath. If necessary, expose the chest for a better assessment. Rule out flail chest or stabilize the flail segment and provide overdrive ventilation (bag-valve masking the breathing patient). Rule out diaphragmatic breathing (associated with cervical spine injury) or provide overdrive ventilation. If the patient complains of dyspnea or if chest excursion or tidal volumes seem limited, auscultate the

Consider the airway to be clear if the patient answers your questions with clear, full, well-articulated sentences.

Consider early intubation if the patient displays any strider, snoring, gurgling, wheezing, or if the gag reflex is absent.

lung fields to identify unilateral diminished or absent breath sounds. Percuss the chest for resonance: A dull sound indicates blood in the pleural space, while hyperresonance indicates air in the pleural space. If you cannot rule out a building tension pneumothorax, consider needle decompression. If you note pneumothorax or decompress a tension pneumothorax, monitor the chest carefully for the development or redevelopment of tension pneumothorax.

If respirations are less than 12 per minute and/or the tidal volume is less than 600 mL per breath in the unconscious patient, consider the use of overdrive ventilation. If the patient is breathing rapidly but ineffectively, you should also consider overdrive ventilation. If the patient is not breathing, ventilate at 12 to 16 times per minute with full breaths (500 to 800 mL) with high-flow, high-concentration oxygen using the bag-valve mask and reservoir. Assure good chest rise in the patient and maintain an oxygen saturation of greater than 95 percent. Also consider the use of capnography to guide your ventilation, especially in the head injury patient.

Circulation

Quickly check the radial pulse for strength, regularity, and rate. A strong tachycardia suggests excitement, while a weak and thready pulse suggests shock compensation. If a radial pulse cannot be palpated, check for a carotid pulse. A rapid, weak carotid pulse suggests serious compensation for hypovolemia, the presence of severe hemorrhage (possibly internal), and the probable need for aggressive fluid resuscitation.

During the pulse check also note the patient's skin condition. Cool, clammy, ashen, or pale skin suggests shock compensation. Perform a capillary refill check. If refill takes more than 3 seconds, that finding supports a possible diagnosis of hypovolemia and compensation. (Please note that other conditions such as smoking, low ambient temperatures, preexisting disease, and use of medications may delay capillary refill as well.)

Make a quick visual sweep of the body, looking for any signs of serious and continuing hemorrhage. Using your analysis of the mechanism of injury, identify probable locations of bleeding and view them or, if the site is hidden from view, carefully pass a gloved hand under the area, looking for blood loss. Also use the mechanism of injury analysis to identify likely locations of internal injury and any associated internal hemorrhage. Use this information to determine the rate of probable blood loss and the priority for rapid transport.

A critical element of the initial assessment is detecting the earliest signs of shock. Remember that internal hemorrhage is the greatest killer of patients who survive the initial impact of trauma. Look carefully at your patient for any early signs of shock. These include a decreased level of consciousness or orientation, anxiety, restlessness, or combativeness. If the patient has consumed alcohol or is otherwise affected by drugs, be especially watchful and wary.

As internal hemorrhage continues, the body employs more drastic measures to compensate for the blood loss, and signs and symptoms become more obvious with the passage of time. The sooner the signs or symptoms develop, the more rapid the internal blood loss and the more quickly the patient is moving through compensated, then uncompensated, then irreversible shock. However, do not wait for these signs and symptoms of later stages of shock to appear. At the first signs of hypovolemic compensation, prioritize the patient for immediate transport to the trauma center. If the patient demonstrates any early signs of shock or the mechanism of injury suggests serious internal injury, initiate the steps of aggressive shock care that are described later in this chapter.

Concluding the Initial Assessment

As you complete the initial assessment, modify your mechanism of injury analysis based on additional evidence gained at the scene such as a bent steering wheel or intrusion into the passenger compartment. Continue to monitor the scene for safety, remaining alert to any alterations in conditions at the scene and assuring that all

A critical element of the initial assessment is detecting the earliest signs of shock.

If the patient has consumed alcohol or is otherwise affected by drugs, be especially watchful and wary.

Consult your local protocols and medical director for your system's position on trauma arrest resuscitation.

providers, patients, and bystanders are protected from scene hazards (including body substance isolation).

At the conclusion of the initial assessment for the trauma patient, you must determine whether the patient merits a rapid trauma assessment or is best served by a focused exam and history. The rapid trauma assessment aims to identify other life threats not revealed during the initial assessment, to provide appropriate rapid intervention, and to assure that the seriously injured trauma patient receives quick transport to the trauma center. The focused exam is used for less seriously injured patients and focuses on the probable injuries and their care. With both these categories of patients, you will also make a preliminary decision about priority for transport. If the patient meets any of the trauma triage criteria, either a mechanism of injury recognized during the scene size-up or a physical condition identified during the initial assessment, consider the patient for rapid transport.

Blunt trauma patients found in cardiac arrest in the prehospital setting rarely survive. This has prompted many EMS systems to institute trauma arrest protocols that permit paramedics to halt resuscitation when presented with a pulseless, nonbreathing blunt trauma patient who displays asystole on the ECG (in two leads). This action prevents the consumption of valuable resources by the EMS system and the generation of anxiety and expense for the family for what would be a fruitless effort. Consult your local protocols and medical director for your system's position on trauma arrest resuscitation.

GENERAL EXAMINATION TECHNIQUES

During the rapid trauma assessment, look at the areas where serious life threats are most likely to occur. These include the head, neck, chest, abdomen, pelvis, extremities, and back. Also quickly study locations of injury suggested either by the mechanism of injury or the symptoms described by the patient. In the focused physical exam, you look specifically at areas where injury is anticipated from the mechanism of injury and patient complaints. Both the rapid trauma assessment and the focused exam use basic techniques of patient questioning, inspection, palpation, auscultation, and percussion to identify signs and symptoms of injury. Both also conclude with a quick, abbreviated patient history and the gathering of a set of baseline vital signs.

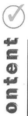

Review

Basic Assessment Techniques

Questioning
Inspection
Palpation
Auscultation
Percussion

Questioning

Before you inspect or palpate a body region, question the patient about any symptoms. Symptoms may include sensations of discomfort, pain, pain on movement, tingling, a pins-and-needles sensation (paraesthesia), numbness or lack of feeling (anesthesia), weakness, inability to move, or other unusual sensations. Also note the patient's response to the complaint. Patient complaints are subjective, and different people have different levels of pain tolerance. Watch how the patient responds to the pain and how easily he is distracted from it. This gives you a good approximation of how significant the pain or sensation is to the patient. Report and record any patient complaint in the patient's own words.

Inspection

As you continue inspecting the patient, look first to the skin color. The skin of a Caucasian with normal circulation will appear light pink. Note any ashen (gray or dusky), cyanotic (bluish), or pale (very light pink or white) colorations. In people of color, look at the coloration of the lips, the conjunctiva of the eyes, the palms of the hands, or soles of the feet. Any discoloration indicates a possible generalized problem like hypovolemia, hypoventilation, or hypothermia. Use the initial coloration you observe as a baseline when you examine specific regions of the body for injury. Look at those regions for erythema, a general reddening of the skin and the first sign of injury. The discoloration of ecchymosis, the "black and blue" normally associated with a contusion, is delayed because it takes the erythrocytes some time to migrate into injured tissue and then lose their oxygen and turn a deeper red or bluish color. A portion of a limb may also change color due to problems with distal circulation. The limb may turn pale (and cold) when arterial circulation is reduced or dark red, dusky, or ashen as circulation stagnates or venous return is halted.

The second element of inspection is looking for deformities. These become most recognizable if you carefully examine and compare limb to limb or one side of the body to the other. Deformity can be either an enlargement of the dimensions of a limb or body region or an abnormal angle or position of a limb or region. Enlargement is usually due to the accumulation of fluid—blood as in a hematoma or plasma and interstitial fluid (edema) as in inflammation associated with a contusion—but it may also be associated with the accumulation of air associated with subcutaneous emphysema. Angulation is the unusual positioning of a limb as with a bend in a bone where a bend would not be expected. Such a condition is most likely associated with a fracture. An unusual bend in a joint, meanwhile, suggests either a fracture or dislocation. Muscle spasm or abnormal retraction of a muscle due to tendon rupture may also cause deformity. Compare any apparent deformity to the opposite limb to better determine the nature and extent of the variance from normal.

The third element of inspection is an examination for disruption of the skin (wounds). Examine for any abrasion of the skin's surface, any tearing of the skin (a laceration), or any signs of skin damage that may be associated with a burn, such as erythema, blistering or gross disruption of the skin, and discoloration. Also look for any penetrations and determine whether they are superficial or deep. Remember that deep wounds that close encourage infection and are often more serious than more grotesque superficial open wounds.

Palpation

After inspection, palpate any area for additional signs of injury. Gently touch the entire surface of the area being evaluated, feeling for general skin and muscle tone, any unusual or warm masses, any grating sensation, or the "rice crispy" feel of subcutaneous emphysema. You should also feel for any muscle spasm (guarding) or pain on palpation (tenderness) that may reflect injury. Determine if that pain is pain on touch (tenderness), pain on movement, or pain on rapid release of pressure (rebound tenderness). Also palpate for relative muscle tone—normal, flaccid, or in spasm.

Auscultation

Auscultate the chest carefully to evaluate for the presence and quality of breath sounds (Figure 12-10 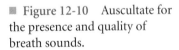). Note side to side, upper lobe to lower lobe, or regional differences. Crackles represent pulmonary edema most commonly related to pulmonary contusion

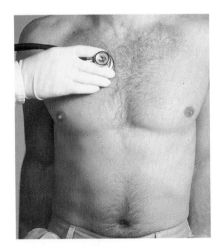

■ Figure 12-10 Auscultate for the presence and quality of breath sounds.

and associated edema in trauma, while side-to-side inequality suggests pneumothorax or tension pneumothorax. Auscultation of the abdomen is not merited in trauma due to the time required to adequately assess for bowel sounds and their poor correlation to injury.

Percussion

Percuss each lobe of the chest for resonance. A dull response suggests fluid or blood accumulating in the pleural space. A hyperresonant response suggests air or air under pressure in the pleural space.

RAPID TRAUMA ASSESSMENT

Use the rapid trauma assessment when you suspect a patient has a serious injury to the body and are inclined to transport him quickly to the trauma center. Such a patient is one who meets the trauma triage criteria. During the rapid trauma assessment, quickly scan the body looking for hemorrhage or evidence of significant injury and examine the patient's head, neck, chest, abdomen, pelvis, extremities, and back. (Order your assessment to limit the movement of the patient. For example, if the patient is found lying face down, quickly assess the back before turning the patient for further assessment and care.) Check the distal function in each limb by noting distal pulse strength, skin temperature and color, capillary refill time, and—as appropriate—sensation and grip strength. If you suspect specific injuries, provide a focused evaluation of the body region using the considerations for that region as specified in the detailed physical exam, discussed later in this chapter. Conclude the rapid trauma assessment by taking a quick patient history and a set of vital signs.

Use the rapid trauma assessment for patients who meet trauma triage criteria or who you suspect to have suffered serious injury.

FOCUSED EXAM AND HISTORY

The focused exam and history is performed on a patient whom you expect has limited injuries. Direct your examination to the location of patient complaint or to any region of injury suggested by the mechanism of injury or by any signs and symptoms noted during the initial assessment. The actual focused exam uses the examination criteria for the body region as specified in the detailed exam. Like the rapid trauma assessment, it concludes with a quick patient history and vital signs.

DETAILED PHYSICAL EXAM

The detailed physical exam is a comprehensive examination of the entire body to locate and identify signs of injury. It is rarely used in the prehospital setting as seriously injured patients receive attention directed at their life-threatening injuries and time becomes a premium as they are rushed to a trauma center. The patient with moderate or minor injuries receives assessment and care directed just at those injuries. The only case where a complete detailed exam may be necessary is in a patient with an altered level of consciousness, limited apparent minor injuries, and a mechanism of injury that suggests possible multiple injury sites. Only perform the detailed exam after you have concluded the initial assessment and stabilized or corrected any life-threatening conditions discovered during it.

While you will rarely use the detailed physical exam in the field, elements of it are used during the focused exam or rapid trauma assessment.

The detailed physical exam is an organized and intensive evaluation of each body area: the head, neck, chest, abdomen, back, pelvis, and extremities. When performing the detailed exam, use the physical assessment techniques of questioning, inspection, palpation, auscultation, and percussion discussed earlier in the chapter. (Using DCAP-BTLS or some other mnemonic or system may help you remember most of the important aspects of the evaluation of a body region.)

Head

When evaluating the head, inspect and palpate its entire surface looking for any deformity, asymmetry, or hemorrhage. In addition to looking for the obvious signs of trauma, direct special attention to the eyes, the auditory canal, the nose and mouth, and the facial region.

Evaluate the eyes for pupillary response. Shade the eyes in a bright environment (or shine a light into them in a dark environment) and note their response. They should dilate (or constrict) briskly, equally, and consensually (together). Check eye movement by having the patient follow your finger as you trace an "H" pattern in front of him; any deficit in the patient's ability to follow your finger suggests either cranial nerve injury or orbital fracture and muscle entrapment. The auditory canal should be clear of fluid and the tympanic membrane should be intact. The nose and mouth should be free of hemorrhage and physical obstruction. Any drainage of fluid from the mouth or nose endangers the airway and suggests skull fracture and the possible leakage of cerebrospinal fluid. Notable signs of basilar skull fracture include bilateral periorbital eccymosis (raccoon eyes) or retroauricular eccymosis (Battle's sign), though both are late signs. Gently palpate the upper jaw and feel for any crepitus or instability, indicative of a Le Fort-type fracture.

Neck

Evaluate the neck for signs of injury, for the position of the trachea, and for the status of the jugular veins. The trachea should be midline in the neck and not moving to one side or tugging with respiration. Displacement to one side suggests tension pneumothorax, although this is a very late sign and not as distinguishable as the other signs of the condition. The jugular veins should be distended in the supine, normovolemic patient and flatten as the patient's torso and head are raised to a 45-degree angle. Extremely distended jugular veins (or ones distended beyond 45 degrees) suggest tension pneumothorax, pericardial tamponade, or traumatic asphyxia. Flat jugular veins in the supine patient suggest hypovolemia. Examine the neck and head for the progressive distortion and crepitus associated with subcutaneous emphysema that may accompany tension pneumothorax. Examine for any open wounds, control any hemorrhage, and cover open wounds with occlusive dressings to prevent air embolism. Anticipate tracheal (airway) compromise that may result from swelling or hemorrhage and consider early intubation (possibly rapid sequence intubation) if serious neck trauma is present.

Chest

In addition to the standard elements of the physical assessment, examine the chest for intercostal or suprasternal retractions, air moving through any open wounds, and paradoxical chest wall motion (Figure 12-11 ■). Carefully observe the surface of the chest for erythema mirroring the structure of the rib cage. When the skin is trapped between an impacting force and the ribs, it contuses and may demonstrate this sign. Auscultate all lung fields of the chest, both anteriorly and posteriorly. Also listen for heart sounds. Apply pressure to the lateral aspect of the rib cage and direct it medially to help identify any fracture site along the ribs. The pressure flexes the ribs, moves the fracture site slightly, and creates local pain. You may feel a grating sensation (crepitus) that also suggests rib or sternal fracture. Palpation may reveal a crackling sensation associated with air under the skin (subcutaneous emphysema).

Abdomen

Observe the abdomen for any asymmetry or apparent pulsing masses. Also look for any indication of compression by the seat belt or other signs of impact. Palpate each quadrant, with one hand placing pressure on the other while you sense any unusual masses

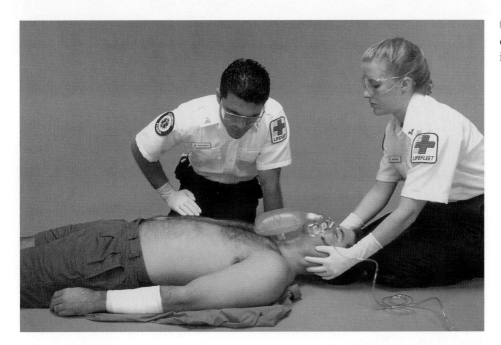

or muscle spasm (guarding). Quickly release the pressure of palpation to detect any rebound tenderness. Always palpate the quadrant with the suspected injury last. Finally, observe and palpate the flanks.

Pelvis

Evaluate the pelvis by placing firm pressure on the iliac crests directed medially and on the pubic bone directed downward. If you notice any crepitus and/or any instability of the pelvis, suspect fracture and serious internal hemorrhage. Examine the inguinal and buttock areas as these locations are often sites of serious injury and hemorrhage. It is essential that you expose these areas if the mechanism of injury suggests injury there because hemorrhage is frequently hidden in jeans or other articles of clothing.

Extremities

Examine each extremity and evaluate its muscle tone, distal pulse, temperature, color, and capillary refill time. Also evaluate for motor response, sensory response, and limb strength. Compare your findings in one limb to those of the opposing limb.

Back

Examine the patient's back during your assessment or when using movement techniques such as a log roll. If spinal injury is suspected, be sure to maintain manual immobilization of the head and neck as you position the patient for examination. Examine the total surface of the back, and palpate the spinal column from top to bottom. Look carefully for any slight deformities, minor reddening, very subtle pain, or tenderness; these may be the only sign or symptom indicative of spinal column injury.

At the conclusion of the rapid trauma assessment, the focused exam, or the detailed assessment, mentally inventory all the suspected injuries you have found. Place them in descending order of priority for care and note the contribution they make to the patient's shock state. Then make your final decision as to the patient's transport status.

TRAUMA PATIENT HISTORY

During the rapid trauma assessment or the focused exam (or, in some cases, the detailed physical exam), conduct an abbreviated patient history. The elements of the *S* component of the SAMPLE history assessment, signs and symptoms, are extensively addressed

The AMPLE elements of the SAMPLE history provide the essential components of a trauma history.

as you perform the physical assessment. Gather the remaining elements of the SAMPLE history—*A*llergies, *M*edications, *P*ast medical history, *L*ast oral intake, and *E*vents leading up to the incident—either while performing your physical examination of the patient or immediately after it.

Allergies

Question the patient about allergies, especially those to medications used commonly in emergency medicine. Such allergies include those to antibiotics, the "-caine" family, analgesics, and tetanus toxoid. If any of these are noted, pass this information on to the emergency department staff.

Medications

Investigate the patient's use of prescription and nonprescription medications as such use may impact response to care or suggest underlying medical problems or disease. For example, drugs, such as beta blockers, reduce the heart's ability to respond to hypovolemia with an increased rate. Be especially watchful for use of aspirin (interferes with clotting), anticoagulants like warfarin (Coumadin), and antibiotics.

Past Medical History

Question the patient about any significant medical history that may impact either his response to shock, your care, or the medications the emergency department is likely to use during treatment. Current medical problems may limit the body's ability to compensate for shock due to trauma and may affect the presentation of signs and symptoms. For example, a heart condition may limit the heart's ability to increase its rate in response to a reduced preload, confounding your assessment. A normally hypertensive patient may present with a normal blood pressure that, in fact, represents hypotension.

Last Oral Intake

The quantity and time since the patient's last fluid and solid oral intake should affect your index of suspicion for abdominal injury and the care a patient will receive in the emergency department. If the patient's bladder, stomach, or bowel was full and strong forces of deceleration or compression were directed to the abdomen, the risk of rupture and peritonitis is increased. Food and liquid in the stomach also pose serious risks should the patient need surgery, because the use of anesthesia may precipitate vomiting, which may result in aspiration and increase mortality and morbidity. You should also be concerned if the trauma patient has recently eaten or drunk because vomiting and aspiration may complicate your prehospital airway care.

Events Leading up to the Incident

The events immediately preceding the incident are very important. They may suggest that the patient's trauma was caused by a medical or other problem such as falling asleep while driving or becoming dizzy just before a fall. (Seeing no skid marks at a scene where an auto has collided with a tree is an important finding and suggests an intentional impact or some other contributing factor.)

VITAL SIGNS

The initial vital signs form a baseline for evaluation against which you can trend changes in the patient's condition.

Complete the rapid trauma assessment or focused exam by collecting a baseline set of vital signs. You can do this either at the scene or during transport as the patient's condition and circumstances allow. These vital signs include pulse rate and quality, blood pressure, respiration rate and quality, and skin temperature and condition. Watch for

Table 12-1	Revised Trauma Score and Glasgow Coma Scale

Revised Trauma Score		Glasgow Coma Scale Score	
Respiratory Rate		**Eye Opening**	
10 to 29 breaths per minute	4	Spontaneous	4
Greater than 29 breaths per minute	3	To voice	3
6 to 9 breaths per minute	2	To pain	2
1 to 5 breaths per minute	1	None	1
No respiration	0	**Verbal Response**	
Systolic Blood Pressure		Oriented	5
Greater than 89	4	Confused (cries, consolable)	4
76 to 89 mmHg	3	Inappropriate words (persistently irritable)	3
50 to 75 mmHg	2	Incomprehensible words (restless, agitated)	2
1 to 49 mmHg	1	None	1
No blood pressure	0	**Motor Response**	
Glasgow Coma Scale		Obeys commands	6
GCS score of 13 to 15	4	Localizes pain	5
GCS score of 9 to 12	3	Withdraws to pain	4
GCS score of 6 to 8	2	Flexes to pain	3
GCS score of 4 or 5	1	Extends to pain	2
GCS score of less than 4	0	None	1

increasing pulse rate and decreasing pulse strength, increasing respiratory rate and decreasing volume, decreasing pulse pressure, and the patient's skin becoming cool and clammy. These changes all suggest increasing compensation for blood loss and shock.

GLASGOW COMA SCALE SCORE

At the end of the initial assessment or concurrent with the rapid trauma assessment or focused assessment and history, determine your patient's Glasgow Coma Scale score. (The GCS is included in Table 12–1.) Record the best eye opening, verbal response, and motor response individually (e.g., E4, V4, M6) along with the initial vital signs. Then track any changes during subsequent ongoing assessments.

TRANSPORT DECISION

The transport decision is made in a preliminary way at the end of the initial assessment and finalized at the end of the rapid trauma assessment or the focused exam and history (Figure 12-12 ■). You will decide whether to provide rapid transport to the trauma center, treat at the scene and then transport to the nearest emergency department, or treat and release as permitted by local protocols.

Rapid Transport

The decision to provide rapid transport to the trauma center is predicated on the trauma triage criteria. If any of the specified mechanisms of injury or the physical signs of injury are present, the patient is a candidate for rapid transport. If the patient demonstrates a significant mechanism of injury but the signs and symptoms and the other results of your initial and rapid trauma assessment do not demonstrate the need

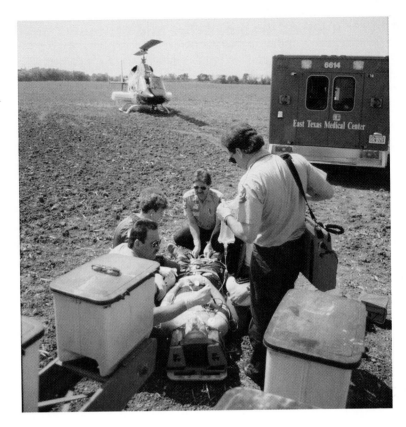

■ Figure 12-12 At the end of the rapid trauma assessment or the focused assessment, make the final decision on whether to provide stabilization on the scene or to expedite transport of the patient.

The revised trauma score combines the Glasgow Coma Scale score with the patient's respiratory rate and systolic blood pressure.

for this level of transport, contact medical direction to possibly transport to a general hospital emergency department instead.

Revised Trauma Score

The revised trauma score is a numeric evaluation of the patient using the elements of the Glasgow Coma Scale (GCS) and the patient's respiratory rate and systolic blood pressure. Some EMS systems use this, or another trauma scoring system, to predict patient outcome and help make the decision on whether the patient requires rapid transport to a trauma center (Table 12–1). Consult your system's medical director and protocols to determine if the revised trauma score is in use in your jurisdiction and to learn what numerical score mandates rapid transport.

Treat and Transport

Provide on-scene care and then transport to the nearest emergency department for any patient who has neither a significant mechanism of injury nor physical signs of serious trauma. Manage the patient's specific injuries on the scene, and transport once your care has stabilized the injuries and the patient is packaged so movement to the ambulance and hospital will not cause further harm. If at any time during your care the patient demonstrates any signs of more serious injury or shock compensation, consider rapid transport to the trauma center.

Treat and Release

Treat and release only those patients with very minor and isolated injuries and do so only if your system's protocols permit it.

Some EMS systems permit care providers to treat patients with minor injuries and then release them to see their personal physician. Provide this service only to the patient with very minor and isolated injuries. Assure that you carefully explain to the patient what care is needed for the injury. Describe the signs that may develop indicating that the injury requires immediate attention and advise the patient that he should call your service again if those signs appear. Finally, tell the patient that he should seek care from a family physician. If possible, provide this information in written form, approved by your system of medical direction, and have the patient acknowledge in writing the receipt of these instructions. If you have any questions about treatment or release of a patient, contact your medical direction physician.

Patient Care Refusals

Some patients suffering trauma will refuse assessment, care, and transport. While this is the patient's right, the situation represents a dilemma for prehospital care providers. The patient may not understand the significance of his injuries, and the early signs of trauma may not clearly reflect its nature or seriousness.

When confronted with a patient refusing care, advise the patient that serious injury may not present with overt or painful symptoms. Try to convince him to permit you to perform an assessment and provide on-scene care. If you are not successful, attempt to have the patient talk with the medical direction physician. Be sure the patient is an adult and is fully conscious, oriented, and able to make a rational decision. Try to use family members to help you encourage the patient to accept your assessment and care. If your attempts to convince the patient fail, suggest that he see a personal physician at the earliest opportunity. Stress that the patient should feel free to call for emergency medical service if additional signs or symptoms develop or existing ones worsen. Be sure to document the refusal thoroughly. Include your recommendation that the patient receive assessment, care, and transport; your warning of the dangers of refusing assessment, care, and transport; your suggestion that the patient see a family physician; and your recommendation to contact emergency medical services again if the problem persists or worsens.

ONGOING ASSESSMENT

The ongoing assessment is important to monitoring and guiding the care you provide. It should be performed every 5 minutes with critically or seriously injured patients and every 15 minutes with other patients. Also perform an ongoing assessment whenever you note any change in the patient's condition or you institute any significant intervention.

During the ongoing assessment, perform the mental, airway, breathing, and circulation status checks of the initial assessment and recheck any significant findings of the rapid trauma assessment or focused exam. Reassess the vital signs—blood pressure; rate, regularity, and strength of the pulse; respiratory rate, volume, and regularity; skin condition; and Glasgow Coma Scale score. With any limb injury, recheck the distal pulse, capillary refill, muscle strength, and sensation. Pay particular attention to an increasing pulse rate, decreasing pulse strength (pulse pressure), increasing respiratory rate, decreasing respiratory volume, increasing capillary refill time, decreasing level of consciousness or orientation, change in skin color or temperature, or increasing anxiety or restlessness. Any of these signs may indicate patient deterioration. Compare results of each ongoing assessment to baseline findings and those from previous ongoing assessments to identify any deterioration or improvement in the patient's condition. Record the results serially so that trending of the patient's signs can continue after arrival at the emergency department.

SHOCK TRAUMA RESUSCITATION

HYPOVOLEMIA/HYPOTENSION/HYPOPERFUSION

Three very important terms are used to describe the status of the cardiovascular system in trauma. They are hypovolemia, hypotension, and hypoperfusion. **Hypovolemia** refers to a reduced volume in the cardiovascular system, caused by hemorrhage, by an excess of fluid loss against inadequate fluid intake, or by losses into third spaces, as with plasma into burns. A relative hypovolemia may occur as the vascular system expands (with spinal injury) and the normal vascular volume is inadequate to fill it.

Review

Steps to Follow If a Patient Refuses Treatment

Suggest strongly that the patient should receive assessment, care, and transport

Warn the patient of the dangers of refusing assessment, care, and transport

Suggest that the patient see a family physician

Encourage the patient to contact EMS again if the problem persists or worsens

Review

Signs of Deterioration During Ongoing Assessment

Increasing pulse rate
Decreasing pulse strength
Narrowing pulse pressure
Increasing respiratory rate
Decreasing respiratory volume
Increasing capillary refill time
Decreasing level of consciousness or orientation
Changes in skin color or temperature
Increasing anxiety or restlessness

hypovolemia *reduced volume in the cardiovascular system.*

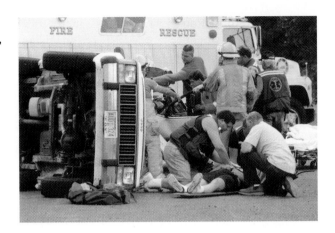

■ Figure 12-13 With a seriously injured trauma patient, employ the aggressive care steps of shock trauma resuscitation. (© *Craig Jackson/In the Dark Photography*)

hypotension *lower than normal blood pressure.*

hypoperfusion *inadequate perfusion of body tissues resulting in inadequate supplies of oxygen and nutrients to body tissue; also called shock.*

 Review

Basic Steps of Shock Trauma Resuscitation

Providing airway protection with endotracheal intubation or rapid sequence intubation

Assuring adequate oxygenation and ventilations

Providing rapid fluid resuscitation with isotonic solution

Performing pleural decompression

Hypotension simply refers to a reduction in blood pressure caused by cardiac, vascular, neurogenic, or volume problems to a level that is lower than normal for the patient. **Hypoperfusion** is a low or inadequate distribution of blood to the body organs and tissues due to cardiac, vascular, neurogenic, or volume problems.

Shock trauma resuscitation is care to rapidly support the seriously injured trauma patient while he is rushed to the trauma center (Figure 12-13 ■). These include:

★ Providing airway protection with endotracheal intubation or rapid sequence intubation

★ Assuring adequate oxygenation and ventilations

★ Providing appropriate fluid resuscitation with isotonic solution

★ Performing pleural decompression

Whenever serious trauma is expected or the signs of shock compensation are evident, consider introducing an endotracheal tube using the digital or oral methods of insertion. Anticipate that the seriously injured patient will deteriorate and be prepared to intubate quickly. Consider using rapid sequence intubation in the extremely agitated or combative patient when shock is evident and the patient demonstrates a steady deterioration.

Apply high-flow, high-concentration oxygen immediately. Consider ventilating the patient (overdrive ventilation with bag-valve mask) if the respirations move less than 600 mL of air or respirations occur less than 12 or more than 30 times per minute.

Initiate two large-bore intravenous sites in large veins and connect at least one nonrestrictive (either trauma or blood tubing) administration set and two 1,000-mL bags of either normal saline or lactated Ringer's solution. If shock is present or expected, choose large veins for cannulation (the anticubital veins). Otherwise, veins in the forearm or hand may suffice. Run the fluid at a to-keep-open rate as long as the patient maintains his blood pressure (pulse pressure) and pulse rate. Be ready to rapidly infuse fluids quickly should the patient begin to show increasing signs and symptoms of serious compensation and shock. Generally, the maximum prehospital fluid volume is 3,000 mL of isotonic solution administered in boluses of 250 to 500 mL. You may adjust this volume based on the size of the patient and the patient's response to infusion. Titrate your infusion rate to assure a systolic blood pressure of 80 mmHg (or 90 mmHg for the suspected head injury patient). Auscultate the lung fields for signs of edema and halt or reduce the rate of fluid administration with the development of any crackles.

Be sure to rule out tension pneumothorax during your assessment. If you cannot, and the patient displays significant dyspnea, decompress the affected side of the chest with a large-bore catheter inserted in the second or third intercostal space, midclavicular line. These steps of shock care are essential to maintain the patient until further, possibly invasive procedures occur at the hospital.

There are several general considerations to keep in mind in shock trauma resuscitation situations. These include preventing hypothermia, providing rapid body splinting, providing rapid transport, and reducing the effects of the fight-or-flight response.

HYPOTHERMIA

Hypothermia is a relatively unappreciated complication of serious trauma and shock. Trauma often initiates the fight-or-flight response, which causes the body to direct its energy away from the internal organs and to the skeletal muscles. When the patient stops his flight (as during your care), the body's energy and heat production decrease dramatically. The problem is further compounded as the body directs its remaining blood volume to critical organs and not to temperature regulation activities. The result is a patient who is very susceptible to hypothermia (Figure 12-14). Caregivers contribute to this problem when they provide rapid fluid resuscitation with fluids that are often at ambient, rather than body, temperature. The result is a rapid infusion of hypothermic fluid and a further lowering of the body's core temperature. In addition, care providers frequently disrobe patients during assessment and fail to recover them adequately with warm blankets. In a normal or cool environment, this behavior only compounds any hypothermia.

Hypothermia can have several negative effects on a patient suffering from injury and shock. The body's natural response to heat loss is increased skeletal muscle activity, specifically shivering. This heat generation consumes the body's energy reserves and increases the impact of injury and shock. A decrease in body temperature also affects blood clotting by inhibiting the clotting cascade and prolonging clotting times. The colder temperature also causes the platelets to release a heparin-like anticoagulant agent that further slows the clotting process.

Hypothermia is a relatively unappreciated complication of serious trauma and shock.

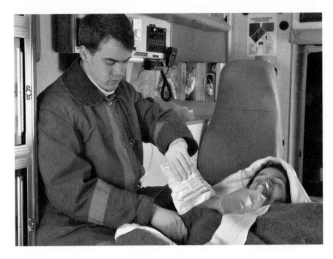

■ Figure 12-14 Hypothermia poses a serious threat to trauma patients. Assure that your care helps the patient maintain his body temperature.

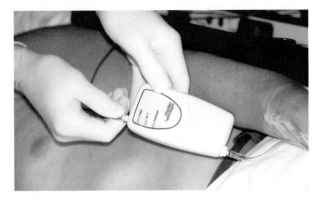

■ Figure 12-15 Use intravenous fluid warmers as necessary.

It is essential to recognize the negative impact a lowering of body temperature has on the patient during shock. Always try to administer fluids that are as close to body temperature as possible, especially in colder environments. Use fluid warmers as necessary (Figure 12-15 ■). Also use more blankets to cover an injured patient than you would use with an uninjured patient in the same environmental conditions.

BODY SPLINTING

The seriously injured trauma patient is likely to have suffered internal injury, life-threatening hemorrhage, and long-bone and possible spinal fractures. To assure rapid transport to the trauma center while not compounding the patient's injuries, splinting must be effective yet must be done quickly. For the seriously injured trauma patient, you can best accomplish this splinting by gently aligning all the limbs and firmly securing the entire patient to a long spine board (Figure 12-16 ■). Movement onto the long board should occur in one coordinated move from the patient's initial location. Body splinting assures that if there is any movement of the limbs while packaging, loading, or transporting the patient, the movement will be limited, thus reducing the chances of aggravating existing injuries.

■ Figure 12-16 Seriously injured patients who require rapid transport may be immobilized to a long spine board for effective splinting of limb fractures. (© *Craig Jackson/In the Dark Photography*)

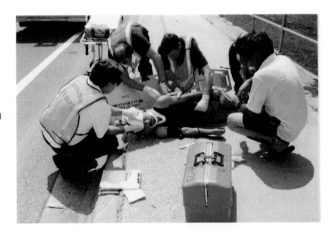

RAPID TRANSPORT

Research has clearly demonstrated that the best way to reduce trauma mortality is to bring the seriously injured patient to surgery as quickly as possible. This presumes that the greatest risk to life is from internal hemorrhage and the only definitive remedy for that risk is surgical repair. Care providers can help meet this objective by providing rapid on-scene assessment, extrication, patient packaging, and transport while maintaining the patient through spinal, airway, ventilatory, and circulatory support. Make every effort to reduce the time at the emergency scene, and limit your actions there so that on-scene time is no more than 10 minutes. Perform procedures such as IV insertion and PASG application while applying spinal immobilization, assuring and supporting the airway and breathing, or controlling hemorrhage or while preparing to move the patient. Otherwise, carry out these procedures in the ambulance during transport. Using air medical service whenever it will substantially reduce transport time is another way of speeding the patient to definitive care.

FIGHT-OR-FLIGHT RESPONSE

When a person is under extreme stress or in fear of bodily harm, the autonomic nervous system responds with the release of adrenaline and an increase in several body functions. These actions induce an increase in heart rate, stroke volume, blood pressure, respiratory rate and volume, and a release of glucose and insulin into the bloodstream. The result is a rapid expenditure of body resources that might be otherwise used for repair and recovery. To reduce the effect of the fight-or-flight response and to make the patient more comfortable with the emergency medical care, try to be calming and reassuring. Clearly tell the patient who you are and that you are there to help. Listen carefully to what the patient says, and describe what will happen during care and why. Let the patient see that you are confident in the care you are about to provide and that your sincere desire is to attend to his injuries. Maintain continuous communication with the patient and try to distract him from concerns over the injuries and the impact they may have on the patient's life. Doing these things will help reduce patient anxiety and the effects of the fight-or-flight response.

NONCRITICAL PATIENTS

Patients needing the services of a trauma center represent only about 10 percent of all trauma patients. While we "overtriage" around twice this number to assure we do not miss individuals with subtle or concealed injuries, noncritical patients account for about 80 percent of trauma responses and receive the largest part of prehospital trauma care. These are patients who do not demonstrate the mechanisms of injury or signs and symptoms detailed in the trauma triage criteria and who receive the focused exam and history.

Noncritical trauma patients receive care directed at their specific injuries. These patients normally require dressing, bandaging, and immobilization of the wound or skeletal injury site and comfortable (and slow) transport to the emergency department of their choice (within reason). With these patients, be careful to monitor distal sensation, motor function, pulses, temperature, and capillary refill to assure there is no neurologic or vascular compromise from the injury or from the bandaging or splinting provided. Should you detect any deficit or any signs or symptoms of developing hypovolemia or shock, increase the patient's priority for transport and consider rerouting to the trauma center.

SPECIAL PATIENTS

Two categories of trauma patients who require special attention are the very young and the old. The pediatric patient is small, growing, and somewhat different anatomically

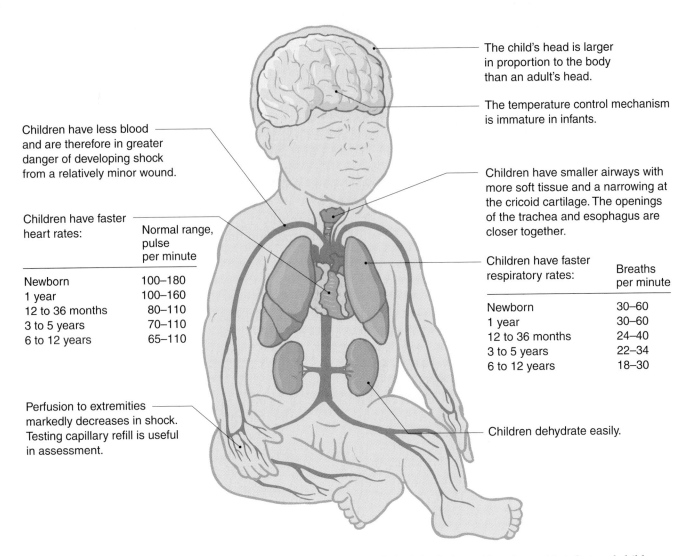

The child's head is larger in proportion to the body than an adult's head.

The temperature control mechanism is immature in infants.

Children have less blood and are therefore in greater danger of developing shock from a relatively minor wound.

Children have smaller airways with more soft tissue and a narrowing at the cricoid cartilage. The openings of the trachea and esophagus are closer together.

Children have faster heart rates:

	Normal range, pulse per minute
Newborn	100–180
1 year	100–160
12 to 36 months	80–110
3 to 5 years	70–110
6 to 12 years	65–110

Children have faster respiratory rates:

	Breaths per minute
Newborn	30–60
1 year	30–60
12 to 36 months	24–40
3 to 5 years	22–34
6 to 12 years	18–30

Perfusion to extremities markedly decreases in shock. Testing capillary refill is useful in assessment.

Children dehydrate easily.

■ Figure 12-17 Anatomical and physiological considerations with infant and child patients.

from the adult. The geriatric patient often has preexisting medical problems and body systems that are not as responsive to the effects of trauma as those of their younger adult counterparts. These patients respond differently to trauma than average adult patients and must be assessed, prioritized, and cared for accordingly.

Pediatric Patients

Pediatric patients are, in many ways, just small adults. They have the same basic anatomy and, for the most part, the same physiology. Because of their smaller size and the dynamics of their growth, however, the effects of trauma on pediatric patients are different from the effects on adults (Figure 12-17 ■). Further, damage to the child's rapidly growing body may have significant, long-lasting effects.

Trauma is the greatest cause of death and disability among pediatric patients after the first year of life. The pediatric patient is most likely to suffer blunt trauma. The most commonly experienced forms of blunt trauma in pediatric patients are auto impacts (including vehicle crashes and pedestrian-vs.-auto and bicycle-vs.-auto collisions), falls, and abuse (in that order). Penetrating trauma (gunshot and knife wounds) is also on the rise in the pediatric population over age 14. Contributing factors to the mortality and morbidity of pediatric trauma are the child's limited life experience and undeveloped recognition of and respect for trauma hazards and their consequences.

The effects of trauma on the pediatric patient are different from those on the adult.

Trauma is the greatest cause of death and disability in the pediatric patient over 1 year of age.

The smaller size and weight of infants and children mean they have a larger ratio of body surface area to volume than adults do. This means that infants and children lose or gain heat from the environment much more quickly than adults. Extensive body surface injuries (like abrasions and burns) become more devastating because of the proportionally greater fluid loss to the injury and the environment. Because of their smaller size, the organs of pediatric patients are closer together, and multisystem trauma is thus more frequent. In pediatric pedestrian-vs.-auto impacts, the energy causing injury is delivered higher on the anatomy. Initial impact is likely to affect the pelvis, abdomen, and chest resulting in greater internal injuries and a smaller incidence of extremity trauma. The impact is also more likely to propel the child ahead of the car where he may be struck again by it or run over.

Some aspects of pediatric anatomy differ significantly from those of adults. The limbs are proportionally shorter than those of the mature adult and less able and effective in protecting children from trunk trauma. Infants and young children have less subcutaneous fat and less-developed muscle masses to protect the internal organs. The heads of infants and children are proportionally larger than those of adults, which results in a greater incidence of blunt head trauma and the application of proportionally greater forces to the neck during acceleration or deceleration. The increased head size also means that when infants or young children are supine the neck is flexed, which may contribute to airway obstruction. The tongues of infants and children fill more of the oral cavity and are more likely to obstruct the airway than in adults. The infant anatomy also means they must breathe through the nose (obligate nasal breathers), thus providing only one airway with no detour around its obstruction. The trachea in infants and children is shorter, more delicate, and more prone to intubation of the right mainstem bronchus and soft-tissue trauma. The mediastinum is more mobile in pediatric patients, which permits greater displacement during tension pneumothorax, resulting in an earlier development of the pathology and a greater restriction of venous return to the heart than in adults.

The pediatric skeletal system grows rapidly. It begins as cartilage and becomes more rigid and stronger with age. This development permits great flexibility and protects the skeleton from fracture. However, the energy of trauma is more easily transmitted through the rib cage, spine, and skull to injure the vital structures beneath. The soft and partial nature of the skull also permits a greater displacement of its contents with hemorrhage or edema and will present with bulging fontanelles with increased intracranial pressure in the child under 18 months of age. This ability of the cranium to expand may also permit intracranial hemorrhage to substantially contribute to hypovolemia, though it, as the sole cause of shock, is very infrequent. The skeleton's flexibility also lessens the incidence, severity, and signs of soft-tissue injury. When injured, the long bones of the skeleton frequently resist fracture until just one side of the bone gives way. The resulting fracture, called a greenstick fracture, provides a relatively stable, though somewhat deformed, limb. However, this type of fracture promotes increased growth on the injured side, causing further angulation of the limb. For this reason, a surgeon often completes a greenstick fracture later in the process of care. Long-bone injury is also likely to occur at the site of bone growth, the epiphyseal plate. This type of injury may damage the growth potential of the limb and create a lifelong disability.

The components of the cardiovascular systems of infants and children are much more vibrant than those in adults. They are very able to compensate for blood loss secondary to trauma and do not show overt signs of compensation as quickly. In fact, a pediatric patient may lose up to 25 percent of his blood volume before any signs appear and may lose 50 percent of his blood volume before compensation fails. However, once the pediatric patient can no longer compensate for blood loss, he moves very quickly toward irreversible shock. The heart of a pediatric patient cannot increase its stroke volume as the heart of an adult does. In hypovolemia and shock, this results in an earlier and more pronounced tachycardia because an increase in heart rate is the only way to significantly increase cardiac output. Additionally, the respiratory system in a pediatric

The pediatric patient may lose up to 25 percent of blood volume before signs of shock appear.

Table 12–2	Normal Vital Signs				
	Pulse (beats per minute)	Respiration (breaths per minute)	Blood Pressure (average mmHg)	Temperature	
Infancy:					
At birth:	100–180	30–60	60–90 systolic	98°–100° F	36.7°–37.8° C
At 1 year:	100–160	30–60	87–105 systolic	98°–100° F	36.7°–37.8° C
Toddler (12 to 36 months)	80–110	24–40	95–105 systolic	96.8°–99.6° F	36.3°–37.9° C
Preschool age (3 to 5 years)	70–110	22–34	95–110 systolic	96.8°–99.6° F	36.3°–37.9° C
School-age (6 to 12 years)	65–110	18–30	97–112 systolic	98.6° F	37° C
Adolescence (13 to 18 years)	60–90	12–26	112–128 systolic	98.6° F	37° C
Early adulthood (19 to 40 years)	60–100	12–20	120/80	98.6° F	37° C
Middle adulthood (41 to 60 years)	60–100	12–20	120/80	98.6° F	37° C
Late adulthood (61 years and older)	+	+	+	98.6° F	37° C

+ Depends on the individual's physical health status.

patient has less of a respiratory reserve, is less able to tolerate stress, and will tire more quickly than an adult's respiratory system.

Pediatric vital signs are very different from those of adults and change quickly during the developmental years (Table 12–2). As infants grow into toddlers, preschoolers, school-age children, and adolescents, their vital signs change, until, in the late teens, their ranges are very similar to those of adults. During these years, blood pressure levels rise and heart and respiratory rates fall. These changing vital signs make accurate assessment of pediatric patients more difficult because you must accurately determine the child's age and vital signs and then compare them to the normal rates for that age. It is helpful to keep a pediatric vital sign table handy when responding to a pediatric trauma emergency.

Psychologically and socially, pediatric patients respond very differently both to injury and to care providers than do adults (Figure 12-18 ■). The responses also change dramatically with the child's growth and development. Please refer to Volume 5, Chapter 7, "Pediatric Emergencies," for a fuller discussion of pediatric growth and development.

As with adults, calculation of a trauma score can help to predict patient outcome and form transport decisions. However, the criteria for pediatric patients are different from the criteria for adults, as shown in Table 12–3.

Pediatric Care Shock trauma resuscitation for pediatric patients follows the same basic processes of assessment and care used with adults, but makes allowances for differences in pediatric anatomy and physiology. Maintain the airway in a neutral position with padding under the shoulders for an infant and limited or no padding under the shoulders or head of a child (depending on the child's anatomic size). To secure the airway, use an appropriately sized oral airway or intubate. Insert the oral airway using a tongue blade, as the normal insertion technique with a 180-degree turn

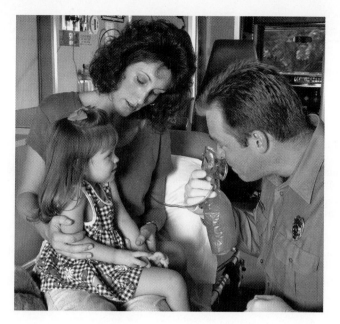

used in adults may injure the delicate soft tissue of the infant or very young child's oral pharynx. Be sure to keep the nasal passage clear in pediatric patients under 6 months of age as they are obligate nasal breathers. If intubation is considered, use an uncuffed endotracheal tube (for patients under 6 years old) that approximates the size of the patient's little finger. Insert the tube gently and pass it only a couple of centimeters beyond the glottis because the pediatric patient is prone to soft-tissue injury and (because of the short trachea) to right mainstem bronchus intubation. Secure the endotracheal tube firmly and carefully monitor the tube's location and the breath sounds because the uncuffed tube may easily be dislodged from the very short trachea.

Initiate intravenous access as with an adult, and be certain to use catheters sized to the patient's veins because you will infuse reduced volumes of fluid. If you cannot obtain normal venous access, consider using the intraosseous site (through the tibia) in patients under 6 years old for administration of both medications and fluid (Figure 12-19 ■). Fluid boluses for volume replacement are usually given as 20 mL/kg boluses. Administer this volume sooner in the pediatric patient than you would in the adult because infants and children can compensate more effectively for fluid loss. (Hence, proportionally more fluid has been lost before you notice it.) This initial bolus may be repeated up to two times for a total of 60 mL/kg.

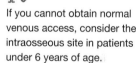

If you cannot obtain normal venous access, consider the intraosseous site in patients under 6 years of age.

Consider less significant mechanisms of injury and more minimal signs of injury than you would with adults as grounds for transporting pediatric patients to the trauma center. Pediatric patients have less protection for internal body organs and are more likely to show fewer signs and symptoms of injury. They have a greater incidence of serious and multisystem trauma than adults. If possible, consider transport to a facility able to accommodate the special needs of pediatric trauma patients, the pediatric trauma center.

Geriatric Patients

The geriatric population is one of the fastest growing demographics in the country. Healthier lifestyles and the advances of modern medicine are extending life and increasing the size of the population older than 65 (Figure 12-20 ■). As this population grows over the next few decades, it will account for more and more trauma emergency responses. Currently trauma accounts for 25 percent of all geriatric mortality and, with the expected growth of this population, will become an even greater proportion of EMS responses.

Table 12–3 | Pediatric Trauma Score and Glasgow Coma Scale Score

Pediatric Trauma Score

Score	+2	+1	−1
Weight	>44 lb (>20 kg)	22–44 lb (10–20 kg)	<22 lb (<10 kg)
Airway	Normal	Oral or nasal airway	Intubated, tracheostomy, invasive airway
Blood pressure	Pulse at wrist > 90 mmHg	Carotid or femoral pulse palpable 50–90 mmHg	No palpable pulse or <50 mmHg
Level of consciousness	Completely awake	Obtunded or any loss of consciousness	Comatose
Open wound	None	Minor	Major or penetrating
Fractures	None	Closed fracture	Open or multiple fractures

Pediatric Glasgow Coma Scale

		> 1 Year	< 1 Year	
Eye opening	4	Spontaneous	Spontaneous	
	3	To verbal command	To shout	
	2	To pain	To pain	
	1	No response	No response	

		> 1 Year	< 1 Year	
Best motor response	6	Obeys		
	5	Localizes pain	Localizes pain	
	4	Flexion-withdrawal	Flexion-withdrawal	
	3	Flexion-abnormal (decorticate rigidity)	Flexion-abnormal (decorticate rigidity)	
	2	Extension (decerebrate rigidity)	Extension (decerebrate rigidity)	
	1	No response	No response	

		>5 Years	2–5 Years	0–23 Months
Best verbal response	5	Oriented and converses	Appropriate words and phrases	Smiles, coos, cries appropriately
	4	Disoriented and converses	Inappropriate words	Cries
	3	Inappropriate words	Cries and/or screams	Inappropriate crying and/or screaming
	2	Incomprehensible sounds	Grunts	Grunts
	1	No response	No response	No response

The geriatric trauma patient often has coexisting problems associated with aging and possible chronic disease. Aging affects virtually every body system (Figure 12-21 ■). Reduced reflexes, hearing, and eyesight result in more injuries in this population, while brittle bones produce fractures with less force. This is especially true of the cervical spine, where the vertebral column becomes more fragile and calcification narrows the spinal foramen, predisposing the geriatric patient to spinal injury. The brain loses mass after middle age and this results in a greater incidence of injury because the brain is freer to move about within and impact the interior of the cranium. Smaller cardiac reserves

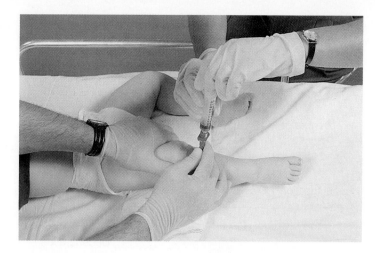

■ Figure 12-19 Consider intraosseous placement in the tibia when administering fluids and medications in children under age 6 if you cannot obtain normal intravenous access.

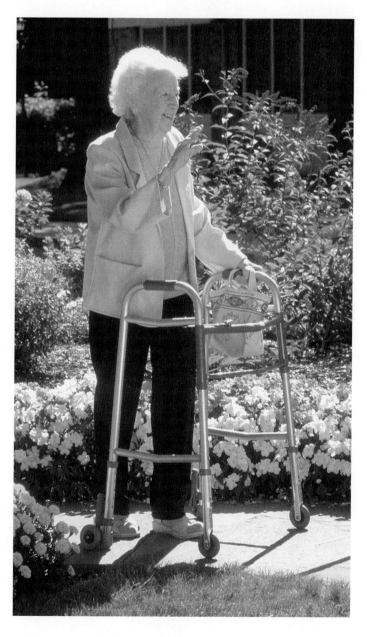

■ Figure 12-20 Geriatric patients represent one of the fastest growing groups requiring emergency medical services.

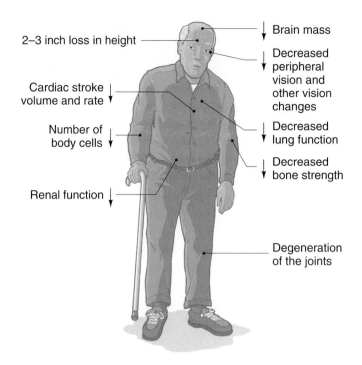

■ Figure 12-21 Age-related changes in geriatric patients.

2–3 inch loss in height

Cardiac stroke volume and rate ↓

Number of body cells ↓

Renal function ↓

Brain mass ↓

Decreased peripheral vision and other vision changes

Decreased lung function

Decreased bone strength

Degeneration of the joints

leave older patients less able to respond to hypovolemia with increases in heart rate or cardiac stroke volume. Reduced fluid reserves limit the amount of fluid the cardiovascular system can draw from body tissues to compensate for fluid lost through burns or hemorrhage. The system also cannot accommodate great fluctuations in fluid volume and is more prone to problems of overhydration with resulting pulmonary edema. The vascular system, especially the venous system, is less able to constrict in response to hypovolemia and restore cardiac preload. In addition, reduced respiratory reserves reduce the ability of older patients to accommodate the problems of diaphragmatic respiration associated with spinal injury, of pneumothorax or tension pneumothorax, and of even the reduction in respiratory movement associated with the pain of rib fractures. A higher pain tolerance and reduced pain perception may also mask the symptoms of serious injury, and poorer temperature regulation may predispose the geriatric patient to hypothermia.

Preexisting diseases are more prevalent in the geriatric population and reduce these patients' abilities to handle the physiological stress of trauma. Cardiovascular disease limits the heart's ability to assist with shock compensation. Chronic respiratory diseases (such as emphysema) increase the cardiac workload and reduce respiratory efficiency and reserves. Many other chronic diseases likewise affect geriatric patients by reducing their ability to compensate for hypovolemia and respond to the stresses of shock. Because of aging and chronic disease, geriatric patients are likely to move more quickly into compensation, then more quickly to uncompensated shock, and then to irreversible shock. They are less able to tolerate the shock state and experience a mortality rate from hypovolemia that is much greater than that of average adults.

Assessment of the geriatric patient is often difficult because the problem that led to the call to EMS is often masked or confused by signs and symptoms of preexisting disease or by a diminished response to pain. However, accurate assessment of these patients is critical because they are less able to tolerate hypovolemia and the stress of shock.

Geriatric Care Initiate shock care early with geriatric patients. Provide that care conservatively, however, to avoid the possibility of fluid overload. Intravenous catheters should be smaller than for normal adults as the catheters must be inserted through

The problem that leads a geriatric patient to call EMS is often masked or confused by signs and symptoms of preexisting disease or by a diminished response to pain.

rather thin yet tough skin and then through veins that tend to be smaller and more delicate than normal adult veins and that also roll more. During any infusion, auscultate the chest frequently for breath sounds and halt fluid flow at the first signs of crackles. Keep the patient warm and watch carefully for any progression of the signs of shock. The use of an ECG is indicated because hypovolemia and shock may initiate dysrhythmias in patients with preexisting cardiac disease. Administer oxygen early to geriatric patients to increase the effectiveness of respirations. Artificial ventilation may be met with greater resistance due to lung stiffness, but excessive ventilation pressures are more likely to lead to pneumothorax. Carefully adjust the bag-valve-mask volume to obtain gentle chest rise. Remember that the elderly are prone to hypothermia, so assure they are well covered in a cool or cold environment.

INTERACTION WITH OTHER CARE PROVIDERS

Emergency medical services often have a tiered structure consisting of progressive levels of care providers attending to the needs of patients. These care providers include the trained or untrained bystanders, certified First Responders, EMT-Basics, EMT-Intermediates, and other EMT-Paramedics. Other members of the system include air medical personnel and the physicians, nurses, and technical personnel in the hospital emergency department, intensive care unit, or surgery. Appropriate interactions among all these members of the EMS system are essential to assure a good continuum of care for the patient. Your interactions with these members also determine how you will be perceived as a care provider and as a professional within the health care system. The information exchanged during these interactions is essential to an effective EMS system and, most importantly, to appropriate patient care (Figure 12-22 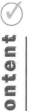).

The initial information you receive from first responders and EMTs about the patient's condition and care as you assume assessment and care responsibilities is vital. This information is essential for developing your initial impression of the patient, and then formulating a management plan for that patient. This information, supplemented by your assessment findings, is equally essential to the emergency department physician or nurse as he assumes responsibility for patient care from you. This information should include a description of the mechanism of injury, the results of your assessment, the interventions performed, and the results of those interventions.

MECHANISM OF INJURY

Concisely describe the mechanism of injury with enough detail to identify the nature and severity of the energy exchange. An example might be "a high-speed frontal impact

✓ Review

Content

Key Elements for the Patient Care Report

Mechanism of injury
Results of assessment
Interventions
Results of interventions

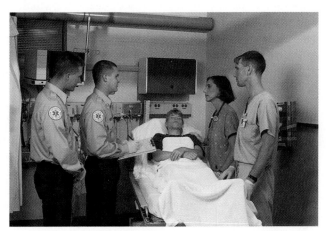

■ Figure 12-22   It is essential that information exchange among care providers be rapid, thorough, and accurate.

with severe vehicle deformity and passenger compartment intrusion of about 10 inches" or "a head-on collision while two football players were running full speed." Also indicate what the patient was doing when the incident occurred—for example, "was the driver." Give the approximate time of the incident (or time since the incident), if known.

RESULTS OF ASSESSMENT

Communicate the results of your assessment, describing the injuries and relating any abnormal or unusual history, vital signs, and other assessment findings to the emergency department staff. Describe any wounds covered by bandages or splints in significant detail so those items need not be removed for immediate assessment. Include in your statement all pertinent patient information such as the patient's age, sex, and weight. Also include any allergies, significant medications, significant medical history, last oral intake, and up-to-date vaccinations such as the last tetanus booster. Finally, identify the last set of vital signs, the Glasgow Coma Scale score, and any trends in patient condition noted from your serial ongoing assessments.

INTERVENTIONS

Identify the care provided by others, then by you, and the results of that care on the patient's condition. Include the size of IV catheters and location of placement; the rate, volume, and type of fluid administered; the dosages, routes, and times of medications administered; and the size and depth of insertion of the endotracheal tube if used.

You should get this information from care providers as you accept responsibility for patient care. If necessary, question the care provider to obtain this information. This information exchange should take only a few moments, and rarely more than a minute. Use this same format and communicate this information to the receiving physician or nurse when you present your patient to the emergency department. If you receive a patient care report from a previous care provider in another format, convert it to this order of information. As you continue to assess and provide care, you will quickly identify whether the information obtained from previous care providers is valid or the patient needs reassessment of both his condition and the care offered up to that point.

It is essential that the information exchange between care providers is rapid and complete or care will suffer. If a care provider does not use a standard, organized format to communicate information, organizing and using the information quickly and efficiently will be difficult. If this happens, talk with the care provider about it after the call and suggest a format to help future exchanges. Be careful to compliment the provider on skills that were performed well and suggest ways that "the both of us" could improve the information exchange and patient care. Also appreciate the role of the emergency department physician as he applies this process to your report and patient care.

As you receive your patient report and begin to assume patient care responsibilities, utilize available basic and advanced life support providers to assist in your patient care. Have them perform manual cervical immobilization, use the bag-valve mask on the patient, and take vital signs. You can also use these personnel to bring equipment from the ambulance and help with patient movement procedures. This leaves you freer to oversee care, provide advanced interventions, and communicate with medical direction. It also makes the other providers feel a part of the response and the overall system. Again, compliment the providers on what they do well and offer constructive and supportive comments on ways to improve their performance. It is rare that you can accomplish all aspects of patient care alone. Having assistance from other providers who feel comfortable working with you improves the coordination and quality of the care at the scene.

BODY SUBSTANCE ISOLATION AT THE TRAUMA SCENE

Many of the materials associated with the emergency response are contaminated with possibly infectious body fluids and substances. These include soiled linens, patient clothing, dressings, and used care equipment, including intravenous needles. It is important that you collect these materials at the scene and dispose of them appropriately to assure your safety as well as the safety of your patients, their families, bystanders, and fellow caregivers. This also protects those who happen on the scene after you leave. Properly dispose of any contaminated materials according to the recommendations outlined below.

For your personal safety, and that of your team, patients, and bystanders, you must dispose of all sharps in a puncture-proof container and all contaminated material in biohazard bags.

★ Handle contaminated materials only while wearing the appropriate personal protective equipment.

★ Place all blood or body fluid contaminated clothing, linens, dressings, and patient care equipment and supplies in a properly marked biological hazard bag and assure it is disposed of properly.

★ Assure that all used needles, scalpels, and other contaminated objects that have the potential to puncture the skin are properly secured in a puncture-resistant and clearly marked sharps container.

★ Do not recap a needle after use, do not stick it into a seat cushion or other object, and do not leave it lying on the ground. These actions increase the risks of an accidental needle stick.

★ Always scan the scene before leaving it to assure that all equipment has been retrieved and all potentially infectious material has been bagged and removed.

★ Contact your service infection control officer if:

  –you are exposed to an infectious disease

  –you have contact with body substances and a route for system entry (such as an open wound on your hand when a glove tears while moving a soiled patient)

  –you receive a needle stick with a contaminated needle.

Following these recommendations will help protect you and the people you care for from the dangers of disease transmission.

AIR MEDICAL TRANSPORT

In recent years, the helicopter has become widely available to EMS systems throughout the country. Helicopters transport patients rapidly (at about 140 mph), bypassing traffic and flying directly to the nearest trauma center (Figure 12-23 ■). Recent studies have demonstrated that medical helicopters may not improve trauma outcomes to the degree once thought. However, since trauma care is often a race against time, air medical service can provide a welcome, lifesaving addition to the prehospital care system. To better interact with this EMS and trauma resource, consider the indications for its use, the criteria for establishing a landing zone, the elements of flight physiology, and how to prepare a patient for air medical transport.

INDICATIONS FOR AIR MEDICAL TRANSPORT

Your system will have its own protocols and procedures for air medical transport, but the following are common considerations. Consider summoning a helicopter when its

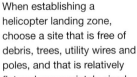

■ Figure 12-23 In recent years, use of helicopters has become widely available to EMS systems throughout the country. (© Mark C. Ide)

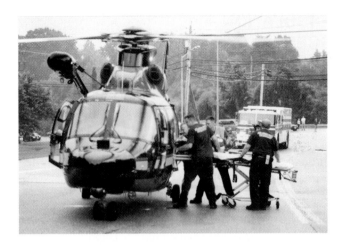

use will significantly reduce transport time for severely injured trauma patients. In making this decision, consider the normal activation and warm-up time for the helicopter (3 to 5 minutes) and the flight time to the scene (about 1 minute for each 2 miles). It is counterproductive to wait 15 minutes at the scene for a helicopter when it will reduce transport time by 10 minutes. However, if the helicopter arrives during a prolonged extrication or during rush hour, the time saved may be very worthwhile. As a general rule, if transport by ground will exceed 30 minutes, request the helicopter. Also consider an intercept en route to the hospital if it will help reduce the patient transport time. Air medical response times can be reduced if flight crews are put on stand-by for serious trauma calls. This permits the crew to get ready and the pilot to warm up the helicopter. If the seriousness of the call is confirmed by police or first responders, you may ask to have the helicopter begin its response. If you arrive at the scene and find that the mechanism of injury and the apparent injuries are less serious than expected, you can then cancel the flight.

While helicopter transport is a very valuable medium for trauma care, it is very expensive and not always available. The service area of a helicopter is rather large and the number of helicopters is usually limited due to their high operational costs. If the helicopter is on a flight, it will not be available for other responses. Weather conditions like fog, heavy rain, or snow may obscure visibility, making it dangerous to take off, fly, or land at an emergency scene. Icing conditions on the ground or at altitude may also endanger the aircraft and restrict its flight. The helicopter is also a maintenance-intensive vehicle and can be out of service for scheduled repairs. These factors may reduce the availability of the service, so be prepared to use ground transport if the helicopter is unavailable.

The helicopter may be able to offer additional services to EMS (Figure 12-24 ■). It can help search rough terrain and can cover great distances quickly when trying to find lost hikers or walk-aways from nursing homes. It can provide vertical patient lift services and help transport patients out of remote areas. With special equipment, the helicopter may also be able to illuminate the scene or use infrared optics to locate patients in wilderness or remote areas at night. Contact your local EMS and police helicopter services to learn what support activities they can provide.

Criteria for the use of air medical transport are listed in Table 12–4.

LANDING ZONE CRITERIA

Direct someone knowledgeable in the appropriate criteria to establish the landing zone at the trauma scene. Assure the landing zone is as level as possible and clear of dust, debris, and snow. Rotor wash—the powerful blast of air that occurs with landing and take

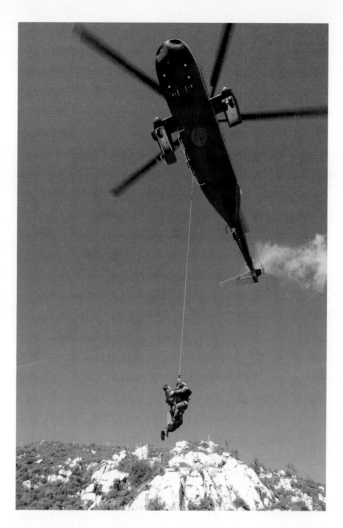

off—can blow debris into the medical care site, onto bystanders, or possibly into the rotors. Dust and snow may turn into clouds that obscure or blind the pilot's vision. A sloping landing zone places the turning rotors closer, possibly dangerously close, to the ground on the uphill side and may make the helicopter unstable as it touches down. It is a good practice to have fire department personnel and equipment on stand-by at the landing zone with a charged fire hose, just in case there is any source of ignition.

Establish a landing zone with minimum sizes of 60 by 60 feet for small helicopters, 75 by 75 feet for medium ones, and 120 by 120 feet for large ones. Assure that the site is free of wires, trees, and other obstructions that may impede landing or interfere with patient loading. If you observe obstructions or other possible hazards, direct someone to radio the information to the incoming pilot. Wires and poles that are visible from the ground may blend into the terrain from aloft and be invisible to the pilot and flight crew.

In daylight, firmly anchor traffic cones or other highly visible objects to mark the corners of the landing zone. At night, illuminate the landing zone with lights pointed at the zone surface. Do not direct lights into the air, at the helicopter, or above the landing zone surface. They may blind the pilot and make a safe landing difficult. Be especially watchful of camera crews looking for a good shot of the helicopter landing. Photo flashes, strobe lights, or high-intensity lighting are particularly blinding. Do not use flares since they may be blown with the rotor wash and ignite leaves, debris, or spilled fuel.

Once the helicopter lands, approach it from the front and only under the direction of the flight crew (Figure 12-25 ■). Frequently, the medical crew will leave the aircraft while the rotors remain turning (a hot off-load). If the patient is properly prepared for

Approach a helicopter only from the front and only under the direction of the flight crew.

Table 12-4	Criteria for Air Medical Transport

Clinical Criteria

General and mechanism considerations
- Trauma score < 12
- Unstable vital signs (e.g., hypotension or tachypnea)
- Significant trauma in patients < 12 years old, > 55 years old, or pregnant patients
- Multisystem injuries (e.g., long-bone fractures in different extremities, injury to more than two body regions)
- Ejection from vehicle
- Pedestrian or cyclist struck by motor vehicle
- Death in same passenger compartment as patient
- Ground provider perception of significant damage to patient's passenger compartment
- Penetrating trauma to the abdomen, pelvis, chest, neck, or head
- Crush injury to the abdomen, chest, or head

Neurologic considerations
- Glasgow Coma Scale score < 10
- Deteriorating mental status
- Skull fracture
- Neurologic presentation suggestive of spinal cord injury

Thoracic considerations
- Major chest wall injury (e.g., flail chest)
- Pneumothorax/hemothorax
- Suspected cardiac history

Abdominal/pelvic considerations
- Significant abdominal pain after trauma
- Presence of a "seat belt" sign or other abdominal wall contusion
- Obvious rib fractures below the nipple line
- Major pelvic fracture (e.g., unstable pelvic ring disruption, open pelvic fracture, or pelvic fracture with hypotension)

Orthopedic/extremity considerations
- Partial or total amputation of a limb (exclusive of digits)
- Finger/thumb amputation when emergent surgical evaluation (i.e., for replantation consideration) is indicated and rapid surface transportation is not available
- Fracture or dislocation with vascular compromise
- Extremity ischemia
- Open long-bone fractures
- Two or more long-bone fractures

Major burns
- >20 Percent body surface area
- Involvement of face, head, hands, feet, or genitalia
- Inhalational injury
- Electrical or chemical burns
- Burns with associated injuries

Immersion injuries
- Patients with near-drowning injuries

Difficult to Access Situations
- Wilderness rescue
- Ambulance egress or access impeded by road conditions, weather, or traffic

Time/Distance Factors
- Transport to trauma center > 15 minutes by ground ambulance
- Transport time to local hospital by ground ambulance greater than transport time to trauma center by helicopter
- Patient extrication time > 20 minutes
- Utilization of local ground ambulance results in absence of ground ambulance coverage for local community

Source: National Association of EMS Physicians Position Paper. Guidelines for Air Medical Dispatch. *Prehospital Emergency Care* 7(2) (2003):265–271.

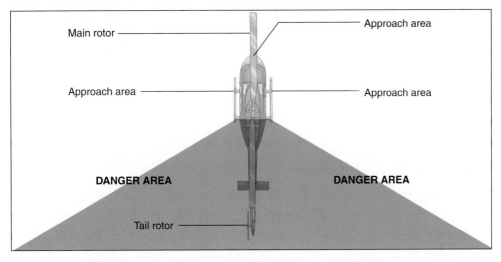

a. Danger areas are those places out of view of the pilot and close to the tail rotor.

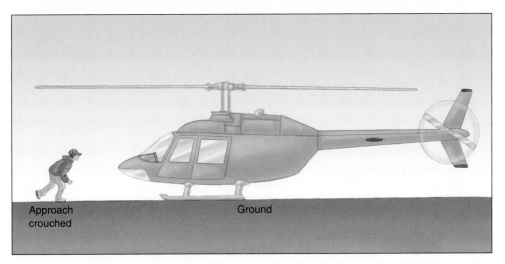

b. When approaching the helicopter, lower all equipment like IV holders and keep your head low.

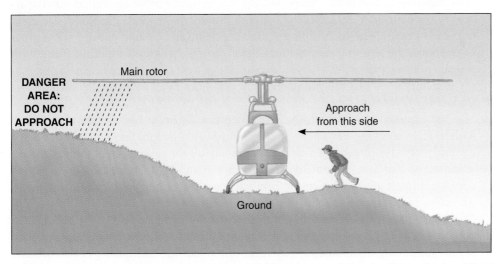

c. Be exceptionally careful with a landing zone on a hillside and approach the aircraft from the downhill side.

■ Figure 12-25 Special considerations with helicopters.

transport and a well-organized patient report is ready, the crew may load the patient while the rotors continue to turn (a hot load). If you are asked to help carry the patient to the helicopter while the rotors are still turning, stay close to the flight crew, keep your head down, and leave any hats or loose clothing behind. Follow the flight crew's instruction carefully and avoid the area of the tail rotor. It spins at speeds in excess of 2,000 rpm and is almost invisible. After you help load the patient, move forward (with your head down) and away from the helicopter, staying in the pilot's clear view.

FLIGHT PHYSIOLOGY

There are some aspects of flight physiology that may impact patient assessment and care and that make air medical service a special aspect of prehospital care. Most notably, as you change altitude you change the height of the column of air above you. This changes the atmospheric pressure around you and has several effects on your patient.

As a helicopter gains altitude, its occupants experience decreased atmospheric pressure. This means that air trapped in body cavities exerts more outward pressure against those cavity walls. You can appreciate this effect on your auditory canal when you go up or down a mountain in a car or up and down an elevator in a tall building. This phenomenon is especially important with a patient who is experiencing a pneumothorax or tension pneumothorax. A rise in altitude increases the relative pressure within the chest and makes the condition worse. Decreasing atmospheric pressure can also increase the severity of asthma and exacerbate COPD as the air trapped within the lungs exerts a greater pressure against the functional alveoli and results in greater effort by the patient to move air in and out. Changing altitude also affects the PASG, the cuff of an endotracheal tube, and air splints used for long-bone injuries. As you increase altitude you decrease the external pressure and effectively increase the pressure within these devices. The reverse is true during descent; as the air pressure increases, it results in a relative decrease of pressure inside the air-filled chambers of both the body and certain equipment.

Another effect of decreasing atmospheric pressure with flight occurs as it changes the pressure driving gases into a liquid. Decreasing pressure pushes less gas into a liquid (think, for example, of the bubbles that appear in a bottle of soda when you first take the top off). In medicine, hyperbaric (enhanced atmospheric) pressure is used to push more oxygen into the bloodstream (and most specifically the plasma) of patients suffering from carbon monoxide poisoning. Decreasing pressure associated with the ascent of the helicopter decreases the pressure driving oxygen into the blood, decreases oxygen saturation, lessens the efficiency of ventilation and circulation, and may further compromise the serious trauma patient. Small changes in altitude for limited lengths of time do not seriously affect a healthy person. If a patient is in shock or is having breathing difficulty or circulation problems, however, these small changes may increase the impact and severity of those problems.

The confined space within the helicopter and the noise and vibration associated with its flight affect the way air medical personnel can function. The structure and aerodynamics of helicopters mean that the space available for patient care is limited and restrictive and that care equipment must be limited and light. Depending on the ship's configuration, it may be difficult to intubate a patient or apply a PASG during flight. The noise and vibration of helicopter flight also reduce a care provider's ability to communicate with and assess and care for the patient. Noise precludes blood pressure auscultation except by using a Doppler stethoscope or automatic blood pressure cuff, and breath sounds are unobtainable. Palpation of a pulse rate and quality is also difficult due to vibration.

Lastly, any patient must be firmly immobilized during flight. The working space within the helicopter is very limited, and the actions of a patient may interfere with the pilot's functions or damage the aircraft's instruments (Figure 12-26 ■). If the patient becomes combative or experiences a seizure during flight, contact with the pilot or he-

Any patient receiving air medical transport must be firmly immobilized during flight.

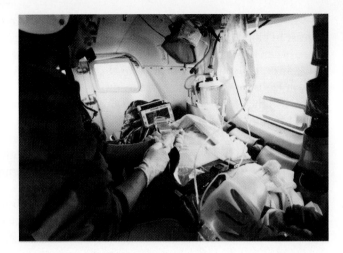

Figure 12-26 The working space in a helicopter is limited, so try to complete all crucial procedures before you load the patient. (© *Mark C. Ide*)

licopter controls is extremely dangerous. Whenever a patient is transported by helicopter, he must be firmly and completely immobilized before flight. Most commonly, this involves complete immobilization to a long spine board. Some aircraft, however, are configured in such ways that use of specially sized litters or spine boards is required.

AIR MEDICAL PATIENT PREPARATION

The principles of flight physiology and the restrictions on care during flight require special preparation of a patient for flight. Any patient who is in shock will likely get worse as the air pressure decreases when the aircraft climbs. You must assure maximal oxygenation and ventilation in preparation for flight. Administer high-flow, high-concentration oxygen to all patients and provide overdrive ventilation for any patient with any significant dyspnea or respiratory embarrassment. (The flight crew will likely use an oxygen-powered ventilator to assure good respirations.) Intubate any marginal patient before flight, possibly using rapid sequence intubation, as needed. Make sure the tube is properly placed, secured firmly, and note its position on the paperwork and in the verbal report you give to the flight crew. Assess for pneumothorax and assure that the patient does not have a tension pneumothorax. If he does, decompress it. If the patient has a pneumothorax, flight protocols may require its decompression also. Establish two good IVs, both with large-bore catheters and at least one with a nonrestrictive fluid administration set. You may establish and maintain the second line with a nonrestrictive saline lock. Secure the IV sites well to assure they are not dislodged during patient loading and flight. Finally, completely secure your patient to the long spine board (or other device approved for use with your local air medical service) so he cannot move about during flight. Provide the flight crew with a complete but abbreviated patient report addressing the elements of a report identified earlier in this chapter. Preparing your patient for flight will speed the transition of care from you to the flight team, reduce the on-scene time, and improve patient care and reduce mortality.

RESEARCH AND TRAUMA

Over the past few years, research has looked carefully at several assessment and care procedures utilized by prehospital emergency care. These include PASG, capillary refill, and rapid isotonic infusion.

Upon its introduction, the PASG was thought to be a great weapon in the fight against shock. It compressed the lower portion of the body, reducing hemorrhage there. It displaced blood from the abdomen and lower extremities into the critical circulation of the chest and head. And it reduced the size of the total vascular space by compressing the venous vessels beneath it. The end result is a relatively reduced hypovolemia and an increase in blood pressure that was thought to benefit the patient in shock. While these effects occur, they do not, however, occur to the degree once thought and, in certain circumstances, are counterproductive to the shock patient's survival. A relatively large study in Houston, Texas, supported by other studies after it, demonstrated that the application of the PASG and the resulting increase in blood pressure also increased the rate and total volume of blood loss in cases of penetrating chest trauma. Since then, numerous studies have determined that the PASG's use in many situations where it was thought to be beneficial is, in fact, detrimental or does not positively impact patient survival. The recommendations of these studies have been summarized in a classification for PASG uses shown in Table 12–5.

The value of capillary refill evaluation has also come into question with recent research. This research points out that refill times by themselves are poor indicators of a patient's circulatory status. Preexisting conditions like caffeine intake, smoking, cold

Table 12–5	Criteria for Use of the Pneumatic Anti-Shock Garment
Class I	Usually indicated, useful and effective ★Hypotension due to ruptured abdominal aortic aneurysm (AAA)
Class IIa	Acceptable, uncertain efficacy, weight of evidence favors usefulness and efficacy ★Hypotension due to suspected pelvic fracture ★Anaphylactic shock (unresponsive to standard therapy)* ★Otherwise uncontrollable lower extremity hemorrhage* ★Severe traumatic hypotension (palpable pulse, BP not obtainable)*
Class IIb	Acceptable, uncertain efficacy, may be helpful, probably not harmful ★Elderly ★Pelvic fracture without hypotension* ★Septic shock* ★Urologic hemorrhage (otherwise controlled)* ★Penetrating abdominal injury ★Paroxysmal supraventricular tachycardia (PSVT) ★Gynecologic hemorrhage (otherwise uncontrolled)* ★Hypothermia-induced hypotension* ★Lower extemity hemorrhage (otherwise controlled)* ★History of congestive heart failure ★Ruptured ectopic pregnancy* ★Spinal shock* ★Assist intravenous cannulation*
Class III	Inappropriate option, not indicated, may be harmful ★Adjunct to CPR ★Penetrating thoracic injury ★To splint fractures of the lower extremities ★Abdominal evisceration ★Cardiac tamponade ★Gravid uterus ★Diaphragmatic rupture ★Pulmonary edema ★Extremity trauma ★Acute myocardial infarction ★Cardiogenic shock

*Data from controlled trials not available. Recommendations were based on other evidence.
Source: *Prehospital Emergency Care*, 1(1):33, 1997.

environmental temperatures, COPD, and many chronic conditions delay refill times well beyond what was previously thought to reflect normal distal skin perfusion. However, capillary refill remains an important diagnostic technique for the status of distal perfusion and is especially useful for trending distal perfusion or for comparing circulation from one limb to another. Increasing capillar refill times reflect a decreasing perfusion while decreasing capillary refill times equate to an increase in distal perfusion.

For reasons similar to the concerns raised about PASG use, the value of rapid infusion of isotonic solutions to the hypovolemic patient in the prehospital setting is being questioned. As with application of the PASG, restoration of fluid volume may increase patient mortality as the increase in blood pressure may dislodge clots and increase the rate and volume of internal hemorrhage. This problem is compounded because isotonic fluid replaces blood, effectively thinning the clotting factors and red blood cells that remain. The guideline for fluid resuscitation still remains at up to 3 liters of fluid for the adult during the normal prehospital care time period.

Research must continue to assure that EMS personnel utilize care procedures that contribute to patient survival. This research may lead to adoption of new techniques that support the chances of trauma patient survival or may reveal that other currently used skills and equipment do not benefit patients. In the future, research will change the way we deliver prehospital emergency care.

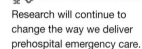

Research will continue to change the way we deliver prehospital emergency care.

Summary

Trauma has remained the number one killer of those below the age of 44 for the past three decades, often taking lives during their most productive years. The EMS system as a whole, and you as a paramedic member of it, must expend resources toward supporting and encouraging injury prevention programs. These programs may be the most effective way to reduce trauma mortality and morbidity. Once serious injury occurs, you must anticipate the nature and severity of the trauma based on the mechanism of injury analysis, then assess and stabilize the cervical spine, airway, breathing, and circulation during the initial assessment. You provide directed assessment and care during the rapid trauma assessment and quickly transport the seriously injured patient to the trauma center. With trauma patients, shock is a critical concern.

You must anticipate shock and look for its earliest signs upon your arrival at the scene and then monitor the patient for any progressive signs or symptoms of hypovolemia compensation during the remainder of your assessment, care, and ongoing assessments. If you suspect shock, you must intervene quickly with rapid fluid infusion, PASG application, aggressive airway care, and pleural decompression, as needed. Assure that your patient is directed to the trauma center as quickly as possible and consider the use of air medical service to reduce the transport time.

You Make the Call

You arrive at an auto collision to find one car significantly deformed around a large tree. Inside there is a young female draped against the steering wheel. She appears to be unconscious.

1. Your scene survey determines the answers to what four questions?

Your questions answered, you move to the patient's side and find her conscious but very confused. She has a weak pulse of 110 beats per minute; her skin is cool, clammy, and ashen in color; and her respirations are 28 and shallow. She complains of general chest pain and speaks in short phrases because she is having "great difficulty breathing." Auscultation of her chest reveals diminished breath sounds on the right and a hyperinflated right hemithorax.

2. You suspect which immediately life-threatening problem?
3. Given your suspicions, what immediate actions should you take with this patient?

See Suggested Responses at the back of this book.

Review Questions

1. All of the following are considered reasons to conduct research in prehospital trauma care except:
   a. to assure that EMS is best serving its patients.
   b. to help assure a future for prehospital emergency care.
   c. to find justifications for longtime mainstay treatments.
   d. to identify areas where injury prevention programs may be beneficial.

2. The demographic group most prone to traumatic injuries and deaths is:
   a. females over the age of 65.
   b. males under the age of 12.
   c. females between the ages of 15 and 20.
   d. males between the ages of 13 and 35.

3. Which of the following groups of criteria is utilized when developing the revised trauma score?
   a. systolic blood pressure, respiratory rate, GCS
   b. GCS, heart rate, and best motor response
   c. best motor response, eye opening, and verbal response
   d. respiratory rate, blood pressure, and capillary refill rate

4. If ground transport time will exceed _____ minutes, helicopter transport may be warranted.
   a. 8
   b. 10
   c. 20
   d. 30

5. All of the following are appropriate steps for shock trauma resuscitation except:
   a. maintaining adequate ventilations.
   b. splinting major long bone fractures.
   c. providing airway maintenance, including endotracheal intubation.
   d. providing rapid fluid resuscitation with hypertonic crystalloid solutions.

6. Of all the care procedures and advanced interventions available to treat the trauma patient, none has more promise for reducing mortality and morbidity than:
   a. early transport.
   b. prevention.
   c. fluid therapy.
   d. air medical transport.

7. All of the following are terms used to describe the status of the cardiovascular system in trauma except:
   a. hypovolemia.
   b. hypothermia.
   c. hypotension.
   d. hypoperfusion.

8. Generally, the maximum prehospital fluid volume is _____ mL of isotonic solution.
   a. 2,000
   b. 3,000
   c. 1,000
   d. 2,500

9. Noncritical patients account for about _____ percent of trauma responses and receive the largest part of prehospital trauma care.
   a. 60
   b. 40
   c. 80
   d. 70

10. In the pediatric trauma patient, fluid boluses for volume replacement are usually given at _____ mL/kg.
   a. 10
   b. 15
   c. 20
   d. 25

See Answers to Review Questions at the back of this book.

Further Reading

American College of Surgeons, Committee on Trauma. *Advanced Trauma Life Support Course: Student Manual.* Chicago: American College of Surgeons, 1997.

American College of Surgeons, Committee on Trauma. *Resources for Optimal Care of the Injured Patient.* Chicago: American College of Surgeons, 1999.

Bates, Barbara, Lynn S. Bickley, and Robert A. Hoekelman. *A Guide to Physical Examination and History Taking.* 8th ed. Philadelphia: J. B. Lippincott, 2003.

Bledsoe, B. E. and D. Clayden. *Prehospital Emergency Pharmacology.* 6th ed. Upper Saddle River, N. J.: Pearson/Prentice Hall, 2005.

Butman, A., S. Martin, R. Vomacka, and N. McSwain. *Comprehensive Guide to Pre-Hospital Skills: A Skills Manual for EMT-Basic, EMT-Intermediate, and EMT-Paramedic.* St. Louis: Mosby, 1996.

Campbell, John E. *Basic Trauma Life Support for Paramedics and Other Advanced Providers.* 5th ed. update. Upper Saddle River, N.J.: Pearson/Prentice Hall, 2004.

McSwain, N. E. and S. B. Frame, eds. *Prehospital Trauma Life Support.* 5th ed. St. Louis, Mosby, 2003.

National Association of EMS Physicians Position Paper. Guidelines for Air Medical Dispatch. *Prehospital Emergency Care* 7(2) (2003):265–271.

New York State Department of Health. *The New York State Trauma System: 1994–1995.* Troy, N.Y.: NYSDOH, 1996.

Rosen, P., and R. Barkin, eds. *Emergency Medicine: Concepts and Clinical Practice.* 5th ed. St. Louis: Mosby, 2002.

Samuels, David, et al. *Air-Medical Crew National Standard Curriculum Instructor Manual.* Pasadena, Calif.: ASHBEAMS, 1998.

On the Web

Visit Brady's Paramedic Website at **www.bradybooks.com/paramedic.**

Precautions on Bloodborne Pathogens and Infectious Diseases

Prehospital emergency personnel, like all health care workers, are at risk for exposure to bloodborne pathogens and infectious diseases. In emergency situations it is often difficult to take or enforce proper infection control measures. However, as a paramedic, you must recognize your high-risk status. Study the following information on infection control carefully.

Infection control is designed to protect emergency personnel, their families, and their patients from unnecessary exposure to communicable diseases. Laws, regulations, and standards regarding infection control include:

★ *Centers for Disease Control and Prevention (CDC) Guidelines.* The CDC has published extensive guidelines on infection control. Proper equipment and techniques that should be used by emergency response personnel to prevent or minimize risk of exposure are defined.

★ *The Ryan White Act.* The Ryan White Act of 1990 allows emergency personnel to find out if they were exposed to an infectious disease while rendering patient care. Employers are required to name a "designated officer" to coordinate communications with the treating hospital.

★ *Americans with Disabilities Act.* This act prohibits discrimination against individuals with disabilities including those with contagious diseases. It guarantees equal employment opportunities and job protection if the infected individual can perform essential job functions and does not pose a threat to the safety and health of patients and coworkers.

★ *Occupational Safety and Health Administration (OSHA) Regulations.* OSHA has enacted a regulation entitled Occupational Exposure to Bloodborne Pathogens that classifies emergency response personnel as being at the greatest risk of occupational exposure to communicable diseases. This regulation requires employers to provide hepatitis B (HBV) vaccinations free of charge, maintain a written exposure control plan, and provide personal protective equipment. These requirements primarily apply to private employers. Applicability to local and state governmental employees varies by locality. Many states have developed their own OSHA plans.

★ *National Fire Protection Association (NFPA) Guidelines.* This is a national organization that has established specific guidelines and requirements regarding infection control for emergency response agencies, particularly fire departments and EMS services.

BODY SUBSTANCE ISOLATION PRECAUTIONS AND PERSONAL PROTECTIVE EQUIPMENT

Emergency response personnel should practice body substance isolation (BSI), a strategy that considers ALL body substances potentially infectious. To achieve this, all emergency personnel should utilize personal protective equipment (PPE). Appropriate PPE should be available on every emergency vehicle. The minimum recommended PPE includes the following:

★ *Gloves.* Disposable gloves should be donned by all emergency response personnel BEFORE initiating any emergency care. When an emergency incident involves more than one patient, you should attempt to change gloves between patients. When gloves have been contaminated, they should be removed as soon as possible. To properly remove contaminated gloves, grasp one glove approximately 1 inch from the wrist. Without touching the inside of the glove, pull the glove halfway off and stop. With that half-gloved hand, pull the glove on the opposite hand completely off. Place the removed glove in the palm of the other glove, with the inside of the removed glove exposed. Pull the second glove completely off with the ungloved hand, only touching the inside of the glove. Always wash hands after gloves are removed, even when the gloves appear intact.

★ *Masks and Protective Eyewear.* Masks and protective equipment should be present on all emergency vehicles and used in accordance with the level of exposure encountered. Masks and protective eyewear should be worn together whenever blood spatter is likely to occur, such as during arterial bleeding, childbirth, endotracheal intubation, invasive procedures, oral suctioning, and cleanup of equipment that requires heavy scrubbing or brushing. Both you and the patient should wear masks whenever the potential for airborne transmission of disease exists.

★ *HEPA and N-95 Respirators.* Due to the resurgence of tuberculosis (TB), prehospital personnel should protect themselves from TB infection through use of an N-95 or a high-efficiency particulate air (HEPA) respirator, as approved by the National Institute of Occupational Safety and Health (NIOSH). It should fit snugly and be capable of filtering out the tuberculosis bacillus. An N-95 or HEPA respirator should be worn when caring for patients with confirmed or suspected TB. This is especially true when performing "high-hazard" procedures such as administration of nebulized medications, endotracheal intubation, or suctioning on such a patient.

★ *Gowns.* Gowns protect clothing from blood splashes. If large splashes of blood are expected, such as with childbirth, wear impervious gowns.

★ *Resuscitation Equipment.* Disposable resuscitation equipment should be the primary means of artificial ventilation in emergency care. Such items should be used once, then disposed of.

Remember, the proper use of personal protective equipment ensures effective infection control and minimizes risk. Use ALL protective equipment recommended for any particular situation to ensure maximum protection.

Consider ALL body substances potentially infectious and ALWAYS practice BSI.

Suggested Responses to "You Make the Call"

The following are suggested responses to the "You Make the Call" scenarios presented in each chapter of Paramedic Care, Volume 4, Trauma Emergencies. Each represents an acceptable response to the scenario but should not be interpreted as the only correct response.

Chapter 1

1. What authority does Janet have regarding the decision to transport her daughter?

Janet is the child's mother, and as such is able to consent to or determine what care and to which hospital her daughter is transported. See Volume 1, Chapter 6, "Medical/Legal Aspects of Advanced Prehospital Care."

2. What will you be telling her regarding your choice for a hospital destination?

You might say the following: "The trauma center is a hospital designated as a destination for trauma patients because it has the commitment, personnel, equipment, and resources to provide optimum care for seriously injured patients like your daughter. Transport to this facility will likely provide immediate access to surgery and any other services necessary for her care. It is where we recommend your daughter be transported and where our protocols suggest she go with the mechanism of injury and the injuries we have found."

Chapter 2

1. What scene hazards would you expect on this call?

The probable scene hazards associated with an auto crash include:

- Broken glass and jagged metal
- Electrocution
- Dangers from spilled fluids
  Caustic—battery acid
  Flammable—gasoline
  Hot—radiator fluid and oil
  Slippery surfaces from oil and transmission fluid
- Traffic hazards

2. What injuries would you suspect?

The forces directed at the driver will likely cause injury to the shoulder, humerus, and pelvis. The lateral impact may also cause the paper bag syndrome (lung injury) and injury to the aorta, aortic tear, or aneurysm. It will also likely cause severe lateral bending and cervical spine injury. The head impact with the window may produce both blunt and penetrating trauma to the scalp, possible skull fracture, and internal head injury. The fractured pelvis or bleeding aorta is likely to cause serious internal bleeding and possibly shock while chest injury may result in pneumothorax and dyspnea. The head injury may reduce the patient's level of responsiveness and may result in intracranial hemorrhage.

3. What care would you expect to provide?

Immobilization of the spine (manual immobilization, cervical collar, vest type immobilization/long spine board, cervical immobilization device)

Airway (high-flow, high-concentration oxygen)

Breathing (positive pressure ventilations as necessary)

Circulation (hemorrhage control and possible shock care)

Rapid splinting of the arm and pelvis (probably by securing them to a long spine board)

Pelvic sling application for the pelvic fracture

Rapid transport to a trauma center

Chapter 3

1. *What is your first concern?*

Your first concern should be scene safety, with special emphasis on the following:

Potential for violence directed toward you—

Have the police secure the scene.

Have the police search the victim for weapons.

Blood- and airborne pathogens—

Body substance isolation precautions

Gloves

Goggles or face shield

Possibly a disposable gown

2. *What information is important to gain from your survey of the scene?*

Information that you should attempt to determine includes:

Gun caliber and type (rifle, shotgun, hand-gun)

Distance from gun to victim

Angle of bullet entry/body position

Number of shots fired/expected entrance and exit wounds;

Chapter 4

1. *What signs suggest hypovolemia and early shock?*

Tachycardia, anxiety, cool and clammy skin.

2. *Does the blood pressure suggest shock? Why or why not?*

No, the body's compensatory mechanisms maintain blood pressure until late in the shock process.

3. *What progressive steps would you take to control the hemorrhage?*

Direct pressure, elevation, use of pressure points, tourniquet.

4. *What supportive care measures would you employ?*

Application of oxygen, elevation of the lower extremities, consider application of the PASG, fluid resuscitation, maintenance of patient's body temperature.

Chapter 5

1. *What type of wound is this and what significance does it have for infection?*

The description of the wound suggests a puncture. Remember that puncture wound mechanisms frequently introduce contaminants, both foreign and infectious material, deep into body tissue. The nature of the wound closes the opening, preventing oxygen from reaching the interior wound site and supporting the growth of anaerobic bacteria. This wound is at significant risk for infection.

2. *What elements of history and specifically vaccinations will be important in assessing this patient?*

It is very important to determine the history of inoculation against tetanus because tetanus is a serious complication of open wounds. If the initial or last tetanus booster was administered more than 10 years ago, a booster will be necessary. It is also important to determine any patient allergies, especially to antibiotics that might be used to care for the potential infection.

3. *What direction would you give this patient if his parents do not wish to have him transported to the local emergency department?*

The boy's parents must be advised of the risks associated with not seeing an emergency physician for this injury. They should be directed to their own physician to receive a tetanus inoculation (or updated booster) and care to prevent infection. You should also speak to both the parents about preventative actions regarding these types of injuries.

Chapter 6

1. *What severity are the burns of the forearm and hand and of the upper arm?*

Forearm and hand—full thickness (third degree) as indicated by the discoloration and anesthesia; upper arm—partial thickness (first and second degree) as indicated by the blistering and pain.

2. *What percentage of the body surface area is burned?*

Rule of nines—full thickness 4½ percent, partial thickness 4½ percent.

3. *What level of acuity would you assign this patient?*

Critical, because of the involvement of the hand in the burn.

Chapter 7

1. *When assessing the injury site, what signs of fracture will you be evaluating?*

Assess for deformity, crepitus, unusual limb placement or asymmetry, and suggestions of soft-tissue injury. You will also consider the six Ps—pain, pallor, paralysis, paresthesia, pressure, and pulses.

2. *What are the three main factors to consider when evaluating distal neurovascular status?*

Pulse, motor function, and sensation.

3. *What steps should you take if you determine the patient is suffering from distal neurovascular impairment and choose to realign the injury?*

Check distal color, temperature, capillary refill, and pulse as well as tactile response and sensation.

4. *How many attempts are permitted when realigning an injury?*

One.

5. *How would you splint this injury once realignment has taken place?*

For an ankle injury you might use an air splint, liberally padded long splints firmly secured to each side of the joint, or a pillow splint.

Chapter 8

1. *What structures are most likely injured?*

Most likely injuries are to the jugular vein (severe flowing but not spurting hemorrhage) and the trachea (air bubbling with expiration).

2. *What care would you employ?*

Assess the mental status and the ABCs. Cover the wound with a sterile occlusive dressing, then apply direct pressure, rapid sequence intubation (try to place tube cuff below the tracheal laceration). Be very careful with the intubation attempt and try not to cause further injury to the trachea. Passing the tube beyond the wound, then inflating the cuff, will protect the lungs from aspiration of blood.

3. *What are serious life threats associated with this injury?*

Airway compromise, blood loss/hypovolemia/shock, air embolism—cardiac arrest and pulmonary embolism.

Chapter 9

1. What additional spinal precautions does this patient require?

Application of a cervical collar, firm immobilization of the trunk to the spine board, then head immobilization to the spine board using the CID. Immobilize him firmly enough to permit board rotation without patient movement if he vomits.

2. What mechanism of injury do you suspect?

Axial loading and flexion from a shallow water dive.

3. What other assessment and care steps does this patient require?

Assessment: motor and sensory assessment of the distal extremities, isolate dermatomes/myotomes, palpate the posterior neck for tenderness and deformity. Also examine for the signs of neurogenic shock—bradycardia, hypotension, warm and dry lower body, and cool and clammy upper body. Care: ABCs, oxygen, maintenance of patient's body temperature.

Chapter 10

1. Considering the mechanism of injury and what is known about the patient, what thoracic pathophysiology may explain the patient's presentation?

The patient has suffered blunt anterior chest trauma and sudden deceleration injury. He has evidence of a flail chest and subcutaneous emphysema of the anterior and lateral left chest suggests a left pneumothorax. In addition, the patient is hypotensive and has JVD. It is also very probable that the patient has pulmonary contusion under the flail segment. Further assessment should rule out possible complications including left tension pneumothorax, pericardial tamponade, great vessel injury, esophageal or tracheobronchial rupture, and left diaphragmatic rupture with abdominal viscera herniation.

2. As the treating paramedic, what is your next step in stabilizing this patient?

An endotracheal tube is indicated as the patient is unconscious and without gag reflex. This will permit intermittent positive pressure ventilation (with supplemental oxygen) and provide effective internal splinting of the flail segment. Also firmly tape a bulky dressing over the flail segment to restrict its movement.

3. What further emergency treatment is likely indicated in the absence of breath sounds on the left side and a relatively normal abdominal exam?

This information strongly suggests the possibility of a left tension pneumothorax. Despite care instituted, the patient still demonstrates hypotension and JVD. The normal abdominal exam makes significant diaphragmatic hernia unlikely. Pleural decompression of the left chest is indicated using a large bore IV catheter inserted in the second intercostal space, midclavicular line.

Chapter 11

1. Given the signs and symptoms, what is the most likely injury and why?

The spleen is frequently injured in left-sided abdominal trauma, especially trauma to the left flank. It often presents with limited signs and symptoms, and blood loss in the supine patient frequently results in diaphragm irritation and referred pain. Blunt trauma may also induce kidney injury.

2. What relation does the right shoulder pain have to the suspected injury?

Shoulder pain is often a referred pain from the abdomen caused by blood irritating the diaphragm.

3. What care will you provide for this patient?

Gentle, rapid transport to the trauma center with aggressive fluid resuscitation initiated en route. Apply high-flow, high-concentration oxygen, ready the PASG, and constantly monitor for the appearance of the signs and symptoms of shock.

Chapter 12

1. *Your scene survey determines the answers to what four questions?*

   What scene hazards are visible or likely (including what body substance isolation precautions are needed)? What was the mechanism of injury and what injuries are expected from it (index of suspicion)? How many patients are there? Do you need any form of additional assistance?

2. *You suspect which immediately life-threatening problem?*

   A developing tension pneumothorax.

3. *Given your suspicions, what immediate actions should you take with this patient?*

   Administration of high-flow, high-concentration oxygen and pleural decompression of the right chest using a large-bore catheter placed through the second intercostal space, midclavicular line.

Answers to Review Questions

The following are the correct answers to the Review Questions presented in each chapter of
Paramedic Care, Volume 4, Trauma Emergencies.

Chapter 1
1. c
2. d
3. d
4. b
5. a
6. a
7. b
8. c
9. c
10. c

Chapter 2
1. b
2. b
3. a
4. d
5. d
6. b
7. b
8. c
9. a
10. b
11. b
12. c
13. c
14. b
15. c
16. a
17. c
18. b

Chapter 3
1. b
2. c
3. d
4. b

5. b
6. a
7. a
8. d
9. d
10. b

Chapter 4
1. a
2. b
3. d
4. b
5. d
6. c
7. b
8. d
9. c
10. d

Chapter 5
1. d
2. b
3. c
4. c
5. c
6. d
7. a
8. a
9. d
10. d
11. a
12. b

Chapter 6
1. b
2. b
3. c

4. b
5. d
6. a
7. c
8. d
9. a
10. b
11. a
12. b

Chapter 7
1. d
2. b
3. d
4. d
5. c
6. c
7. a
8. a
9. b
10. b
11. c
12. d
13. d
14. b
15. d

Chapter 8
1. a
2. b
3. d
4. a
5. c
6. b
7. b
8. a
9. c

10. d
11. a
12. c
13. d
14. d
15. d

Chapter 9

1. a
2. c
3. a
4. b
5. d
6. d
7. c
8. a
9. a
10. a
11. b
12. d

13. b
14. d
15. d

Chapter 10

1. d
2. c
3. b
4. c
5. d
6. a
7. d
8. a
9. b
10. d

Chapter 11

1. c
2. d

3. d
4. a
5. b
6. c
7. c
8. c
9. d
10. c

Chapter 12

1. c
2. d
3. a
4. d
5. d
6. b
7. b
8. b
9. c
10. c

Glossary

abduction movement of a body part away from the midline.

abrasion scraping or abrading away of the superficial layers of the skin; an open soft-tissue injury.

abruptio placentae a condition in which the placenta separates from the uterine wall.

acceleration the rate at which speed or velocity increases.

acute retinal artery occlusion a nontraumatic occlusion of the retinal artery resulting in a sudden, painless loss of vision in one eye.

adduction movement of a body part toward the midline.

adrenocorticotropic hormone hormone secreted by the anterior lobe of the pituitary gland that is essential to the function of the adrenal cortex, including production of glucocorticoids.

aerobic metabolism second stage of metabolism, requiring the presence of oxygen, in which the breakdown of glucose (in a process called the Krebs or citric acid cycle) yields a high amount of energy.

afterload the resistance a contraction of the heart must overcome in order to eject blood; in cardiac physiology, defined as the tension of cardiac muscle during systole (contraction).

aggregate to cluster or come together.

aldosterone hormone secreted by the adrenal cortex that increases sodium reabsorption by the kidneys; it plays a part in regulation of blood volume, blood pressure, and blood levels of potassium, chloride, and bicarbonate.

alpha radiation low-level form of nuclear radiation; a weak source of energy that is stopped by clothing or the first layers of skin.

ampere basic unit for measuring the strength of an electric current.

amphiarthrosis joint that permits a limited amount of independent motion.

amputation severance, removal, or detachment, either partial or complete, of a body part.

anaerobic able to live without oxygen.

anaerobic metabolism the first stage of metabolism, which does not require oxygen, in which the breakdown of glucose (in a process called glycolysis) produces pyruvic acid and yields limited energy.

anaphylactic shock form of distributive shock in which histamine causes general vasodilation, precapillary sphincter dilation, capillary engorgement, and fluid movement into the interstitial compartment.

anemia a reduction in the hemoglobin content in the blood to a point below that required to meet the oxygen requirements of the body.

aneurysm a weakening or ballooning in the wall of a blood vessel.

angiotensin a vasopressor hormone that causes contraction of the smooth muscles of arteries and arterioles, produced when renin is released from the kidneys; angiotensin I is a physiologically inactive form, while angiotensin II is an active form.

anterior cord syndrome condition that is caused by bony fragments or pressure compressing the arteries of the anterior spinal cord and resulting in loss of motor function and sensation to pain, light touch, and temperature below the injury site.

anterior medial fissure deep crease along the ventral surface of the spinal cord that divides the cord into right and left halves.

anterograde amnesia inability to remember events that occurred after the trauma that caused the condition.

antidiuretic hormone (ADH) hormone released by the posterior pituitary that induces an increase in peripheral vascular resistance and causes the kidneys to retain water, decreasing urine output, and also causes splenic vascular constriction.

appendicular skeleton bones of the extremities, shoulder girdle, and pelvis (excepting the sacrum).

aqueous humor clear fluid filling the anterior chamber of the eye.

arachnoid membrane middle layer of the meninges.

arteries vessels that carry blood from the heart to the body tissues.

arteriole a small artery.

arthritis inflammation of a joint.

articular surface surface of a bone that moves against another bone.

ascending reticular activating system a series of nervous tissues keeping the human system in a state of consciousness.

ascending tracts bundles of axons along the spinal cord that transmit signals from the body to the brain.

atelectasis collapse of a lung or part of a lung.

autonomic hyperreflexia syndrome condition associated with the body's adjustment to the effects of neurogenic shock; presentations include sudden hypertension, bradycardia, pounding headache, blurred vision, and sweating and flushing of the skin above the point of injury.

autoregulation   process that controls blood flow to brain tissue by causing alterations in the blood pressure.

avulsion   forceful tearing away or separation of body tissue; an avulsion may be partial or complete.

axial loading   application of the forces of trauma along the axis of the spine; this often results in compression fractures of the spine.

axial skeleton   bones of the head, thorax, and spine.

axon   extension of a neuron that serves as a pathway for transmission of signals to and from the brain; major component of white matter.

ballistics   the study of projectile motion and its interactions with the gun, the air, and the object it contacts.

baroreceptor   sensory nerve ending, found in the walls of the atria of the heart, vena cava, aortic arch, and carotid sinus, that is stimulated by changes in pressure.

beta radiation   medium-strength radiation that is stopped with light clothing or the uppermost layers of skin.

bilateral periorbital ecchymosis   black-and-blue discoloration of the area surrounding the eyes. It is usually associated with basilar skull fracture. (Also called *raccoon eyes*.)

blast wind   the air movement caused as the heated and pressurized products of an explosion move outward.

blepharospasm   twitching of the eyelids.

blunt trauma   injury caused by the collision of an object with the body in which the object does not enter the body.

body surface area (BSA)   amount of a patient's body affected by a burn.

brainstem   the part of the brain connecting the cerebral hemispheres with the spinal cord. It is comprised of the medulla oblongata, the pons, and the midbrain.

Brown-Séquard syndrome   condition caused by partial cutting of one side of the spinal cord resulting in sensory and motor loss to that side of the body.

bursa   sac containing synovial fluid that cushions adjacent structures.

bursitis   acute or chronic inflammation of the small synovial sacs.

calcaneus   the largest bone of the foot; the heel.

caliber   the diameter of a bullet expressed in hundredths of an inch. (.22 caliber = 0.22 inches); the inside diameter of the barrel of a hand gun, shotgun, or rifle.

callus   thickened area that forms at the site of a fracture as part of the repair process.

cancellous   having a lattice-work structure, as in the spongy tissue of a bone.

capillary   one of the minute blood vessels that connect the ends of arterioles with the beginnings of venules; where oxygen is diffused to body tissue and products of metabolism enter the bloodstream.

cardiac output   the amount of blood pumped by the heart in 1 minute (computed as stroke volume × heart rate).

cardioacceleratory center   a sympathetic nervous system center in the medulla oblongata, controlling the release of epinephrine and norepinephrine.

cardiogenic shock   shock resulting from failure to maintain the blood pressure because of inadequate cardiac output.

cardioinhibitory center   a parasympathetic center in the medulla oblongata, controlling the vagus nerve.

carpal bones   bones of the wrist.

cartilage   connective tissue providing the articular surfaces of the skeletal system.

catecholamine   a hormone, such as epinephrine or norepinephrine, that strongly affects the nervous and cardiovascular systems, metabolic rate, temperature, and smooth muscle.

cavitation   the outward motion of tissue due to a projectile's passage, resulting in a temporary cavity and vacuum.

central cord syndrome   condition usually related to hyperflexion of the cervical spine that results in motor weakness, usually in the upper extremities and possible bladder dysfunction.

cerebellum   portion of the brain located dorsally to the pons and medulla oblongata. It plays an important role in the fine control of voluntary muscular movements.

cerebral perfusion pressure (CPP)   the pressure moving blood through the brain.

cerebrospinal fluid   fluid surrounding and bathing the brain and spinal cord (the elements of the central nervous system).

cerebrum   largest part of the brain. It consists of two hemispheres separated by a deep longitudinal fissure. It is the seat of consciousness and the center of the higher mental functions such as memory, learning, reasoning, judgment, intelligence, and emotions.

chemoreceptor   sense organ or sensory nerve ending located outside the central nervous system that is stimulated by and reacts to chemical stimuli.

chemotactic factors   chemicals released by white blood cells that attract more white blood cells to an area of inflammation.

Cheyne-Stokes respirations   respiratory pattern of alternating periods of apnea and tachypnea.

chyme   semifluid mixture of ingested food and digestive secretions found in the stomach and small intestine.

circumduction   movement at a synovial joint where the distal end of a bone describes a circle but the shaft does not rotate.

citric acid cycle   *see* Krebs cycle.

clavicle   bone that holds the scapula and shoulder joint at a fixed distance from the sternum and permits the shoulder to move up and down (shrug).

closed fracture   a broken bone in which the bone ends or the forces that caused it do not penetrate the skin.

clotting   the body's three-step response to stop the loss of blood.

coagulation   the third step in the clotting process, which involves the formation of a protein called fibrin that forms a network around a wound to stop bleeding, ward off infection, and lay a foundation for healing and repair of the wound.

coagulation necrosis   the process in which an acid, while destroying tissue, forms an insoluble layer that limits further damage.

collagen   tough, strong protein that comprises most of the body's connective tissue.

comminuted fracture   fracture in which a bone is broken into several pieces.

co-morbidity   associated disease process.

compartment syndrome   muscle ischemia that is caused by rising pressures within an anatomical fascial space.

compensated shock   hemodynamic insult to the body in which the body responds effectively. Signs and symptoms are limited, and the human system functions normally.

concussion   a transient period of unconsciousness. In most cases, the unconsciousness will be followed by a complete return of function.

conjunctiva   mucous membrane that lines the eyelids.

consensual reactivity   the response of both eyes to changes in light intensity that affect only one eye.

contrecoup injury   occurring on the opposite side; an injury to the brain opposite the site of impact.

contusion   closed wound in which the skin is unbroken, although damage has occurred to the tissue immediately beneath.

cornea   thin, delicate layer covering the pupil and the iris.

coup injury   an injury to the brain occurring on the same side as the site of impact.

cramping   muscle pain resulting from overactivity, lack of oxygen, and accumulation of waste products.

cranium   vaultlike portion of the skull encasing the brain.

cricothyrostomy   the introduction of a needle or other tube into the cricothyroid membrane, usually to provide an emergency airway.

cricothyrotomy   a surgical incision into the cricothyroid membrane, usually to provide an emergency airway.

crumple zone   the region of a vehicle designed to absorb the energy of impact.

crush injury   mechanism of injury in which tissue is locally compressed by high pressure forces.

crush syndrome   systemic disorder of severe metabolic disturbances resulting from the crush of a limb or other body part.

current   the rate of flow of an electric charge.

Cushing's reflex   response due to cerebral ischemia that causes an increase in systemic blood pressure, which maintains cerebral perfusion during increased intracranial pressure.

Cushing's triad   the combination of increasing blood pressure, slowing pulse, and erratic respirations in response to increased intracranial pressure.

deceleration   the rate at which speed or velocity decreases.

decompensated shock   continuing hemodynamic insult to the body in which the compensatory mechanisms break down. The signs and symptoms become very pronounced, and the patient moves rapidly toward death.

degloving injury   avulsion in which the mechanism of injury tears the skin off the underlying muscle, tissue, blood vessels, and bone.

denature   alter the usual substance of something.

dermatome   topographical region of the body surface innervated by one nerve root.

dermis   true skin, also called the corium; it is the layer of tissue producing the epidermis and housing the structures, blood vessels, and nerves normally associated with the skin.

descending tracts   bundles of axons along the spinal cord that transmit signals from the brain to the body.

devascularization   loss of blood vessels from a body part.

diaphysis   hollow shaft found in long bones.

diarthrosis   a synovial joint.

diastolic blood pressure   pressure exerted against the arterial walls during relaxation of the left ventricle of the heart.

diffuse axonal injury   type of brain injury characterized by shearing, stretching, or tearing of nerve fibers with subsequent axonal damage.

digestive tract   internal passageway that begins at the mouth and ends at the anus.

diplopia   double vision.

direct pressure   method of hemorrhage control that relies on the application of pressure to the actual site of the bleeding.

dislocation   complete displacement of a bone end from its position in a joint capsule.

distributive shock   shock that results from mechanisms that prevent the appropriate distribution of nutrients and removal of metabolic waste products.

drag   the forces acting on a projectile in motion to slow its progress.

dura mater   tough layer of the meninges firmly attached to the interior of the skull and interior of the spinal column.

dyspnea   labored or difficult breathing.

ecchymosis   blue-black discoloration of the skin due to leakage of blood into the tissues.

electrical alternans   alternating amplitude of the P, QRS, and T waves on the ECG rhythm strip as the heart swings in a pendulumlike fashion within the pericardial sac during tamponade.

emboli   undissolved solid, liquid, or gaseous matter in the bloodstream that may cause blockage of blood vessels.

emergent phase   first stage of the burn process that is characterized by a catecholamine release and pain-mediated reaction.

energy   the capacity to do work in the strict physical sense.

epicardium   serous membrane covering the outer surface of the heart; the visceral pericardium.

epidermis   outermost layer of the skin comprised of dead or dying cells.

epidural hematoma   accumulation of blood between the dura mater and the cranium.

epiphyseal fracture   disruption in the epiphyseal plate of a child's bone.

epiphyseal plate   area of the metaphysis where cartilage is generated during bone growth in childhood. Also called the *growth plate*.

epiphysis   end of a long bone, including the epiphyseal, or growth plate, and supporting structures underlying the joint.

epistaxis   bleeding from the nose resulting from injury, disease, or environmental factors; a nosebleed.

epithelialization   early stage of wound healing in which epithelial cells migrate over the surface of the wound.

erythema   general reddening of the skin due to dilation of the superficial capillaries.

erythrocyte   peripheral blood cell that contains hemoglobin; responsible for transport of oxygen to the cells.

erythropoietin   one of a specialized group of proteins that is produced by the kidneys and spurs production of red blood cells in the bone marrow.

eschar   hard, leathery product of a deep full thickness burn; it consists of dead and denatured skin.

esophageal varices   enlarged and tortuous esophageal veins.

evisceration   a protrusion of organs from a wound.

exsanguination   the draining of blood to the point at which life cannot be sustained.

extravascular space   the volume contained by all the cells (intracellular space) and the spaces between the cells (interstitial space).

fascia   a fibrous membrane that covers, supports, and separates muscles and may also unite the skin with underlying tissue.

fasciculations   involuntary contractions or twitchings of muscle fibers.

fasciculus   small bundle of muscle fibers.

fatigue   condition in which a muscle's ability to respond to stimulation is lost or reduced through overactivity.

fatigue fracture   break in a bone associated with prolonged or repeated stress.

femur   large bone of the proximal lower extremity.

fibrin   protein fibers that trap red blood cells as part of the clotting process.

fibroblasts   specialized cells that form collagen.

fibula   the small bone of the lower leg.

flail chest   defect in the chest wall that allows for free movement of a segment. Breathing will cause paradoxical chest wall motion.

flechettes   arrow-shaped projectiles found in some military ordnance.

fluid shift phase   stage of the burn process in which there is a massive shift of fluid from the intravascular to the extravascular space.

full thickness burn   burn that damages all layers of the skin; characterized by areas that are white and dry; also called third-degree burn.

galea aponeurotica   connective tissue sheet covering the superior aspect of the cranium.

gamma radiation   powerful electromagnetic radiation emitted by radioactive substances with powerful penetrating properties; it is stronger than alpha and beta radiation.

gangrene   deep space infection usually caused by the anaerobic bacterium *Clostridium perfringens*.

Glasgow Coma Scale   scoring system for monitoring the neurological status of patients with head injuries.

glucagon   hormone that increases the blood glucose level by stimulating the liver to change stored glycogen to glucose.

glucocorticoids hormones released by the adrenal cortex that increase glucose production and reduce the body's inflammation response.

glycogen a polysaccharide; one of the forms in which the body stores glucose.

glycogenolysis the process by which the body converts glycogen into glucose.

glycolysis the first stage of the process in which the cell breaks apart an energy source, commonly glucose, and releases a small amount of energy.

Golden Hour the 60-minute period after a severe injury; it is the maximum acceptable time between the injury and initiation of surgery for the seriously injured trauma patient.

gout inflammation of joints and connective tissue due to buildup of uric acid crystals.

granulocytes white blood cells charged with the primary purpose of neutralizing foreign bacteria.

Gray a unit of absorbed radiation dose equal to 100 rads.

gray matter areas in the central nervous system dominated by nerve cell bodies; central portion of the spinal cord.

great vessels large arteries and veins located in the mediastinum that enter and exit the heart.

greenstick fracture partial fracture of a child's bone.

growth hormone hormone secreted by the anterior pituitary gland that promotes the uptake of glucose and amino acids in the muscle cells and stimulates protein synthesis.

guarding protective tensing of the abdominal muscles by a patient suffering abdominal pain; may be a voluntary or involuntary response.

hairline fracture small crack in a bone that does not disrupt its total structure.

haversian canals small perforations of the long bones through which the blood vessels and nerves travel through the bone itself.

hematemesis the vomiting of blood.

hematochezia blood in the stool; passage of stools containing red blood.

hematocrit the percentage of the blood consisting of the red blood cells, or erythrocytes.

hematoma collection of blood beneath the skin or trapped within a body compartment.

hematuria blood in the urine.

hemoglobin an iron-based compound found in red blood cells that binds with oxygen and transports it to body cells.

hemopneumothorax condition where air and blood are in the pleural space.

hemoptysis coughing (expectoration) of blood that has origin in the respiratory tract.

hemorrhage an abnormal internal or external discharge of blood.

hemostasis the body's natural ability to stop bleeding; the ability to clot blood.

hemothorax blood within the pleural space.

histamine substance released during the degranulation of mast cells and basophils that increases blood flow to the injury site due to vasodilation and increased permeability of capillary walls.

homeostasis the natural tendency of the body to maintain a steady and normal internal environment.

humerus the single bone of the proximal upper extremity.

hydrostatic pressure the pressure of liquids in equilibrium; the pressure exerted by or within liquids.

hypermetabolic phase stage of the burn process in which there is increased body metabolism in an attempt by the body to heal the burn.

hyphema blood in the anterior chamber of the eye, in front of the iris.

hypoperfusion inadequate perfusion of body tissues resulting in inadequate supplies of oxygen and nutrients to body tissue; also called *shock*.

hypotension lower than normal blood pressure.

hypothalamus portion of the brain important for controlling certain metabolic activities, including regulation of body temperature.

hypovolemia reduced volume in the cardiovascular system.

hypovolemic shock shock caused by loss of blood or body fluids.

hypoxic drive mechanism that increases respiratory stimulation when PaO$_2$ falls and inhibits respiratory stimulation when PaO$_2$ climbs.

iliac crest lateral bony ridge that is a landmark of the pelvis.

ilium large, flat innominate bone.

impacted fracture break in a bone in which the bone is compressed on itself.

impaled object foreign body embedded in a wound.

incendiary an agent that combusts easily or creates combustion.

incision very smooth or surgical laceration, frequently caused by a knife, scalpel, razor blade, or piece of glass.

index of suspicion the anticipation of injury to a body region, organ, or structure based on analysis of the mechanism of injury.

inertia tendency of an object to remain at rest or in motion unless acted upon by an external force.

inflammation complex process of local cellular and biochemical changes as a consequence of injury or infection; an early stage of healing.

innominate   one of the structures of the pelvis.

insertion   attachment of a muscle to a bone that moves when the muscle contracts.

insulin   pancreatic hormone needed to transport simple sugars from the interstitial spaces into the cells.

integumentary system   skin, consisting of the epidermis, dermis, and subcutaneous layers.

interstitial space   the space between cells.

intervertebral disk   cartilaginous pad between vertebrae that serves as a shock absorber.

intracerebral hemorrhage   bleeding directly into the tissue of the brain.

intracranial pressure (ICP)   pressure exerted on the brain by the blood and cerebrospinal fluid.

intravascular space   the volume contained by all the arteries, veins, and capillaries and other components of the circulatory system.

ionization   the process of changing a substance into separate charged particles (ions).

iris   pigmented portion of the eye. It is the muscular area that constricts or dilates to change the size of the pupil.

irreversible shock   final stage of shock in which organs and cells are so damaged that recovery is impossible.

ischemia   a blockage in the delivery of oxygenated blood to the cells.

ischial tuberosity   one of the bony knobs of the posterior pelvis.

ischium   irregular innominate bone.

Jackson's theory of thermal wounds   explanation of the physical effects of thermal burns.

joint   area where adjacent bones articulate.

Joule's law   the physical law stating that the rate of heat production is directly proportional to the resistance of the circuit and to the square of the current.

keloid   a formation resulting from overproduction of scar tissue.

kinetic energy   the energy an object has while it is in motion. It is related to the object's mass and velocity.

kinetics   the branch of physics that deals with motion, taking into consideration mass, velocity, and force.

Krebs cycle   process of aerobic metabolism that uses carbohydrates, proteins, and fats to release energy for the body; also known as the citric acid cycle.

laceration   an open wound, normally a tear with jagged borders.

lacrimal fluid   liquid that lubricates the eye.

lactic acid   compound produced from pyruvic acid during anaerobic glycolyis.

laminae   posterior bones of a vertebra that help make up the foramen, or opening, of the spinal canal.

Le Fort criteria   classification system for fractures involving the maxilla.

leukocyte   one of the white blood cells, which plays a key role in the body's immune system and inflammatory (infection-fighting) responses.

ligaments   bands of connective tissue that connect bone to bone and hold joints together.

ligamentum arteriosum   cordlike remnant of a fetal vessel connecting the pulmonary artery to the aorta at the aortic isthmus.

liquefaction necrosis   the process in which an alkali dissolves and liquefies tissue.

lumen   opening, or space, within a needle, artery, vein, or other hollow vessel.

lymphangitis   inflammation of the lymph channels, usually as a result of a distal infection.

lymphocyte   white blood cell that specializes in humoral immunity and antibody formation.

macrophage   immune system cell that has the ability to recognize and ingest foreign pathogens.

malleolus   the protuberance of the ankle.

mandible   the jawbone.

mass   a measure of the matter that an object contains; the property of a physical body that gives the body inertia.

maxilla   bone of the upper jaw.

mechanism of injury   the process and forces that cause trauma.

medulla oblongata   lower portion of the brainstem containing the respiratory, cardiac, and vasomotor centers.

medullary canal   cavity within a bone that contains the marrow.

melena   black, tarlike feces due to gastrointestinal bleeding.

meninges   three membranes that surround and protect the brain and spinal cord. They are the dura mater, pia mater, and arachnoid membrane.

mesentery   double fold of peritoneum that supports the major portion of the small bowel, suspending it from the posterior abdominal wall.

metabolism   the total changes that take place in an organism during physiological processes.

metacarpals   bones of the palm.

metaphysis   growth zone of a bone, active during the development stages of youth. It is located between the epiphysis and the diaphysis.

metatarsal   one of the bones forming the arch of the foot.

microcirculation   blood flow in the arterioles, capillaries, and venules.

midbrain   portion of the brain connecting the pons and cerebellum with the cerebral hemispheres.

motion   the process of changing place; movement.

muscle   contractile tissue organized in large bundles that provides locomotion and movement for the body.

myocardium   the cardiac muscle tissue of the heart.

myotome   muscle and tissue of the body innervated by spinal nerve roots.

nares   the openings of the nostrils.

necrosis   tissue death, usually from ischemia.

neovascularization   new growth of capillaries in response to healing.

neurogenic shock   type of shock resulting from an interruption in the communication pathway between the central nervous system and the rest of the body leading to decreased peripheral vascular resistance.

neutron radiation   powerful radiation with penetrating properties between that of beta and gamma radiation.

oblique   having a slanted position or direction.

oblique fracture   break in a bone running across it at an angle other than 90 degrees.

obstructive shock   shock resulting from interference with the blood flowing through the cardiovascular system.

ohm   basic unit for measuring the strength of electrical resistance.

Ohm's law   the physical law identifying that the current in an electrical circuit is directly proportional to the voltage and inversely proportional to the resistance.

olecranon   proximal end of the ulna.

open fracture   a broken bone in which the bone ends or the forces that caused it penetrate the surrounding skin.

opposition   pairing of muscles that permits extension and flexion of limbs.

orbit   the eye socket.

ordnance   military weapons and munitions.

origin   attachment of a muscle to a bone that does not move (or experiences the least movement) when the muscle contracts.

orthostatic hypotension   a decrease in blood pressure that occurs when a person moves from a supine or sitting to an upright position.

osteoarthritis   inflammation of a joint resulting from wearing of the articular cartilage.

osteoblast   cell that helps in the creation of new bone during growth and bone repair.

osteoclast   bone cell that absorbs and removes excess bone.

osteocyte   bone-forming cell found in the bone matrix that helps maintain the bone.

osteoporosis   weakening of bone tissue due to the loss of essential minerals, especially calcium.

overdrive respiration   positive pressure ventilation supplied to a breathing patient.

overpressure   a rapid increase, then decrease, in atmospheric pressure created by an explosion.

oxidizer   an agent that enhances combustion of a fuel.

parasympathetic nervous system   division of the autonomic nervous system that is responsible for controlling vegetative functions.

partial thickness burn   burn in which the epidermis is burned through and the dermis is damaged; characterized by redness and blistering; also called a second-degree burn.

pedicles   thick, bony struts that connect the vertebral bodies with the transverse processes and help make up the opening for the spinal canal.

pelvic space   division of the abdominal cavity containing those organs located within the pelvis.

pelvis   skeletal structure where the lower extremities attach to the body.

penetrating trauma   injury caused by an object breaking the skin and entering the body.

perforating canals   structures through which blood vessels enter and exit the bone shaft.

pericardial tamponade   filling of the pericardial sac with fluid, which in turn limits the filling and function of the heart.

pericardium   fibrous sac that surrounds the heart.

periosteum   the tough exterior covering of a bone.

peripheral vascular resistance   the resistance of the vessels to the flow of blood; it increases when the vessels constrict and decreases when the vessels relax.

peristalsis   wavelike muscular motion of the esophagus and bowel that moves food through the digestive system.

peritoneal space   division of the abdominal cavity containing those organs or portions of organs covered by the peritoneum.

peritoneum   fine fibrous tissue surrounding the interior of most of the abdominal cavity and covering most of the small bowel and some of the abdominal organs.

peritonitis   inflammation of the peritoneum caused by chemical or bacterial irritation.

phagocytosis   process in which a cell surrounds and absorbs a bacterium or other particle.

phalanges   bones of the fingers and toes.

pia mater   inner and most delicate layer of the meninges. It covers the convolutions of the brain and spinal cord.

pinna   outer, visible portion of the ear.

platelet   one of the fragments of cytoplasm that circulates in the blood and works with components of the coagulation system to promote blood clotting. Platelets also release serotonin, a vasoconstrictive substance.

platelet phase   second step in the clotting process in which platelets adhere to blood vessel walls and to each other.

pneumatic anti-shock garment (PASG)   garment designed to produce uniform pressure on the lower extremities and abdomen; used with shock and hemorrhage patients in some EMS systems.

pneumothorax   collection of air or gas in the pleural cavity between the chest wall and lung.

pons   process of tissue responsible for the communication interchange between the cerebellum, the cerebrum, midbrain, and the spinal cord.

portal system   part of the circulatory system consisting of the veins that drain some of the digestive organs. The portal system delivers blood to the liver.

posterior medial sulcus   shallow longitudinal groove along the dorsal surface of the spinal cord.

precordium   area of the chest wall overlying the heart.

preload   the pressure within the ventricles at the end of diastole; the volume of blood delivered to the atria prior to ventricular diastole.

pressure wave   area of overpressure that radiates outward from an explosion.

profile   the size and shape of a projectile as it contacts a target; it is the energy exchange surface of the contact.

prognosis   the anticipated outcome of a disease or injury.

pubis   irregular innominate bone.

pulmonary hilum   central medial region of the lung where the bronchi and pulmonary vasculature enter the lung.

pulse pressure   difference between the systolic and diastolic blood pressures.

pulsus paradoxus   drop of greater than 10 mmHg in the systolic blood pressure during the inspiratory phase of respiration that occurs in patients with pericardial tamponade.

puncture   specific soft-tissue injury involving a deep, narrow wound to the skin and underlying organs that carries an increased danger of infection.

pupil   dark opening in the center of the iris through which light enters the eye.

rad   basic unit of absorbed radiation dose.

radius   bone on the thumb side of the forearm.

rebound tenderness   pain on release of the examiner's hands, allowing the patient's abdominal wall to return to its normal position; associated with peritoneal irritation.

red bone marrow   tissue within the internal cavity of a bone responsible for the manufacture of erythrocytes and other blood cells.

reduction   returning of displaced bone ends to their proper anatomic orientation.

remodeling   stage in the wound healing process in which collagen is broken down and relaid in an orderly fashion.

resiliency   the connective strength and elasticity of an object or fabric.

resistance   property of a conductor that opposes the passage of an electric current.

resolution phase   final stage of the burn process in which scar tissue is laid down and the healing process is completed.

respiratory shock   shock resulting from failure of the respiratory system to supply oxygen to the alveoli or remove CO_2 from them.

retina   light- and color-sensing tissue lining the posterior chamber of the eye.

retinal detachment   condition that may be of traumatic origin and present with patient complaint of a dark curtain obstructing a portion of the field of view.

retroauricular ecchymosis   black-and-blue discoloration over the mastoid process (just behind the ear) that is characteristic of a basilar skull fracture. (Also called *Battle's sign.*)

retrograde amnesia   inability to remember events that occurred before the trauma that caused the condition.

retroperitoneal space   division of the abdominal cavity containing those organs posterior to the peritoneal lining.

rhabdomyolysis   acute pathologic process that involves the destruction of skeletal muscle.

rheumatoid arthritis   chronic disease that causes deterioration of peripheral joint connective tissue.

rouleaux   group of red blood cells that are stuck together.

rule of nines   method of estimating the amount of body surface area burned by a division of the body into regions, each of which represents approximately 9 percent of total BSA (plus 1 percent for the genital region).

rule of palms   method of estimating amount of body surface area burned that sizes the area burned in comparison to the patient's palmar surface.

scapula   triangular bone buried within the musculature of the upper back.

sclera   the "white" of the eye.

sebaceous glands   glands within the dermis secreting sebum.

sebum   fatty secretion of the sebaceous gland that helps keep the skin pliable and waterproof.

semicircular canals   the three rings of the inner ear. They sense the motion of the head and provide positional sense for the body.

septic shock   form of distributive shock caused by massive infection in which toxins compromise the vascular system's ability to control blood vessels and distribute blood.

serous fluid   a cellular component of blood, similar to plasma.

sesamoid bone   bone that forms in a tendon.

shock   a state of inadequate tissue perfusion.

spasm intermittent or continuous contraction of a muscle.

spinal canal opening in the vertebrae that accommodates the spinal cord.

spinal cord central nervous system (CNS) pathway responsible for transmitting sensory input from the body to the brain and for conducting motor impulses from the brain to the body muscles and organs.

spinal nerves 31 pairs of nerves that originate along the spinal cord from anterior and posterior nerve roots.

spinous process prominence at the posterior part of a vertebra.

spiral fracture a curving break in a bone as may be caused by rotational forces.

sprain tearing of a joint capsule's connective tissues.

Starling's law of the heart the law that an increase in cardiac output occurs in proportion to the diastolic stretch of the heart muscle fibers.

strain injury resulting from overstretching of muscle fibers.

stroke volume the amount of blood ejected by the heart in one cardiac contraction.

subcutaneous tissue body layer beneath the dermis.

subdural hematoma collection of blood directly beneath the dura mater.

subglottic referring to the lower airway.

subluxation partial displacement of a bone end from its position in a joint capsule.

sudoriferous glands glands within the dermis that secrete sweat.

superficial burn a burn that involves only the epidermis; characterized by reddening of the skin; also called a first-degree burn.

supine hypotensive syndrome inadequate return of venous blood to the heart, reduced cardiac output, and lowered blood pressure resulting from pressure on the inferior vena cava by the fetus and uterus late in pregnancy.

supraglottic referring to the upper airway.

sutures pseudo-joints that join the various bones of the skull to form the cranium.

sympathetic nervous system division of the autonomic nervous system that prepares the body for stressful situations.

synarthrosis a joint that does not permit movement.

synovial fluid substance that lubricates synovial joints.

synovial joint type of joint that permits the greatest degree of independent motion.

systolic blood pressure pressure exerted against the arterial walls during contraction of the left ventricle of the heart.

tendonitis inflammation of a tendon and/or its protective sheath.

tendons bands of connective tissue that attach muscle to bone.

tension lines natural patterns in the surface of the skin revealing tensions within.

tension pneumothorax buildup of air under pressure within the thorax. The resulting compression of the lung severely reduces the effectiveness of respirations.

thalamus switching station between the pons and the cerebrum in the brain.

thoracoabdominal pump process by which respirations assist blood return to the heart.

tibia the larger bone of the lower leg that articulates with the femur.

tilt test drop in the systolic blood pressure of 20 mmHg or an increase in the pulse rate of 20 beats per minute when a patient is moved from a supine to a sitting position; a finding suggestive of a relative hypovolemia.

tone state of slight contraction of muscles that gives them firmness and keeps them ready to contract.

tourniquet a constrictor used on an extremity to apply circumferential pressure on all arteries to control bleeding.

tracheobronchial tree the structures of the trachea and the bronchi.

trajectory the path a projectile follows.

transection a cutting across a long axis; a cross-sectional cut.

transverse fracture a break that runs across a bone perpendicular to the bone's orientation.

transverse process bony outgrowth of the vertebral pedicle that serves as a site for muscle attachment and articulation with the ribs.

trauma a physical injury or wound caused by external force or violence.

trauma center a hospital that has the capability of caring for acutely injured patients; trauma centers must meet strict criteria to use this designation.

trauma registry a data retrieval system for trauma patient information, used to evaluate and improve the trauma system.

trauma triage criteria guidelines to aid prehospital personnel in determining which trauma patients require urgent transportation to a trauma center.

tunica adventitia outer fibrous layer of the blood vessels that maintains their maximum size.

tunica intima smooth interior layer of the blood vessels that provides for the free flow of blood.

tunica media the middle, muscular layer of the blood vessels that controls the vessel lumen size.

ulna bone on the little finger side of the forearm.

vagus nerve the 10th cranial nerve that monitors and controls the heart, respiration, and much of the abdominal viscera.

vascular phase step in the clotting process in which smooth blood vessel muscle contracts, reducing the vessel lumen and the flow of blood through it.

vasomotor center center in the medulla oblongata that controls arterial and, to a degree, venous tone.

vein a blood vessel that carries blood toward the heart.

velocity the rate of motion in a particular direction in relation to time.

ventricular filling the forcing of blood into the ventricle by the contraction of the atrium.

vertebra one of 33 bones making up the vertebral column.

vertebral body short column of bone that forms the weight-bearing portion of a vertebra.

vitreous humor clear watery fluid filling the posterior chamber of the eye. It is responsible for giving the eye its spherical shape.

voltage the difference of electric potential between two points with different concentrations of electrons.

washout release of accumulated lactic acid, carbon dioxide (carbonic acid), potassium, and rouleaux into the venous circulation.

white matter material that surrounds gray matter in the spinal cord; made up largely of axons.

xiphisternal joint union between xiphoid process and body of the sternum.

yaw swing or wobble around the axis of a projectile's travel.

yellow bone marrow tissue that stores fat in semiliquid form within the internal cavities of a bone.

zone of coagulation area in a burn nearest the heat source that suffers the most damage and is characterized by clotted blood and thrombosed blood vessels.

zone of hyperemia area peripheral to a burn that is characterized by increased blood flow.

zone of stasis area in a burn surrounding the zone of coagulation that is characterized by decreased blood flow.

zygoma the cheekbone.

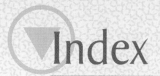

Index

The paramedic index includes entries for all five volumes in the Paramedic Care series. Each reference presents volume number followed by page reference in that volume. The sample entry Abdominal cavity, 4:437 refers to Volume 4, page 437.

Cytosol, 1:168
Cytotoxic T cells, 1:236
Cytoxan, 1:358

D₅W, 1:194, 1:410
D₅₀W, 1:355
D post, 5:411
DAI, 4:294
Daily stress, 1:37
Dalton's law, 3:516
Dam, 5:400
Damage pathway (penetrating trauma), 4:64–66
DAN, 3:523
Dandruff, 2:54
Dangerous crowds, 5:463
"Dangerous" placard, 5:433
Dantrium, 1:325
Dantrolene, 1:325
Date rape drug, 3:452, 5:218
DC countershock, 3:112
DCAP-BTLS, 2:203
Dead space volume (V_D), 1:522, 4:386
Deafness, 5:226–229
Death and dying, 1:29–33, 1:501
Death in the field, 1:135
Debridement, 1:251
Decadron, 3:343
Deceleration injury, 4:393, 4:403
Decerebrate posture, 3:269
Deci-, 1:450
Decision making. *See* Clinical decision making
Decision-making algorithm. *See* Algorithms
Decompensated shock, 1:213, 4:110–111, 5:100–101
Decompensation, 1:173
Decompression illness, 3:519–521
Decontamination, 3:420–421, 5:445–449
Decontamination methods, 3:553–554
Decontamination of equipment, 1:27–28
Decorticate posture, 3:269
Decubitus ulcers, 5:183–184
Decubitus wounds, 5:256
Deep frostbite, 3:511
Deep pitting edema, 2:133
Deep venous thrombosis (DVT), 3:201
Deerfly fever, 5:515
Defamation, 1:124
Defendant, 1:115
Defense wounds, 4:66
Defensive strategies, 1:33
Defibrillation, 3:162–166
Defibrillator, 3:162
Degenerative disk disease, 3:295
Degenerative joint disease, 4:240
Degenerative neurological disorders, 3:290–294
ALS, 3:292
Alzheimer's disease, 3:290
Bell's palsy, 3:292
central pain syndrome, 3:292

dystonia, 3:291
MD, 3:291
MS, 3:291
myoclonus, 3:292
Parkinson's disease, 3:291–292
polio, 3:293
spina bifida, 3:292–293
Degloving injury, 4:139, 4:140
Degranulation, 1:242–243, 3:337
Dehydration, 1:183, 3:503, 5:111
Deka-, 1:450
Delayed effects, 5:442
Delayed hypersensitivity, 1:236, 3:337
Delayed hypersensitivity reactions, 1:254
DeLee suction trap, 5:10, 5:17
Delirium, 3:605, 5:177–178
Delirium tremens (DTs), 3:454
Delivery, 3:671–683. *See also* Pregnancy
abnormal presentations, 3:677–680
APGAR score, 3:675, 3:676
breech presentation, 3:677, 3:678
cephalopelvic disproportion, 3:680
field, 3:671–674
limb presentation, 3:678
maternal complications, 3:681–683
meconium staining, 3:681
multiple births, 3:680
neonatal care, 3:674–677
neonatal resuscitation, 3:675–677
normal (vertex position), 3:672–673
occiput posterior position, 3:678–680
precipitous, 3:680–681
prolapsed cord, 3:677–678, 3:679
shoulder dystocia, 3:681
Delta cells, 3:310, 3:311
Delta wave, 3:141
Deltoid, 1:403, 1:404, 4:230, 4:231
Delusions, 3:606
Demand pacemaker, 3:136, 3:138
Demand valve resuscitator, 1:605–606
Demargination, 3:464
Dementia, 3:605, 5:178–179
Dendrites, 3:250
Dental injury, 4:300, 4:327
Deontological method, 1:146
Depakote, 1:305, 1:309
Dependent personality disorder, 3:612
Depersonalization, 3:611
Depo-Provera, 3:634
Depolarization, 3:83–84
Depolarization impulse, 3:99
Deposition, 1:116
Depression, 2:21, 3:608–609, 5:194–195

Dermatologic drugs, 1:362
Dermatome, 3:257, 3:259, 4:343
Dermatome chart, 2:151, 2:152, 3:352
Dermis, 4:131–132, 4:179–180
Descending colostomy, 5:282
Descending loop of Henle, 3:385
Descending tracts, 4:340
Descriptive statistics, 1:619
Descriptive studies, 1:614
Desensitization, 3:345
Desensitization techniques, 1:255
Desipramine, 1:308
Desired dose, 1:453
Desmopressin, 1:351
Destination log, 5:368–369
Detached retina, 2:66
Detailed physical examination, 2:221–228. *See also* Physical exam
Devascularization, 4:220
Developmental stages. *See* Life-span development
Developmentally disabled patients, 5:235–236
Dexamethasone, 3:343
Dexedrine, 1:306
Dextran, 1:193, 1:409
Dextroamphetamine, 1:306
Dextromethorphan, 1:345
Dextrose, 4:324
Diabetes, 1:352–355, 3:314–317, 5:180
adult onset, 3:317
cultural considerations, 3:314
emergencies, 3:318
gestational, 1:353, 3:665–666
glucose metabolism, 3:315–316
hyperglycemic agents, 1:350
hypoglycemic agents, 1:350
IDDM, 1:353, 3:317
insulin preparations, 1:353–354
NIDDM, 1:353, 1:355, 3:317
peripheral circulation, 5:255
pregnancy, 3:665–666
regulation of blood glucose, 3:316
type I, 3:317
type II, 3:317
Diabetes insipidus, 3:308
Diabetes mellitus. *See* Diabetes
Diabetic ketoacidosis, 3:318–320, 5:112, 5:113
Diabetic retinopathy, 5:229
Diabetogenic effect of pregnancy, 3:665
Diabinese, 1:355
Diagnostic and Statistical Manual of Mental Disorders, Fourth Edition (DSM-IV), 3:604
Dialysate, 3:404
Dialysis, 3:403–405
Dialysis shunts, 5:277
Diamox, 3:524
Diapedesis, 1:247, 3:464

Diaphragm, 3:5, 3:12, 3:18, 3:73, 3:634, 4:382–383
Diaphragmatic excursion, 2:83–85
Diaphragmatic hernia, 5:27–28
Diaphragmatic injury, 4:440
Diaphragmatic perforation, 4:409
Diaphragmatic rupture, 4:409
Diaphragmic hernia, 5:8
Diaphysis, 4:220
Diapid, 1:351
Diarrhea, 1:348
children, 5:111
newborns, 5:33–34
Diarthroses, 4:222
Diastole, 2:88, 3:79
Diastolic blood pressure, 2:35, 4:103
Diazepam, 1:570, 3:161, 3:285, 3:620, 4:264, 4:323
Diazoxide, 1:355
Dibenzyline, 1:324
DIC, 3:485–486
Diencephalon, 3:254
Diesel hybrid ambulance, 1:66
Diet-induced thermogenesis, 3:494
Diet supplements, 1:362–363
Differential diagnosis, 5:295
Differential field diagnosis, 2:5, 2:242
Differentiation, 1:168
Difficult child, 1:489
Diffuse axonal injury (DAI), 4:294
Diffuse injuries, 4:294
Diffusion, 1:186–188, 1:289, 1:519, 3:15–16
DiGeorge syndrome, 1:258
Digestion, 1:349
Digestive system, 2:93, 2:94
Digestive tract, 4:430, 4:431
Digibind, 5:190
Digital communications, 2:267–268
Digital intubation, 1:563–566, 4:315–316
Digitalis, 3:161–162, 5:190
Digitalis glycosides, 1:337
Digitoxin, 1:337
Digoxin, 1:331, 1:332, 1:337–338, 3:161–162, 5:190
Digoxin toxicity, 5:190
Dihydropyridines, 1:336
Dilantin, 1:305, 1:330
Dilatation, 3:668
Dilation, 1:175
Diltiazem, 1:331, 1:338, 3:113, 3:162
Dimenhydrinate, 1:345
Diphenhydramine, 1:307, 1:310, 1:345, 3:342
Diphtheria-pertussis-tetanus (DPT), 3:576
Diphtheria-tetanus toxoid (Td), 3:583
Diphtheria-tetanus toxoid, pertussis (DTP), 3:583

Extrapyramidal symptoms (EPS), 1:307
Extrauterine, 5:6
Extravasation, 1:425
Extravascular space, 4:183
Extremities, 4:68
  children, 5:52, 5:123
  lower, 4:227–228
  physical exam, 2:105–123
  upper, 4:225–227
Extrication/rescue unit, 5:369
Extrinsic pathway, 1:245, 1:246
Exudate, 1:247
Eye
  anatomy, 4:282–284
  drugs, 1:349
  head injury, 4:299, 4:326–327
  physical exam, 2:60–67
Eye contact, 1:471, 2:6
Eye protection, 5:383
Eyedrop administration, 1:378–379
Eyewear, 1:24
EZ-IO, 1:444, 1:445

Face, 4:280–284. See also Head, facial, and neck trauma
Face mask, 1:602
Facial bones, 2:57, 2:58, 4:274, 4:275, 4:281
Facial dislocations/fractures, 4:300–301
Facial injury, 4:299–304
  dislocations/fractures, 4:300–301
  dislodged teeth, 4:327
  ear injury, 4:302, 4:326
  eye injury, 4:302, 4:326–327
  nasal injury, 4:301–302
  neck injury, 4:303–304
  soft-tissue injury, 4:299–300
Facial nerve, 2:138, 2:141, 2:146, 3:260, 4:279, 4:280
Facial paralysis, 3:266–267
Facial soft-tissue injury, 4:299–300
Facilitated diffusion, 1:188, 1:289, 3:387
Facilities unit, 5:360
Facsimile machine (fax), 2:268
Factitious disorders, 3:610–611
Factor VIII, 3:485
Failsafe franchise, 1:72
Fainting, 3:285, 5:175
Fall, 4:47–48
  children, 5:116–117
  elderly persons, 5:152–153
Fallopian tubes, 3:630–631
Fallout, 5:507
False assurance, 1:474
False imprisonment, 1:130
False labor, 3:666
False ribs, 4:382
Falx cerebri, 4:277
Family history, 1:201–205
Famotidine, 1:346
Farm machinery, 5:489–491
FAS, 5:237
Fasciae, 4:133

Fasciculations, 4:322, 5:509
Fasciculus, 4:229
Fasciculus cutaneous, 4:341
Fasciculus gracilis, 4:341
Fast-break decision making, 5:446–447
F.A.S.T.1, 1:444, 1:445
Fat embolism, 4:238
Fatigue, 4:234
Fatigue fracture, 4:238
Fatty change, 1:179
Fatty necrosis, 1:180
Fax, 2:268
FBAO, 1:587, 5:68, 5:75, 5:95–96, 5:99
FCC, 2:272
FDA approval, 1:282–285
FDA pregnancy categories, 1:287
FDA standards, 1:282
Febrile nonhemolytic reaction, 3:473
Febrile seizures, 5:108
Fecal-oral diseases, 3:544, 3:545
Fecal-oral route, 3:544
Federal Communications Commission (FCC), 2:272
Federal court system, 1:115
Federal Food, Drug and Cosmetic Act, 1:280–281
Feed-or-breed system, 3:261
Feedback, 1:172–173
Feedback techniques, 1:473–474
Feeding tubes, 5:280–281
Feet. See Foot
Female genitalia, 2:99–100, 3:627–631
Female reproductive system, 1:355–357, 2:95
Female urethra, 3:384, 3:389
Female urinary system, 3:384
Femoral nerve, 3:258, 4:342
Femur, 4:227, 4:228
Femur fracture, 4:255–256
Fentanyl, 1:570, 3:160, 4:264, 4:324
Fernotrac traction splint, 4:251
Fertilization, 3:646, 3:647
Fertilizer, 5:491
Fetal alcohol syndrome (FAS), 5:237
Fetal circulation, 3:652–653
Fetal development, 3:650–652
Fetal heart tones (FHTs), 3:651, 3:656
Fetal stage, 3:651
FEV, 1:523, 3:14
FEV$_1$, 3:14
Fever, 3:468, 3:503–504
Fever (newborns), 5:31
Fexofenadine, 1:345
FHTs, 3:651, 3:656
Fibrin, 1:244, 4:86
Fibrinogen, 3:470
Fibrinolysis, 3:470
Fibrinolytic agents, 3:160–161
Fibrinolytic therapy, 3:279
Fibrinolytic agents (fibrinolytics), 1:340, 3:160–161

Fibroblasts, 1:250, 4:143
Fibrosis, 5:163
Fibula, 4:227, 4:228
Fibular fractures, 4:257
Fick Principle, 1:209
Fiddleback spider, 3:441
Field assessment, 2:172–235. See also Physical examination
  airway assessment, 2:190–194
  breathing assessment, 2:194–196
  circulation assessment, 2:196–199
  DCAP-BTLS, 2:203
  detailed physical exam, 2:221–228
  focused history and physical exam, 2:200–221
  initial assessment, 2:186–200. See also Initial assessment
  isolated-injury trauma patient, 2:211
  major trauma patient, 2:201–211
  one-minute cranial nerve exam, 2:216
  ongoing assessment, 2:228–232
  rapid medical assessment, 2:220
  rapid trauma assessment, 2:203–210
  responsive patient, 2:212–219
  SAMPLE history, 2:210, 2:211
  scene size-up, 2:176–186. See also Scene size-up
  unresponsive patient, 2:219–221
Field contamination, 5:447–449
Field delivery, 3:671–674
Field diagnosis, 2:238, 2:293
Field ECG, 3:152–156, 3:232, 3:237–241
Field extubation, 1:579–580
15-lead ECG, 3:226
Fight-or-flight response, 3:261, 4:106, 4:485
Filtrate, 3:386
Filtration, 1:189, 1:290
Finance/administration section, 5:360
Financial considerations (Medicare payments, etc.), 5:335
Financially-challenged patients, 5:244–245
Finasteride, 1:357
Finger clubbing, 3:29, 3:41
Finger dislocation/fracture, 4:262–263
Fingernails, 2:55–57
Fingerprints, 5:473
FiO$_2$, 1:520
Firearms, 4:61–63. See also Weapons
FIRESCOPE, 5:349
Firewall, 5:411
First-degree, 4:191, 4:199
First-degree AV block, 3:116–117, 3:226
First-pass effect, 1:292

First Responder, 1:59–60
First Responder patch, 1:60
Fissure, 2:54
Fixed-rate pacemaker, 3:136
Fixed-wing aircraft, 5:335
Flaccidity, 2:148
Flaccidity, 2:148
Flagella, 1:168
Flagyl, 1:359, 3:587
Flail chest, 1:526, 2:206, 3:18, 4:398–399, 4:418
Flame/flash protection, 5:384
Flame hemorrhages, 2:67
Flammable/explosive limits, 5:439
Flanks, 3:384
Flash point, 5:439
Flash protection, 5:384
Flashback chamber, 1:416
Flashover, 4:195
Flat affect, 3:606
Flat sound, 2:32
Flat terrain, 5:414
Flat-water rescue, 5:400–404
Flecainide, 1:330
Flechettes, 4:41
Flexeril, 1:324
Flexibility, 1:17–18
Flexion, 4:223
Flexion injury, 4:346
Flexion-rotation injury, 4:346
Flexor carpi, 4:231
Floating ribs, 4:382
Florinef Acetate, 1:352
Flow regulator, 1:413
Flow-restricted, oxygen-powered ventilation device, 1:605
Flowcharts. See Algorithms
Flu (influenza), 3:573–574
Flu vaccine, 1:362
Fludrocortisone, 1:352
Fluency disorders, 5:232
Fluid bolus resuscitation, 5:30
Fluid intake/output, 1:182–183
Fluid replacement, 1:192
Fluid resuscitation, 4:117–119
Fluid shift phase, 4:183
Fluid therapy/management
  children, 5:84, 5:120–121
  electrolytes. See Electrolytes
Fluid volume over time, 1:456–457
Flumadine, 3:574
Flumazenil, 1:304, 3:285
Flunitrazepam, 3:452
Fluorouracil, 1:358
Fluoxetine, 1:308
Fluoxymesterone, 1:357
Focal clonic seizure, 5:30
Focal motor seizure, 3:282
Focal sensory seizure, 3:282
Focused history and physical exam, 2:200–221
Foley catheter, 5:279
Folic acid, 1:363
Folk remedies, 1:279
Follicle stimulating hormone (FSH), 3:305
Fontanelle, 1:487, 2:161